Review of Family Medicine

4ᵗʰ EDITION

Edward T. Bope, MD, FAAFP

Residency Director
Riverside Methodist Family Practice Residency
Riverside Methodist Hospital
Clinical Professor
Department of Family Medicine
The Ohio State University College of Medicine
Columbus, Ohio

SAUNDERS

ELSEVIER

SAUNDERS
ELSEVIER

1600 John F. Kennedy Boulevard, Suite 1800
Philadelphia, PA 19103–2899

REVIEW OF FAMILY MEDICINE, FOURTH EDITION   ISBN-13: 978-1-4160-3064-5

Notice

Knowledge and best practice in this field are constantly changing. As new research and experience broaden our knowledge, changes in practice, treatment and drug therapy may become necessary or appropriate. Readers are advised to check the most current information provided (i) on procedures featured or (ii) by the manufacturer of each product to be administered, to verify the recommended dose or formula, the method and duration of administration, and contraindications. It is the responsibility of the practitioner, relying on his or her own experience and knowledge of the patient, to make diagnoses, to determine dosages and the best treatment for each individual patient, and to take all appropriate safety precautions. To the fullest extent of the law, neither the Publisher nor the Editor assumes any liability for any injury and/or damage to persons or property arising out or related to any use of the material contained in this book.

Library of Congress Cataloging-in-Publication Data

Review of family medicine / [edited by] Edward T. Bope. – 4th ed.
       p. ; cm.
   Companion vol. to: Textbook of family practice.
   Rev. ed. of: Saunders review of family practice.
   ISBN 1-4160-3064-6
   1. Family medicine–Case studies.   2. Family medicine—Examinations, questions, etc.   I. Bope, Edward T.   II. Textbook of family practice.
III. Saunders review of family practice.
   [DNLM: 1. Family Practice–Examination Questions.   2. Comprehensive Health Care–Examination Questions.   WB 18.2 R454 2007]
RC46.T327 Suppl.
610–dc22

                                                                                    2006033513

Acquisitions Editor: Rolla Couchman
Developmental Editor: Pamela Hetherington
Design Direction: Karen O'Keefe Owens

Printed in the United States of America.

Last digit is the print number: 9 8 7 6 5 4 3 2 1

I dedicate this edition to my mother and father for their
encouragement and support.

Contributors

Chelley K. Alexander, MD

Assistant Professor, Assistant Dean for Graduate Medical Education, Residency Director, College of Community Health Sciences, The University of Alabama, Tuscaloosa, Alabama

Ann M. Aring, MD

Assistant Program Director, Riverside Family Practice Residency Program; Clinical Assistant Professor, Department of Family Medicine, The Ohio State University College of Medicine, Columbus, Ohio

Ravi Balasubrahmanyan, MD

Co-Chair, Department of Primary Care, United Hospital; Associate Director, United Family Medicine Residency Program, St. Paul, Minnesota

Katherine T. Balturshot, MD

Assistant Clinical Professor, Family Medicine, The Ohio State University College of Medicine, Columbus, Ohio

Gina M. Basello, DO

Assistant Director of Family Practice Residency Program, Mount Sinai Family Medicine Residency Program, Jamaica Hospital Medical Center; Adjunct Clinical Instructor, Mount Sinai School of Medicine, Jamaica, New York

Diane K. Beebe, MD

Professor and Interim Chairman and Residency Director, Department of Family Medicine, University of Mississippi Medical Center, Jackson, Mississippi

Edward T. Bope, MD, FAAFP

Residency Director, Riverside Methodist Family Practice Residency, Riverside Methodist Hospital; Clinical Professor, Department of Family Medicine, The Ohio State University College of Medicine, Columbus, Ohio

Pamela J. Boyers, PhD

ACGME Designated Institutional Official, Executive Director/Chief Academic Officer, Center for Medical Education and Innovation, Medical Education, Riverside Methodist Hospital – OhioHealth, Columbus, Ohio

Chad A. Braun, MD

Assistant Professor of Clinical Family Medicine, Department of Family Medicine, University of Illinois-Chicago, Chicago, Illinois

Darrin Bright, MD, Diplomate, American Board of Family Practice, Certificate of Added Qualification in Sports Medicine

Clinical Assistant Professor, Family Medicine, The Ohio State University College of Medicine; Clinical Assistant Faculty, Family Medicine, Riverside Methodist Hospital, Columbus, Ohio

Lance C. Brunner, MD

Assistant Clinical Professor, Department of Family Medicine, University of California, Irvine, Orange, California; Assistant Clinical Chief, Assistant Program Director, Department of Family Medicine, Orange County Family Medicine Residency Program, Kaiser Permanente Anaheim Hills, Anaheim, California

Paul Callaway, MD

Clinical Associate Professor, Department of Family & Community Medicine, Kansas University School of Medicine–Wichita; Program Director, Wesley Family Medicine Residency Program, Wesley Medical Center, Wichita, Kansas

James F. Calvert, Jr, MD

Associate Professor, Department of Family Medicine, Oregon Health and Science University; Medical Director, Department of Family Medicine, Merle West Medical Center, Klamath Falls, Oregon

James S. Campbell, MD

Assistant Professor, Department of Family Medicine, Louisiana State University Health Sciences Center, New Orleans, Louisiana

Julie S. Cantrell, MD

Department of Family Medicine, Riverside Methodist Hospital; Staff Physician, Worthington Industries Family Medical and Wellness Center, Columbus, Ohio

Miriam Chan, RPh, PharmD

Clinical Assistant Professor of Family Medicine, College of Medicine and Public Health, The Ohio State University College of Medicine, Director of Pharmacy Education, Riverside Family Practice Center, Riverside Methodist; Clinical Assistant Professor of Pharmacy, College of Pharmacy, The Ohio State University, Columbus, Ohio

Ronald L. Cook, DO, MBA

Program Director, Family Medicine Residency Program, Family & Community Medicine, Texas Tech Health Sciences Center, Lubbock, Texas

William C. Crow, MD

Assistant Professor, Department of Clinical
Family Medicine, University of Virginia School of
Medicine, Charlottesville, Virginia; Director of
Scholarly Activity, Lynchburg Family Medicine
Residency; Staff Physician, Lynchburg General Hospital,
Staff Physician, Virginia Baptist Hospital,
Lynchburg, Virginia

Douglas DiOrio, MD

Clinical Adjunct Faculty, Department of Family
Practice, The Ohio State University College of
Medicine; Fellowship Director, Riverside Sports
Medicine Fellowship, Department of Family
Medicine, Riverside Methodist Hospital,
Columbus, Ohio

Charles E. Driscoll, MD

Clinical Professor, Family Medicine, University of
Virginia, Charlottesville, Virginia; Clinical Professor,
Family Medicine, Medical College of Virginia;
Richmond, Virginia; Director, Family Medicine
Residency, CentraHealth, Inc., Lynchburg, Virginia

Mary Frances Duggan, MD

Assistant Professor of Family Medicine, Department
of Family and Social Medicine, Albert Einstein
College of Medicine; Attending Physician/Faculty/
Program Director Family Medicine Residency,
Family Medicine, Montefiore Medical Center,
Bronx, New York

Brian L. Elkins, MD, FAAFP

Assistant Professor, Department of Family Medicine and
Comprehensive Care, Louisiana State University Health
Sciences Center, Shreveport, Louisiana

Bill G. Gegas, MD

Clinical Assistant Professor, Department of Family
Medicine, The Ohio State University College of
Medicine; Medical Director, Worthington Industries,
Family Medical and Wellness Center, Columbus, Ohio

Dean G. Gianakos, MD, ABIM

Associate Director, Lynchburg Family Medicine
Residency, Lynchburg, Virginia; Associate Professor
of Clinical Family Medicine, Director of Internal
Medicine & Critical Care Education. University of
Virginia School of Medicine, Charlottesville, Virginia

Curtis Gingrich, MD, FAAFP

Associate Program Director, Riverside Methodist Hospital
Family Practice Residency Program; Chair, Department
of Family Medicine, Riverside Methodist Hospital,
Columbus, Ohio

Joseph M. Ginty, MD

Clinical Assistant Professor of Family Medicine,
Department of Family Medicine, The Ohio State
University College of Medicine; Clinical Preceptor,
Department of Family Medicine, Riverside Methodist
Hospital, Columbus, Ohio; Family Physician,
Department of Family Medicine, Fairfield Medical
Center, Lancaster, Ohio

Wanda Gonsalves, MD

Medical Director, University Family Medicine Center,
Assistant Professor of Family Medicine, Medical
University of South Carolina, Charleston, South Carolina

David S. Gregory, MD, FAAFP

Assistant Professor of Clinical Family Medicine, University
of Virginia, Charlottesville, Virginia; Director of
Pediatric Education, Lynchburg Family Medicine
Residency, Lynchburg, Virginia

Kenneth J. Griffiths, MD

Associate Professor, Department of Family Medicine,
University of California San Diego, San Diego, California

Nikhil Hemady, MD, FAAFP

Clinical Assistant Professor, Department of Family Medicine,
Wayne State University, Detroit, Michigan; Program
Director, Family Medicine Residency Program, North
Oakland Medical Centers, Pontiac, Michigan

Joyce C. Hollander-Rodriguez, MD

Assistant Professor, Department of Family Medicine,
Oregon Health and Science University, Portland,
Oregon; Associate Program Director, Cascades East
Family Practice Residency, Klamath Falls, Oregon

Jonathan D. Hollister, MD

Geriatrician, Department of Family Medicine, Licking
Memorial Hospital; Geriatrician, Department of
Geriatrics, Licking Memorial Health Professionals,
Newark, Ohio

Christine D. Hudak, MD

Assistant Director, Riverside Family Medicine Residency;
Assistant Clinical Professor, Department of Family
Medicine, The Ohio State University College of
Medicine, Columbus, Ohio

Abbie Jacobs, MD

Clinical Associate Professor/Director, Family Medicine
Residency Program, Family Medicine, UMDNJ/New
Jersey Medical School, Newark, New Jersey; Attending
Physician/Director, Family Medicine Residency Program,
Family Medicine, Hoboken University Medical Center,
Hoboken, New Jersey

Daniel A. Knight, MD

Associate Professor/Acting Chairman/Program Director, Department of Family and Preventive Medicine, University of Arkansas for Medical Sciences; UAMS Hospital, Family and Preventive Medicine, University of Arkansas for Medical Sciences, Little Rock, Arkansas

Ronald H. Labuguen, MD, FAAFP

Assistant Clinical Professor; Assistant Medical Director for Urgent Care Services, Family and Community Medicine, University of California, San Francisco, Physician-in-Charge, Adult Urgent Care Center, San Francisco General Hospital Medical Center, San Francisco, California

Dennis A. LaRavia, MD, FAAFP, Diplomate, ABFM

Professor and Director, Rural Family Medicine Residency, Department of Family Medicine, Louisiana State University Health Sciences Center – New Orleans, Staff Member, Department of Family Medicine, Bogal Medical Center, Bogal, Louisiana

James R. Little, MD

Clinical Assistant Professor, Department of Family Medicine, Oregon Health Sciences University, Portland, Oregon; Medical Director, Family Physicians Group, Vancouver, Washington

Glenn Loomis, MD, FAAFP

Program Director, Mercy Health System Family Medicine Residency Program, Janesville, Wisconsin

Stephen E. Markovich, MD, MBA

Senior Vice President–Operations, Riverside Methodist Hospital; Clinical Assistant Professor, Department of Family Medicine, Ohio State University College of Medicine, Commander, 121st Medical Group, Ohio Air National Guard, Rickenbacker IAP, Columbus, Ohio

William J. Martin, III, MD

PGY 1 Resident, Department of Family Medicine, Mercy Health System, Janesville, Wisconsin

Jeffrey W. Milks, MD

Clinical Assistant Professor, Department of Family Medicine; Geriatrics Coordinator, Department of Family Medicine Residency Program, The Ohio State University College of Medicine, Columbus, Ohio

William F. Miser, MD, MA

Associate Professor, Department of Family Medicine, The Ohio State University College of Medicine, Columbus, Ohio

Jennifer J. Mitchell, MD, FAAFP

Associate Professor of Medicine, Department of Family and Community Medicine; Associate Director, Family Medicine Residency Program, Texas Tech University Health Sciences Center School of Medicine, Lubbock, Texas

Kelly Mitchell, MD

Assistant Professor, Department of Ophthalmology, Texas Tech University Health Sciences Center School of Medicine, Lubbock, Texas

Paul Moglia, PhD

Assistant Clinical Professor, Department of Psychiatry and Behavioral Sciences, New York Medical College, Valhalla, New York; Associate Residency Director, Director of Behavioral and Faculty Education, Department of Family Medicine, South Nassau Communities Hospital, Oceanside, New York

Peter Nalin, MD, FAAFP

Associate Dean for Graduate Medical Education, Associate Professor of Clinical Family Medicine, Indiana University School of Medicine; Active Medical Staff, Department of Family Medicine, Clarian Health Partners, Indiana Clarian Methodist Hospital, Indianapolis, Indiana; President 2004-2005, Association of Family Medicine Residency Directors

Jeri A. O'Donnell, MA, LPCC

Director, Clinical Behavioral Science, Doctors Hospital Family Practice, Department of Family Medicine, Columbus, Ohio

Cheyn Onarecker, MD

Program Director, Family Medicine Residency, St. Anthony Hospital, Oklahoma City, Oklahoma

Trish Palmer, MD

Assistant Professor, Co-Director Primary Care Sports Medicine Fellowship, Departments of Family Medicine and Orthopedic Surgery, Rush University Medical Center, Chicago, Illinois

Patricia Pletke, MD, CAQ Geriatrics

Clinical Assistant Professor, Department of Family Medicine, University of Virginia, Charlottesville, Virginia; Faculty, Director of Geriatric Training, Lynchburg Family Medicine Residency, Lynchburg, Virginia

Roger Michael Ragain, MD, MSEd

Chairman, Family and Community Medicine, Texas Tech University Health Sciences Center School of Medicine;

Chief of Service, Family Medicine, University Medical Center, Lubbock, Texas

Ann Riehl, RDLD, CDE

Registered Dietitian, Certified Diabetes Educator, Department of Nutrition, Riverside Family Practice Center/Riverside Methodist Hospital, Columbus, Ohio

Alan R. Roth, DO, FAAFP

Chairman and Residency Director, Department of Family Medicine, Jamaica Hospital Medical Center Jamaica, New York; Assistant Professor, Community and Preventive Medicine, Mt. Sinai School of Medicine, New York, New York

Michael P. Rowane, DO, MS, FAAFP, FAAO

Associate Clinical Professor of Family Medicine and Psychiatry, Case Western Reserve University, Cleveland, Ohio; Director of Medical Education, University Hospitals Richmond Medical Center, Richmond Heights, Ohio; Director of Osteopathic Medical Education, University Hospitals Case Medical Center, Cleveland, Ohio

David R. Rudy, MD, MPH

Professor, Department of Family and Preventive Medicine, The Chicago Medical School of the Rosalind Franklin University of Medicine and Science; Attending Staff, Department of Family Medicine, Highland Park Hospital, Highland Park, Illinois; Attending Staff, Department of Family Medicine, Swedish Covenant Hospital, Chicago, Illinois

Kristen B. Rundell, MD

Assistant Program Director, Riverside Family Practice Residency Program, Riverside Methodist Hospital; Clinical Teaching Faculty, The Ohio State University College of Medicine, Columbus, Ohio

Dennis F. Ruppel, MD

Clinical Assistant Professor, Family Medicine, The Ohio State University College of Medicine; Program Director, Family Medicine Residency, Medical Education, Mount Carmel Health System Columbus, Ohio; Clinical Assistant Professor, Family Medicine, Wright State University Boonshoft School of Medicine, Dayton, Ohio

Samuel A. Sandowski, MD

Director, Family Medicine Residency Program, South Nassau Communities Hospital, Oceanside, New York

James E. Schmidt, MSW, LISW

Director, Clinical Behavioral Science, Riverside Family Medicine Residency Program, Riverside Methodist Hospital, Columbus, Ohio

Quincy Scott, DO, FAAFP

Associate Professor, Department of Family and Community Medicine, Southern Illinois University – Carbondale Family Medicine Residency Program, Carbondale, Illinois

Mrunal Shah, MD, ABFP

Vice President, Physician IT Services, OhioHealth; Assistant Program Director, Medical Education Information Systems Liaison, Riverside Methodist Hospital Family Practice Residency Program; Clinical Assistant Professor, Department of Family Medicine, The Ohio State University College of Medicine, Columbus, Ohio

Daniel L. Stulberg, MD, FAAFP

Associate Professor, Department of Family Medicine, University of Colorado Hospital, Denver, Colorado

Penelope K. Tippy, MD, FAAFP

Professor and Program Director, Department of Family and Community Medicine, Southern Illinois School of Medicine; Staff Physician, Department of Family Medicine, Memorial Hospital of Carbondale, Carbondale, Illinois

Bruce T. Vanderhoff, MD, MBA, FAAFP, ABFM

Clinical Associate Professor, Assistant Dean for Medical Education, Department of Family Medicine; Clinical Associate Professor, Vice President for Medical Education, Quality, and Patient Safety, Grant Medical Center, Columbus, Ohio

William A. Verhoff, RN, BSN

Nurse Manager, Riverside Family Practice Center, Riverside Hospital, Columbus, Ohio

George C. Wortley, MD

Clinical Assistant Professor of Family Medicine, University of Virginia, Charlottesville, Virginia; Clinical Assistant Professor of Family Medicine, Medical College of Virginia, Richmond, Virginia; Director of Rural Services, Lynchburg Family Medicine Residency, CentraHealth, Inc., Lynchburg, Virginia

Preface to the Fourth Edition

This edition marks my first as the sole editor of this review book. It seems fitting for me to recognize the past co-editors who helped me in the previous editions. Alvah Cass, MD and Michael Hagen, MD met with me as we launched this companion study guide for the *Textbook of Family Practice*. I want to thank them for their friendship and dedication to the earlier editions. Also deserving of thanks would be Robert Rakel, MD, who asked me to tackle this project and to our mentor, Nicholas J. Pisacano, MD, who inspired us to do our best for family medicine.

A new name, *The Review of Family Medicine*, signals the changes we will also see in Dr. Rakel's book, in recertification, and in our specialty. Family Medicine, our new specialty name, takes pride both in being the first to require recertification and in being a leader in its evolution to Maintenance of Certification (MOC). MOC is now required by all of the American Board of Medical Specialties (ABMS) boards, and family medicine is recognized for setting the example for life-long learning.

This book can help you in at least two important ways. It can provide a test to see how well you understood and committed to memory the important material you just read in the *Textbook of Family Medicine*. Students, residents, and practicing physicians will find this function useful in building a good fund of medical knowledge. Those preparing for an examination will also find it a useful review of the body of core family medicine knowledge.

Each question is written by a family physician or family physician educator who has carefully studied Dr. Rakel's text. They have created questions similar to board questions and have provided a page reference for more reading and a summary critique for each item.

I hope that you will find this book to be a great addition to your library, and I hope that the corners become tattered from use. Finally I hope that this book will add to your medical knowledge. The family physician must have the highest fund of medical knowledge, and this is one way to test and add to yours.

Edward T. Bope, MD, FAAFP

Foreword

Curiosity is one of the permanent and certain characteristics of a vigorous intellect.

Samuel Johnson

The glory of medicine is that it is constantly moving forward, that there is always more to learn.

William J. Mayo

Family physicians have a continuing enthusiasm for learning and derive great satisfaction from remaining current with advances in medicine. Ours is a comprehensive discipline that covers the entire breadth of clinical medicine as presented in the 7th edition of the *Textbook of Family Medicine*. Dr. Bope has compiled a variety of questions related to the content of the textbook in a manner that is both challenging and informative. He and the authors he selected, in addition to giving the correct response to each question, provide a critique explaining why each option is correct or incorrect and reference the location in the *Textbook of Family Medicine* that deals with the issue more thoroughly.

Persistent curiosity and an enthusiasm for learning are traits of all successful family physicians. Testing and retesting have been a component of our specialty since the formation of the American Board of Family Medicine in 1969. We thrive on the variety of challenges and problems that confront us daily in practice. We realize how much we learn from these challenges and recognize how repeated testing keeps our knowledge sharp and up to date.

This review will be of greatest value to family physicians preparing for examination by the American Board of Family Medicine, whether it be for initial certification or to maintain certification. However, it is also of value to all health professionals engaged in primary care who wish to be knowledgeable and remain current. This is especially true for family nurse practitioners (FNPs), physician assistants (PAs), and physicians in other specialties called upon to provide primary care.

To paraphrase Samuel Johnson, persistent curiosity is the sign of a vigorous intellect. This review book will nourish the curiosity of outstanding health professionals and help sustain enthusiasm for the practice of medicine.

Robert E. Rakel, MD

Contents

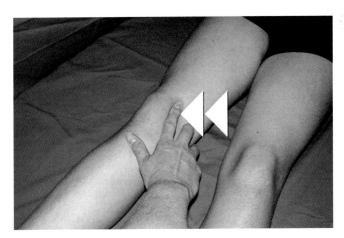

Color Plate 42-4 Copyright Mark R. Hutchinson, MD. In Rakel RE, editor: *Textbook of family medicine,* ed 7, Philadelphia, WB Saunders, 2007.

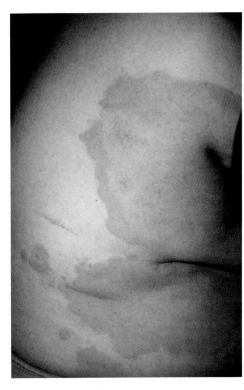

Color Plate 44-2 In Rakel RE, editor: *Textbook of family medicine,* ed 7, Philadelphia, WB Saunders, 2007.

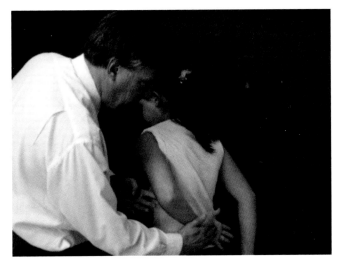

Color Plate 42-6 Copyright Mark R. Hutchinson, MD. In Rakel RE, editor: *Textbook of family medicine,* ed 7, Philadelphia, WB Saunders, 2007.

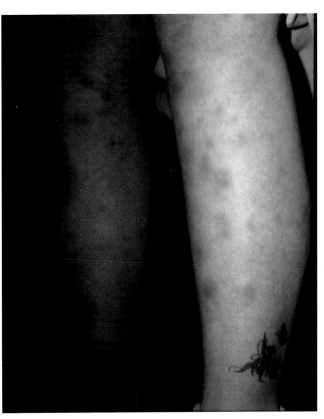

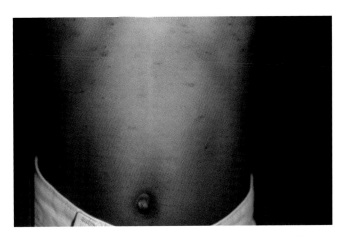

Color Plate 44-1 In Rakel RE, editor: *Textbook of family medicine,* ed 7, Philadelphia, WB Saunders, 2007.

Color Plate 44-3 In Rakel RE, editor: *Textbook of family medicine,* ed 7, Philadelphia, WB Saunders, 2007.

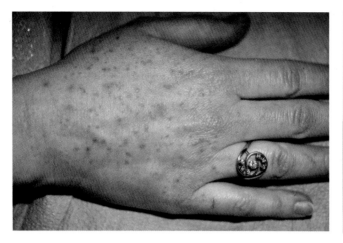

Color Plate 44-4 In Rakel RE, editor: *Textbook of family medicine,* ed 7, Philadelphia, WB Saunders, 2007.

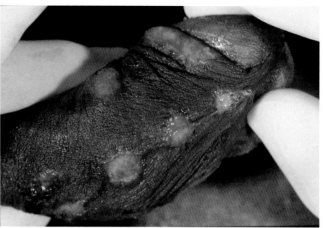

Color Plate 44-6 In Rakel RE, editor: *Textbook of family medicine,* ed 7, Philadelphia, WB Saunders, 2007.

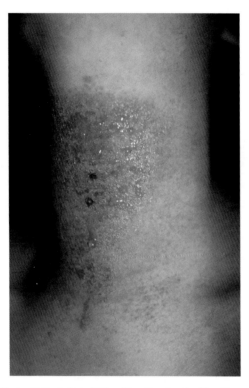

Color Plate 44-5 In Rakel RE, editor: *Textbook of family medicine,* ed 7, Philadelphia, WB Saunders, 2007.

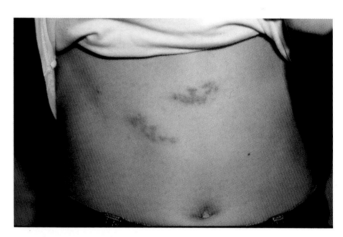

Color Plate 44-7 In Rakel RE, editor: *Textbook of family medicine,* ed 7, Philadelphia, WB Saunders, 2007.

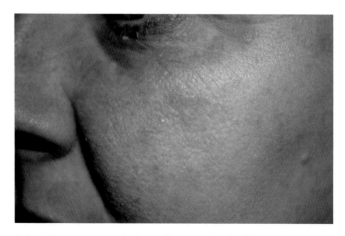

Color Plate 44-8 In Rakel RE, editor: *Textbook of family medicine,* ed 7, Philadelphia, WB Saunders, 2007.

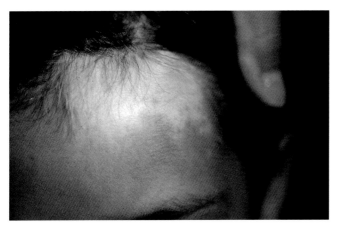

Color Plate 44-9   In Rakel RE, editor: *Textbook of family medicine,* ed 7, Philadelphia, WB Saunders, 2007.

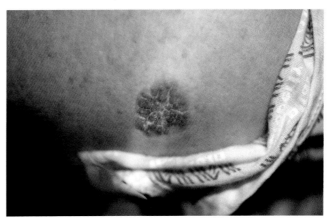

Color Plate 44-11   In Rakel RE, editor: *Textbook of family medicine,* ed 7, Philadelphia, WB Saunders, 2007.

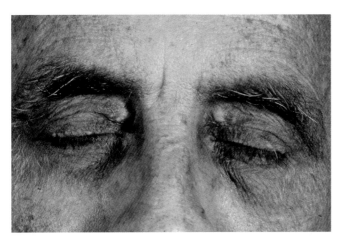

Color Plate 44-10   In Rakel RE, editor: *Textbook of family medicine,* ed 7, Philadelphia, WB Saunders, 2007.

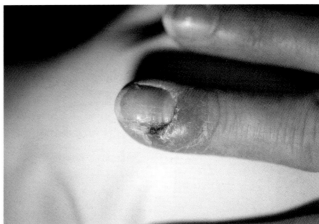

Color Plate 44-12   In Rakel RE, editor: *Textbook of family medicine,* ed 7, Philadelphia, WB Saunders, 2007.

Preparing for Examinations

Edward T. Bope

Preparing for an examination—particularly a certification examination—will be one of the most important efforts of your life. The first step is to contact the organization giving the examination to check dates, locations, and requirements for taking it. Often the deadline for registration will be months ahead of the actual testing date. A visit to the Web site of the organization will be beneficial for obtaining registration information and for reviewing the description of the examination. It will tell you how many parts and how many questions to expect. In some cases, it will give sample test items and perhaps even some practice questions. It is also possible that a "blueprint" of the test will be included, giving you a clue about the test's content.

THE TYPES OF QUESTIONS THAT ARE USED

The most popular question used today is the multiple-choice question with one correct answer. With this question style, there is a body of information (the stem) followed by four or five possible answers (the options). Your task as a test taker is to carefully read the stem and then choose the one correct option and mark it on the answer sheet (or enter it if you are taking an online examination). This question type is the most reliable and time tested, and it is preferred by most test takers. A new type question has surfaced that is similar to the multiple-choice question; it is called the "un-cued" question. For this question type, there is the standard stem, but the answers are not listed. The test taker must come up with the answer and then look for it in a taxonomy that is provided. This new style of question avoids misleading the test taker with nearly correct or confusing options. Sometimes the multiple true-or-false question format is used on examinations. This style of question has a stem like a multiple-choice question, but each option must be read and determined to be true or false. The question may require that all options are answered correctly to count as correct, or the options may be scored as individual items. Always be sure to read the instructions carefully before answering a question.

HOW TO PREPARE FOR AN EXAMINATION

1. *Set up a schedule for studying, and make it realistic.* You will be frustrated if the actual study time falls short of your expectations. For some, a commitment of time each day, Monday through Friday, will be better than a block of time on the weekend. Others will plan marathon sessions or even retreats to cover large amounts of material without interruption. Early in the year, you will want to consider whether you will attend a board review course. The American Academy of Family Physicians sponsors several review courses throughout the year, and they are of equal quality, regardless of site. Whatever time you set aside will reward you with new knowledge. Be honest and earnest in your approach so that you will walk into the testing site with confidence.

2. *Choose the material you want to review.* A resource of questions like this book provides breadth and depth of the field and provides teaching in the form of critiques for each question. There are several board review books on the market. Alternatively, you may choose a journal to review for the last year. In that case, choosing one that has review questions would provide some test-taking practice in addition to knowledge acquisition. This review book offers the opportunity to read the *Rakel Textbook of Family Medicine* and then check your knowledge.

3. *Collect a list of items that are difficult for you to remember but that you feel sure will be on the test.* This is the list that you will review the night before the examination. Room has been left at the end of each chapter in this book for you to record this information for rapid review. You will have a sense of things that are usually asked on an examination. Make a list of those items, and mark the ones that you need to review. For example, you would not have gone to the MCAT or Step 1 of USMLE without reviewing the Krebs cycle. Use that same intuition for these important certification examinations.

4. *Reserve time to accelerate your review for a week or two before the examination.* If possible, save some time for study just before the test. If you have not reserved the time, you might find yourself panicked as the test nears. Because your schedule is very busy, planning ahead will save you from test-week panic.

5. *Stop studying the day before the examination.* Make this the day you review the hard-to-remember and frequently asked material that you have recorded. It is too

late to review a book or read a journal. On the day before the examination, your energy is best spent preparing your attitude and demeanor.

6. *Have a relaxing evening the night before the examination, and get to bed a little early.* You have a big day ahead of you, and hopefully you can reward yourself for preparing in a responsible way. Make dinner plans with someone who listens well, and tell them about the test and how you have prepared. Go over your schedule with them so that they know what your day will be like. Reviewing the schedule will also help you make sure that you get to the right site at the right time.

7. *Allow enough time to get to the test site so that you are not frazzled by being late.* You are responsible for arriving at the testing site on time. Remember that tires still go flat and alarms sometimes fail. Be sure to have your usual breakfast; there are no snack breaks.

8. *Use your lucky pencil or wear your lucky shirt if it has helped you before.* Many people find comfort with these items. If they are important to you, by all means, use them.

9. *Answer every question.* You get no credit if no answer is selected. On the other hand, using your best guess could get you a point. If you are uncertain, mark your best choice, and flag the item so that you can return to it if time permits. The computerized examination allows for the review of questions.

10. *After the test, reward yourself with a treat that will be well deserved.* Plan a celebration dinner or a favorite activity. You have worked hard, and you deserve to celebrate your effort and anticipated success.

TESTMANSHIP: TIPS FOR ANSWERING INDIVIDUAL QUESTIONS

Test questions are designed to determine a physician's cognitive knowledge about the discipline of family practice. Each question has a set of answers from which the examinee must pick the correct answer. In this section, we look at specific suggestions for answering questions: in other words, we recommend ways to improve your "testmanship."

TIP 1   *Read the questions and answers carefully.*

One common error is to be in a hurry or anxious and to misread the question. Key words or phrases in many of the questions must not be missed. "Except," "contraindicated," "the first step," "most likely," and "least likely" are common examples.

Answers also have some important words buried in them. Because medicine is not black or white, words such as "always," "at all times," "never," and "exactly" should cause the examinee to eliminate these answers as potential choices. Do not confuse these terms with the frequently used "None of the above" and "All of the above," which can be correct answers.

TIP 2   *Look for the principle of the question.*

Test questions are written to assess your knowledge about a specific principle. If you can determine the underlying principle of the question, you will be able to more successfully answer it. The principle is not often stated, but it is implied through a short case scenario. As you read the stem, recognize that the written words in the scenario are purposefully leading you to the principle.

As an example, the following question was designed to determine whether the examinee knew that a functional assessment is fundamental to the field of geriatrics:

Sample question: An 85-year-old woman is admitted after a fall resulting in the fracture of her right hip. After the repair of her hip and in-hospital physical therapy, she is scheduled for discharge. She lives alone in a second-floor apartment and must negotiate three steps to get to her bedroom. She has two daughters who live in the community, and both have jobs that occupy their daytime hours. What is the first step in planning her discharge?

A. Discuss the patient's needs with her daughters.
B. Determine the patient's financial abilities.
C. Determine the patient's functional status.
D. Arrange for necessary home care services.
E. Plan to send the patient to a skilled nursing facility for further rehabilitation.

The correct answer is C. All of the answers are good ideas, but functional assessment is the underlying principle's first step. When reading the stem, do not get lost in some of the details (e.g., that the patient has to navigate three steps or that her daughters work).

TIP 3   *Avoid getting angry about questions, and avoid using anecdotal or local issue information as you look for answers.*

Many questions appear confusing or to not have answer options that appear to you to be correct. The test question's author believes that there is a right answer, and, for the purpose of passing the examination, the examinee must determine which answer to choose. Anger about questions is counterproductive to finding the best solution, and it will linger into future questions. Do not use anecdotal information or local issues when answering questions; search for the underlying principle.

Sample question: A 42-year-old man is being maintained on ventilatory support because of end-stage amyotrophic lateral sclerosis. He is bedbound, and his movement is limited entirely to his eyes. He communicates by eye motions using a letter board. He requests that you, as his physician, disconnect his mechanical ventilator, but his family does not agree with this request. Which of the following are you responsible for doing?

A. Asking for an opinion from legal counsel
B. Beginning therapy with an antidepressant
C. Refusing to turn off the mechanical ventilator
D. Working with the family and staff to plan for discontinuing the ventilator
E. Removing yourself from the case

This question presents a difficult and potentially contentious problem. Many examinees are angry that there is not a choice about involving an ethics committee, or they may choose the option involving legal counsel because of a case they have encountered in practice. The standard principle that this question addresses, however, is patient rights to decision making at the end of life.

TIP 4   For questions with long stems, read the answers first.

Many questions—particularly the clinical set problems—have long stems that detail a clinical scenario and that are followed by a set of answers. It is best in these instances to read the answers first; doing so will enable you to better focus your reading of the stem, and it will reduce your need to reread it.

TIP 5   Eliminate answers that you know are incorrect to improve your guessing odds.

One of the fundamentals of testmanship is to find and eliminate wrong answers. Most multiple-choice questions have five answers, so you have a 20% chance of getting the question correct with a guess. If you can find two or three incorrect answers and eliminate them from your guessing options, you significantly improve your chances of guessing correctly.

TIP 6   Do not pick choices that are unfamiliar but that sound correct.

As test writers develop questions, they must create incorrect answers. One of the ways to create a good incorrect answer is to make up something that sounds good but that is not correct. Do not select answers that are not familiar to you.

Sample multiple true-or-false question: Which of the following are commonly used to manage patients with erectile dysfunction?

A. Intraurethral implant of a prostaglandin medication
B. Intracorporal injection of vasoactive medication
C. Oral medication that increases cGMP
D. Transdermal vasoactive medication
E. Surgical insertion of an erectile implant
F. External vacuum-assistive device

All of these answers are true except D. That answer sounds correct, but such a transdermal system is not available.

TIP 7   Analyze similar answers carefully.

In some questions, two or three answers look alike but have important variations; these answers should catch the attention of the examinee. One of these answers is frequently the correct one, but simple alterations have been made to change it into an incorrect answer.

Sample question: Which of the following is the most common location for the Christmas-tree–like rash of pityriasis rosea?

A. Lower extremity
B. Dorsal aspect of the forearm
C. Anterior aspect of the trunk
D. Posterior aspect of the trunk
E. Scalp

The correct answer is D, but a good wrong answer is the opposite of this: the anterior aspect of the trunk. In addition, a common way to alter a good answer is to change a correct answer that includes a number to an incorrect answer by changing the number. In this manner, the question writer is trying to find out if the examinee knows the correct number.

Another use of similar answers in test writing is to create two wrong answers. If a test writer creates an incorrect answer that seems to be a reasonable choice, then a simple change in that answer will make a second reasonable incorrect answer.

Sample question: A 65-year-old man is admitted for antibiotic therapy for diverticulitis. On the second day of hospitalization, he complains of an acute onset of right lateral chest pain and shortness of breath. On examination, he is found to be tachycardic and tachypneic, and he has splinting respiratory effort. His chest x-ray is clear, his electrocardiogram shows a deep S wave in lead I, and his arterial blood gas values show a marked hypoxia and hypercapnia. Which of the following statements is correct?

A. This clinical picture is characteristic of a rupture of his diverticula and should be treated with emergency surgery.
B. This clinical picture is characteristic of a rupture of his diverticula and should be treated with intravenous triple antibiotic therapy.
C. This patient needs emergent treatment with an intravenous thrombolytic.
D. This is a classic description of a pulmonary embolus.
E. This is most likely a rib fracture from an undiagnosed metastatic colon malignancy.

The correct answer to this question is D. Answers A and B are written similarly, but are both incorrect.

TIP 8   For answers with numbers or percentages, pick a midrange answer.

If you are strictly guessing about a question with answers that are numbers, pick a midrange value. Correct-number answers are commonly placed in the center of a list with smaller and larger flanking numbers.

TIP 9 For answers containing numbers or percentages, pick those that look like other answers.

Another way to approach a question with numbers or percentages is to pick a choice from answers that appear to be similar.

Sample question: Which of the following is a positive purified protein derivative reading as read by the induration of the placed test at 48 hours in a patient with known human immunodeficiency disease?

A. 2 mm
B. 5 mm
C. 8 mm
D. 10 mm
E. 5 cm

In this question, the correct answer is B. The answer that is unlike the rest—E—should be eliminated if you are guessing. Answers A through D are similar (i.e., they are all measurements in millimeters), and, if you are guessing, then this is the group from which you should choose.

TIP 10 Look for answers that support family physician tenets, and avoid answers that have poor values.

This is an examination written by family physicians for family physicians, and it will expose the values that are considered important for family physicians. If an answer does not support the tenets of our specialty, then it should be eliminated from your options.

Sample question: A 23-year-old female presents with complaints of a year-long history of intermittent chest pain associated with a rapid heart rate and a feeling of doom. Her examination is normal. Which of the following is appropriate management at this time?

A. Refer her to a psychiatrist to treat her anxiety.
B. Order an electrocardiogram, a chest x-ray, a chemistry panel, a lipid panel, and a computed tomography scan.
C. Discuss with her that these complaints are common in patients with a borderline personality.
D. Obtain an electrocardiogram to look for a shortened PR interval.
E. Prescribe an anxiolytic and have her return for reevaluation in 6 months.

The correct answer is D. The other answers are all exaggerated to show how you could write answers that do not fit with good values for family physicians to have.

ACKNOWLEDGMENT

The author wishes to thank Lanyard K. Dial, MD, for the 10 test-taking tips at the end of this chapter.

Part I

Principles of Family Medicine

Chapter

1

The Family Physician

Edward T. Bope

1. Which of the following is an attribute that contributes to patient satisfaction?

   A. A modern office
   B. Good listening skills
   C. Hospital privileges
   D. X-ray on site
   E. A physician who efficiently judges each situation

   Review this! ❏

2. Physicians practicing which specialty are the most likely to be satisfied with their careers?

   A. Family medicine
   B. Obstetrics/gynecology
   C. Internal medicine
   D. Otolaryngology
   E. Ophthalmology

   Review this! ❏

3. Which of the following is the strongest predictor of decreasing satisfaction for physicians?

   A. Malpractice costs
   B. Long work hours
   C. Decreasing income
   D. Loss of clinical autonomy

   Review this! ❏

4. Which of the following is true about the American Board of Family Medicine (ABFM)?

   A. The first diplomats were certified without a test.
   B. The ABFM was formed in 1966.
   C. The ABFM requires 100 hours of continuing medical education (CME) each year.
   D. It was the first board to require recertification.

   Review this! ❏

5. What percentage of Americans report a family physician as their usual source of care?

   A. 16%
   B. 62%
   C. 70%
   D. 54%

   Review this! ❏

6. Of the following words starting with the letter C, which one has *not* been used to describe care given by family doctors?

   A. Comprehensive
   B. Coordination
   C. Cost effective
   D. Continuity

   Review this! ❏

7. Which of the following is true about continuity of care?

   A. It is not related to improved quality of care.
   B. It is a core attribute of family medicine.
   C. It can interfere with the care of patients with emotional problems.
   D. It is an adult patient concept.

   Review this! ❏

8. Which of the following is true about families who receive continuity of care from a family doctor?

   A. They have more hospitalizations.
   B. They have the same number of operations.
   C. They visit the physician more often.
   D. They spend less money on health care.

   Review this! ❏

9. What percentage of patients with diabetes mellitus receive their care from a primary care physician?

Things to remember for the test.

A. 90%
B. 75%
C. 50%
D. 20%

Review this! ❑

10. For patients who have been hospitalized with pneumonia, which one of the following is true about care provided by a family physician versus that provided by a hospitalist?

   A. The hospital stay is longer with a family doctor.
   B. The cost of the hospital stay is greater with a family doctor.
   C. The family physician uses more resources.
   D. There is no difference in quality.

Review this! ❑

11. True or false: When the balance of the physicians shifts from primary care to specialist, the outcomes are worse and mortality increases.

   A. True
   B. False

Review this! ❑

12. How does the care of low-risk obstetric patients differ for family physicians versus obstetricians?

   A. Obstetricians have fewer Cesarean sections.
   B. Obstetricians have fewer episiotomies.
   C. Both types of physicians have the same neonatal outcomes.
   D. Obstetricians use epidural anesthesia less often.

Review this! ❑

13. True or false: The cost of health care is projected to be at 18% of the gross domestic product by 2012.

   A. True
   B. False

Review this! ❑

14. Which of the following statements is true about the underinsured citizens of America?

   A. This population numbers about 50 million.
   B. The size of the group is shrinking.
   C. These individuals are unemployed.
   D. These individuals are considered poor.

Review this! ❑

15. True or false: The United States is the only developed country that does not have health coverage for all of its citizens.

   A. True
   B. False

Review this! ❑

16. All of the following are called for by the Institute of Medicine (IOM) as requirements for care to be given by 2010, except:

   A. Universal coverage.
   B. Continuity of care.
   C. Specialty delivered care.
   D. Affordable care.
   E. High-quality care.

Review this! ❑

17. True or false: Family physicians provide only a small number of office visits each year as compared with the other, larger specialties.

   A. True
   B. False

Review this! ❑

18. Five percent of visits to a family doctor result in a referral. Which group of specialists receives the most referrals?

   A. Medical specialists
   B. Obstetricians/gynecologists
   C. Psychiatrists
   D. Surgical specialists

Review this! ❑

19. True or false: Primary care physicians manage an average of three problems during each visit.

   A. True
   B. False

Review this! ❑

20. Family physicians are making more house calls recently because of which one of the following factors?

   A. Reimbursement has dramatically improved.
   B. There is an increase in the population of homebound elderly.
   C. They are mandated by Medicare to do so.
   D. Children can be better cared for at home.

Review this! ❑

Chapter

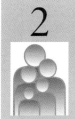

2

Promoting Optimal Healing in Family Medicine

David R. Rudy

According to Jonas and Rakel, practitioners of family medicine have in their special expertise and at their disposal the opportunity to provide the optimal healing environment (OHE). For Questions 1–5, match the following numbered ingredients of the OHE with the examples given in the lettered phrases. Lettered choices may applied more than once or not at all.

1. Relationship-centered care
2. Healing space
3. Self-care
4. Intention and awareness
5. Wholism

   A. The doctor focuses on the patient's numerous atherosclerotic risk factors but asks about and deals with the ongoing adaptation of the patient to timely preventive measures and his work and home environments.

   B. The patient has chosen the doctor in great part because he feels comfortable talking about sensitive issues and feels as if he is listened to and that his concerns are validated.

   C. The patient likes visiting her physician because the office is open and airy, and this helps the patient to feel relaxed before and after her visit with the doctor.

   D. The doctor regularly instructs and exhorts the patient to lose and control weight to prevent the development of insulin resistance and diabetes. At the same time, the doctor is near the ideal weight for his height and shares the fact that he has had to work at the mainte-nance of this weight.

   E. The patient feels, when in the presence of the doctor in the examination or consultation room, that the doctor is focused entirely on her (the patient) rather than on his own personal pro-blems, other patients' problems, or administrative concerns.

Review this! ❏

Questions 6–8 are a continuation of the same theme that applied to Questions 1–5: match a numbered ingredient of the OHE with a lettered example of that ingredient.

6. Collaborative care
7. Lifestyle and empowerment
8. Spiritual meaning and purpose

   A. The patient feels sorry for the doctor because of the apparent overbearing time urgency. The patient feels con-strained to make suggestions for increasing a sense of acceptance of patients' problems at the reception area.

   B. During a patient's developing divorce, she has descended into a recurrence of endogenous depression. The doctor has prescribed a serum serotonin reuptake-inhibiting antidepressant while discuss-ing the behavioral aspects of the depression, and he refers the patient to a clinical psychologist with whom he communicates on a regular basis.

   C. A 42-year-old male patient has gained a further 15% of his previous, mildly elevated weight since his last visit 1 year ago. The doctor verbalizes that the patient has two first-degree relatives with type 2 diabetes mellitus. The doctor then discusses the fact that this ex-athlete can expect a slowing in metabolism and a changing philosophy of living with advancing years as he moves into the fifth decade of life, resulting in certain weight gain in the absence of a change in food intake and/ or an increase in regular, modest exercise.

   D. A patient feels that specific problems are usually solved during his visits with the doctor. However, today he has a vague sense of illness at ease, because his position at his work seems less stable with the prospect of an upcoming merger with a larger corporation.

Things to remember for the test.

E. The doctor, while discussing a patient's hypertension, dissatisfaction at work (involving technical work with machines), and increased weight, notes the patient's stated love of working with people. While adjusting the patient's antihypertensive medication and counseling him with regard to weight loss and exercise, the doctor suggests that the patient take a look at becoming a sales representative of the company or industry in which he has developed expertise after several years' experience.

Review this! ❏

9. Each of the following is an example of what may result from an OHE, except:

A. The development of personal insight on the part of a patient into his ostensible problem.
B. A resolution as opposed to a suppression of symptoms.
C. The recruitment of internal resources to facilitate healing.
D. An increase in the use of health care resources.
E. A minimalization of long-term cost.

Review this! ❏

10. Jonas and Rakel have identified characteristics that should be present in a health care team to prepare the ground for the development of an OHE. The authors pose rhetorical questions about whether these characteristics are confirmed by more specific occurrences. Which of the characteristics of the OHE is identified by the following occurrences in the personal lives of the group: mind-body activities, spiritual and community activities, self-improvement workshops, exercise programs, and weight control?

A. The health care team provides continuous contact with patients.
B. The team is trained in professional communication skills.
C. Healers engage in self-care practices.
D. The team has received training in management and in skills of compassion.
E. Appropriate access to the community is provided to the patients by the team.

Review this! ❏

11. Along the same line as the theme addressed in Question 10, to which of the character-

istics do the following occurrences pertain: complementary medical practitioners networks, community services available, religious and social support, family involvement in care, and community service performed?

A. There is the existence of a process for facilitating access to the community.
B. There is the existence of emotional management and skills of compassion.
C. There are opportunities for continuous contact with the health care team.
D. The mission statement contains a commitment to healing.
E. The health care team provides continuous contact with patients.

Review this! ❏

12. Jonas and Rakel have pointed out that the integration of mind and body, in terms of broadening the narrow band of conscious awareness to gain greater insight into one's motivations, may lead to important benefits by allowing a measure of behavioral control of certain psychophysiological processes. The "mind"-conscious concept in this theme refers to the cognitive and emotional aspects of the brain as opposed to direct volitionally controlled actions of the body emanating from the brain. Conversely, the "body" functions considered here are the largely autonomic aspects of somatic function. This concept does not refer to pathologic situations that depend on direct volitional pathological conditions, such as smoking, alcohol abuse, and other lifestyle issues (which are addressed by other behavioral approaches). Each of the following is an example of a technique that can be used to enhance mind-body integration, except:

A. Yoga
B. Tai chi
C. Qigong
D. Serum serotonin reuptake inhibiting agents
E. Biofeedback

Review this! ❏

13. Consider the information presented in Question 12. Each of the following is an example of a common medical condition. Which of these is the least likely to respond to techniques for the integration of mind and body in the light of today's medical knowledge?

A. Hypertension
B. Irritable bowel syndrome
C. Lupus erythematosus
D. Reactive airway disease
E. Prinzmetal's angina

Review this! ❏

14. Jonas and Rakel cite three components for the development of awareness and intention: (1) education, (2) creation of expectancy through rituals, suggestions, and imagery (by the doctor), and (3) mindfulness (techniques used by the patients for the self-actualization of awareness of one's own needs and motivations). Each of the following is an example of the techniques of creation of expectancy, except:

A. The doctor tells a patient who suffered a "whiplash"-induced cervical strain that the injury will be completely healed 3 weeks after the time of the accident.
B. The patient practices meditation to gain answers to questions involving connections between physical symptoms and psychological makeup.
C. The physician notices dilated flank veins, palmar erythema, and telangiectasias on a 45-year-old male patient. A week later, the results of the patient's laboratory tests show elevations of AST (SGOT) and ALT (SGPT) to 150 U/L and 75 U/L, respectively. They also show that, although the alkaline phosphatase level is within normal limits, the GGT is elevated to 80 U/L (twice the normal

level). The doctor points out that this pattern is typical of alcoholic cirrhosis.
D. The clinical psychologist places the hypertensive patient under light hypnosis and evokes thoughts of tension-producing events in the patient's daily life. He then leads the patient through an analysis of whether the catastrophic interpretation of most of these events is necessary or rational.
E. The physician has diagnosed in her own mind that the patient's tachycardia is the result of a panic disorder. However, this is not mentioned with certainty to the patient until after a thorough physical examination and a revelation to the patient that thyroid function tests, standard comprehensive profile, complete blood count, and urinalysis are within normal limits.

Review this! ❏

15. Poor social connectivity, alienation, and loneliness are discussed by Jonas and Rakel as sharing a common theme. Which of the following conditions, according to Jonas and Rakel, is most clearly a sequela of these behavioral deficits?

A. Cardiac dysrhythmias
B. Dyslipidemia
C. Hypertension
D. Peptic ulcer disease
E. Premature death

Review this! ❏

Things to remember for the test.

11

3

The Family's Influence on Health

Mary Frances Duggan

1. A family is defined as any group of people related in the following way(s):

   A. Biologically
   B. Legally
   C. Emotionally
   D. Either biologically, legally, or emotionally
   Review this! ❑

2. True or false: There is strong evidence in the medical literature that shows that social support affects morbidity and mortality.

   A. True
   B. False
   Review this! ❑

3. True or false: The relationship that has the strongest impact on physical health is marriage.

   A. True
   B. False
   Review this! ❑

4. True or false: The prognosis of a person's chronic illness is not associated with the quality of his or her marital relationship.

   A. True
   B. False
   Review this! ❑

5. True statements about partner support and smoking cessation include all of the following, except:

   A. Partner support predicts successful smoking cessation.
   B. Partner criticism is not associated with failure to quit.
   C. According to the Agency for Healthcare Quality and Research, an effective smoking cessation program should include family and social support interventions.

   D. Studies of family and social support interventions fail to show an impact of partner support on smoking cessation.
   Review this! ❑

6. True statements about partner support and obesity treatment include all of the following, except:

   A. Couples interventions have been shown to improve weight loss during obesity treatment programs, but the differences in outcomes are not seen at 2- and 3-year follow-up appointments.
   B. Patients with higher marital satisfaction lose more weight.
   C. Couples interventions have been shown to increase partner support and to promote positive partner behaviors for weight loss.
   D. Partner criticism is predictive of little or no weight loss in obesity treatment programs.
   Review this! ❑

7. True or false: Family interventions and parental involvement have not been shown to improve weight loss for children in pediatric obesity programs.

   A. True
   B. False
   Review this! ❑

8. True or false: The morbidity and mortality rates for family caregivers are equal to their age-matched controls.

   A. True
   B. False
   Review this! ❑

9. True or false: Families—not health care providers—are the primary caretakers of patients with chronic illnesses.

   A. True
   B. False
   Review this! ❑

10. Which of the following is true about the psychoeducational intervention developed by Mittleman for family caregivers of patients with Alzheimer's disease?

    A. It was mainly intended to provide emotional support to families.
    B. It was not shown to improve the physical or emotional health of the family caregivers.
    C. It provided individual and group problem-solving sessions to teach caregivers how to manage the difficult behaviors of patients with Alzheimer's.
    D. It was not cost-effective.

    Review this! ❏

11. True or false: The course of a chronic illness is affected by the ability of the family to cope and adapt to the illness.

    A. True
    B. False

    Review this! ❏

12. Which of the following is not one of the three components of the stress process?

    A. The stressors (the environmental events experienced by an individual)
    B. The physiologic response to the stressors
    C. The health consequences of the stressors
    D. The change in an individual's function as a result of the stressors

    Review this! ❏

13. Studies using the Holmes and Rahe life-event scale have shown which of the following?

    A. An increase in stressful life events does not precede the development of disease.
    B. Life events that are viewed to be out of the individual's control do not have a negative effect on their health.
    C. Life events that are perceived negatively have the most adverse effect on health.
    D. Very few of the most stressful life events on the scale involve the family.

    Review this! ❏

14. True or false: Family life events have not been shown to have an impact on children's health.

    A. True
    B. False

    Review this! ❏

15. True or false: Normal changes in the family life cycle stage represent some of the most stressful life events on the Holmes and Rahe scale.

    A. True
    B. False

    Review this! ❏

16. True or false: Individual family members often experience divorce similarly.

    A. True
    B. False

    Review this! ❏

17. True or False: Divorce is always harmful, especially for children.

    A. True
    B. False

    Review this! ❏

18. When treating couples with marital distress who are contemplating divorce, what is the role of the family physician?

    A. To make appropriate referrals for marriage counseling or additional help
    B. To decrease the psychological risks for patients
    C. To promote healthy methods of coping with stress
    D. All of the above

    Review this! ❏

19. True or false: Marital discord is the most powerful sociodemographic predictor of stress-related illness.

    A. True
    B. False

    Review this! ❏

20. As compared with married men, divorced men have which of the following?

    A. A lower rate of suicide
    B. Decreased immune functioning
    C. Less risk of being a victim of violence
    D. A lower rate of physical illness

    Review this! ❏

21. How many years after divorce do most adults "recover" and develop a stable life?

    A. 5 years
    B. 1 year
    C. 2 years
    D. It is highly variable for each individual

    Review this! ❏

Things to remember for the test.

Things to remember for the test.

22. Research shows that the effects of divorce on children are more traumatic for which of the following?

    A. Boys
    B. Girls
    C. There is no gender difference

    Review this! ❑

23. Which of the following statements about children's reactions to their parents' divorce is false?

    A. Children between the ages of 12 and 18 years commonly react with anger and resentment, and they blame themselves for their parent's divorce.
    B. Children younger than 3 years old usually exhibit developmental delay and more intense separation anxiety.
    C. Children between the ages of 4 and 6 years are likely to experience developmental delay and behavior regression.
    D. Children between the ages of 6 and 11 years often respond with sadness and report reconciliation fantasies.

    Review this! ❑

24. During the first 2 years after a divorce, discipline and parenting practices are less effective as a result of all of the following, except:

    A. Parents feeling guilt about the divorce.
    B. Parents experiencing role overload.
    C. Children being more compliant and responsive to their parents.
    D. Family structures and routines being disrupted.

    Review this! ❑

25. True or false: Children in stable stepfamilies have the same rate of behavior problems as children in nuclear families.

    A. True
    B. False

    Review this! ❑

26. True or false: It is not necessary to screen every member of the family for unhealthy behaviors.

    A. True
    B. False

    Review this! ❑

27. Family physicians can help children recover from their parents' divorce with all of the following interventions, except:

    A. Allowing the child to talk about his or her perceptions of and feelings about the divorce.
    B. Recognizing signs that the child may be at risk for serious emotional or developmental problems and referring the child for professional intervention.
    C. Support the parents in the way they have chosen to present the divorce to the child.
    D. Encouraging both parents to be involved in monitoring and supporting the child.

    Review this! ❑

28. True or false: Family physicians can help families cope with stressful life events by listening empathetically and providing support and education to mobilize family resources and strengths.

    A. True
    B. False

    Review this! ❑

4 Psychosocial Influences on Health

Chad A. Braun

1. Which of the following statements is not considered an imperative for providing care that is responsive to psychosocial issues?

   A. The physician sees the person first, conceptualizing his or her symptoms and behaviors in both social and psychological contexts and responding with sensitivity to the patient's experiences and priorities.
   B. The physician evaluates the dynamic nature of multiple biopsychosocial variables to respond in a timely manner that optimizes positive results.
   C. The physician fosters a supportive and empathic doctor-patient relationship to provide the foundation for gathering information and for intervening effectively.
   D. The physician evaluates the patient on the basis of biomedical factors and formulates a treatment plan designed to best treat the patient's condition in accordance with the assumptions of mind-body dualism, biologic reductionism, and linear causality.
       Review this! ❏

2. In what year did George Engel propose the biopsychosocial model, which included social and psychological variables as crucial determinants of disease and illness?

   A. 1952
   B. 1977
   C. 1965
   D. 1984
       Review this! ❏

3. Which of the following is not a conceptual model or perspective cited to emphasize different dimensions of the psychosocial influence on health?

   A. The systems approach
   B. The biomedical model
   C. The ethnomedical cultural model
   D. The life-span perspective
   E. The stress and coping model
       Review this! ❏

4. Which of the following statements is true about the life-span perspective?

   A. Every encounter between a patient and physician is a cross-cultural transaction.
   B. Use of this perspective in clinical encounters is accomplished through the LEARN acronym.
   C. To adequately conceptualize a person in health or illness requires a systems approach that encompasses a patient's complexity.
   D. This perspective emphasizes the importance of where a person is on his or her personal developmental trajectory.
       Review this! ❏

5. Which of the following is not a component of the LEARN acronym?

   A. *L*isten with empathy and understanding to a patient's perception of his or her problem by eliciting the patient's explanatory model for the illness.
   B. *E*xplain your perceptions or explanatory model in language that the patient can understand.
   C. *A*ffirm the patient's independence in the medical decision-making process
   D. *R*ecommend treatment that you decide is optimal within your explanatory model.
   E. *N*egotiate treatment with the patient, seeking a compromise that is acceptable to the patient, that is consistent with your ethical standards, and that makes use of the patient's social network, when necessary.
       Review this! ❏

Things to remember for the test.

6. True or false: The LEARN acronym was designed by Engel in 1977 as a part of the biopsychosocial conceptual model.

   A. True
   B. False

   Review this! ❑

7. Which of the following is not a component of the family APGAR developed by Smilkstein as part of the systems approach conceptual model?

   A. Adaptation
   B. Planning
   C. Growth
   D. Affection
   E. Resolve

   Review this! ❑

8. True or false: As part of Engel's biopsychosocial model, the physician was encouraged to "observe biochemical and morphologic changes in relation to a patient's emotional patterns, life goals, attitudes toward illness, and social environment."

   A. True
   B. False

   Review this! ❑

9. Which of the following is not one of the three assumptions that Engel's biopsychosocial model is based on?

   A. Patients can be seen in distinct biologic, psychologic, and social categories, and problems can then be expressed as a set of scientific principles from which diagnosis and treatment can be derived.
   B. Clinical care needs to go beyond biomedicine, because illness can be fully understood only in the context of psychological and social factors.
   C. The three domains—biological, psychological, and social—are interrelated.
   D. Effective treatment requires attention to complex interactions and to the integration of the biopsychosocial factors.

   Review this! ❑

10. Which of the following is not considered a pillar of the biopsychosocially oriented clinical practice as cited by Burrell-Carrio?

    A. Self-awareness
    B. Active cultivation of trust
    C. Using informed intuition

D. Communicating clinical evidence to foster dialogue
E. None of the above

   Review this! ❑

11. Which of the following is not one of Sarafino's five types of personal control?

    A. Behavioral control
    B. Cognitive control
    C. Decisional control
    D. Intuitive control
    E. Retrospective control

    Review this! ❑

12. True or false: Cognitive control involves the ability to use thought processes or strategies to modify the impact of a stressor.

    A. True
    B. False

    Review this! ❑

13. Which of the following is not one of the three "Cs" of hardiness as defined by Kobasa?

    A. Control
    B. Compassion
    C. Commitment
    D. Challenge

    Review this! ❑

14. Which of the following is not recognized as a variety of social support that can be experienced by a patient?

    A. Emotional support
    B. Esteem support
    C. Financial support
    D. Instrumental support
    E. Information support

    Review this! ❑

15. True or false: The "direct effects" hypothesis suggests that social support affects health by protecting the person against negative effects of stress, perhaps by affecting the cognitive appraisal of stress.

    A. True
    B. False

    Review this! ❑

16. Which of the following is not considered to be a key point in the psychosocial database?

A. Family composition
B. Health insurance status
C. Physical environment
D. Sexual orientation
E. All of the above are considered key points.

Review this! ❑

17. Which of the following strategies are commonly used to supplement biopsychosocial information gathered from interviewing the patient?

A. Health questionnaires
B. Interviews with family members
C. Consultations with cultural informants and translators
D. Home visits
E. All of the above are used.

Review this! ❑

18. Which of the following is not a recommended intervention for family physicians working with patients using the biopsychosocial model?

A. Directly reduce stress.
B. Enhance social support resources.
C. Manage the patient independently rather than referring him or her to another provider.
D. Reinforce positive stress appraisal and coping.

Review this! ❑

19. Which of the following is not considered an important time for psychosocial intervention?

A. When there are transitions in the family life cycle
B. When compliance issues affect health
C. When there are dramatic changes in patient symptoms
D. When significant new diagnoses are present
E. All of the above

Review this! ❑

20. Which of the following is not an emotionally charged issue that people with chronic illness inevitably confront?

A. Anger
B. Abandonment
C. Bargaining
D. Stigma
E. Isolation

Review this! ❑

21. True or false: Managed care has introduced significant challenges to the implementation of the biopsychosocial model in clinical practice.

A. True
B. False

Review this! ❑

Things to remember for the test.

5 Practicing Biopsychosocial Medicine

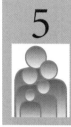

James E. Schmidt

1. In what year did the American medical education community adopt the university model, thereby bringing medical schools into the more traditional higher education graduate school format?

   A. 1863
   B. 1910
   C. 1944
   D. 1960

   Review this! ❏

2. True or false: In the university model, medical investigators began performing scholarly inquiry as dictated by the tenets of the scientific method.

   A. True
   B. False

   Review this! ❏

3. True or false: The traditional reductionistic approach treats diseases as independent entities that are amenable to categorization and presumed to have a specific cause.

   A. True
   B. False

   Review this! ❏

4. Physicians have multiple responsibilities, including the need to understand the biomedical condition and its associated factors. Which of the following factors is not one of their fields of responsibility?

   A. Behavioral factors
   B. Social factors
   C. Empirical factors
   D. Cultural factors

   Review this! ❏

5. True or false: The physician's awareness of the impact of stress on the overall number of problems presented by a patient is critical for determining the appropriate course of treatment.

   A. True
   B. False

   Review this! ❏

6. Which of the following powers are not attributed to physicians (and thus singularly qualify them to influence their patients)?

   A. Reward power
   B. Subjective power
   C. Expert power
   D. Referent power
   E. Legitimate power

   Review this! ❏

7. The physician can capably employ certain skills to decrease stress and to enable patients to deal more effectively with those things that are contributing to their misery. Which of the following is not considered a major common component of psychotherapy?

   A. The expectation of receiving help
   B. The therapeutic relationship
   C. Obtaining an internal perspective
   D. Encouraging a corrective experience
   E. The opportunity to test reality repeatedly

   Review this! ❏

8. True or false: The BATHE technique that is used to assess a patient's psychosocial situation and then react accordingly stands for the following:

   - *Background*
   - *Affect*
   - *Trouble*
   - *Handling*
   - *Empathy*

   A. True
   B. False

   Review this! ❏

9. The physician's inquiry into the patient's psychosocial status is designed to do the following, except:

    A. To produce an enhanced comprehension on the part of the physician of the overall dimensions of a patient's presenting problem.
    B. To allow the physician to assume responsibility for the patient's particular situation.
    C. To assess the patient's situation so that therapeutic suggestions can be made.
    D. To enable the patient to deal with his or her problem more effectively.
       Review this! ❏

10. True or false: The physician empowers the patient by giving advice or directly solving a problem.

    A. True
    B. False
       Review this! ❏

11. True or false: Patients must learn to differentiate among thoughts, feelings, and behavior.

    A. True
    B. False
       Review this! ❏

12. Which of the following statements does not describe the physician's role in helping patients explore options when the patients become overwhelmed by the circumstances of their lives?

    A. The physician's suggestion that there are options to be explored moves the patient in a positive direction.
    B. It is the physician's task to generate these options.
    C. The physician communicates the expectation that the patient can and will follow the identified option.
    D. The physician expects the patient to report back the results to him or her.
       Review this! ❏

13. Which of the following four options for handling a bad situation is unhealthy?

    A. Leaving the situation
    B. Ignoring the situation
    C. Changing the situation
    D. Reframing the situation
       Review this! ❏

14. True or false: Therapeutic talk is direct conversation that focuses patients on their strengths and choices and that makes patients feel like someone cares about them.

    A. True
    B. False
       Review this! ❏

15. Which of the following stereotypes of difficult patients are common triggers of negative feelings in physicians?

    A. Dependent clingers
    B. Manipulative help-rejecters
    C. Entitled demanders
    D. Self-destructive deniers
    E. All of the above
       Review this! ❏

16. Which of the following is the most appropriate amount of time to spend with a patient who arouses negative emotions in the physician?

    A. Less than 15 minutes
    B. 15–30 minutes
    C. 30–45 minutes
    D. 45–60 minutes
       Review this! ❏

17. True or false: Hypochondriacs do not believe "good health" means being relatively "symptom free," which accounts for these patients' numerous somatic complaints and resistance to reassurance.

    A. True
    B. False
       Review this! ❏

18. True or false: There are no real differences between hypochondriacs and chronic complainers.

    A. True
    B. False
       Review this! ❏

19. True or false: Depression that is not diagnosed or treated by the primary care physician often results in long-lasting symptomatology, decreased quality of life, and suicide.

    A. True
    B. False
       Review this! ❏

Things to remember for the test.

Things to remember for the test.

20. Which of the following principles of survival is essential for the physician who is practicing biopsychosocial medicine?

    A. Do not take responsibility for things that you cannot control.

    B. Take care of yourself, or you cannot take care of anyone else.
    C. Recognize that you have to start where the patient is.
    D. All of the above

    Review this! ❑

6 Domestic Violence: Child Abuse, Rape, Spouse Abuse, and Elder Abuse

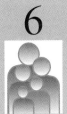

Jeri A. O'Donnell

ELDER MISTREATMENT

1. True or false: Elder abuse first achieved notable recognition within the U.S. social work literature during the late 1970s.

   A. True
   B. False

   Review this! ❑

2. True or false: Numerous studies have confirmed the fact that elderly females are far more likely to be victims of abuse then elderly males.

   A. True
   B. False

   Review this! ❑

3. Pregnancy triggers violence for all of the following reasons, except:

   A. The male is no longer central to his partner's life.
   B. There is more involvement with the female's family than the male wants.
   C. Pathological jealousies.
   D. Marital status.

   Review this! ❑

INTIMATE PARTNER VIOLENCE

4. All are violence markers, except:

   A. Marriage.
   B. Pregnancy.
   C. Being female.
   D. Age.

   Review this! ❑

5. True or false: Younger white women are more likely than older women to use both formal and informal resources when seeking help.

   A. True
   B. False

   Review this! ❑

6. True or false: Violence is a less common risk factor for pregnant women than conditions as preeclampsia, gestational diabetes, and placenta previa.

   A. True
   B. False

   Review this! ❑

7. All are barriers to communication between the physician and the abused adult patient, except:

   A. The patient's belief that the physician lacks time and interest in discussing abuse.
   B. The patient is an adult and therefore can determine when it is the best time to ask for help.
   C. The patient fears legal ramifications and loss of confidentiality.
   D. The physician's own discomfort with feeling capable of effectively dealing with abuse issues.

   Review this! ❑

8. True or false: Research indicates that, in half of households in which a batterer beats a partner, child abuse is also occurring, especially among children between the ages of 3 and 6 years.

   A. True
   B. False

   Review this! ❑

9. True or false: Research has noted that male batterers are not too different from nonviolent men.

   A. True
   B. False

   Review this! ❑

10. Demographics associated with those who attempt suicide include which of the following?

A. Being female
B. Alcoholism
C. Being separated and having children
D. Clinical depression

Review this! ❑

11. True or false: The average age of husbands who murder their wives is 46 years, whereas the average age of wives who murder their husbands is 57 years.

A. True
B. False

Review this! ❑

12. The following are among the risk factors for being a victim of intimate partner violence (IPV) homicide, except:

A. A history of forced sex.
B. Firearm(s) in the home.
C. Being a black female.
D. An increasing frequency of violence.

Review this! ❑

13. True or false: Often a family physician is the doctor to both the victim of violence and the perpetrator. Because of this relationship, the family physician can more effectively counsel the couple.

A. True
B. False

Review this! ❑

14. True or false: There is clear evidence to demonstrate that physician screening, counseling, and referral improve the clinical outcome of the victim who is experiencing IPV.

A. True
B. False

Review this! ❑

CHILD ABUSE

15. True or false: All states agree that, beyond the obvious evidence of physical harm, even suspected child abuse is cause enough for a physician to report to a children's services agency.

A. True
B. False

Review this! ❑

16. True or false: Thankfully, the media has brought to everyone's attention the significant number of child maltreatment cases involving day care centers and foster care homes, which has been reported as being well over 7% of these cases.

A. True
B. False

Review this! ❑

17. True or false: Rape and sexual assault are highest among nonmarried women and women under the age of 35 who are raped by someone unknown to them.

A. True
B. False

Review this! ❑

18. True or false: Despite the best emergency room efforts and media educational attempts, injured victims of rape and sexual assault do not receive medical care for their injuries nor do they report their attacks to a law-enforcement agency.

A. True
B. False

Review this! ❑

19. True or false: Sexual dysfunction occurs among more than 50% of sexual assault victims and should be a definite red flag for the physician.

A. True
B. False

Review this! ❑

20. True or false: The definition of rape includes that it is an act of forceful, non-consensual, sexual contact.

A. True
B. False

Review this! ❑

21. True or false: Typically, the emotional reaction of a female to rape is the "expressed style," whereas, among male victims of rape, the "controlled style" is more frequently seen.

A. True
B. False

Review this! ❑

7 Care of the Elderly

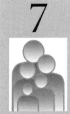

Jeffrey W. Milks

1. Which of the following is false?

   A. Currently, approximately 1 out of every 10 people in the world is 60 years old or older.
   B. By 2050, 1 out of every 3 people in the world will be 60 years old or older.
   C. The number of working-age persons (15–64 years old) per older persons (65 years old or older) is referred to as the "dependency burden."
   D. It is anticipated that the dependency burden will lessen substantially within the next 50 years.

   Review this! ❏

2. Which of the following can affect function in the geriatric patient? (Function is defined as the ability to adapt to the environment and to perform activities of daily living.)

   A. Poor health habits
   B. Poor nutrition
   C. Polypharmacy
   D. All of the above

   Review this! ❏

3. Which one of the following is an important part of an effective geriatric health questionnaire?

   A. General health questions that might include a self-rated health assessment
   B. Assessment of activities of daily living and instrumental activities of daily living
   C. Assessment of pain
   D. All of the above

   Review this! ❏

4. Which of the following would not be used specifically to evaluate a patient's cognitive function?

   A. The Hamilton Depression Rating Scale
   B. The Folstein Mini-Mental Status Examination
   C. The Mini-Cog Test
   D. The Trail-Making Test

   Review this! ❏

5. Which of the following is not a part of the Folstein Mini-Mental Status Examination?

   A. The subtraction of serial 7s or spelling the word *world* backwards
   B. Naming the current president of the United States
   C. Writing a sentence
   D. Following a three-step command

   Review this! ❏

6. True statements about dementia include all of the following, except:

   A. In North America, up to 10% of persons 65 years old and older have dementia, and two thirds of those cases are the result of Alzheimer's disease.
   B. Four and a half million persons in the United States suffer from Alzheimer's disease, and this number is projected to climb to 13.2 million by the year 2050.
   C. Dementia represents a significant clinical problem, and it is frequently difficult to diagnose in routine daily practice.
   D. Patients with dementia often complain of memory loss.

   Review this! ❏

7. The diagnosis of dementia, according to *Diagnostic and Statistical Manual of Mental Disorders, Fourth Edition* criteria, requires all of the following except:

   A. The patient with dementia must have multiple cognitive deficits, one of which is memory impairment.
   B. The patient with dementia needs to have evidence of at least one of the following categories of deficits: aphasia, apraxia, agnosia, or executive function disturbance.

Things to remember for the test.

C. To establish a diagnosis of dementia, the cognitive deficits of the patient need to have significant social or occupational impairment consequences and to not just be present in the delirious state.

D. The diagnostic criteria for dementia require that there be a gradual onset and continuing decline of the cognitive impairment.

Review this! ❑

8. Which of the following is not a true statement about the Folstein Mini-Mental State Examination?

A. The diagnostic criteria for Alzheimer's disease require that the dementia be of a gradual onset and show decline of the cognitive impairment over time. The Folstein Mini-Mental State Examination provides a tool with which to document this progression.

B. One of the strengths of the Folstein Mini-Mental State Examination is that testing is not subject to variation in education or age.

C. The Folstein Mini-Mental State Examination provides an 87% sensitivity rate and an 82% specificity rate when testing for dementia in white populations, with a cutoff of 24.

D. Although the progression of dementias such as Alzheimer's disease is quite variable, a loss of approximately 2 points on the Folstein Mini-Mental State Examination can be expected each year among these patients.

Review this! ❑

9. Which of the following is not true about the clock-drawing test?

A. A perfect score on this test is a 6.

B. The numbering (organization), the clock's hour and minute hand placement, and the visual-spatial orientation are all aspects that must be evaluated.

C. A score of 3 represents a cognitive deficit.

D. The only equipment required for this exercise is a writing utensil and a piece of paper.

Review this! ❑

10. Which of the following would be unusual for a patient presenting with dementia?

A. An insidious onset of the disorder

B. Self-reporting of the problem

C. Clear consciousness

D. The condition being present for months or years before presentation

Review this! ❑

11. Appropriate laboratory testing for the initial investigation of dementia includes all of the following, except:

A. Syphilis serology.

B. Thyroid studies.

C. Vitamin B_{12} levels.

D. Apolipoprotein E epsilon 4 allele.

Review this! ❑

12. Which of the following pharmacologic treatments of Alzheimer's disease has shown evidence of effectiveness for the management of dementia?

A. Cholinesterase inhibitors: donepezil (Aricept), rivastigmine (Exelon), galantamine (Razadyne [formerly Reminyl]), tacrine (Cognex)

B. *N*-methyl-D-aspartate (NMDA) receptor antagonist: memantine (Namenda)

C. Antibiotics

D. All of the above

Review this! ❑

13. Which of the following statements is not true?

A. Screening for cognitive impairment is a cost-effective task that should be performed on all geriatric patients.

B. When caregivers describe cognitive decline in an individual, these observations should be taken seriously, and cognitive assessment and careful follow-up are indicated.

C. It is critical to identify and treat general medical conditions that may be responsible for or that may contribute to the dementia or associated behavioral symptoms.

D. Cholinesterase inhibitor treatment of patients with clinically detected mild to moderate Alzheimer's disease provides minimal impact on functional status but a modest tendency in some patients to stabilize cognition.

Review this! ❑

14. All of the following are true about falls among the aged population, except:

Things to remember for the test.

A. About one third of community-dwelling persons over the age of 65 years fall each year.

B. Half of fallers will fall again in a given year.

C. Each year, about 50% of persons over the age of 80 years and about 50% of nursing home residents will fall.

D. Women fall with the same frequency as men, but men tend to have less mortality as the result of falling.

Review this! ❏

15. Which of the following statements is true?

A. Physical restraint use in the nursing home and hospital settings does not reduce the risk of falling, and it is actually associated with an increased risk of injury.

B. Only medications that sedate an individual—including benzodiazepines, antipsychotics, and antihistamines—increase fall risk.

C. Only after a patient has sustained recurrent, significant falls should that patient be labeled a faller and an evaluation into the potential causes of falling be undertaken.

D. Up to 80% of older persons have orthostatic hypotension.

Review this! ❏

16. Which of the following interventions has been shown to reduce the risks of falls among the aged?

A. Modification of environmental hazards in the home

B. Discontinuation of psychotropic drugs

C. Supervised exercise programs that improve gait, balance, and strength

D. All of the above

Review this! ❏

17. Which of the following statements is true?

A. The presence of falls alone is a strict contraindication to anticoagulation for atrial fibrillation.

B. Multifactorial interventions designed to decrease the risk of falling are not likely to succeed among the cognitively impaired.

C. Cardiac pacing for fallers with cardio-inhibitory carotid sinus hypersensitivity does not reduce the risk of falling.

D. Interventions for the management of orthostatic hypotension have not been shown to decrease the frequency of falls in the geriatric population. Some of these interventions include discontinuing diuretics, wearing supportive stockings, instructing patients to rise carefully and ensure balance before ambulating, and liberalizing salt and fluid in the diet.

Review this! ❏

18. Which of the following statements is not true about the "get up and go" test?

A. The patient is asked to stand up from a seated position, walk about 10 feet (3 meters), turn around, walk back, and sit down again.

B. The test is the quick and easy to perform.

C. The test can be used as an overall assessment of the patient's gait, stability, balance, and strength.

D. The test would not likely be helpful for the evaluation of a patient with a single fall.

Review this! ❏

19. All of the following are true about depression among the aged, except:

A. Depression is a clinical diagnosis that is made entirely on the basis of an adequate patient interview.

B. Most older patients with depression will also have at least one or more specific depressive symptoms, such as depressed mood, feelings of guilt or worthlessness, anhedonia, or thoughts of suicide.

C. Grief after the death of a spouse or another loved one rarely produces the symptoms of a major depressive disorder.

D. Depression and dementia are often comorbid conditions rather than one disease mimicking the other.

Review this! ❏

20. With regard to depression in the patient with Alzheimer's disease, which of the following is true?

A. The diagnosis of depression among patients with Alzheimer's disease is less difficult than it is among older patients without dementia, because their clinical manifestations of depression are more exaggerated.

B. Guilt and suicidal thoughts are uncommon in the patient with Alzheimer's disease, and, although suicidal feelings are rare, the risk still needs to be thoroughly evaluated.

C. Psychotic symptoms, such as delusions and hallucinations, are less likely to accompany depression among patients with Alzheimer's disease than among patients without dementia.

D. The Geriatrics Depression Scale is valid and reliable only for individuals with Mini-Mental State Examination scores of 25 or more.

Review this! ❏

21. Which of the following would be the poorest choice for the initial treatment of a mild depression in a geriatric patient?

A. Watchful waiting
B. Sertraline (Zoloft and others)
C. Amitriptyline (Elavil and others)
D. Mirtazapine (Remeron)

Review this! ❏

22. Which of the following is frequently an underlying cause of depression?

A. Hypothyroidism
B. Diabetes
C. Malignancy, especially pancreatic cancer
D. Glucocorticoid excess

Review this! ❏

23. Which of the following is not true about suicide among the geriatric population?

A. Rates of suicide increase markedly among Americans over the age of 75 years, especially among white men.
B. The co-occurrence of alcohol-use disorders and depression increases suicide risk.
C. Late-life suicide is characterized by less warning, higher lethality, and greater prevalence of depression and physical illness.
D. Older people usually commit suicide by less-violent means than younger people, and firearms are infrequently used during suicide attempts.

Review this! ❏

24. Which of the following is false with regard to the bladder among older adults?

A. Bladder capacity declines with age.
B. Post-void residual increases with age.
C. The presence of involuntary bladder contractions increases with age.
D. Urinary incontinence should be considered part of normal aging.

Review this! ❏

25. Reversible causes of acute incontinence include which of the following?

A. Urinary tract infection
B. Fecal impaction
C. Hyperglycemia
D. All of the above

Review this! ❏

26. Which of the four forms of urinary incontinence would be primarily responsible for incontinence in a patient with severe dementia?

A. Stress
B. Urge
C. Overflow
D. Functional

Review this! ❏

27. Which of the following tests should be performed routinely as part of the initial evaluation of a patient with urine incontinence?

A. Computed tomography of the pelvis
B. Post-void residual
C. Voiding cystourethrogram
D. Intravenous pyelogram

Review this! ❏

28. Because incontinence among older patients is often multifactorial in nature, evaluation and treatment proceed in tandem with potential problems being addressed as they are revealed. With this approach in mind, there are a number of nonspecific treatments that should be implemented for most patients with chronic incontinence, regardless of the cause. Which of the following should be recommended?

A. Patients should be encouraged to void frequently during the day and always before bedtime.
B. For patients with nocturnal problems, fluids should be avoided 3 or 4 hours before bedtime.

C. Patients should be educated about the use of protective undergarments, incontinence pads, and environmental modifications (e.g., bedside commodes, urinals).
D. All of the above

Review this! ❏

29. Which one of the following statements is not a best-evidence recommendation regarding urinary incontinence among older patients?

A. Hormone replacement therapy (estrogen alone or estrogen plus progestin) in menopausal women is associated with a decreased risk of all types of urinary incontinence, and it should be used for the prevention and treatment of incontinence.
B. Pelvic floor muscle training is effective for reducing urinary incontinence among women with stress- or mixed-type incontinence.
C. Bladder training is effective for reducing the symptoms of urge-type incontinence, and it is also effective for mixed incontinence in combination with pelvic floor exercises.
D. Laparoscopic colposuspension, retropubic colposuspension, and tension-free vaginal tape are surgical interventions that have shown benefit for treating stress incontinence.

Review this! ❏

30. Rational drug prescribing requires knowledge of which of the following?

A. Pharmacokinetics
B. Functional status and life expectancy of the patient
C. Current medications, including prescriptions, over-the-counter drugs, vitamins, and herbal treatments
D. All of the above

Review this! ❏

31. Which of the following statements is true about elder mistreatment?

A. In 1996, it was been reported that nearly 550,000 adults over the age 60 years were victims of abuse in a domestic setting and that about 80% of such cases were reported.
B. States with mandatory reporting laws that require physicians to report elder mistreatment have a lower incidence of elder abuse.
C. The privilege of confidential communications between doctors and patients supersedes the obligation to report elder abuse.
D. Elder mistreatment, like other forms of domestic violence, tends to escalate if interventions are not initiated.

Review this! ❏

Things to remember for the test.

8 Care of the Dying Patient

Paul Callaway

1. Proper strategies for dealing with terminal patients include which of the following?

   A. Avoid sharing the true prognosis if the results might be frightening to the patient or to his or her family.
   B. Plan hospital rounds at an early morning time, when the patient and his or her family are less likely to discuss details.
   C. Provide honest information while focusing on the patient's needs.
   D. Advise the patient to not worry about the disease process.

   Review this! ❑

2. Regarding the discussion of religion and spiritual issues, the physician should do which of the following?

   A. Steer the conversation toward lighter topics, such as sports or current events.
   B. Listen respectfully, allowing the patient to discuss his or her concerns.
   C. Avoid the topic entirely, and ask the hospital clergy to visit with the patient.
   D. Ask permission to leave religious tracts in the patient's room.

   Review this! ❑

3. Modern medical science and technology have allowed for a longer duration of life, often despite terminal illness. The focus of the physician managing the dying patient should incorporate which attitude?

   A. When cure is no longer possible, care should focus on the comfort of the patient and of his or her family.
   B. It is unethical to allow a patient to die without exhausting all treatment options available.
   C. Concentrate on quantity of life, despite current patient suffering.
   D. Provide adequate nutrition, including tube feedings, to allow natural defense mechanisms to work.

   Review this! ❑

4. Pain management represents a major challenge for the physician who is caring for the terminally ill. Select the management strategy that is most effective for breaking the cycle of uncontrolled pain.

   A. Analgesic medication should be given as needed in a large enough dose to control pain.
   B. Analgesic medication should be given on a regular schedule in amounts that are adequate to control pain. Booster doses of analgesics may also be necessary.
   C. Avoid high doses of opioids initially, allowing larger doses to be added later, during the final days of life.
   D. Referring the patient to a pain specialist will allow the primary physician to avoid Drug Enforcement Administration scrutiny for prescribing narcotic analgesics.

   Review this! ❑

5. Which statement best reflects the proper use of nonpharmacologic techniques of pain management?

   A. Nonpharmacologic techniques should only be used as an adjunct to opioids.
   B. Herbal therapy should be tried before opioid pain relievers.
   C. Appropriate nonpharmacologic techniques of pain management may include relaxation techniques, massage, hypnosis, and biofeedback.
   D. Heat therapy is particularly useful for neuropathic pain.

   Review this! ❑

6. Which of the following is the opioid agent that represents good initial effectiveness for cancer pain?

A. Meperidine (Demerol), which has oral and parenteral preparations and a long duration of action

B. Hydrocodone or oxycodone, which cause only temporary sedation and require the use of a laxative

C. Pentazocine (Talwin), which is more potent than codeine and has a low incidence of side effects

D. Ibuprofen (Motrin, Advil), which may alleviate the pain associated with bone lesions

Review this! ❑

7. Which statement best reflects the management of the distressing symptom of dyspnea?

A. Even in the absence of signs of acute infection, antibiotics are indicated when the terminal patient develops a breakthrough in the symptom of dyspnea.

B. Booster dosing of narcotic analgesics is an effective way to control breakthrough dyspnea, and it carries a low risk of significant respiratory depression.

C. The presence of dyspnea suggests toxicity from the analgesic, thus requiring a reduction in the dosage of narcotics.

D. The use of oxygen is always superior to the use of narcotics for the management of dyspnea.

Review this! ❑

8. Treatment of constipation in the terminally ill patient includes all of the following, except:

A. Senna (Senokot), one to four tablets daily.

B. Sorbitol 70%, two to three times daily.

C. Bulk laxative (Metamucil, Citrucel), 2 tablespoons one to two times daily.

D. Bisacodyl (Dulcolax), 10 mg suppositories as needed.

Review this! ❑

9. Treatment of persistent nausea and vomiting in the dying patient includes all of the following, except:

A. Searching for and, if possible, correcting treatable causes of the symptom (e.g., nonsteroidal anti-inflammatory drug-induced gastritis, constipation).

B. Using steroids when increased intracranial pressure is suspected.

C. Subcutaneously infusing metoclopramide, haloperidol, and an opioid.

D. Combining antiemetic agents to control symptoms, thereby allowing for the continuation of tube feeding.

Review this! ❑

10. Cancer patients often lose their appetites and experience a reduction in body weight. Current understanding of nutrition, calorie supplementation, and clinical outcomes support which of the following statements?

A. The routine use of parenteral nutrition for patients undergoing chemotherapy should be discouraged.

B. The causes of cancer cachexia are well understood.

C. For patients with either small-cell carcinoma of the lung or colorectal cancer, total parenteral nutrition in combination with chemotherapy results in a longer life.

D. Oral protein supplement among older patients produces a small yet consistent weight gain, and it is associated with an improvement in clinical outcome and reduced hospital stay.

Review this! ❑

11. The treatment of chronic pain, especially in the cancer patient, often requires a booster dose of an opioid pain reliever. Which agent below would be an appropriate choice for use as a booster?

A. Morphine sulfate SR (MS Contin)

B. Methadone

C. Pentazocine (Talwin)

D. Morphine solution (Roxanol)

Review this! ❑

12. Persistent hiccups can occur from a variety of causes. Effective options for treatment include all of the following, except:

A. Chlorpromazine (Thorazine), 25–50 mg orally every 4–6 hours

B. Metoclopramide (Reglan), 10–20 mg orally every 6–8 hours

C. Escitalopram (Lexapro), 10–20 mg orally every day

D. Haloperidol (Haldol), 1–2 mg orally every 4–6 hours

Review this! ❑

Things to remember for the test.

13. Terminally ill patients often cannot tolerate oral opioids or antiemetics as a result of nausea, vomiting, or extreme weakness. In the setting of cachexia in a terminal cancer patient, which of the following is the best option to consider?

    A. Hydromorphone (Dilaudid) given intramuscularly
    B. Fentanyl transdermal (Duragesic patch)
    C. Hydromorphone (Dilaudid) given via subcutaneous infusion
    D. Morphine sulfate intravenously given via infusion pump

    Review this! ❏

14. A hospice program provides palliative and supportive care for the dying patient and his or her family. To qualify for Medicare funding of hospice, the patient life expectancy is less than which of the following?

    A. 6 months
    B. 4 weeks
    C. 12 months
    D. 3 months

    Review this! ❏

15. An advance directive is a legal document that allows competent adults to express their intentions regarding medical treatment in the event of a terminal illness in which they have lost their decision-making capacity. Which of the following statements is true about advance directives?

    A. A living will expresses the individual's choice for a medical power of attorney.
    B. A living will is a comprehensive document that is an effective tool when dealing with multiple state laws.
    C. The majority of Americans have a living will in place.
    D. A durable power of attorney designates a person to make health, financial, and legal decisions if the patient is unable to do so.

    Review this! ❏

16. Physicians use many different styles of communication. When caring for the terminally ill patient, which of the following questions or strategies is most likely to bring about a greater understanding of the patient's needs and wishes?

    A. "As your physician, I will recommend the most effective treatment plan for you."
    B. "What is your highest priority now? How can I help you achieve this? What is your greatest fear about this illness?"
    C. Give the patient the greatest independence by not asking questions that are probing. Allow the patient to ask only the questions that he or she wants answered.
    D. Avoid the discussion of religion and spiritual issues.

    Review this! ❏

17. When delivering bad news, which strategy will set the stage for an optimum physician-patient relationship during the ensuing time?

    A. Deliver the news on the phone, as soon as possible, to allow for the immediate initiation of possible treatment options.
    B. To avoid a possible Health Insurance Portability and Accountability Act violation, deliver the news in person but without any family members present. The patient may inform appropriate family members at a later time.
    C. Allow for uninterrupted time, with honest but not blunt information. Have a family member present to serve as another set of ears.
    D. Deliver the news in an authoritarian manner, keeping a professional distance.

    Review this! ❏

18. Understanding oral morphine equivalent potencies is useful when using oral opioid agents. Accurate statements about morphine equivalents include all of the following, except:

    A. Hydromorphone (Dilaudid) is a potent agent—a 2-mg dose of this drug is equivalent to a 10-mg dose of oral morphine.
    B. A 5-mg dose of hydrocodone plus a 1.5-mg dose of homatropine (Hycodan) is a potent combination drug that is more potent than oxycodone (5 mg/5 mL dose of Roxicodone).
    C. A fentanyl patch delivering 50 g of the drug per hour is more potent than 5 mg of oxycodone plus 325 mg of acetaminophen (Percocet) given every 4 hours.

D. A 30-mg dose of codeine plus a 300-mg dose of acetaminophen (Tylenol No. 3) is equivalent in potency to a 5-mg dose of hydrocodone plus a 500-mg dose of acetaminophen (Vicodin).

Review this! ❏

19. Evaluating pain on a scale of 1 to 10 is a useful way to quantify the severity of pain and the effectiveness of treatment. Which of the following statements is true about pain scale use?

A. Any pain should be considered to be severe; the target level of pain should always be 0.
B. Anxiety can worsen the perception of pain. Therefore, the patient's pain scale rating can never be trusted.
C. For chronic and severe pain (4–10 on the pain scale), potent medication should be given on an as-needed basis.
D. Target levels of pain relief can be negotiated with the patient, but, in general, they should be less than 4.

Review this! ❏

20. Which of the following is the most accurate statement about pain control?

A. Slow-release morphine is an appropriate first choice for controlling severe pain.
B. When opioids do not relieve pain without intolerable side effects, switching to a benzodiazepine is appropriate.
C. Adding a laxative to regular opioid use is only necessary if the patient complains of constipation.
D. When opioids are titrated to relieve pain or dyspnea, the risk of addiction or respiratory depression is very low.

Review this! ❏

21. True or false: Patients with chronic disease and those who are terminally ill will benefit most from good supportive care.

A. True
B. False

Review this! ❏

22. True or false: A major fear of the terminally ill patient is abandonment.

A. True
B. False

Review this! ❏

23. True or false: Decreased interest in eating may be a symptom of oral candidiasis.

A. True
B. False

Review this! ❏

24. True or false: For the burning, stabbing, or shooting pain caused by nerve damage, a nonsteroidal anti-inflammatory drug such as ibuprofen (600–800 mg three times a day) is the treatment of choice.

A. True
B. False

Review this! ❏

25. True or false: Assisted suicide is illegal throughout the United States.

A. True
B. False

Review this! ❏

Things to remember for the test.

9

Ethics in Family Practice

James S. Campbell

Things to remember for the test.

1. The quality of the modern-day physician-patient relationship is threatened by which of the following?

   A. Third-party intervention
   B. A misunderstanding of patient autonomy
   C. A and B
   D. None of the above

   Review this! ❑

2. Which of the following statements about health care delivery is not correct?

   A. Physicians have an obligation to practice medicine within professional standards of care.
   B. Physicians have the right to avoid violation of their own religious convictions.
   C. Health maintenance should serve as the primary common goal of the physician-patient relationship.
   D. Medical decision making should not be influenced by third-party payer intervention.

   Review this! ❑

3. The purpose of a pre-employment examination is to do which of the following?

   A. Determine fitness for work and protect workers from illness and injury
   B. Protect employers from the costs of preventable job-related illnesses and injuries
   C. Collect data for future use
   D. A and B
   E. All of the above

   Review this! ❑

4. True or false: Physicians should restrict their evaluations of school absenteeism to medically related facts.

   A. True
   B. False

   Review this! ❑

5. The emphasis on patient confidentiality has changed from the withholding of information to restricted information sharing as a result of which of the following?

   A. Deviations from the basic principles of the Hippocratic Oath
   B. American Medical Association guidelines
   C. Changes in health care delivery models
   D. Decreased emphasis on the patient's right to privacy

   Review this! ❑

6. The release of patient information without consent is acceptable in which of the following situations?

   A. When there is a need for a work release
   B. When the patient is in a communicable disease state
   C. When there is third-party payer demand
   D. When there is a family inquiry during hospitalization

   Review this! ❑

7. The approach to the confidentiality of information is clear for all of the following patients, except:

   A. Pediatric patients.
   B. Adolescent patients.
   C. Competent adult patients.
   D. Incompetent adult patients.

   Review this! ❑

8. The term *informed consent* first appeared in what year?

   A. 1937
   B. 1957
   C. 1977
   D. 1997

   Review this! ❑

9. Which of the following is a recognized exception to the need for informed consent?

A. Emergency exception
B. Therapeutic privilege
C. A and B
D. None of the above

Review this! ❑

10. The principle of informed consent has which of the following characteristics?

A. It applies to all medical interventions.
B. It applies to invasive procedures only.
C. It is not valid without a signed document.
D. It is a legal principle with little or no clinical benefit.

Review this! ❑

11. The concept of providing consent information that reasonable medical practitioners would normally provide to patients under similar circumstances is referred to as which of the following?

A. The professional practice standard
B. The reasonable professional standard
C. The reasonable person standard
D. The professional person standard

Review this! ❑

12. True or false: When defining informed consent, most courts use the reasonable person standard.

A. True
B. False

Review this! ❑

13. Which of the following is considered an essential element of informed consent?

A. Risks/benefits of treatment
B. Alternative treatment
C. Costs of treatment
D. A and B
E. All of the above

Review this! ❑

14. Most cases of patient noncompliance involve which of the following?

A. Communication breakdown
B. Value conflict between physician and patient
C. Patient incompetence
D. A and B
E. All of the above

Review this! ❑

15. With respect to medication noncompliance, physicians should do which of the following?

A. Avoid frank discussion about costs for fear of embarrassing the patient.
B. Consider less optimal, cheaper medications.
C. Decide which medication side effects are acceptable based on a review of the medical literature.
D. Be prepared to quickly acknowledge medication noncompliance as an inevitable consequence of medical practice.

Review this! ❑

16. With respect to patient referrals, which of the following statements is true?

A. After a referral, the consultant assumes full responsibility for the quality of care.
B. The principles of informed consent have little or no impact on referral decisions.
C. The referral process is complete after the consultant has seen the patient.
D. None of the above

Review this! ❑

17. Individual physician well-being is contingent upon which of the following?

A. The avoidance of mistakes
B. The recognition and expression of emotions
C. Placing career ahead of family
D. Deprofessionalizing the physician–patient relationship

Review this! ❑

18. Which of the following statements is true?

A. Most Americans oppose the legalization of assisted death.
B. Public support of assisted death has increased over the past decade.
C. Most terminally ill patients defer palliative care.
D. Physicians practicing in teaching hospitals are the most comfortable with death.

Review this! ❑

19. Which of the following statements is not true?

A. The American Medical Association opposes efforts to legalize euthanasia.

B. In the Netherlands, the government does not prosecute physicians who adhere to strict criteria for euthanasia.

C. Physician-assisted suicide is not legal in the United States.

D. Patient requests for physician-assisted suicide, where legal, must be repeated and confirmed before the procedure.

Review this! ❏

20. True or false: As a result of advances in pain and symptom management, the under-treatment of pain among the terminally ill is now uncommon.

A. True
B. False

Review this! ❏

21. Which of the following parties exercised intervention in the Terri Schiavo life-support case?

A. The state legislature
B. The president of the United States
C. Congressional physicians
D. A and B
E. All of the above

Review this! ❏

22. Public opinion over right-to-die issues has been shaped by which of the following historical landmark cases?

A. Terri Schiavo
B. Karen Quinlan
C. Nancy Beth Cruzan
D. A and B
E. All of the above

Review this! ❏

23. On the basis of national consensus standards, which of the following statements is not true?

A. A patient has the right to refuse treatment, even if the physician disagrees.

B. Competent patients have the right to refuse hydration and nutritional needs.

C. Incompetent patients do not have the right to refuse life-saving medical treatment.

D. Surveys show that 70% to 80% of Americans would prefer not to be kept alive in a persistent vegetative state.

Review this! ❏

24. Which of the following is a result of the Patient Self-Determination Act?

A. All U.S. citizens are required to designate a durable power of attorney for health care.

B. State and federal legislatures have the power to intervene in end-of-life cases.

C. Hospice agencies have the power to make end-of-life decisions.

D. Medical clinics and hospitals are required to offer advance directives.

Review this! ❏

25. To avoid burnout, physicians must learn to distinguish between which of the following?

A. Competence and incompetence
B. Alcoholism and workaholism
C. Compassion and sentimentalism
D. None of the above

Review this! ❏

Part II

Family Medicine in the Community

10 Periodic Health Examination

Wanda Gonsalves

CHILDREN

1. True or false: There is strong evidence to support the use of annual complete physical examinations for asymptomatic patients over the age of 35 years.

   A. True
   B. False

   Review this! ❏

2. Which of the reason(s) for not performing a complete physical examination in asymptomatic patients is/are valid?

   A. Financial cost to the patient and use of the physician's time
   B. High false-positive rate, with potentially harmful follow-up evaluations
   C. False sense of security provided to patients with normal findings
   D. All of the above

   Review this! ❏

3. The Denver Developmental Screening Test is a tool used to assess a child's development. Which one of following is not evaluated using this screening test?

   A. Gross motor movement
   B. Fine motor movement
   C. Sensation to touch
   D. Social and language development

   Review this! ❏

4. True or false: The measurement of height, weight, and head circumference should be obtained for all infants until they are 2 to 3 years old.

   A. True
   B. False

   Review this! ❏

5. Blood pressure screening is recommended to begin at which of the following ages?

   A. 5 years
   B. 7 years
   C. 3 years
   D. 4 years

   Review this! ❏

6. True or false: The U.S. Preventive Services Task Force (USPSTF) finds sufficient evidence to recommend annual visual acuity testing in children who are more than 5 years old.

   A. True
   B. False

   Review this! ❏

7. True or false: Universal newborn hearing screening before hospital discharge is now required by law for all states.

   A. True
   B. False

   Review this! ❏

8. Newborn blood screening as recommended by the American Academy of Pediatrics (AAP) and the American Academy of Family Physicians (AAFP) include all of the following, except:

   A. Maple syrup urine disease.
   B. Phenylketonuria.
   C. Hemoglobinopathies.
   D. Hypothyroidism.

   Review this! ❏

9. At what age do the AAP, the Centers for Disease Control and Prevention (CDC), and the USPSTF recommend lead screening for certain high-risk children?

   A. 9 months
   B. 12 months
   C. 15 months
   D. 24 months

   Review this! ❏

10. At what age should screening for hyperlipidemia begin in children?

Things to remember for the test.

A. 3 years
B. 2 years
C. 5 years
D. 10 years

Review this! ❏

11. True or false: Although there has been a recent resurgence in the number of tuberculosis cases, screening is not recommended except for that of certain high-risk individuals, new immigrants from endemic areas, and individuals who are otherwise suspected of having active tuberculosis.

A. True
B. False

Review this! ❏

12. The following counseling recommendations have been shown to be effective for injury prevention, except:

A. Advising parents to "baby-proof" their homes to remove potential dangers.
B. Encouraging the use of bicycle helmets.
C. Advising the reduction of hot water heater temperatures to below 120°F.
D. Applying "Mr. Yuck" stickers to medications.

Review this! ❏

13. Secondhand smoke has been shown to increase the risk of all diseases below, except:

A. Preterm labor.
B. Sudden infant death syndrome.
C. Respiratory infections.
D. Otitis media.

Review this! ❏

14. Which one of the following is the leading cause of death of school-aged and adolescent children?

A. Cardiovascular disease
B. Accidental death
C. Lung disease
D. Malignant neoplasms

Review this! ❏

15. True or false: The USPSTF and the AAFP strongly recommend screening all sexually active females and males age 25 years old or younger for chlamydia.

A. True
B. False

Review this! ❏

16. A 16-year-old female has had two sexual partners within the last year. She has had no previous sexually transmitted disease, and her immunizations are up to date. All of the following screening tests are recommended, except:

A. Gonorrhea.
B. Chlamydia.
C. Human immunodeficiency virus serology.
D. Papanicolaou (Pap) smear.

Review this! ❏

17. True or false: *HEADS* is a mnemonic that is used to help identify topics of concern for adolescents.

A. True
B. False

Review this! ❏

18. A 16-year-old male is new to your practice. Which of the following would be the most appropriate?

A. Conducting the interview with a parent in the room
B. Performing a complete physical examination and checking laboratory results for anemia
C. Conducting a hearing and vision screening
D. Assessing the risk for accidental injury

Review this! ❏

19. You are seeing a 12-year-old girl for a sports physical. You learn that she had chicken pox at the age of 4 years. Which of the following immunizations are required for this patient?

A. Tetanus booster
B. Pneumonia vaccine
C. Varicella vaccine
D. IPV vaccine

Review this! ❏

ADULTS

20. True or false: The USPSTF strongly recommends screening all adults yearly for hypertension.

A. True
B. False

Review this! ❏

21. Your 55-year-old female patient plans to begin a vigorous exercise class. She has no cardiovascular risk factors. Which one of the following should you recommend to her before she starts her exercise program?

    A. An echocardiogram
    B. A resting echocardiogram
    C. A stress echocardiogram
    D. None of the above

    Review this! ❑

22. True or false: Mr. Jones, a 55-year-old diabetic patient, visits your office every 3 months for uncontrolled diabetes. He denies chest pain and numbness or tingling of the extremities. You should perform an ankle-brachial index during his next visit to screen for peripheral vascular disease (PVD).

    A. True
    B. False

    Review this! ❑

23. True or false: Ultrasound of the abdomen to screen for abdominal aortic aneurysm should be obtained at least once for male smokers or past smokers between the ages of 65 and 75 years.

    A. True
    B. False

    Review this! ❑

24. The USPSTF strongly recommends screening all adults for the following conditions, except:

    A. Cholesterol for males older than 35 years old and for females older than 45 years old
    B. Hypertension
    C. PVD
    D. Chlamydia

    Review this! ❑

25. True or false: Screening for diabetes is strongly recommended by the USPSTF and the American Diabetes Association for those asymptomatic adults with a family history of diabetes.

    A. True
    B. False

    Review this! ❑

26. The primary tool available for screening for osteoporosis is the dual-energy x-ray absorptiometry scan. Which of the following T-scores at the femoral neck correlates well with the risk of hip fracture?

    A. −3.0
    B. −2.75
    C. −2.5
    D. −3.5

    Review this! ❑

27. The USPSTF recommends against screening for all of the following, except:

    A. Cholesterol.
    B. Thyroid function.
    C. Asymptomatic PVD.
    D. Coronary artery disease.

    Review this! ❑

28. True or false: The *CAGE* mnemonic is a diagnostic tool used for the detection of alcohol abuse.

    A. True
    B. False

    Review this! ❑

29. True or false: As many as one third of adults are overweight. The USPSTF and the AAFP recommend screening for obesity by observing the change in weight over a period of time.

    A. True
    B. False

    Review this! ❑

30. Which one of the following is an actual USPSTF recommendation for breast cancer screening?

    A. Mammography should be performed on all women beginning at the age of 50 years.
    B. Mammography should be discontinued at the age of 70 years.
    C. Performing clinical breast examination and teaching self breast examination are highly recommended.
    D. Women with a family history that is suggestive of BRCA1 or BRCA2 mutations should be offered genetic testing and counseling.

    Review this! ❑

31. True or false: Women who have had a hysterectomy for uterine fibroids do not need Pap screening.

    A. True
    B. False

    Review this! ❑

32. Which of the following statements about the sensitivity of screening studies for colon cancer is true?

    A. A single fecal occult blood test has a sensitivity as high as 80%.
    B. Sigmoidoscopy has a sensitivity of 60%.
    C. Virtual colonoscopy has a sensitivity of approximately 70%.
    D. Colonoscopy has a sensitivity of almost 100%.

    Review this! ❑

33. True or false: The USPSTF strongly recommends that patients be screened for colorectal cancer beginning at the age of 50 years. However, no recommendation is made for the use of any particular screening strategy.

    A. True
    B. False

    Review this! ❑

34. True or false: The mortality rate of patients with prostate cancer depends on the grade of differentiation of the cancer rather than the stage of the cancer at diagnosis.

    A. True
    B. False

    Review this! ❑

35. Which of the following statements about prostate screening is false?

    A. It is likely that some percentage of patients would benefit from the early detection of prostate cancer screening.

    B. Sufficient evidence does not exist to determine whether screening for prostate cancer is more likely to harm or help patients who are offered screening.
    C. Prostate cancer screening reduces mortality caused by prostate cancer.
    D. Methods used for prostate cancer screening include the digital rectal examination and the serum prostate-specific antigen test.

    Review this! ❑

36. True or false: Although specific screening tests exist for lung and ovarian cancers, they are not recommended by the USPSTF.

    A. True
    B. False

    Review this! ❑

37. For which of the following behaviors has counseling caused a decrease in the associated mortality rate?

    A. Smoking
    B. Alcohol use
    C. Exercise
    D. Dietary practices

    Review this! ❑

38. Immunizations recommended for adults include all but which one of the following?

    A. Annual influenza vaccination for those more than 50 years old
    B. One-time pneumonia vaccine for those more than 65 years old
    C. Tetanus-diphtheria booster every 10 years
    D. Measles-mumps-rubella vaccine for those born after 1960

    Review this! ❑

11 Preventive Health Care

Brian L. Elkins

Things to remember for the test.

1. Screening for the early detection of a disease among individuals who are asymptomatic but who are at risk for the disease is considered which of the following?

   A. Primary prevention
   B. Secondary prevention
   C. Tertiary prevention

   Review this! ❑

2. Characteristics of a good screening test include all of the following, except:

   A. The condition being screened for should be an uncommon health problem.
   B. There should be a detectable early stage of the disease.
   C. Treatment at an early stage should be of more benefit than treatment at a later stage.
   D. The risks—both physical and psychological—should be fewer than the benefits.
   E. The costs should be balanced with the benefits.

   Review this! ❑

3. Screening for which of the following diseases has not been shown to result in reduced morbidity and/or mortality?

   A. Breast cancer
   B. Prostate cancer
   C. Cervical cancer
   D. Colorectal cancer

   Review this! ❑

4. Which of the following is the intervention with the greatest potential impact for decreasing morbidity and mortality and improving the quality of life across diverse populations?

   A. Changing the health behaviors of the population
   B. Achieving 100% screening of all individuals for diseases for which they are at risk

   C. Immunizing all eligible children and adults with appropriate vaccinations
   D. Increasing aspirin use among patients with cardiovascular diseases

   Review this! ❑

5. The proportion of the tested population without the disorder who have a negative test refers to which of the following of the test's characteristics?

   A. Its sensitivity
   B. Its specificity
   C. Its positive predictive value
   D. Its negative predictive value

   Review this! ❑

6. Improving the quality, delivery, and effectiveness of prevention in the family physician's office is best achieved by which of the following?

   A. Continuing medical education in the area of prevention
   B. Changes in the office system
   C. Better prevention-oriented patient education

   Review this! ❑

7. Which of the following is a true statement about clinical preventive services?

   A. Because screening occurs in healthy, asymptomatic patients, the standard of evidence for proposed prevention strategies is low.
   B. All interventions, including preventive services, have harms.
   C. Intermediate outcomes, such as improvements in laboratory test results, are reasonably good measures of the effectiveness of preventive services.

   Review this! ❑

8. "The proportion of a defined group of people who have a condition or disease at

any given point in time" best defines which of the following terms?

A. Prevalence
B. Incidence
C. Morbidity
D. Mortality

Review this! ❏

9. True or false: In a population with a low prevalence of a specific disease, a positive test result is likely to represent a false positive, even for a test with high specificity.

A. True
B. False

Review this! ❏

10. True or false: The sensitivity of colonoscopy for large polyps is 100%.

A. True
B. False

Review this! ❏

11. According to the U.S. Preventive Services Task Force (USPSTF), acceptable screening strategies for colorectal cancer include all of the following, except:

A. Fecal occult blood testing.
B. Flexible sigmoidoscopy.
C. Colonoscopy.
D. Double-contrast barium enema.
E. Digital rectal examination.

Review this! ❏

12. Which group describes the population for which the USPSTF recommends colorectal cancer screening?

A. Men more than 50 years old and women more than 60 years old
B. Men more than 40 years old
C. Men more than 50 years old
D. Men and women more than 50 years old

Review this! ❏

13. Which of the following is the most important risk factor for cervical cancer?

A. Cigarette smoking
B. Human papillomavirus
C. Early onset of sexual intercourse
D. Greater number of sexual partners

Review this! ❏

14. According to the USPSTF recommendation, all of the following women should have cervical cancer screening, except:

A. An 18-year-old female who became sexually active at the age of 15 years.
B. A 23-year-old sexually active woman with a cervix.
C. A 30-year-old woman who had a hysterectomy last year as a result of bleeding uterine fibroids.
D. A 60-year-old woman who had a hysterectomy at the age of 40 years as a result of cervical cancer.

Review this! ❏

15. Which of the following screening measures has been shown to reduce mortality as a result of breast cancer?

A. Self breast examination
B. Clinical breast examination
C. Mammography
D. Breast ultrasound

Review this! ❏

16. True or false: The USPSTF recommends lung cancer screening for individuals who have smoked for more than 10 years.

A. True
B. False

Review this! ❏

17. The USPSTF recommends screening for which of the following cancers?

A. Lung cancer
B. Ovarian cancer
C. Prostate cancer
D. Cervical cancer

Review this! ❏

18. True or false: The USPSTF recommends combined screening for prostate cancer with both prostate-specific antigen testing and digital rectal examination.

A. True
B. False

Review this! ❏

19. True or false: The USPSTF recommends screening all adults for high blood pressure.

A. True
B. False

Review this! ❏

20. The USPSTF recommends screening adults for all of the following risk factors for cardiovascular disease, except:

    A. Hypertension.
    B. Hyperlipidemia.
    C. Tobacco use.
    D. Elevated C-reactive protein.

    Review this! ❏

21. True or false: There is no evidence that counseling is an effective intervention for the promotion of smoking cessation.

    A. True
    B. False

    Review this! ❏

22. True or false: The USPSTF recommends against using electrocardiography, exercise testing, or computed tomography scanning to screen low-risk adults for coronary heart disease.

    A. True
    B. False

    Review this! ❏

23. According to the USPSTF recommendation, which of the following individuals should receive screening for abdominal aortic aneurysm?

    A. A 70-year-old female who is a current smoker
    B. A 65-year-old male who is a former smoker
    C. A 60-year-old male who is a current smoker
    D. None of the above

    Review this! ❏

24. The USPSTF recommends against routine screening for which of the following problems?

    A. Tobacco use
    B. Alcoholism
    C. Depression
    D. None of the above

    Review this! ❏

25. According to the USPSTF recommendation, which of the following asymptomatic individuals should be screened for chlamydia?

    A. A 25-year-old sexually active male with multiple sexual partners
    B. A 23-year-old sexually active female in a monogamous relationship
    C. A 35-year-old sexually active female in a monogamous relationship
    D. A 20-year-old female who has never been sexually active
    E. None of the above

    Review this! ❏

26. The USPSTF recommends against any screening for which of the following infectious diseases?

    A. Chlamydia
    B. Gonorrhea
    C. Syphilis
    D. Human immunodeficiency virus
    E. Hepatitis B and C

    Review this! ❏

27. According to the USPSTF recommendation, all of the following individuals should be offered screening for type 2 diabetes, except:

    A. A 60-year-old healthy male
    B. A 30-year-old obese female with medication-controlled hypertension
    C. A 50-year-old female with medication-controlled hyperlipidemia
    D. A 40-year-old male smoker with uncontrolled hypertension

    Review this! ❏

28. According to the USPSTF recommendation, all of the following patients should be screened for osteoporosis, except:

    A. A 63-year-old female smoker
    B. A 60-year-old female whose mother suffered an osteoporotic hip fracture
    C. A 50-year-old female who had a hysterectomy last year
    D. A 65-year-old healthy female

    Review this! ❏

29. The USPSTF recommends postmenopausal hormone replacement therapy for the prevention of which of the following conditions?

    A. Osteoporosis
    B. Coronary heart disease
    C. Dementia
    D. None of the above

    Review this! ❏

Things to remember for the test.

30. Which of the following is the area of preventive services for children with the largest evidence base?

    A. Immunizations
    B. Screening for genetic disorders such as phenylketonuria and cystic fibrosis
    C. Counseling to prevent injuries
    D. Counseling to prevent alcohol, tobacco, and drug use

    Review this! ❏

31. Important topics for anticipatory guidance and screening in adolescents include which of the following?

    A. Sexual activity
    B. Alcohol, tobacco, and drug use
    C. Healthy eating and physical activity
    D. Injury prevention
    E. All of the above

    Review this! ❏

12 Evidence-Based Medicine

Curtis Gingrich

1. What is the ultimate goal of evidence-based medicine (EBM)?

   A. To improve patient outcomes by considering the most current and valid clinical research evidence when making patient care decisions
   B. To only make clinical decisions that are based on hard evidence as described in the scientific literature
   C. To provide a medicolegal basis for patient care decisions that will prevent lawsuits
   D. To do away with individual physician experience or logic and thus allow any individual to make medical decisions

   Review this! ❏

2. Which of the following is not a hallmark of a well-done, randomized, controlled trial (RCT)?

   A. Double-blinded
   B. Concealed allocation assignment
   C. Intention-to-treat analysis
   D. Not including patients lost to follow-up in the final study outcome measures

   Review this! ❏

3. Which of the following properly represents the correct ascending hierarchy of EBM?

   A. Expert opinion, cohort studies, meta-analysis, RCTs
   B. Meta-analysis, expert opinion, RCTs, cohort studies
   C. Expert opinion, cohort studies, RCTs, meta-analysis
   D. RCTs, meta-analysis, cohort studies, expert opinion

   Review this! ❏

4. Identify the correct order of the classic steps of EBM.

   A. Conduct a systematic search of the medical literature; formulate a clear, answerable, clinical question; critically appraise the article; integrate the findings into the clinical decision-making involving the patient
   B. Formulate a clear, answerable, clinical question; conduct a systematic search of the medical literature; critically appraise the article; integrate the findings into the clinical decision-making involving the patient
   C. Formulate a clear, answerable, clinical question; critically appraise the article; integrate the findings into the clinical decision-making involving the patient; conduct a systematic search of the medical literature
   D. Integrate the findings into the clinical decision-making involving the patient; conduct a systematic review of the medical literature; form a clear, answerable, clinical question; critically appraise the article

   Review this! ❏

5. Which of the following statements regarding the non–evidence-based approaches to clinical decision-making is true?

   A. The apprentice model is demonstrated when an experienced physician shows or tells a less-experienced physician how he or she practices and the less-experienced physician learns to emulate the teacher.
   B. In the apprentice model, it is easy for the apprentice to distinguish between helpful and harmful practices and to only incorporate the helpful practices into his or her own patterns.
   C. Deferral to authority implies a physician who changes his or her practice patterns when an evidenced-based piece of information is brought to light.
   D. Clinical experience is clearly superior to EBM when it comes to making informed decisions.

   Review this! ❏

Things to remember for the test.

6. Which of the following statements regarding empiricism is true?

   A. Empiricism in medicine has its roots in the early nineteenth century.
   B. EBM is one of the many expressions of empiricism in medicine in that it uses actual observations in real patient populations using careful and replicable methods.
   C. When solid empirical evidence is in conflict with prevailing pathophysiological theory, the empirical evidence should be discarded.
   D. The experiment conducted among 10 British sailors in 1747 demonstrating that eating limes prevented scurvy is an example of anti-empiricism.

   Review this! ❏

7. When considering RCTs, which of the following statements is false?

   A. The first RCTs were conducted in grain fields in the 1920s.
   B. The first medical RCT proved that streptomycin was superior to standard therapy for the treatment of pulmonary tuberculosis.
   C. RCTs are considered the gold standard for the evaluation of preventive and treatment interventions.
   D. RCTs are the strongest form of EBM available.

   Review this! ❏

8. Which of the following is not a commonly used EBM resource?

   A. InfoRetriever
   B. DynaMed
   C. Cochrane Review
   D. DynaMap

   Review this! ❏

9. Which of the following statements about patient-oriented evidence that matters (POEM) is true?

   A. POEM is usually less relevant than disease-oriented evidence (DOE).
   B. The fact that a medicine has been shown to decrease a person's low-density lipoprotein level by 30% is an example of a POEM.
   C. A decrease in mortality is an example of a POEM.
   D. InfoRetriever is a resource that concentrates on analyzing and publicizing DOE.

   Review this! ❏

10. Which of the following statements about Clinical Inquiries is false?

    A. Clinical Inquiries is a part of the Family Physicians Inquiries Network developed by family physicians to answer 80% of the practicing family physicians' questions at the point of care.
    B. Questions discussed in this format are actual questions developed through web-based voting by groups of family physicians.
    C. Each clinical inquiry is reviewed by at least four peer reviewers.
    D. Clinical Inquiries has an exhaustive list of questions in its database for review.

    Review this! ❏

11. What type of study involves identifying patients who have the outcome of interest (cases) and patients without the same outcome (controls) and looking back to see if they had the exposure of interest?

    A. Cohort study
    B. RCT
    C. Case-control study
    D. Retrospective case series

    Review this! ❏

12. Define allocation concealment.

    A. The study participant does not know to which group he or she has been assigned.
    B. The person enrolling a participant into a clinical trial is unaware whether the next participant to be enrolled will be allocated to the intervention group or the control group.
    C. The people evaluating the effect of the intervention do not know if the participant is in the control group or the intervention group.
    D. Participants are assigned to either the treatment group or the control group through a random process.

    Review this! ❏

13. Which of the following is not an example of a systematic review?

    A. A summary of the medical literature that uses explicit methods to perform a comprehensive literature search and the critical appraisal of individual studies and that uses appropriate statistical techniques to combine these valid studies

    B. A meta-analysis of the effects of vitamin E on mortality

    C. A textbook chapter reviewing the diagnosis and treatment of atrial fibrillation

    D. A Cochrane review of treatment for dementia of Alzheimer's type

    Review this! ❑

14. Which of the following is defined as "a method of analysis in which all patients randomly assigned to one of the treatment groups are analyzed together, regardless of whether or not they completed or received that treatment, to preserve randomization"?

    A. Incidence
    B. Summary statistic
    C. Meta-analysis
    D. Intention-to-treat analysis

    Review this! ❑

15. Which answer is the best definition of *confidence interval*?

    A. The percentage of accuracy as a result of the study design

    B. The range of values within which one can expect the true value for the whole population to reside

    C. The range of values in which the result is not related to the treatment being studied

    D. The proportion of patients in the experimental treatment group who are observed to experience the outcome of interest

    Review this! ❑

16. Which of the following is defined as "the number of patients who need to be treated to prevent one bad outcome"?

    A. Number needed to treat
    B. Number needed to harm
    C. Negative predictive value
    D. Odds ratio

    Review this! ❑

17. Original research by family physicians has shown repeatedly that the findings conducted on populations of patients referred to other specialists often do not apply to the patient population seen by family physicians. What type of bias is this?

    A. Treatment bias
    B. Selection bias
    C. Allocation bias
    D. Publication bias

    Review this! ❑

18. When researching a clinical question about treatment, which of the following would be the best type of article to look for?

    A. An RCT
    B. A cohort study
    C. A case-control trial

    Review this! ❑

19. When researching a clinical question about diagnosis, what type of study will provide the best information?

    A. An RCT
    B. A cohort study
    C. A case-control trial

    Review this! ❑

20. Which of the following is not a distinguishing characteristic of EBM?

    A. Standardized critical appraisal
    B. Designation of levels of evidence
    C. Verifiable findings
    D. Treating all studies as equal, regardless of design or type

    Review this! ❑

Things to remember for the test.

13 Interpreting the Literature

Ronald H. Labuguen

1. Which of the following can prevent family physicians in practice from applying evidence-based medicine (EBM)?

   A. Lack of time or expertise to answer critically the questions that arise in practice
   B. Lack of evidence that is pertinent to an individual patient
   C. Lack of quick access to information at the point of care
   D. All of the above

   Review this! ❏

2. Which of the following can prevent the use of EBM in practice?

   A. The difficulty for family physicians to keep up with the growing body of evidence surrounding common primary care problems
   B. The broad scope of family medicine
   C. Potential negative impact on the art of medicine
   D. All of the above

   Review this! ❏

3. Which of the following is not an example of an observational study?

   A. Unblinded case series
   B. Case-control study
   C. Cohort study
   D. Randomized, controlled trial (RCT)

   Review this! ❏

4. On the basis of several cases that have been reported in the post-marketing surveillance of an antibiotic, drug A, investigators wish to determine whether female patients of childbearing age who have taken drug A are at increased risk of bearing children with congenital heart defects. Which of the following is the best type of study to use to answer this question?

   A. Case series
   B. Case-control study
   C. Cohort study
   D. RCT
   E. Meta-analysis

   Review this! ❏

5. Suppose that investigators wish to determine whether the use of a new drug-eluting coronary artery stent results in fewer cases of coronary artery restenoses than the currently used non–drug-eluting stents. Which type of study would provide the most valid evidence to answer this question?

   A. Case-control study
   B. Cohort study
   C. RCT
   D. Meta-analysis
   E. Systematic review

   Review this! ❏

6. A group of investigators wishes to determine whether treatment X decreases the intensity of musculoskeletal low back pain. Several studies have been performed to address this question. The most valid approach for the investigators to take to determine what is currently known about this topic is to conduct which of the following types of studies?

   A. Case series
   B. Case-control study
   C. Cohort study
   D. RCT
   E. Systematic review

   Review this! ❏

7. Which of the following is not a characteristic of case-control studies?

   A. They are relatively inexpensive and rapidly completed.
   B. They are always looking forward in time (prospective).

C. Their results are commonly affected by recall bias.

D. Recall bias results from errors involving accurately determining whether both cases and controls were exposed to the factor being studied.

Review this! ❏

8. Which of the following is not a characteristic of cohort studies?

A. They are generally more expensive and take longer to complete than case-control studies.

B. They observe outcomes in groups, but they do not assign participants to a particular exposure or treatment.

C. Small numbers of participants are usually sufficient to show significant differences among groups.

D. The primary statistical measure is relative risk.

Review this! ❏

9. Which of the following is true about statements #1 and #2 below?

Statement #1: The results of cohort studies are commonly affected by "healthy-user bias."

Statement #2: "Healthy-user bias" occurs when participants who choose an exposure or treatment also tend to make healthier lifestyle decisions that may also prevent the measured outcome.

A. Only statement A is true.

B. Only statement B is true.

C. Both statements are true.

D. Neither statement is true.

Review this! ❏

10. Which of the following statements is true about reviews and meta-analyses?

A. Structured reviews often summarize the results of a number of studies.

B. Meta-analysis combines data from a series of studies using statistical techniques.

C. An advantage of meta-analysis is that it allows increased statistical power to determine the weight of evidence from a series of studies.

D. All of the above

Review this! ❏

11. Which of the following is not a characteristic of RCTs?

A. Randomization maximizes differences between treatment and control groups to make it more likely for study results to achieve statistical significance.

B. Study participants are randomly allocated to two or more groups.

C. Groups of study participants are assigned to receive either an intervention or no active treatment (placebo or usual care).

D. Study design helps eliminate many biases that affect observational studies.

Review this! ❏

12. Which of the following statements is true about the statistical significance of study results?

A. Relative risk is a summary measure of differences between the treatment and placebo groups.

B. Relative risk is calculated as the ratio of the incidence rate for the placebo group divided by the incidence rate for the treatment group.

C. The incidence rate for each group of study participants (treatment vs. placebo) is the ratio of the number of patients in the group divided by the number of outcomes in the group over a specific period of time.

D. When relative risk is reported as the summary result of a study, the 95% confidence interval cannot be used instead of the P value to describe the level of statistical significance of the result.

Review this! ❏

13. Which of the following represent a statistically significant difference between the treatment and control groups?

A. A P value greater than .05

B. A 95% confidence interval for relative risk that includes 1

C. A number needed to treat (NNT) of 2

D. A number needed to harm (NNH) of 500

E. None of the above

Review this! ❏

14. All of the following statements are true about statistical significance, except:

Things to remember for the test.

A. Statistical significance is not always associated with clinical significance.

B. The *P* value describes the statistical probability that the observed difference between the study groups was a result of chance alone.

C. A relative risk reported as 1.9 with a 95% confidence interval of 0.96 to 3.4 is considered to be statistically significant.

D. Just because a study shows statistical significance in a single measure does not mean that appropriate patient-oriented outcomes were considered.

Review this! ❏

15. Which of the following best measures the clinical significance of a statistically significant difference in observed outcomes between a treatment (intervention) group and a control (placebo or usual care) group in an RCT?

A. Relative risk
B. Absolute risk difference
C. NNT
D. *P* value
E. 95% confidence interval

Review this! ❏

16. What factors help determine whether the results of a study should lead to a change in clinical practice?

A. Whether all relevant patient-oriented outcomes were considered
B. Whether important harms (risks) were measured
C. The acceptability of the intervention to patients
D. Whether appropriate competing alternatives for treatment were assessed
E. All of the above

Review this! ❏

17. Which of the following is an example of clinically significant outcomes?

A. Physiologic outcomes
B. Intermediate outcomes
C. Patient-oriented outcomes
D. All of the above

Review this! ❏

18. Examples of patient-oriented outcomes include which of the following?

A. Follicle-stimulating hormone level
B. Mortality rate

C. Both A and B
D. Neither A nor B

Review this! ❏

19. Which of the following does not affect the power of a study?

A. The number of patients in the study
B. The number of patients excluded from the study
C. The magnitude of the effect of the intervention
D. The variability of the effect of the intervention from one subject to another

Review this! ❏

20. Which of the following is true about reviews?

A. Systematic reviews use rigorous attempts to uncover all studies, published and unpublished, in English and other languages.
B. Meta-analyses use formal mathematical methods to combine the results of studies.
C. Qualitative reviews synthesize data according to an author's overall judgment.
D. All of the above

Review this! ❏

21. How can clinicians hone critical appraisal skills and solidify their grasp of basic EBM concepts?

A. Through involvement with local journal clubs
B. By working with the Family Practice Inquiries Network
C. By assisting with the development of Clinical Inquiries or patient-oriented evidence that matters (POEMs)
D. By attending an information mastery or EBM workshop
E. All of the above

Review this! ❏

22. Which of the following is not an example of secondary sources of clinical information?

A. Evidence-based summaries
B. Systematic reviews
C. Clinical guidelines
D. Evidence-based databases
E. RCT

Questions 23 through 32 refer to the following study:

In an RCT, drug X, an agent that reduces blood cholesterol levels, is studied to determine whether patients taking drug X experience fewer heart attacks. A total of 4400 patients are randomized to the treatment group, whereas 4200 are randomized to the placebo group. At the end of the 2-year study, 22 patients in the treatment group and 42 patients in the placebo group suffered heart attacks. A total of 110 patients in the treatment group and 30 patients in the placebo group experienced clinically significant abdominal pain (i.e., pain significant enough for them to stop taking the medication).

23. What is the incidence rate of heart attacks in the treatment group?

    A. 0.50%
    B. 1.0%
    C. 2.5%
    D. 5.2%
    E. 0.25%

    Review this! ❑

24. What is the incidence rate of heart attacks in the placebo group?

    A. 0.25%
    B. 0.50%
    C. 1.0%
    D. 2.5%
    E. 5.2%

    Review this! ❑

25. What is the incidence rate of clinically significant abdominal pain in the treatment group?

    A. 0.71%
    B. 2.5%
    C. 5.0%
    D. 10%
    E. 52%

    Review this! ❑

26. What is the incidence rate of clinically significant abdominal pain in the placebo group?

    A. 0.35%
    B. 0.68%
    C. 0.71%
    D. 5.0%
    E. 10%

    Review this! ❑

27. What is the relative risk of heart attacks in the treatment group?

    A. 0.068
    B. 0.13

C. 0.25
D. 0.26
E. 0.50

Review this! ❑

28. What is the relative risk of clinically significant abdominal pain in the treatment group?

    A. 0.68
    B. 1.3
    C. 2.6
    D. 3.5
    E. 5.0

    Review this! ❑

29. True or false: Assuming that the 95% confidence interval for the relative risk of heart attacks in the treatment group is 0.16 to 0.70, the study finds a statistically significant difference.

    A. True
    B. False

    Review this! ❑

30. What is the absolute risk difference (or attributable risk) of heart attacks between the treatment and placebo groups for this 2-year study?

    A. 0.0008
    B. 0.005
    C. 0.25
    D. 0.50
    E. 7.0

    Review this! ❑

31. What is the NNT for 1 year to prevent one heart attack?

    A. 200
    B. 300
    C. 400
    D. 700
    E. 1229

    Review this! ❑

32. What is the NNH for 1 year to cause one patient to have clinically significant abdominal pain?

    A. 20
    B. 56
    C. 112
    D. 123
    E. 140

    Review this! ❑

14 Electronic Medical Record

William Verhoff

1. Computer use in the family medicine office can be helpful in which of the following three general areas?

   A. Internet access, performance reviews, and schedule management
   B. Communications, clinical/business information management, and knowledge management
   C. Evidence-based medicine, word processing, and calendar maintenance

   Review this! ❏

2. Which of the following is probably the most powerful tool invented by humankind?

   A. Magnetic resonance imaging
   B. The automobile
   C. The spaceship
   D. The Internet

   Review this! ❏

3. Which of the following is a benefit of a fully implemented electronic health record (EHR)?

   A. Information is automatically updated during the patient's care process.
   B. Information is organized in a way that is easy to access.
   C. Entering the information one time makes it available in many parts of the EHR.
   D. All of the above

   Review this! ❏

4. True or false: An office note can be embedded into the EHR by dictation/transcription, voice recognition, keyboard entry, data point selector, or a combination of all of these methods.

   A. True
   B. False

   Review this! ❏

5. Which of the following is the technology item that has revolutionized instant access to medical information?

   A. The telephone
   B. The desktop personal computer
   C. The personal digital assistant
   D. The digital camera

   Review this! ❏

6. True or false: The EHR and the computerized practice management systems have not shown any improvements with regard to accuracy, efficiency, or the timely submission of bills to the appropriate payer.

   A. True
   B. False

   Review this! ❏

7. Which of the following statements is true about the impact of the EHR on office workflow?

   A. The EHR has increased the time it takes for messages to get routed to the appropriate caregiver.
   B. The EHR can only be accessed by one person at a time.
   C. The EHR can be accessed remotely.
   D. The overall time saved over the use of the paper chart as compared with the EHR is minimal.

   Review this! ❏

8. True or false: The continuity of care record is a document standard for basic health information using XML (extensible markup language)?

   A. True
   B. False

   Review this! ❏

9. The EHR will improve the quality and safety of patient care by doing which of the following?

A. It will provide an office system that delivers reliable health care outcomes and that supports excellent customer service.
B. It will include functionality that helps physicians manage both health maintenance and chronic illness.
C. It will track and report laboratory results, which are then seamlessly integrated into the flow of patient care.
D. All of the above

Review this! ❏

10. The complex process of transforming to a paperless office can be made easier by all the following, except:

A. A lack of leadership and change management.
B. A project team with a positive attitude toward change.
C. Good individualized training and implementation strategies.
D. The use of available resources to provide guidance.

Review this! ❏

Things to remember for the test.

15 Clinical Problem Solving

Mrunal Shah

1. During the course of a busy practice day, a physician who uses mindlines to make a decision is using which of the following?

   A. Peer-reviewed, original-research–based recommendations
   B. A preconceived, conceptualized, and standardized approach to a clinical scenario based on early training
   C. Patient-oriented evidence
   D. Disease-oriented evidence

   Review this! ❑

2. True or false: The best way to practice medicine is to develop as many mindlines as one can early on during the process of training and to maintain that knowledge throughout one's practice.

   A. True
   B. False

   Review this! ❑

3. A shared clinical decision can be reached by which of the following?

   A. Telling the patient what the clinician is going to do
   B. Telling the patient what the clinician is going to do and obtaining consent
   C. Asking the patient what he or she wants to do and proceeding in order to avoid litigation
   D. Integrating medical evidence with the patient's preferences

   Review this! ❑

4. True or false: Retrospective studies have confirmed that clinicians seek answers to most questions that arise in clinical practice.

   A. True
   B. False

   Review this! ❑

5. After a knowledge gap is identified, it is important to ask an answerable clinical question to close that gap. Which of the following are two types of clinical questions?

   A. True and false
   B. Background and foreground
   C. Evidence-based and expert opinion
   D. Disease-oriented evidence and patient-oriented evidence

   Review this! ❑

6. All of the following are components of a focused clinical question, except:

   A. The patient's specific problem.
   B. The intervention.
   C. The reference impact factor.
   D. The comparison or control.
   E. The outcome of interest.

   Review this! ❑

7. All of the following statements are examples of patient-oriented outcomes, except:

   A. Sulfonylureas reduce diabetic nephropathy.
   B. Sulfonylureas reduce fasting plasma glucose.
   C. ACE inhibitors reduce diabetic nephropathy.
   D. ACE inhibitors reduce exacerbations of congestive heart failure.

   Review this! ❑

8. True or false: Original research is the least available form of evidence.

   A. True
   B. False

   Review this! ❑

9. True or false: Original research requires the clinician to have significant knowledge of statistical methods and study design.

   A. True
   B. False

   Review this! ❑

10. Systematic reviews and meta-analyses are which of the following?

    A. Clinicians reading many original research articles and forming conclusions
    B. Studies that take a single topic and attempt to draw conclusions from the volume of previously reported data
    C. Studies that take multiple topics and draw comparisons among them
    D. Statistical methods

    Review this! ❏

11. The acronym *POEMs* describes which of the following?

    A. Four or five lines of text that rhyme
    B. Practice outcome evidence measures
    C. Patient-oriented evidence that matters
    D. The least useful form of evidence in the literature

    Review this! ❏

12. True or false: POEMs are available for any clinical question.

    A. True
    B. False

    Review this! ❏

13. Which statement below is the most accurate?

    A. MEDLINE uses POEMs exclusively.
    B. The National Library of Medicine only keeps review articles on file.
    C. PubMed searches MEDLINE, which is a database of 15 million articles, through the National Library of Medicine.
    D. PubMed is the National Library of Medicine.

    Review this! ❏

14. Which one of the following types of evidence would be most useful for answering a typical clinical question about a therapeutic intervention?

    A. Original research article from MEDLINE
    B. Meta-analysis from PubMed

    C. POEM from InfoRetriever
    D. Clinical guidelines from the Agency for Healthcare Research and Quality

    Review this! ❏

15. In today's society, patients prefer to do which of the following?

    A. Make their own decisions and avoid their physicians' advice
    B. Share decision-making with their physicians
    C. Hear the options but ask their physicians to make the decision
    D. Blindly trust the decisions of their physicians, without knowledge about options

    Review this! ❏

16. True or false: There is no evidence to suggest that increased patient involvement increases trust, satisfaction, or compliance.

    A. True
    B. False

    Review this! ❏

17. Which of the following determines the usefulness of shared decision-making?

    A. Risk
    B. Number of alternatives
    C. Involvement of moral beliefs
    D. Patient preferences
    E. All of the above

    Review this! ❏

18. True or false: Clinical decision-making is the intersection of the science of evidence-based medicine and the art of shared decision-making occurring within the bounds of the health care system.

    A. True
    B. False

    Review this! ❏

Things to remember for the test.

55

16 Complementary and Alternative Medicine Techniques

Diane K. Beebe

1. Which of the following statements is the most accurate?

   A. The terms *integrative, holistic, complementary,* and *alternative medicine* can be used interchangeably to refer to the same nonconventional medical practices.
   B. Integrative medicine combines mainstream medical therapies and complementary and alternative medicine (CAM) therapies for which there is some high-quality scientific evidence of safety and effectiveness.
   C. Alternative and complementary medicine are both practiced in place of conventional medicine.
   D. Holistic medicine and homeopathy are not included among CAM therapies.
   Review this! ❑

2. Which of the following persons are most likely to use CAM therapies?

   A. Men more than women
   B. Persons with lower educational and socioeconomic levels
   C. Persons hospitalized during the past year
   D. Persons dissatisfied with conventional medicine
   Review this! ❑

3. Regarding the use of CAM therapy, which of the following statements is true?

   A. In a 2004 published study, approximately 20% of U.S. adults were using at least one CAM therapy during the preceding 12 months.
   B. Most CAM users discuss their use of alternative medicine with their primary physicians.
   C. There are no reliable published studies regarding CAM use in the United States.
   D. Visits to CAM practitioners by English-speaking adults in the United States rose to 629 million in 1997.
   Review this! ❑

4. The White House Commission on CAM Policy was formed to address which of the following?

   A. The regulation of insurance payments to cover CAM therapy
   B. The expansion of CAM practice into other countries
   C. The education and training of health care practitioners in CAM
   D. The introduction of new CAM therapies that are in practice around the world
   Review this! ❑

5. True statements about acupuncture include all of the following, except:

   A. Health is determined by a balanced flow of energy.
   B. There are approximately 100 acupoints that can be stimulated along the qi meridians.
   C. Studies show efficacy of this therapy for treating adult postoperative and chemotherapy nausea and vomiting.
   D. Acupuncture is one modality that is included in the practice of traditional Chinese medicine.
   Review this! ❑

6. Which of the following statements is true about yoga?

   A. It was first practiced by the ancient Chinese monarchs.
   B. It is a risky practice during pregnancy, and it has led to increased preterm labor and stillbirths.
   C. It has been shown to decrease preterm labor when practiced during pregnancy.
   D. It must be taught only by medical professionals certified through the Yoga Alliance.
   Review this! ❑

7. Which of the following statements is true about Ayurveda?

A. It involves the use of laxatives and enemas to cleanse the system.

B. It is based on the law of similars, and it makes use of small mixtures of herbal remedies.

C. It involves hydrotherapy to calm the body systems and to stimulate the circulation.

D. It involves the doshas of alpha, omega, and aqua.

Review this! ❏

8. Which of the following statements is true about homeopathy?

A. It is based on the theory that the more dilute the remedy, the more potent its effect.

B. It is based on the theory that megadoses of vitamins will cure disease.

C. It has a large base of evidence suggesting its initial use for numerous medical conditions.

D. It makes use of bioengineered chemicals similar to those found in nature but at smaller doses.

Review this! ❏

9. Which of the following statements about chelation is false?

A. Chelation removes toxic metals from the bloodstream through urinary filtration.

B. Chelation removes wastes from the body through the P450 system of the liver.

C. Chelation can be used to treat lead poisoning.

D. Chelation is being used to treat arteriosclerosis.

Review this! ❏

10. When patients seek information about CAM therapies, physicians should do which of the following?

A. Discourage their use; they are unproven and dangerous.

B. Refer the patient to another practitioner whose malpractice covers such therapies.

C. Tell the patient that all practice of these therapies is illegal in the United States.

D. Be willing to listen, learn, and explore options.

Review this! ❏

11. Which of the following is considered a form of energy therapy?

A. Reiki
B. Yoga
C. Ayurveda
D. Massage

Review this! ❏

12. Which of the following statements is true about Reiki?

A. Therapeutic ultrasound is used to stimulate muscle fibers to promote healing.

B. The process involves rhythmic deep breathing in cycles of 10 to quiet the mind.

C. The practice is often used in conjunction with conventional medical treatments.

D. The practice involves a series of relaxation techniques followed by the visualization of peaceful images.

Review this! ❏

13. Which of the following statements is true about tai chi?

A. It is a form of exercise.
B. It is a form of self-defense.
C. It is a CAM therapy.
D. All of the above

Review this! ❏

14. Which of the following best describes the body scan?

A. It is computerized tomography scanning of the brain to map out stress excitation areas.

B. It is a breathing technique used to achieve a relaxed state by focusing on different body parts.

C. It is a full body massage to loosen muscles and create relaxation.

D. It is self-hypnosis using images of relaxed muscles throughout the body.

Review this! ❏

15. Which of the following statements about biofeedback is true?

A. It originated in ancient times.

B. It requires that the patient control his or her breathing in response to imagery.

C. It requires electrical monitoring of the autonomic response.

D. It involves small electrical shock stimulation in response to negative images.

Review this! ❏

16. An anti-inflammatory diet consists of which of the following?

    A. A decreased ratio of omega-6 to omega-3 fatty acids
    B. An increased intake of omega-6 fatty acids
    C. Taking a nonsteroidal anti-inflammatory drug daily to decrease inflammation in the body
    D. A decreased intake of omega-3 fatty acids

    Review this! ❏

17. Which of the following statements is true about gua sha?

    A. It involves pressing the skin with a hard, round-edged instrument to create petechiae.
    B. It involves creating a vacuum in a cup and applying the vacuum to the skin.
    C. It involves the insertion of needles into various points along the qi meridians.
    D. It involves the burning of moxa on or near meridian points.

    Review this! ❏

18. Which of the following are practitioner-based CAM therapies?

    A. Acupuncture, biofeedback, and naturopathy
    B. Acupuncture, chelation therapy, and qigong
    C. Chelation therapy, naturopathy, and tai chi
    D. Chelation therapy, naturopathy, and Reiki

    Review this! ❏

19. Which of the following statements about transcendental meditation is true?

    A. It focuses on postures and breathing exercises.
    B. It is practiced by an Eastern religious sect of Buddhism.
    C. It involves repeating a mantra to avoid distracting thoughts.
    D. It involves burning incense and chanting to connect with the spiritual world.

    Review this! ❏

20. Which of the following statements about CAM research problems and potentials is true?

    A. Patients are eager to participate in studies that assess CAM therapies, because so many are using them already.
    B. Rigorously designed clinical trials are simply not possible with therapies outside of conventional medicine.
    C. Developing appropriate placebo controls for CAM therapies is difficult.
    D. Studies with herbal medicines are among the most accurate because of the standardization of dosing.

    Review this! ❏

21. Which of the following describes a difference between naturopathy and homeopathy?

    A. There is no difference; the terms are used interchangeably.
    B. Naturopathy uses drugs found in nature to treat disease, whereas homeopathy uses home remedies handed down from ancient times.
    C. Naturopathy believes that the body is able to heal itself, whereas homeopathy is based on the law of similars.
    D. Both use vitamin and mineral therapy to cure disease: naturopathy uses high doses, whereas homeopathy uses very small doses of the same compounds.

    Review this! ❏

22. All of the following CAM therapies include movement and breathing exercises, except:

    A. Transcendental meditation.
    B. Tai chi.
    C. Qigong.
    D. Feldenkrais.

    Review this! ❏

23. Excluding the use of megavitamin therapy and prayer, CAM therapy is most frequently used in the United States for which of the following conditions?

    A. Arthritis
    B. Anxiety/depression
    C. Back pain
    D. Neck pain

    Review this! ❏

24. In descending order of use, which of the following were the most common CAM therapies reported in 2002 in the United States?

A. Prayer, chiropractic, diets, massage
B. Prayer, chiropractic, massage, diets
C. Diets, prayer, massage, chiropractic
D. Chiropractic, diets, massage, prayer

Review this! ❏

25. When was the National Center for Complementary and Alternative Medicine (NCCAM) established?

A. 1978
B. 1998
C. 2000
D. 2005

Review this! ❏

26. Which of the following statements is true about prayer?

A. It is not considered a part of CAM, because it is a private, very personal matter.
B. It is only included in CAM therapy if individuals practice group prayer and meditation.
C. It takes several forms in CAM therapy, including individual, centered, and group prayer.
D. It should only be included in CAM therapy if an individual practices a Christian religion.

Review this! ❏

27. An anti-inflammatory diet consists of which of the following?

A. Eating more walnuts and green, leafy vegetables
A. Eating a low-carbohydrate, high-protein diet
B. Eating more oils from corn, soybeans, and sunflowers
C. Increasing the dairy and poultry intake

Review this! ❏

Things to remember for the test.

28. Which of the following statements about hypnosis is true?

A. It is a technique of mind–body medicine.
B. It involves the use of hallucinogenic agents to promote a dreamlike state.
C. It facilitates a person's ability to critically judge situations that have been bothering him or her.
D. It is practiced only by licensed clinical psychologists.

Review this! ❏

29. Which of the following statements about traditional Chinese medicine is true?

A. The five elements of wood, fire, earth, sky, and water have competing influences on various body parts.
B. Acupuncture, moxibustion, and rose blossom are all considered therapeutic practices in this discipline.
C. A specific diagnosis is needed for therapy to be effective.
D. Pain is the result of blocked qi.

Review this! ❏

30. Which of the following statements about therapeutic touch is true?

A. It includes Swedish massage and deep-tissue massage.
B. It involves the use of the hands to balance chakra function in the body.
C. It is considered a manipulative and body-based therapy.
D. It involves the use of magnets to change the flow of energy in the body.

Review this! ❏

17

Herbs and Supplemental Therapy

Miriam Chan

1. Which one of the following statements about the Dietary Supplements Health and Educations Act of 1994 is true?

   A. It defines dietary supplements as drugs to be evaluated for safety and efficacy by the U.S. Food and Drug Administration.
   B. It was created to ensure the potency and purity of nutritional supplements.
   C. It allows the sale of botanical and other natural products as dietary supplements.
   D. It was created to avoid false claims of specific health benefits of dietary supplements.

   Review this! ❑

2. According to a telephone survey conducted by Kelly and colleagues, which of the following best represents the prevalence of the use of herbal therapies by adults in the United States in 2002?

   A. 14.2%
   B. 18.8%
   C. 33.5%
   D. 52.7%

   Review this! ❑

3. Regarding supplement use, which of the following statements is false?

   A. Product safety and standardization of supplements are often variable.
   B. The sheer number of available products and advertising claims can lead to the confusion of both patients and health care professionals.
   C. The National Center for Complementary and Alternative Medicine is funded by supplement manufacturers to gather important supplement data.
   D. Research may be of poor quality or difficult to interpret.

   Review this! ❑

4. Many people do not share information about their supplement use with their physicians because of all the following reasons, except:

   A. They feel that their doctors are prejudiced against the use of supplements.
   B. They feel that their doctors have limited knowledge about such products.
   C. They often do extensive research regarding supplements, and they value their independence with regard to making decisions about taking them.
   D. They feel that their doctors are not interested in whether they are using supplements or not.

   Review this! ❑

5. All of the following statements about supplement use are true, except:

   A. "Natural" does not mean "safe."
   B. Clinicians may not be aware of any potential drug–supplement interactions and their adverse effects.
   C. "Proprietary blend" combination products are of higher quality than single ingredient, non-patented formulations.
   D. The use of dietary supplements should be avoided among pregnant and lactating women.

   Review this! ❑

6. All of the following are considered when reviewing a supplement's packaging, except:

   A. The ingredients of the product should be listed on the label.
   B. The specific indication of use can be found on the supplement's label.
   C. The product's contents should be standardized.
   D. The manufacturer's name and address should be seen on the label.

   Review this! ❑

7. Why is birthwort (*Aristolochia* spp.) considered unsafe and to be avoided?

   A. It causes heart attacks and strokes.
   B. It causes central nervous system excitation.
   C. It causes liver damage.
   D. It causes kidney failure.

   Review this! ❏

8. Liver damage has been associated with which of the following herbs?

   A. Comfrey, chaparral, germander, and kava
   B. Chaparral, germander, kava, and milk thistle
   C. Comfrey, ephedra, germander, and kava
   D. Chaparral, germander, kava, and saw palmetto

   Review this! ❏

9. All of the following herbs are rated as likely hazardous, except:

   A. Yohimbe.
   B. Yucca.
   C. Pennyroyal oil.
   D. Skullcap.

   Review this! ❏

10. Based on the latest research data about vitamin E, which of the following statements is false?

    A. Vitamin E at doses of more than 400 IU should be avoided.
    B. Vitamin E does not reduce the incidence of cancer or major cardiovascular events.
    C. Vitamin E supplementation may prevent Parkinson's disease.
    D. Vitamin E may increase the risk of heart failure among patients with vascular disease or diabetes.

    Review this! ❏

11. St. John's wort has been shown to induce the cytochrome P450 isoenzymes and to decrease the blood levels of all of the following, except:

    A. Indinavir.
    B. Oral contraceptives.
    C. Cyclosporine.
    D. Selective serotonin reuptake inhibitors (SSRIs).

    Review this! ❏

12. Which of the following herbs does not increase the potential for hemorrhage?

    A. Garlic
    B. Stinging nettle
    C. Dong quai
    D. Ginkgo leaves

    Review this! ❏

13. All of the following herbs may lower blood glucose, except:

    A. Ginseng.
    B. Dehydroepiandrosterone (DHEA).
    C. Bitter melon.
    D. Fenugreek.

    Review this! ❏

14. Which of the following herbs can lower blood pressure?

    A. American ginseng.
    B. Ginger.
    C. Black cohosh.
    D. Licorice.
    E. Cayenne.

    Review this! ❏

Questions 15 through 19: Match each of the following herbs with its commonly used formulation.

15. Cranberry
16. Ginger root
17. Dried feverfew
18. Chamomile tea
19. Ginseng

    A. Crude herb
    B. Juice
    C. Infusion
    D. Dry herb
    E. Decoction

    Review this! ❏

20. Black cohosh, dong quai, evening primrose, and soy are commonly used for which of the following conditions?

    A. Insomnia
    B. Depression
    C. Menopausal symptoms
    D. Arthritis

    Review this! ❏

Questions 21 through 26: Match each of the following herbs with its "possibly effective" use.

21. Echinacea
22. Feverfew
23. Ginkgo
24. Hawthorn
25. St. John's wort
26. Saw palmetto

   A. Dementia and intermittent claudication
   B. Stage I or II heart failure
   C. Migraine prevention
   D. Benign prostatic hypertrophy
   E. Upper respiratory infections
   F. Mild to moderate depression

Review this! ❑

27. Which of the following symptoms is a side effect of Panax ginseng?

   A. Decreased libido
   B. Hyperglycemia
   C. Morning drowsiness
   D. Increase in blood pressure

Review this! ❑

28. Which of the following symptoms is a side effect of valerian?

   A. Decreased libido
   B. Hyperglycemia
   C. Morning drowsiness
   D. Increase in blood pressure

Review this! ❑

29. Which of the following precautions should patients be given about garlic?

   A. Discontinue taking it at least 7 days before surgery.
   B. It may be taken with drugs that affect platelets.
   C. Do not operate heavy machinery or drive after ingestion.
   D. It should be used with caution in the presence of *Helicobacter pylori* infection.

Review this! ❑

30. Which of the following statements about vitamins is false?

   A. Folic acid supplementation is needed for patients with high homocysteine levels.
   B. Beta-carotene, a pro-vitamin A compound, has been shown to increase mortality among smokers with coronary heart disease. It may also increase cancer risk among smokers.
   C. Metformin may reduce the activity of vitamin B_1.
   D. Vitamin B_3 can reduce the risk of myopathy when it is given with statins.
   E. The level of vitamin B_6 is reduced with isoniazid use.

Review this! ❑

31. Which of the following statements about chromium is false?

   A. It can cause cognitive, sensory, and motor problems.
   B. It can cause hyperglycemia.
   C. It may cause weight gain among women.
   D. It may cause anemia, hemolysis, thrombocytopenia, and liver dysfunction when given at high doses.

Review this! ❑

32. Which of the following statements about creatine is true?

   A. It can precipitate manic episodes among bipolar patients, and it may augment serotonergic effects of SSRIs and meperidine.
   B. It can raise androgen and estrogen levels, and it may possibly increase the risk of hormone-sensitive cancers.
   C. It may cause sleepiness, headaches, mood changes, drops in blood pressure, and hyperglycemia among patients with type 1 diabetes.
   D. It has been linked to dehydration and heat intolerance; it may also cause muscle cramping and breakdown.

Review this! ❑

33. Which of the following statements about DHEA is true?

   A. It can precipitate manic episodes among bipolar patients, and it may augment the serotonergic effects of SSRIs and meperidine.
   B. It can raise androgen and estrogen levels, and it may possibly increase the risk of hormone-sensitive cancers.
   C. It may cause sleepiness, headaches, mood changes, drops in blood pressure, and hyperglycemia among patients with type 1 diabetes.
   D. It may alter drug effects on glucose levels, and it may have more side effects when taken with diuretics.

Review this! ❑

Things to remember for the test.

34. Which of the following statements about glucosamine is true?

    A. It can precipitate manic episodes among bipolar patients, and it may augment the serotonergic effects of SSRIs and meperidine.
    B. It can cause amnesia and decrease muscle tone, and it has been linked to 122 reports of serious adverse reactions.
    C. It may cause sleepiness, headaches, mood changes, drops in blood pressure drops, and hyperglycemia among patients with type 1 diabetes.
    D. It is well tolerated; however, it may worsen asthma symptoms and alter the effects of drugs on glucose levels.

    Review this! ❏

35. Which of the following statements about melatonin is true?

    A. It can precipitate manic episodes among bipolar patients, and it may augment the serotonergic effects of SSRIs and meperidine.

    B. It can cause amnesia and decrease muscle tone, and it has been linked to 122 reports of serious adverse reactions.
    C. It may cause sleepiness, headaches, mood changes, drops in blood pressure, and hyperglycemia among patients with type 1 diabetes.
    D. Use of this supplement may be linked to eosinophilia myalgia syndrome.

    Review this! ❏

36. Which of the following statements about *S*-adenosyl-L-methionine (SAMe) is true?

    A. It can precipitate manic episodes among bipolar patients, and it may augment the serotonergic effects of SSRIs and meperidine.
    B. It can cause amnesia and decrease muscle tone, and it has been linked to 122 reports of serious adverse reactions.
    C. It has antithrombotic effects, and it should not be used with anticoagulants or antiplatelet drugs.
    D. Use of this supplement may be linked to eosinophilia myalgia syndrome.

    Review this! ❏

Part III

Communication in Family Medicine

20 Interviewing Techniques

William Verhoff

1. Which of the following statements is true?

   A. It is the quantity of time spent with the patient that enhances the physician–patient relationship.
   B. It is the plan of care that is critical to the patient experience.
   C. Awareness of the verbal cues from the patient will be adequate to complete the examination.
   D. It is the perceived quality of time that is paramount to a positive patient experience.

   Review this! ❏

2. Ritter and Wilson[1] noted that listening is a key element for the establishment of the three Rs of interviewing. Which one of the following is not one of the three Rs?

   A. Reality
   B. Rapport
   C. Relationship
   D. Respect

   Review this! ❏

3. The listening environment—which includes the physical environment of the room, the physician's body position and eye contact, and the patient's sense of having the physician's attention—helps to create which one of the following?

   A. Reverence
   B. Rapport
   C. Resistance
   D. Responsibility

   Review this! ❏

4. The conversational give and take during the interview provides the opportunity for the physician to learn which of the following?

   (1) The biopsychosocial understanding of the patient

   (2) The plans for the patient's future financial success
   (3) The context of the patient's life and relationships
   (4) The correlation between health and wealth

   A. 1 and 2
   B. 2 and 4
   C. 1 and 3
   D. 2 and 3

   Review this! ❏

5. True or false: When the physician explains the diagnosis and recommendation, it is best to get the patient to be in compliance with the plan of care.

   A. True
   B. False

   Review this! ❏

6. Which of the following is not a time demand barrier to effective communication?

   A. The patient hiding an agenda
   B. Open-access scheduling
   C. Work-in or same-day appointment visits
   D. Adequate time for dictation and/or documentation

   Review this! ❏

7. All of the following can create barriers to effective physician–patient communication, except:

   A. Patients who use or want to discuss the use of complimentary and alternative medicine.
   B. Technological advances, such as electronic health records and personal digital assistants.
   C. The physician informing the patient of what he or she is doing when viewing or entering data into the computerized health record.

Things to remember for the test.

1. Ritter RH, Wilson PA: Developing the fine art of listening. *Texas Bar J* 64:897-900, 2001.

D. Interruptions in the continuous flow of information during the medical interview.

Review this! ❏

8. A recent survey indicated that 43% of adults would welcome a discussion of spiritual matters with their physicians. However, what percentage reported ever being asked by their physician about their faith and its impact on their health?

A. 5%
B. 10%
C. 20%
D. 30%

Review this! ❏

9. A brief spiritual interview assessment tool developed by Pulchaski and Romer[2] is abbreviated as **FICA.** Match the letters with the correct spiritual areas being assessed.

F _____ (1) Community
I _____ (2) Alignment
C _____ (3) Faith
A _____ (4) Attitude
(5) Inspiration
(6) Address
(7) Fundamental
(8) Church
(9) Inquisitive
(10) Freedom
(11) Importance
(12) Character

Review this! ❏

10. In 2002, Prochaska, Di Clemente, and Norcross[3] published their newest model for understanding the stages people go through when making a change. Put those stages in the proper order of occurrence.

_____ Preparation
_____ Maintenance
_____ Precontemplation
_____ Termination
_____ Contemplation
_____ Action

Review this! ❏

2. Pulchalski C, Romer A: Taking a spiritual history allows clinicians to understand patients more fully. *J Palliat Med* 3:129-137, 2000.
3. Prochaska and colleagues (2002).

11. The CAGE screening method for determining the possibility of problems associated with drugs and alcohol has a sensitivity and specificity of what percentages?

A. 60% and 80%, respectively
B. 90% and 90%, respectively
C. 50% and 50%, respectively
D. 70% and 90%, respectively

Review this! ❏

12. Match the various techniques for establishing and maintaining rapport, respect, and relationships with the appropriate age group or patient type.

A. Infants and babies
B. Toddlers and children
C. Adolescents
D. Adult patients
E. Elderly patients
F. Elderly patients with dementia
G. The difficult patient
H. The somatizing patient

_____ The HEADSSS technique is a helpful tool for structuring the interview for this group of patients.

_____ This group requires the physician to be attentive to any visual or auditory acuity problems and to adjust speech, rate, and tone accordingly.

_____ Future behavior during physician appointments is in part determined by the cumulative experience of each office visit; try to avoid unpleasant portions of examinations when clinically acceptable.

_____ Frequent, regularly scheduled visits are very helpful. They allow the patient to feel that he or she is being followed closely, and this decreases the need for emergency room visits.

_____ When talking with the patient's caregiver about the reason for the visit, observe the patient for his or her level of activity and for developmental milestones.

_____ Avoid a judgmental attitude. View these patients' behaviors as opportunities to learn more about their needs and concerns.

_____ Briefly review the patient's records before entering the room; it is important that he or she knows that you are at least somewhat familiar with his or her history.

_____ If possible, address the patient rather than the caregiver, and ask the patient's permission before you begin talking with the caregiver about the patient.

Review this! ❏

13. Which of the following is the Ritter paradigm mnemonic for interviewing and assessment?

A. INTERVIEW
B. LISTEN
C. RAPPORT
D. HISTORY

Review this! ❏

Things to remember for the test.

Part IV

Practice of Family Medicine

21 Pain Management

Joyce C. Hollander-Rodriguez and James F. Calvert, Jr.

1. Which of the following laboratory tests is recommended before starting medication for pain?

   A. Serum creatinine
   B. Complete blood cell count
   C. Thyroid-stimulating hormone
   D. Urinalysis
   E. Acetylneuraminic acid

   Review this! ❏

2. A patient that describes his or her pain as "burning and stabbing" most likely has which type of pain?

   A. Visceral pain
   B. Neuropathic pain
   C. Musculoskeletal pain
   D. Nociceptive pain

   Review this! ❏

3. When initiating a treatment program for a patient with chronic nonmalignant pain, what goal should be clearly established between the patient and the physician?

   A. Complete relief of pain
   B. Use of medications without initial side effects
   C. Improvement in functional status
   D. Achieving euphoria

   Review this! ❏

4. A 46-year-old man gives a history of nausea and vomiting along with itching after receiving morphine intravenously. Which of the following statements is true?

   A. He has an allergy to morphine, so hydromorphone should be used instead.
   B. He should be given Benadryl (diphenhydramine) before any intravenous use of opioids and warned that he will not develop tolerance to this reaction.
   C. He will have the same response with any opioid of the same class.

   D. Itching and nausea are common side effects of opioids, but the patient does not have a true allergy to them.

   Review this! ❏

5. When choosing a dosing schedule for a patient with continuous chronic pain, which of the following would be best?

   A. Start as-needed dosing of a short-acting opioid every 4–6 hours.
   B. Start as-needed dosing of a long-acting opioid every 8–12 hours.
   C. Start a scheduled opioid three times daily at 7 AM, 3 PM, and 11 PM.
   D. Start a scheduled opioid four times daily.

   Review this! ❏

6. Which opiate blocks the reuptake of norepinephrine and serotonin in addition to its effect on opioid receptors?

   A. Hydrocodone
   B. Morphine
   C. Methadone
   D. Hydromorphone

   Review this! ❏

7. The term *maldynia* refers to which of the following?

   A. Acute pain syndromes
   B. Chronic pain syndromes
   C. Nociceptive pathways
   D. Peripheral sensitization

   Review this! ❏

8. A 49-year-old woman with rheumatoid arthritis was placed on one tab of Vicodin (hydrocodone/APAP 5/500) by mouth four times daily for pain. She has always been on time with appointments and refills. Today, she says that her pain improves when she takes her pills but that it is not controlled throughout the day. On careful questioning,

Things to remember for the test.

you discover that she is in pain about 1 to 2 hours before her next dose, and she sometimes forgets to take the medication regularly when she is busy with her day. What is the best approach to her pain regimen?

A. Increase her dose to two tabs of Vicodin (hydrocodone/APAP) by mouth four times daily.
B. Change her medication to Percocet (oxycodone/APAP) for better pain control.
C. Change her dosing schedule to every 4 to 6 hours so that she can take the next dose earlier.
D. Change her medication to MS Contin (morphine sulfate sustained release) 15 mg by mouth twice daily.
E. Add acetaminophen for breakthrough pain.

Review this! ❏

9. Which of the following agents has a toxic nonopioid metabolite?

A. Codeine
B. Meperidine
C. Fentanyl
D. Oxycodone

Review this! ❏

10. Nonsteroidal anti-inflammatory drugs (NSAIDs) should be used with caution in patients with which of the following conditions?

A. Creatinine clearance of 45 mL/min
B. Liver failure and ascites
C. Congestive heart failure
D. Diabetes
E. All of the above

Review this! ❏

11. Which of the following is true about acetaminophen toxicity?

A. The maximum daily dosage of acetaminophen is 2000 mg/24 hours.
B. Toxicity does not occur at doses of less than 4000 mg/24 hours.
C. Chronic use of alcohol should be avoided with chronic acetaminophen use.
D. Toxic doses of acetaminophen usually occur with prescription combination products rather than over-the-counter preparations.

Review this! ❏

12. Which of the following pain disorders is not likely to respond to an antidepressant?

A. Acute musculoskeletal pain
B. Dysmenorrhea
C. Chronic low back pain
D. Diabetic neuropathy

Review this! ❏

13. A 39-year-old man is being treated with opioids for chronic pain. He has been maintained on a very strict medication regimen and warned by his provider that he cannot have higher doses of medications, despite complaints of inadequate pain control. Lately, he has become anxious, and he is preoccupied with getting his prescriptions at each visit. His behavior is an example of which of the following?

A. Drug seeking
B. Pseudoaddiction
C. Tolerance
D. Drug addiction

Review this! ❏

14. When starting chronic pain treatment for a patient with a mental health disorder, which of the following is true?

A. Their mental health issues are unlikely to affect their pain issues.
B. Affective disorders (e.g., depression, anxiety) are important to pain treatment, but thought disorders (e.g., schizophrenia) will not affect a treatment regimen.
C. The physician prescribing the pain medications should not also treat the mental health disorders.
D. The experience of chronic pain can cause mental health issues, even in patients without any prior history.

Review this! ❏

15. How do skeletal muscle relaxants work?

A. They act on the neuromuscular junction.
B. They slow neuromuscular transmission and excitability.
C. They have a direct relaxant effect on the skeletal muscle.
D. They are nonspecific sedatives and depressants that affect polysynaptic pathways.

Review this! ❏

16. A 75-year-old woman with a creatinine clearance of 30 mL/min is being started on a medication for pain after inadequate control with over-the-counter acetaminophen. Which of the following is the best choice for her medication?

    A. Propoxyphene/APAP (Darvocet)
    B. Meperidine (Demerol)
    C. Oxycodone (Roxicodone)
    D. Indomethacin (Indocin)

    Review this! ❏

17. Which approach to constipation for patients receiving chronic opioid therapy is the most appropriate?

    A. Warn patients that it is unlikely to become a chronic problem as the mu–2 receptors develop tolerance.
    B. Start every patient on a prophylactic bowel regimen at the time of his or her initial opioid prescription.
    C. Use prophylactic stool softeners for those opioids that are most associated with constipation, such as codeine.
    D. Use regular laxatives only when prescribing high doses of opioids.

    Review this! ❏

18. Which of the following is true about nausea and vomiting with opioids?

    A. Prophylactic antiemetics will worsen sedation and should not be used.
    B. Tolerance usually develops in 5 to 10 days.
    C. Nausea and vomiting are signs of allergy to opioids.
    D. Nausea and vomiting occur in less than 10% of people who have initiated opioid therapy.

    Review this! ❏

19. What is the role of a medication contract for prescribing chronic opioids?

    A. Contracts are legally required in all states.
    B. Contracts create an adversarial relationship between the patient and the physician, so they should only be used for patients who are behaving inappropriately.
    C. Contracts are only useful if substance abuse is suspected.
    D. Contracts allow patient and physician expectations to be addressed explicitly.

    Review this! ❏

20. Which of the following is true about opioid receptors?

    A. Mu2 receptors are primarily responsible for non-analgesic effects.
    B. Mu1 receptors mediate analgesia and chemical dependency.
    C. Kappa receptors within the intestinal tract are responsible for constipation.
    D. Kappa and delta receptors are not involved in mediating analgesic effects.

    Review this! ❏

21. How is chronic pain different from acute pain?

    A. Chronic pain does not respond to opioids, whereas acute pain does.
    B. Chronic pain involves changes in the nervous-system processing of pain signals.
    C. Acute pain is characterized by hyperalgesia and allodynia.
    D. Chronic pain is defined as pain that has lasted for more than 6 months.

    Review this! ❏

22. The correct use of short-acting opioids in chronic pain includes which of the following?

    A. The use of a limited number of pills per month for breakthrough pain
    B. One or two pills every 4 hours as needed for pain, allowing the patient to regulate their own medication
    C. Patients making appointments only when they need refills of their medication
    D. Short-acting opioids never being prescribed along with long-acting opioids

    Review this! ❏

23. Which of the following statements about fentanyl is true?

    A. A small percentage of the fentanyl released from the transmucosal form of the drug is absorbed in the gastrointestinal tract.
    B. Abuse is less common with the transmucosal form of fentanyl than with the transdermal form, making it a better choice for generalist physicians.
    C. Placing the patch over an area of the body with heavy adipose distribution gives the best results.
    D. The rotation of application sites is desirable for the transdermal patch.

    Review this! ❏

Things to remember for the test.

81

24. Which of the following statements about oxycodone is true?

    A. The extended-release formulation of the drug includes acetaminophen.
    B. The extended-release form gives a uniform drug level over a 12-hour period.
    C. The immediate-release form has a peak effect in 1 hour and duration of 4 hours.
    D. The drug has a strong mu1 effect, which causes euphoria and the potential for abuse.

    Review this! ❏

25. Which of the following statements about propoxyphene is false?

    A. It is in the same chemical class as methadone.
    B. It has a cardiotoxic metabolite that may cause arrhythmias.
    C. The efficacy of the drug is decreased in smokers.
    D. The drug causes good analgesia, and euphoria is unusual.

    Review this! ❏

26. Regarding opioids in general, which of the following statements is false?

    A. Opioids are in pregnancy category C.
    B. Among elderly persons, the cytochrome P450 system is upregulated compared with younger persons; this increases drug levels.
    C. Urinary retention may be a problem in the elderly.
    D. Opioids may lower the seizure threshold.

    Review this! ❏

27. Which of the following statements about tramadol is true?

    A. The time of onset depends on the dose.
    B. The drug should be taken on an empty stomach.
    C. It is a controlled substance in the same U.S. Food and Drug Administration/

Drug Enforcement Administration category as hydrocodone.
    D. There is no need to adjust the dose for renal failure.

    Review this! ❏

28. Which of the following statements about morphine is true?

    A. The drug is primarily excreted via the hepatic route.
    B. Epidural analgesia may last up to 48 hours.
    C. The peak analgesic effect of the oral extended-release form is 60 minutes.
    D. Many people taking the oral extended release-form require dosing three times daily.

    Review this! ❏

29. Which of the following statements about oxymorphone is true?

    A. It is currently available in an oral sustained-release form.
    B. The drug is metabolized in the liver and excreted in the kidneys.
    C. Peak analgesic effect by the rectal route is 60 minutes.
    D. The duration of analgesia by the intravenous route is 8 to 10 hours.

    Review this! ❏

30. Which of the following statements about hydromorphone is false?

    A. It is available in a controlled release form in the United States.
    B. The onset of action parenterally is up to 15 minutes.
    C. The time to peak analgesic effect is 60 minutes.
    D. It is excreted renally.

    Review this! ❏

31. Which of the following is a COX-2 inhibitor?

    A. Diclofenac
    B. Etoricoxib
    C. Abciximab
    D. Meloxicam

    Review this! ❏

22 Infectious Diseases

Chelley K. Alexander

1. Emerging challenges in infectious disease include which of the following?

   A. The emergence of community-acquired methicillin-resistant *Staphylococcus aureus*
   B. The increasing resistance of *Escherichia coli* to antibiotics
   C. The increasing resistance of *Streptococcus pneumoniae* to commonly used antibiotics
   D. Bioterrorism
   E. All of the above

   Review this! ❏

2. To take the best care of a patient with a potential infectious disease, the physician should do which of the following?

   A. Take a careful history, including travel and sick contacts
   B. Begin empiric antibiotic therapy before diagnostic tests in life-threatening situations
   C. Drain any abscesses and remove all foreign bodies
   D. Be aware of local antibiotic sensitivity patterns
   E. All of the above

   Review this! ❏

3. Which of the following is true?

   A. The majority of fevers of unknown origin have infectious causes.
   B. Fever of unknown orgin, by definition, requires an illness lasting longer than 3 weeks, a fever of more than 101°F, and an uncertain diagnosis after 1 week of study in the hospital
   C. Tuberculosis, endocarditis, and abdominal abscesses make up a significant proportion of fevers of unknown origin caused by infection.
   D. Newborns with a fever may be treated based on clinical appearance if their fever responds to Tylenol.
   E. None of the above

   Review this! ❏

4. Which of the following is true about a patient who presents with cough?

   A. Cough that is productive of purulent sputum should usually be treated with antibiotics.
   B. Postnasal drip, asthma, and gastroesophageal reflux disease cause the vast majority of cases of chronic cough.
   C. Empiric treatment with β-agonists reduces the length of cough in patients who present with cough and symptoms of an upper respiratory infection.
   D. Patients with cough of less than 2 weeks' duration should be treated with antibiotics that cover atypical organisms.
   E. None of the above

   Review this! ❏

5. Which of the following is the treatment of choice for mild acute exacerbations of chronic bronchitis?

   A. Amoxicillin or doxycycline
   B. A fluoroquinolone with enhanced activity against drug-resistant *S. pneumoniae*
   C. Supportive care for viral illness
   D. Treatment based on sputum culture results
   E. None of the above

   Review this! ❏

6. The treatment of pneumonia should be tailored to cover the suspected pathogen based on clinical presentation. Which of the following statements about treatment for pneumonia is false?

   A. Patients without comorbidities and with no recent antibiotic therapy who can be treated as outpatients should be covered with azithromycin, clarithromycin, doxycycline, or a respiratory fluoroquinolone.

B. Patients with comorbidities or recent antibiotic therapy should receive a respiratory fluoroquinolone or a combination therapy with a β-lactam plus either a macrolide or doxycycline for at least 5 days and until the patient has been afebrile for 48 to 72 hours.

C. Patients with pneumonia who are admitted to the intensive care unit should be treated with combination therapy with a β-lactam plus either an advanced macrolide or a respiratory fluoroquinolone.

D. Patients admitted to the intensive care unit should be treated with coverage for *Pseudomonas*.

E. All of the above are true.

Review this! ❑

7. According to the Pneumonia Severity Index, factors that significantly increase the risk of mortality in a patient presenting with pneumonia include which of the following?

A. Comorbidity with neoplastic disease
B. Acidosis, with pH of <7.35
C. Advanced age
D. Altered mental status
E. All of the above

Review this! ❑

8. Which of the following results of a tuberculin skin tests indicates a positive result?

A. 12 mm of induration in a patient with no risk factors for tuberculosis
B. 12 mm of induration in a child from a homeless shelter
C. 12 mm of erythema in a patient from a group home
D. 5 mm of erythema in a patient with human immunodeficiency virus (HIV)
E. None of the above

Review this! ❑

9. Which of the following would be appropriate treatment for a health care worker whose purified protein derivative (PPD) has converted from negative to positive during the last year?

A. Isoniazid, 300 mg orally daily, for a total duration of 9 months
B. Isoniazid, 300 mg orally daily for a total duration of 9 months, plus pyridoxine, 25 mg daily

C. A chest x-ray; if it is negative, no treatment
D. Isoniazid, 300 mg orally daily, and Rifampin, daily for 6 months
E. No treatment is necessary if the patient is asymptomatic.

Review this! ❑

10. Which of the following patients should not receive antibiotic prophylaxis to prevent endocarditis?

A. A patient with a prosthetic heart valve undergoing routine teeth cleaning
B. A patient with a previous history of endocarditis undergoing tooth abstraction
C. A patient with a cyanotic congenital heart disease having a cavity filled
D. A patient with surgically constructed systemic-pulmonary shunts and conduits undergoing routine teeth cleaning
E. A patient with a physiologic heart murmur undergoing routine teeth cleaning

Review this! ❑

11. Which of the following statements is true?

A. Spontaneous bacterial peritonitis (SBP) is the most commonly observed infection in cirrhotic patients who are Child-Pugh class B or C.
B. Patients presenting with SBP invariably present with peritoneal signs.
C. Patients who have an ascetic fluid white blood cell count of >250 cells/mm^3 who later have a negative culture of the ascitic fluid do not have SBP.
D. SBP is nearly always caused by a mix of bacterial flora.
E. The antibiotic treatment of choice for SBP is one that covers anaerobes.

Review this! ❑

12. All of the following statements about acute cholecystitis are true, except:

A. Antibiotics that cover enteric gastrointestinal flora should be given to patients with underlying comorbidities.
B. Infection is thought to precipitate most cases.
C. Definitive treatment consists of decompression or removal of the gallbladder.
D. The mechanical obstruction of bile drainage is thought to precipitate most cases.

E. The gallbladder is best imaged using ultrasound and hepato-iminodiacetic acid scanning.

Review this! ❏

13. All of the following statements about diverticulitis are true, except:

A. The clinical presentation is typically that of an elderly patient with left lower quadrant pain, diarrhea, fever, and leukocytosis.
B. Empiric antibiotics should cover gram-negative enteric and anaerobic organisms.
C. A colonoscopy is advisable at the time of admission to rule out underlying colon cancer.
D. Surgical treatment is reserved for patients who are not responding to conservative therapy.
E. All of the above

Review this! ❏

14. Traveler's diarrhea is characterized by which of the following?

A. The majority of cases are caused by *Salmonellae, Shigellae,* or vibrios and should be treated with antibiotics.
B. Many cases are caused by enterotoxigenic *E. coli* and should be treated with antibiotics.
C. Treatment with a short course of a fluoroquinolone is appropriate if enterohemorrhagic *E. coli* is suspected.
D. Treatment with a short course of Bactrim is appropriate if diarrhea is severe and accompanied by fever or bloody diarrhea.
E. Many cases are caused by enterotoxigenic *E. coli,* and supportive care should be sufficient.

Review this! ❏

15. Which of the following statements about antibiotic-associated diarrhea is true?

A. The major offending antibiotics are clindamycin and the cephalosporins.
B. *Clostridium difficile* is the major etiologic agent in the majority of cases of antibiotic-associated colitis.
C. The clinical presentation includes diarrhea, abdominal pain or cramping, and

fever in a patient who has previously used antibiotics.
D. Leukocytosis is common and may be marked.
E. All of the above

Review this! ❏

16. Which of the following patients should be treated for a urinary tract infection (UTI)?

A. A patient with a long-term indwelling catheter with bacteruria and dysuria
B. A pregnant patient with bacteruria but no symptoms
C. A patient with 2 to 5 white blood cells per high-powered field on a centrifuged specimen with dysuria and polyuria
D. None of the above
E. All of the above

Review this! ❏

17. Which of the following statements about UTIs is false?

A. Constipation, taking broad-spectrum antibiotics, and infrequent voiding are all factors that may contribute to the development of UTIs in children.
B. Every febrile infant or young child with a first UTI should have imaging of the urinary tract performed.
C. A chronic prostatic focus is the most common cause of recurrent UTIs among men.
D. Pregnant patients with UTIs should be treated with fluoroquinolones.
E. Simple interventions, such as drinking cranberry juice, voiding immediately after sexual intercourse, and using a contraceptive method other than a diaphragm and spermicide may help decrease the frequency of UTIs.

Review this! ❏

18. Which of the following sexually transmitted infections can be diagnosed based on history and physical examination alone?

A. Herpes simplex
B. Gonorrhea
C. Syphilis
D. Chlamydia
E. None of the above

Review this! ❏

Things to remember for the test.

19. Which of the following is true about vaginal infections?

    A. The three most common causes of vaginal discharge are trichomoniasis, bacterial vaginosis, and candidiasis.
    B. Bacterial vaginosis is best treated with metronidazole or clindamycin.
    C. The treatment of the sexual partners of women with recurrent candidiasis may be necessary.
    D. Candidiasis may be treated with oral or intravaginal imidazoles; both are equally effective.
    E. All of the above

    Review this! ❏

20. A brain computed tomography scan before lumbar puncture is necessary for which of the following patients?

    A. A patient with papilledema
    B. A patient with focal neurologic findings
    C. A patient who is HIV-positive
    D. A patient in whom subarachnoid hemorrhage is suspected
    E. All of the above

    Review this! ❏

21. A 58-year-old diabetic patient presents with 3+ pitting edema and cellulitis of the right lower extremity. Appropriate treatment would include which of the following?

    A. The mobilization of edema fluid
    B. Antibiotics covering gram-positive cocci
    C. Antibiotics covering gram-positive aerobes, gram-negative anaerobes, and anaerobes
    D. A and B
    E. A and C

    Review this! ❏

22. A 35-year-old white male presents with a furuncle on the nape of his neck. His history is significant for two previous skin infections with methicillin-resistant *S. aureus* during the last 3 months. Appropriate treatment includes which of the following?

    A. A 10- to 14-day course of Bactrim
    B. An extended (>14 days) course of Clindamycin
    C. Careful handwashing after contact with the lesion; washing the bed sheets daily in hot water

    D. A and C
    E. B and C

    Review this! ❏

23. All of the following are characteristics of a non–limb-threatening diabetic ulcer, except:

    A. Superficial ulcer with cellulitis <2 cm from the portal of entry
    B. No systemic toxicity
    C. No limb ischemia
    D. Infection with group B streptococci, Enterobacteriaceae, anaerobes, and bacteroides
    E. All of the above are characteristics of non–limb-threatening diabetic ulcers.

    Review this! ❏

24. Which of the following is not typical of osteomyelitis in children?

    A. The metaphysis of the long bones is the most common location.
    B. Blood cultures are positive in up to 50% of cases.
    C. Osteomyelitis in children is most often the result of trauma.
    D. *S aureus* is responsible for up to 90% of cases among healthy children.
    E. All of the above are typical of osteomyelitis in children.

    Review this! ❏

25. Which of the following is not typically treated with doxycycline?

    A. Rocky Mountain spotted fever
    B. Ehrlichiosis
    C. Babesiosis
    D. Lyme disease
    E. All of the above are treated with doxycycline.

    Review this! ❏

26. Which of the following is true?

    A. The most frequent pathogen in dog and cat bites is *Pasteurella multocida*.
    B. Human bites have a higher complication rate than do animal bites.
    C. Bite wounds involving the hands should be evaluated by a hand surgeon.
    D. Augmentin for 7 to 14 days is an appropriate treatment for bite wounds.
    E. All of the above

    Review this! ❏

Things to remember for the test.

27. A child with chickenpox is highly contagious and should not return to school until which of the following occurs?

    A. The patient is afebrile for 24 hours.
    B. All vesicles are crusted over.
    C. It has been 14 days since the initial vesicle formation.
    D. Crops of lesions are in multiple stages of healing.
    E. None of the above

    Review this! ❏

28. All of the following statements are true about infectious mononucleosis, except:

    A. Epstein-Barr virus is an infection of the T lymphocytes.
    B. Fever and lymphadenopathy are present in up to 90% of patients.
    C. Splenomegaly is present in half of the cases.
    D. Treatment with corticosteroids should be considered for severe complications.
    E. Cytomegalovirus causes 20% of infectious mononucleosis, and it is clinically indistinguishable from Epstein-Barr virus.

    Review this! ❏

29. Which of the following is spread by the fecal–oral route?

    A. Hepatitis A
    B. Hepatitis B
    C. Hepatitis C
    D. Hepatitis D
    E. None of the above

    Review this! ❏

30. The following patients have risk factors for acquiring hepatitis A, except:

    A. Those in a lower socioeconomic group.
    B. Daycare workers.
    C. Illicit drug users.
    D. Consumers of raw shellfish.
    E. Recipients of multiple blood transfusions.

    Review this! ❏

31. Which of the following is true about hepatitis B infection?

    A. Most children with acute hepatitis B progress to chronic infection.
    B. The consumption of raw shellfish is a risk factor.
    C. Hepatitis B causes the majority of cases of acute icteric hepatitis in the United States.
    D. Hepatitis B vaccine is available only to health personnel who are at a high risk of exposure.
    E. All of the above

    Review this! ❏

32. Which of the following is true about hepatitis C infection?

    A. It usually results in chronic hepatitis.
    B. It is spread by parenteral transmission.
    C. The major long-term risk is progression to cirrhosis and hepatocellular carcinoma.
    D. It was a common cause of transfusion-associated hepatitis before screening.
    E. All of the above

    Review this! ❏

23

Care of the Adult HIV-1–Infected Patient

Kenneth J. Griffiths

Things to remember for the test.

1. Currently, in the United States, which of the following is not a risk factor for human immunodeficiency virus (HIV) transmission?

   A. Male–male sex
   B. Injection drug use
   C. Blood transfusions
   D. Perinatal transmission

   Review this! ❏

2. In developing countries, HIV is most frequently transmitted through which of the following?

   A. Intravenous drug use
   B. Heterosexual sex
   C. Homosexual sex
   D. Perinatal transmission

   Review this! ❏

3. On average, at what length of time after exposure to HIV may a patient present to a physician with acute symptoms?

   A. 3 days
   B. 1 week
   C. 2–4 weeks
   D. 8 weeks

   Review this! ❏

4. What percentage of patients will experience acute symptomatic illness after infection?

   A. 10%
   B. 25%
   C. 50%
   D. 75%

   Review this! ❏

5. Common signs and symptoms of acute HIV infection include all of the following, except:

   A. Fever.
   B. Lymphadenopathy.
   C. Maculopapular rash.
   D. Cough.

   Review this! ❏

6. A 29-year-old male presents to your office with symptoms that are suggestive of acute HIV infection. The HIV antibody screen is negative. What test may be ordered to diagnose his primary infection?

   A. CD4 count
   B. CD8 count
   C. HIV viral load
   D. Complete blood cell count

   Review this! ❏

7. What is the average length of time from infection to a positive HIV antibody test?

   A. 1 month
   B. 2 months
   C. 4 months
   D. 6 months

   Review this! ❏

8. The HIV test is a test for antibodies to HIV. Which of the following cannot be used to test for HIV?

   A. Urine
   B. Oral fluids
   C. Blood
   D. Hair

   Review this! ❏

9. A patient has a positive HIV enzyme-linked immunosorbent assay (ELISA) test. What test is performed to confirm the diagnosis?

   A. Western blot
   B. Eastern blot
   C. Northern blot
   D. Southern blot

   Review this! ❏

10. A patient has a Western blot that is read as indeterminate. What is a reasonable recommendation?

A. Do nothing.
B. Repeat the ELISA.
C. Repeat the Western blot immediately.
D. Repeat the Western blot in 3 to 6 months.

Review this! ❏

11. Which health care occupational exposure requires consideration for postexposure medication prophylaxis?

A. Saliva
B. Urine
C. Non-bloody feces
D. Needlestick

Review this! ❏

12. Which of the following vaccines should not be given to a patient with HIV?

A. Influenza
B. Varicella
C. Pneumococcus
D. Adult diphtheria/tetanus

Review this! ❏

13. A patient who has been recently diagnosed with HIV comes to your office for an initial visit. Which of the following is not recommended?

A. Chest x-ray
B. Complete history and physical examination
C. Complete blood cell count and chemistry profile
D. CD4 and HIV viral load

Review this! ❏

14. True or false: Patients with HIV should be checked for serum hepatitis A and B antibodies before immunization is offered.

A. True
B. False

Review this! ❏

15. A patient with HIV presents to discuss treatment. Her CD4 count is 400, and her HIV viral load is 30,000. Which of the following do you recommend?

A. Continued monitoring every 3 to 4 months
B. Considering therapy
C. Initiating antiretroviral therapy
D. Doing nothing and following up as needed

Review this! ❏

16. True or false: Patients with a CD4 count of less than 200 and those with symptomatic HIV infection should take antiretroviral medications in combination.

A. True
B. False

Review this! ❏

17. What is the standard number of drugs used to treat HIV?

A. One
B. Two
C. Three
D. Four

Review this! ❏

18. Which of the following is a class of HIV medication?

A. Nucleoside reverse transcriptase inhibitors (NRTIs)
B. Non-nucleoside reverse transcriptase inhibitors (NNRTIs)
C. Protease inhibitors
D. All of the above

Review this! ❏

19. Which of the following is a common side effect of protease inhibitors?

A. Gastrointestinal distress
B. Arthralgia
C. Myalgia
D. Insomnia

Review this! ❏

20. How often should a patient be seen after he or she is stable on HIV therapy?

A. Every 6 months
B. Every 3 months
C. Every 2 months
D. Every month

Review this! ❏

21. Which of the following is the major reason for the failure of HIV medication?

A. Potency of the drug
B. Adherence to the drug
C. Pretreatment CD4 count
D. Drug interactions

Review this! ❏

22. Which class of medication may elevate serum triglycerides?

Things to remember for the test.

A. NRTIs
B. NNRTIs
C. Protease inhibitors
D. Fusion inhibitors

Review this! ❑

23. At what CD4 count is *Pneumocystis carinii* pneumonia (PCP) prophylaxis recommended?

    A. <500
    B. <400
    C. <300
    D. <200

    Review this! ❑

24. Which of the following medications is the first-line recommendation for PCP prophylaxis?

    A. Trimethoprim-sulfamethoxazole
    B. Dapsone
    C. Clindamycin
    D. Fluconazole

    Review this! ❑

25. For a patient with HIV, a tuberculin skin test is positive at what measurement?

    A. ≥1 mm
    B. ≥5 mm
    C. ≥10 mm
    D. ≥15 mm

    Review this! ❑

26. True or false: PCP prophylaxis may be discontinued after the CD4 count has been greater than 200 for 3 months.

    A. True
    B. False

    Review this! ❑

27. Toxoplasmosis gondii tends to affect which of the following body systems?

    A. The cardiovascular system
    B. The respiratory system
    C. The renal system
    D. The central nervous system

    Review this! ❑

28. Which of the following viruses is associated with chorioretinitis among patients with advanced HIV or acquired immunodeficiency syndrome (AIDS)?

    A. Herpes simplex virus
    B. Cytomegalovirus
    C. Varicella zoster virus
    D. Hepatitis B virus

    Review this! ❑

29. Current therapies for oral thrush include which of the following?

    A. Nystatin oral suspension
    B. Mycelex troche
    C. Diflucan
    D. All of the above

    Review this! ❑

30. True or false: Human papillomavirus is felt to be the most important etiologic factor for cervical and anal neoplasia.

    A. True
    B. False

    Review this! ❑

31. What is the recommended schedule for Pap smears for a woman with HIV?

    A. Every 6 months
    B. Every 1 year
    C. Every 6 months for 1 year, then yearly if normal
    D. Every 4 months for 1 year, then yearly if normal

    Review this! ❑

32. True or false: All patients with HIV should be screened for hepatitis C infection.

    A. True
    B. False

    Review this! ❑

33. The greatest increase in HIV cases in the United States has occurred in which of the following groups?

    A. Men
    B. Women
    C. Gay men
    D. Intravenous drug users

    Review this! ❑

34. Antiretroviral therapy during pregnancy reduces vertical transmission by what fraction?

    A. ¼
    B. ⅓
    C. ½
    D. ⅔

    Review this! ❑

35. Which of the following drugs is the most teratogenic?

    A. Sustiva
    B. Viramune
    C. Crixivan
    D. Zidovudine

    Review this! ❏

36. True or false: HIV-positive women should be counseled to breast-feed their children.

    A. True
    B. False

    Review this! ❏

Things to remember for the test.

Things to remember for the test.

1. Even simple physician advice to quit smoking provides the marginal benefit of what percentage of patients quitting successfully?

   A. 2.5%
   B. 6.4%
   C. 11%
   D. 21%

   Review this! ❏

2. The Legacy Foundation reports that ex-smokers have an average of how many quit attempts before ultimately sustaining a tobacco-free lifestyle?

   A. 2
   B. 4
   C. 6
   D. 8

   Review this! ❏

3. True or false: Vocal fremitus and tactile fremitus are increased in lung consolidation.

   A. True
   B. False

   Review this! ❏

4. The diagnosis of obstructive lung disease is best made by which of the following?

   A. Demonstrating an FEV_1/FVC ratio (or FEV_1/FEV_6) of <70%
   B. Clinical examination
   C. Decrease in FEV_1
   D. Hyperinflation on chest radiograph

   Review this! ❏

5. True or false: An improvement in FEV_1 of at least 12% and of at least 200 mL from prebronchodilator to postbronchodilator is considered evidence of the reversibility of airway obstruction.

   A. True
   B. False

   Review this! ❏

6. Cough may be the only symptom experienced by some patients with asthma (cough-variant asthma). Other causes of persistent cough include which of the following?

   A. Pertussis
   B. Gastroesophageal reflux disease
   C. Angiotensin-converting enzyme inhibitors
   D. All of the above

   Review this! ❏

7. True or false: A meta-analysis of controlled trials showed that handheld metered-dose inhalers with a spacer device are at least as effective as a nebulizer for delivering albuterol and for achieving a clinical response.

   A. True
   B. False

   Review this! ❏

8. When low-dose inhaled corticosteroids are not providing a patient with complete remission, the clinician may add a second medication or increase the inhaled steroid dose to moderate levels. Which of the following is the second medication of choice?

   A. Leukotriene inhibitor
   B. Theophylline
   C. Long-acting β_2-agonist
   D. Mast cell stabilizer

   Review this! ❏

9. True or false: It's important to educate patients about the methods of dust-mite removal.

   A. True
   B. False

   Review this! ❏

10. True or false: Smoking cessation is the only intervention that has been proven to slow the long-term rate of decline in FEV$_1$ among patients with chronic obstructive pulmonary disease.

    A. True
    B. False

    Review this! ❏

11. All of the following decreased exacerbation rates by 20% to 25% in patients with moderate to severe chronic obstructive pulmonary disease, except:

    A. Inhaled corticosteroids.
    B. Long-acting ß$_2$-agonists (e.g., salmeterol, formoterol).
    C. The long-acting anticholinergic agent tiotropium.
    D. Theophylline.

    Review this! ❏

12. An especially serious form of respiratory failure called adult respiratory distress syndrome may occur in patients with which of the following?

    A. Trauma
    B. Sepsis
    C. Aspiration pneumonia
    D. All of the above

    Review this! ❏

13. Which of the following statements about bronchiectasis is true?

    A. It is characterized by reversible airflow obstruction.
    B. It is seen in patients with cystic fibrosis.
    C. It responds well to amoxicillin.
    D. It responds well to inhaled steroids.

    Review this! ❏

14. Which of the following is a common cause of acute bronchitis?

    A. Influenza
    B. Pseudomonas
    C. Group A streptococcus
    D. Anaerobes

    Review this! ❏

15. Causes of atypical pneumonia include all of the following, except:

    A. Pseudomonas.
    B. Adenovirus.
    C. Chlamydia.
    D. Mycoplasma.

    Review this! ❏

16. True or false: The most important risk factor for developing tuberculosis is living in a household with or having close contact with an individual who has active tuberculosis.

    A. True
    B. False

    Review this! ❏

17. True or false: A 9-month course of isoniazid or a 4-month course of rifampin is effective for preventing the development of active tuberculosis in asymptomatic patients with positive purified protein derivative testing and negative chest x-ray (i.e., latent infection), even for patients with human immunodeficiency virus coinfection.

    A. True
    B. False

    Review this! ❏

18. A 42-year-old truck driver presents with fever, chills, and cough. He tells you that Arizona was his last destination. Fungal infections to consider include which of the following?

    A. Histoplasmosis
    B. Coccidiomycosis
    C. Blastomycosis
    D. Aspergillosis

    Review this! ❏

19. True or false: A 32-year-old female presents with the acute onset of shortness of breath. Oxygen saturation on room air is 99%. This normal oxygen saturation level rules out pulmonary embolus.

    A. True
    B. False

    Review this! ❏

20. Secondary causes of pulmonary hypertension include which of the following?

    A. Mitral stenosis
    B. Pulmonary fibrosis
    C. Sleep apnea
    D. All of the above

    Review this! ❏

Things to remember for the test.

21. A 40-year-old male smoker presents with hemoptysis, cavitary infiltrates, chronic sinusitis, and hematuria. Which of the following is the most likely diagnosis?

    A. Tuberculosis
    B. Endocarditis
    C. Wegener's granulomatosis
    D. Aspergilloma

    Review this! ❏

22. Pulmonary complications of sickle cell disease include which of the following?

    A. Pulmonary hypertension
    B. Acute chest syndrome
    C. Pneumonia
    D. All of the above

    Review this! ❏

23. True or false: Lung cancer is the leading cause of death among both men and women.

    A. True
    B. False

    Review this! ❏

24. All of the following are important for preventing lung cancer, except:

    A. Beta carotene
    B. Smoking cessation
    C. Spiral computed tomography scanning of the chest
    D. All of the above

    Review this! ❏

25. The differential diagnosis for bilateral hilar adenopathy includes which of the following?

    A. Sarcoidosis
    B. Coccidiomycosis
    C. Lymphoma
    D. All of the above

    Review this! ❏

26. All of the following can cause interstitial lung disease, except:

    A. Sarcoidosis.
    B. Chronic obstructive pulmonary disease.
    C. Rheumatoid arthritis.
    D. Progressive systemic sclerosis.

    Review this! ❏

27. All of the following are associated with transudative pleural effusions, except:

    A. Nephrotic syndrome.
    B. Congestive heart failure.
    C. Alcoholic cirrhosis.
    D. Pancreatitis.

    Review this! ❏

28. A 42-year-old obese male who does not smoke presents with bilateral peripheral edema and polycythemia. His chest x-ray is normal. Which of the following is the most likely diagnosis?

    A. Congestive heart failure
    B. Cirrhosis
    C. Sleep apnea
    D. Nephrotic syndrome

    Review this! ❏

29. For obese patients with sleep apnea, treatment includes which of the following?

    A. Weight reduction
    B. Alcohol avoidance
    C. Avoid supine sleep position
    D. All of the above

    Review this! ❏

30. True or false: All patients with persistent asthma (daytime symptoms more than twice a week or nocturnal symptoms more than twice a month) should be treated with daily long-term control medication, preferably an inhaled corticosteroid.

    A. True
    B. False

    Review this! ❏

25 Otolaryngology

Ronald L. Cook

1. The signs and symptoms of epiglottitis include which of the following?

   A. Sore throat
   B. High fever
   C. Thumbprint sign on lateral neck x-ray
   D. Drooling
   E. All of the above

   Review this! ❏

2. True or false: The use of a tongue blade in a patient suspected of having epiglottitis is contraindicated during the physical examination.

   A. True
   B. False

   Review this! ❏

3. A peritonsillar abscess is the accumulation of pus in the space that surrounds the tonsil. Typical signs and symptoms include which of the following?

   A. Dysphagia
   B. Peritonsillar swelling and displacement of the uvula
   C. Trismus
   D. "Hot potato" voice
   E. All of the above

   Review this! ❏

4. True or false: An adult presenting with the signs and symptoms of a peritonsillar abscess may be treated in the outpatient setting.

   A. True
   B. False

   Review this! ❏

5. Which of the following statements is false?

   A. The most common location for an esophageal foreign body to lodge is just inferior to the cricopharyngeal muscle.
   B. The most common foreign objects are coins.

   C. Disk-type batteries may be treated conservatively (i.e., waiting for them to pass in the stool).
   D. Plain radiographs, including lateral films, are usually diagnostic.
   E. Foreign body ingestion is many times unwitnessed, and other diagnostic techniques are frequently necessary.

   Review this! ❏

6. A child presents to your office with new-onset wheezing with no previous history of airway disease. All of the following statements are true about this case, except:

   A. Your differential diagnosis should include the aspiration of a foreign body.
   B. After a choking or coughing spell, there may have been a symptom-free period of time before the wheezing began.
   C. Most foreign bodies in the trachea are radiolucent, and x-rays can be normal.
   D. Treat the patient with bronchodilators, and give the parents reassurance.
   E. Definitive therapy is direct laryngoscopy or rigid bronchoscopy.

   Review this! ❏

7. Bleeding from the anterior nasal cavity is the most common, and it originates from what plexus of vessels?

   A. Heimlich's plexus
   B. Kiesselbach's plexus
   C. Froelich's plexus
   D. Friedman's plexus
   E. Kiolbassa's plexus

   Review this! ❏

8. Which of the following is the initial step in the management of epistaxis?

Things to remember for the test.

A. Cauterization with silver nitrate
B. Direct pressure on the nose
C. Airway stabilization
D. Two large-bore IVs of lactated Ringer's solution
E. Blood draw for coagulation studies

Review this! ❏

9. When packing the nose for epistaxis, the following procedures should be followed, except:

A. Remembering that the nasal cavity widens posteriorly rather than superiorly.
B. Hydrating the pack before placement may be helpful.
C. Removing the pack in 2 to 5 days.
D. Expanding the pack until the nasal ala blanch.
E. All of the above

Review this! ❏

10. Posterior nasal bleeds are more serious than anterior nasal bleeds. All of the following statements about posterior epistaxis are true, except:

A. An anterior pack that continues to bleed may be a sign of a posterior bleed.
B. If bleeding is controlled, no ear, nose, and throat consultation is necessary.
C. Necrosis of the nasal ala, septum, and palate may occur.
D. Posterior packing is usually painful and may require judicious amounts of narcotics.
E. Supplemental oxygen and monitoring are appropriate during the procedure.

Review this! ❏

11. A patient presents to your emergency center after a motor vehicle collision. She has obvious head and neck trauma. The stabilization of a compromised airway should be accomplished as soon as possible for all of the following reasons, except:

A. A muffled quality of voice that may be the result of an expanding hematoma.
B. Carbon dioxide retention, which is an early sign of airway obstruction.
C. Airway obstruction, which may progress rapidly.

D. The prevention of facial edema and ecchymosis.
E. The prevention of significant blood loss.

Review this! ❏

12. When examining the tympanic membrane (TM), the normal light reflex is seen in which of the following areas?

A. The anterior-inferior portion of the TM
B. The anterior-superior portion of the TM
C. The posterior-inferior portion of the TM
D. The posterior-superior portion of the TM
E. None of the above

Review this! ❏

13. Both the Weber's test and the Rinne's test are used to determine laterality in hearing loss. Which of the following best describes the placement of the tuning fork when performing the Weber's test?

A. The vibrating tuning fork is placed on the mastoid process of the side with suspected hearing loss.
B. The non-vibrating tuning fork is placed on the mastoid process of the side without suspected hearing loss.
C. The vibrating tuning fork is placed on the forehead of the patient.
D. The vibrating tuning fork is placed in front of the ear.
E. The vibrating tuning fork is placed on the tip of the nose.

Review this! ❏

14. Sensation of the ear is supplied by a combination of all of the following cranial nerves, except:

A. VII
B. V
C. X
D. IX
E. VIII

Review this! ❏

15. True vertigo most often indicates aberrant function of which of the following?

A. The eustachian tube
B. The middle ear
C. The external auditory canal
D. The inner ear
E. The ossicles

Review this! ❏

16. A typical Ménière's attack produces all of the following symptoms, except:

A. Severe vertigo, often with nausea and vomiting.
B. A high-frequency hearing loss.
C. Attacks that often last between 2 and 36 hours.
D. Roaring tinnitus.
E. A sensation of aural fullness.

Review this! ❑

17. Treatment for Ménière's disease may include which of the following?

    A. A low-sodium diet
    B. Dyrenium/hydrochlorothiazide (Dyazide) diuretics
    C. Minimal caffeine and alcohol intake
    D. Intratympanic gentamycin
    E. All of the above

Review this! ❑

18. All of the following are true about benign positional vertigo, except:

    A. It is the most common cause of the peripheral vertigo.
    B. It is caused by displaced otoconia particles in the utricle or the saccule.
    C. It is more common in males than females.
    D. Movement of the head makes the symptoms worse.
    E. Treatment includes repositioning of the otoconia.

Review this! ❑

19. Which of the following is a viral infection that causes pain and vesicular eruptions around the auricle and the external ear canal?

    A. Ramsay–Hunt syndrome
    B. Labyrinthitis syndrome
    C. Vestibular neuronitis
    D. Vertiginous otolithiasis

Review this! ❑

20. True or false: In general, if tinnitus is bilateral (rather than pulsatile) and associated with symmetric hearing loss, it is likely a result of the hearing loss itself.

    A. True
    B. False

Review this! ❑

21. All of the following are true about external otitis, except:

A. Fungal infections make up less than 10% of the cases.
B. Most common bacterial infections are from *Pseudomonas* or *Staphylococcus* species.
C. Pain is a more common complaint of patients with fungal ear infections.
D. Oral antifungal medicines may be added if topical medicines are ineffective.
E. Impacted cerumen, seborrheic dermatitis, and psoriasis call affect the external ear canal.

Review this! ❑

22. Foreign objects in the external auditory canal can be quite challenging to remove. Which of the following items should not be irrigated when trying to remove it?

    A. A bean
    B. Popcorn
    C. A battery
    D. All of the above

Review this! ❑

23. True or false: The ear canal is self-cleaning.

    A. True
    B. False

Review this! ❑

24. Ear, nose, and throat consultation for cerumen impaction removal is indicated in which of the following situations?

    A. When the cerumen is in direct contact with the tympanic membrane
    B. When the tympanic membrane is perforated
    C. When the cerumen is hard, black, and adherent to the canal
    D. When tepid or warm water irrigation has no effect
    E. When mild bleeding occurs after curettage

Review this! ❑

25. Which of the following factors plays a role in acute otitis media?

    A. Bacterial colonization
    B. Eustachian tube dysfunction
    C. *Staphylococcus pneumoniae*
    D. Childcare outside of the home, parental smoking
    E. All of the above

Review this! ❑

26. Middle-ear effusion is one of the three criteria needed to confirm the diagnosis of acute otitis media. The condition can be diagnosed by which of the following?

    A. The visualization of an air-fluid level behind the TM
    B. A bulging TM
    C. A flat tympanogram
    D. All of the above

    Review this! ❏

27. Which of the following is the antibiotic of choice for the treatment of otitis media for a patient who is not allergic to penicillin?

    A. Bactrim
    B. Cefuroxime
    C. Augmentin
    D. Amoxicillin
    E. None of the above

    Review this! ❏

28. Otolaryngologic evaluation of chronic otitis media includes all of the following, except:

    A. Culture-directed antibiotic therapy.
    B. Magnetic resonance imaging.
    C. Computed tomography scanning.
    D. Otomicroscopy and audiometry.
    E. Surgery.

    Review this! ❏

29. True or false: A cholesteatoma is composed of cholesterol deposits.

    A. True
    B. False

    Review this! ❏

30. True or false: Otitis media with effusion is best diagnosed with pneumatic otoscopy.

    A. True
    B. False

    Review this! ❏

31. Which of the following best describes recurrent otitis media?

    A. 6 episodes in 9 months
    B. 3 episodes in 6 months or 4 episodes in 12 months
    C. 1 episode per month for 6 months
    D. 1 episode every other month for 12 months

E. None of the above

Review this! ❏

32. Match the following types of hearing loss with the appropriate dysfunction:

    A. Conductive hearing loss
    B. Sensorineural hearing loss
    C. Mixed hearing loss
    D. Central hearing loss

    1. A dysfunction of the inner ear
    2. A loss or failure of the normal propagation of acoustic energy in the ossicles
    3. A loss from ischemic or traumatic brain injury
    4. A loss of both conductive and sensorineural functions

    Review this! ❏

33. True or false: A sudden sensorineural hearing loss is an otologic emergency.

    A. True
    B. False

    Review this! ❏

34. Which of the following examinations should be performed during the evaluation of an acoustic neuroma?

    A. Complete otolaryngologic and neurologic examination
    B. Tuning fork examination
    C. Magnetic resonance imaging of the head with gadolinium
    D. Audiogram
    E. All of the above

    Review this! ❏

35. Which of the following statements about hearing loss from acoustic energy is true?

    A. Acute exposure to loud noise can cause conductive loss.
    B. Acute exposure to loud noise can case sensorineural loss.
    C. The conductive loss may be surgically corrected, or a hearing aid may be used for nonsurgical candidates.
    D. If the loss is sensorineural, a hearing aid is the only option.
    E. All of the above

    Review this! ❏

Things to remember for the test.

36. Which of the following statements represents the most appropriate treatment for idiopathic Bell's palsy?

    A. Amoxicillin/clavulanate and steroids
    B. Amoxicillin/clavulanate and acyclovir
    C. Acyclovir and steroids
    D. Acyclovir and Cortisporin eardrops
    E. Cortisporin eardrops and steroids

    Review this! ❏

37. Which of the following statements is true?

    A. Mucus production of the sinuses is about 100 mL each day.
    B. The turbinates (inferior, medial, and superior) can be easily seen during the nasal examination with an otoscope.
    C. The majority of the mucus produced each day drains via the superior meatus just inferior to the middle turbinate.
    D. Most people have a mild septal deviation.
    E. All of the above

    Review this! ❏

38. True or false: Magnetic resonance imaging is helpful for evaluating sinusitis.

    A. True
    B. False

    Review this! ❏

39. True or false: Nasal decongestant sprays are very effective for treating severe nasal congestion. Rhinitis medicamentosa (rebound congestion) only occurs after long-term chronic use.

    A. True
    B. False

    Review this! ❏

40. All of the following statements about nasal polyps are true, except:

    A. They are the result of nasal mucosal inflammation and edema.
    B. They may predispose the patient to sinusitis.
    C. They often cause anosmia.
    D. If present unilaterally, they may represent a sinonasal tumor.
    E. In children, their presence is a normal variant.

    Review this! ❏

41. The diagnosis of allergic rhinitis is made by which of the following?

    A. Primarily by history
    B. By the finding of a nasal crease
    C. By eosinophils seen on a nasal smear
    D. By pale-pink to blue, boggy mucosa
    E. All of the above

    Review this! ❏

42. The diagnosis of acute rhinosinusitis can be very difficult. Which of the following is the most common cause?

    A. Bacterial
    B. Viral
    C. Allergy mediated
    D. Foreign body
    E. All of the above

    Review this! ❏

43. Which of the following signs and symptoms of sinusitis require urgent treatment and evaluation?

    A. Altered mental status
    B. Increasing or severe headache
    C. A periorbital erythema
    D. High fever
    E. All of the above

    Review this! ❏

44. Malignant tumors of the nose include all of the following, except:

    A. Adenocarcinoma.
    B. Adenoid cystic carcinoma.
    C. Osteosarcoma.
    D. Squamous papilloma.
    E. Hemangiopericytoma.

    Review this! ❏

45. Nasal polyps are often associated with the term **asthma triad,** which refers to which of the following?

    A. Nasal polyps, chronic urticaria, and penicillin allergy
    B. Nasal polyps, asthma, and penicillin allergy
    C. Asthma, penicillin allergy, and chronic urticaria
    D. Asthma, polyps, and aspirin sensitivity
    E. Aspirin sensitivity, chronic urticaria, and penicillin allergy

    Review this! ❏

46. Which of the following is the antibiotic of choice for group A β-hemolytic streptococcal pharyngitis?

Things to remember for the test.

A. Cefpodoxime (Vantin)
B. Cefaclor (Ceclor)
C. Amoxicillin/clavulanate (Augmentin)
D. Penicillin
E. All of the above

Review this! ❑

47. Which of the following describes an indication for tonsillectomy (with respect to streptococcal pharyngitis)?

A. 10 episodes within 1 year or 3 to 4 episodes within 2 years
B. 3 to 4 episodes within 1 year or 6 to 7 episodes within 2 years
C. 6 episodes within 1 year or 3 to 4 episodes within 2 years
D. 6 episodes within 18 months or 6 to 7 episodes within 2 years
E. 3 to 4 episodes within 1 year or 6 to 7 episodes within 18 months

Review this! ❑

48. Which of the following statements about obstructive sleep apnea is true?

A. It affects more men than women.
B. Snoring is a common symptom.
C. Adults with sleep apnea are typically overweight and stocky.
D. Symptoms may include daytime sleepiness, morning headache, hypertension, and depression.
E. All of the above

Review this! ❑

49. True or false: The most common midline neck mass is a branchial cleft cyst.

A. True
B. False

Review this! ❑

26 Allergy

Dennis A. LaRavia

1. All of the following statements are true, except:

   A. Allergic asthma has an allergic etiology.
   B. Intrinsic asthma has nonallergic etiologies.
   C. Anaphylaxis is always mediated by immunoglobulin E.
   D. Rhinitis may be either allergic or non-allergic.

   Review this! ❏

2. All of the following symptoms are almost always present in a patient with seasonal allergic rhinitis, except:

   A. Episodes of paroxysmal sneezing.
   B. Watery nasal discharge with congestion.
   C. Nasal pruritus.
   D. Sinus headaches.

   Review this! ❏

3. Seasonal allergic rhinitis is commonly associated with all of the following, except:

   A. An upward thrust of the palm against the nares to relieve itching and to open the nasal airways.
   B. Dennie's lines or wrinkles beneath the lower eyelid.
   C. Sleep disruption as a result of nasal obstruction and mouth breathing.
   D. Persistent and recurrent bacterial otitis media.

   Review this! ❏

4. All of the following are true about perennial allergic rhinitis, except:

   A. Nasal congestion, itching, and frequent sniffing are common findings.
   B. There is no effect on hearing among patients with this disorder.
   C. A loss of the senses of taste and smell is not uncommon.
   D. Paroxysms of sneezing and rhinorrhea may result from changes in ambient temperature, head movement, odors from perfume, and exposure to small quantities of antigen.

   Review this! ❏

5. Which one of the following statements about allergic rhinitis is false?

   A. The nasal turbinates are usually swollen and edematous, and they may be mistaken for nasal polyps.
   B. More than 90% of children with allergic rhinitis have eustachian tube obstruction with resultant serous otitis.
   C. Among patients with intact tympanic membranes, tympanometry can be used to measure middle-ear pressures, which may provide an indirect measure of eustachian tube function.
   D. Up to one third of patients with allergic rhinitis may have a lower respiratory tract component, including exercise-induced asthma and mild persistent asthma.

   Review this! ❏

6. The environmental control of allergens can play a part in the treatment of allergic patients. All of the following statements are true, except:

   A. It is the family's responsibility to deal with the control of bacteria, fibrous material, human epidermis, food remnants, fungi, insect debris, and animal debris in the home.
   B. Dust mites are commonly found in the home in bedding, mattresses, carpeting, and upholstered furniture.
   C. High-efficiency particulate air filters are helpful in general, but they are not particularly helpful with regard to the removal of dust and animal dander.
   D. The use of fans should be avoided in homes with allergic patients.

   Review this! ❏

Things to remember for the test.

Things to remember for the test.

7. Antihistamines are often helpful for patients with symptoms of rhinitis. All of the following statements are true, except:

   A. For optimal results, antihistamines should be used before exposure to allergens.
   B. Second-generation antihistamines are usually preferred because they generally do not penetrate into the central nervous system, thereby reducing the side effect of sedation.
   C. Fexofenadine (Allegra) is a safe and dependable second-generation antihistamine that may also diminish airway inflammation.
   D. Cetirizine (Zyrtec) is extremely effective as an antihistamine, and it is normally is less sedating than desloratadine (Clarinex).

   Review this! ❏

8. Which of the following statements is true?

   A. Beclomethasone and fluticasone are extremely effective as topical intranasal agents, even when used sporadically.
   B. The use of nasal saline is ineffective as a moisturizing agent when it is used with intranasal steroids.
   C. The intranasal glucocorticoids may take 1 to 3 weeks to be maximally effective.
   D. Intramuscular long-acting steroids are the first-line therapy for the treatment of routine allergic rhinitis.

   Review this! ❏

9. Which of the following statements is true?

   A. Immunotherapy as determined by skin testing is reliable and usually helpful for the treatment of seasonal allergic rhinitis.
   B. The efficacy of immunotherapy is more than 95% for the treatment of molds and house dust among patients with perennial allergic rhinitis.
   C. Immunotherapy is usually not well tolerated among children with seasonal allergic rhinitis.
   D. The use of immunotherapy for the treatment of allergic rhinitis has not been found to be helpful for preventing the development of asthma among children.

   Review this! ❏

10. Which of the following statements about nasal polyps is true?

    A. Perennial allergic rhinitis is rarely associated with nasal polyps.
    B. In adults, the presence of nasal polyps may be associated with sensitivity to aspirin manifested by the aggravation of rhinitis, asthma, and even shock.
    C. Nasal polyps only develop in the presence of prolonged allergic problems.
    D. The size of nasal polyps may be reduced by systemic glucocorticoids, but it is not affected by the use of topical glucocorticoids.

    Review this! ❏

11. All of the following statements about sinusitis are true, except:

    A. Chronic allergic rhinitis predisposes to a patient sinus disease, although sinus disease can develop in the absence of allergy.
    B. Acute sinusitis often presents with persistent rhinorrhea, postnasal drip, purulent drip, or discharge after an upper respiratory infection.
    C. The most commonly infected sinuses in children and adults are the frontal sinuses.
    D. Periorbital edema, facial pallor, and circles under the eyes may be striking presentations of acute sinusitis in a patient with allergic rhinitis.

    Review this! ❏

12. True or false: Some patients with perennial rhinitis are not atopic according to history or skin testing.

    A. True
    B. False

    Review this! ❏

13. True or false: Chronic nasal obstruction is the predominant symptom among patients with eosinophilic nonallergic rhinitis.

    A. True
    B. False

    Review this! ❏

14. True or false: Although there is no evidence of allergy by skin testing, numerous eosinophils are present in patients with eosinophilic nonallergic rhinitis, and the diagnosis is readily made by examining the nasal secretions for eosinophils and eosinophilic cationic protein.

A. True
B. False

Review this! ❑

15. True or false: The most effective treatment for eosinophilic nonallergic rhinitis is second-generation antihistamines.

A. True
B. False

Review this! ❑

16. All of the following statements are true, except:

A. Conjunctivitis is the usual ocular reaction to airborne allergens.
B. Vernal conjunctivitis is so called because of its occurrence during the spring and summer.
C. Vernal conjunctivitis usually starts during adolescence, and it routinely continues through most of the adult life.
D. Olopatadine (Patanol) and ketorolac (Acular) are excellent topical medications for the treatment of vernal conjunctivitis.

Review this! ❑

17. True or false: The three elements critical to the diagnosis of asthma include reversible airway obstruction, airway inflammation, and increased airway responsiveness to a variety of stimuli.

A. True
B. False

Review this! ❑

18. All of the following statements are true, except:

A. Asthma is a chronic inflammatory disorder of the airways.
B. Inflammation may result in acute infection, irreversible obstructive changes, and hyperresponsiveness to brompheniramine.
C. Pulmonary function testing is the gold standard of testing for the diagnosis and management of asthma.
D. Spirometry and the measurement of FEV_1 are extremely helpful for the diagnosis of asthma and for the assessment of airflow obstruction, respectively.

Review this! ❑

19. The diagnosis of asthma includes all of the following stages, except:

A. Suggestive symptoms referable to the chest with precipitating factors should raise the possibility of asthma.
B. Chest films (including PA and lateral views) revealing hyperexpansion of the lungs are diagnostic proof of asthma for a typical subject who has chest symptoms.
C. Further testing should be performed to confirm the diagnosis in the patient who has chest symptoms.
D. The patient should have symptomatic improvement with the appropriate asthma therapy.

Review this! ❑

20. All of the following statements are true, except:

A. It is helpful to use albuterol when performing spirometry. Improvement of FEV_1 by 12% or 200 mL after bronchodilator use suggests significant reversibility of the airway obstruction.
B. With the use of home peak flow meters, three zones are set on the meter using green, yellow, and red. The green zone is 70% to 90% of the personal best when the patient is in the recovery phase of an asthmatic attack.
C. Asthma is frequently found in the presence of atopic dermatitis in children.
D. The classification of asthma includes mild intermittent asthma, mild persistent asthma, moderate persistent asthma, and severe persistent asthma.

Review this! ❑

21. True or false: Mild persistent asthma is characterized by the intermittent use of inhaled corticosteroids and the regular use of short-acting β_2-agonists at least three times a week.

A. True
B. False

Review this! ❑

22. True or false: Moderate persistent asthma is defined as having daily symptoms of asthma requiring the daily use of bronchodilator medications, the development of asthmatic attacks that interfere with activity, nocturnal awakenings more than once per week, or a peak expiratory flow rate of 60% to 80% of normal.

A. True
B. False

Review this! ❏

A. True
B. False

Review this! ❏

23. True or false: Severe persistent asthma is defined when patients are awakened from sleep four to seven times per night; when they have frequent asthma exacerbations from their daily routines; when they have an FEV_1 below 60% of predicted; and when they are unable to achieve normal lung function despite appropriate treatment.

24. True or false: Exercise-induced broncho-spasm usually occurs within 5 to 10 minutes after stopping the physical activity, and it usually resolves completely within 5 minutes without treatment.

A. True
B. False

Review this! ❏

27 Parasitology

William F. Miser

1. Which of the following is not a principal factor responsible for the reemergence of parasitic diseases seen in developed countries?

   A. Improved methods of detection
   B. Increase in worldwide travel
   C. Increase in immunodeficiency as a result of the human immunodeficiency virus or iatrogenic causes
   D. Increased immigration

   Review this! ❏

2. Which of the following is the most common protozoan cause of enteritis?

   A. *Ascaris lumbricoides*
   B. *Entamoeba histolytica*
   C. *Enterobius vermicularis*
   D. *Giardia lamblia*
   E. *Toxoplasma gondii*

   Review this! ❏

3. Which of the following statements about the transmission of giardiasis is false?

   A. Transmission of infection is usually by water or food.
   B. *G. lamblia* cysts are sensitive to the low-level chlorination of water supplies and/or swimming pools.
   C. Day care centers are a major source of the spread of giardiasis.
   D. Groups at highest risk for giardiasis include infants and young children, travelers, and those who are immuno-compromised.

   Review this! ❏

4. Which of the following is usually not part of the spectrum of illness caused by giardiasis?

   A. Asymptomatic carrier state
   B. Acute nausea, vomiting, and fever
   C. Acute diarrhea with abdominal pain, flatulence, and lassitude
   D. Chronic diarrhea with malabsorption, steatorrhea, and weight loss

   Review this! ❏

5. Which one of the following statements about giardiasis is true?

   A. The average interval between infection and the development of symptoms is about 30 days.
   B. Most symptomatic patients will require treatment to resolve their illness.
   C. One of the first-line agents to treat giardiasis is tinidazole (Tindamax).
   D. Metronidazole (Flagyl) is approved by the U.S. Food and Drug Administration to treat giardiasis.

   Review this! ❏

6. Which of the following is the most common parasitic infection worldwide?

   A. *Ascaris lumbricoides*
   B. *Entamoeba histolytica*
   C. *Enterobius vermicularis*
   D. *Giardia lamblia*
   E. *Toxoplasma gondii*

   Review this! ❏

7. Which of the following is the most common cause of serious morbidity and mortality among people infected with ascariasis?

   A. Cognitive impairment as a result of infestation of the central nervous system
   B. Pneumonitis as a result of invasion of the trachea and pulmonary branches
   C. Obstruction of the biliary tree by a few adult worms
   D. Intestinal obstruction by large number of adult worms

   Review this! ❏

8. Which of the following is the best treatment for ascariasis?

Things to remember for the test.

A. Mebendazole (Vermox) 100 mg orally twice daily for 7 days
B. Mebendazole (Vermox) 500 mg orally once
C. Albendazole (Albenza) 400 mg orally twice daily for 7 days
D. Pyrantel pamoate (Antiminth) 1000 mg intravenously once

Review this! ❑

9. Which of the following is the most common cause of death from parasitic infection (after schistosomiasis and malaria)?

A. *Ascaris lumbricoides*
B. *Entamoeba histolytica*
C. *Enterobius vermicularis*
D. *Giardia lamblia*
E. *Toxoplasma gondii*

Review this! ❑

10. Which of the following parasites produces a classic "flask-shaped" ulcer?

A. *Ascaris lumbricoides*
B. *Entamoeba histolytica*
C. *Enterobius vermicularis*
D. *Giardia lamblia*
E. *Toxoplasma gondii*

Review this! ❑

11. You are providing care to a middle-aged man who just returned from a business trip to a developing country. He is currently febrile with right upper quadrant abdominal pain, leukocytosis, and abdominal tenderness on examination. Which of the following parasitic infections should you suspect as the cause of this illness?

A. *Ascaris lumbricoides*
B. *Entamoeba histolytica*
C. *Enterobius vermicularis*
D. *Giardia lamblia*
E. *Toxoplasma gondii*

Review this! ❑

12. Which of the following is not a recommended treatment for amebiasis?

A. Metronidazole (Flagyl) 750 mg orally three times a day for 5–10 days
B. Tinidazole (Tindamax) 800 mg orally three times a day for 5 days
C. Iodoquinol (Yodoxin) 650 mg orally three times a day for 5 days

D. Paromomycin (Humatin) 25–35 mg/kg per day divided three times daily for 5–10 days

Review this! ❑

13. Which of the following is the most common helminth infection in the developed world?

A. *Ascaris lumbricoides*
B. *Entamoeba histolytica*
C. *Enterobius vermicularis*
D. *Giardia lamblia*
E. *Toxoplasma gondii*

Review this! ❑

14. Which of the following populations are not at increased risk for enterobiasis?

A. Those living in poverty or who have a lower socioeconomic status
B. Children in day care
C. Institutionalized persons
D. Families with small children

Review this! ❑

15. Which of the following can be diagnosed by placing a piece of cellophane tape on perianal skin and then examining it under a microscope?

A. *Ascaris lumbricoides*
B. *Entamoeba histolytica*
C. *Enterobius vermicularis*
D. *Giardia lamblia*
E. *Toxoplasma gondii*

Review this! ❑

16. Which of the following statements about the treatment of enterobiasis is false?

A. Mebendazole (Vermox) 100–200 mg orally taken just one time is an effective treatment.
B. There is no need to treat family members or other close contacts unless they too are symptomatic.
C. Albendazole (Albenza) 200–400 mg orally taken just one time is an effective alternative treatment.
D. Thorough cleaning of bedding and clothing reduces the risk of transmission.

Review this! ❑

17. Which one of the following infections can be caused by ingesting raw or poorly prepared fish?

A. Anisakiasis
B. Ascariasis
C. Enterobiasis
D. Giardiasis
E. Trichinosis

Review this! ❑

18. Which one of the following methods will kill anisakid larvae in infected fish?

A. Freezing at −20°C for 24 hours
B. Salting
C. Smoking
D. Marinating

Review this! ❑

19. Which of the following statements about anisakiasis is false?

A. Symptoms may be severe enough to mimic a surgical abdomen.
B. Angioedema and anaphylaxis may occur.
C. Treatment with an antiparasitic is almost always required for cure.
D. Upper gastrointestinal endoscopy is usually necessary to confirm the diagnosis of gastric anisakiasis.

Review this! ❑

20. In which one of the following ways can a human become infected with babesiosis?

A. Mosquito bite
B. Tick bite
C. Consumption of raw fish
D. Walking barefoot on a sandy beach

Review this! ❑

21. Which of the following statements about babesiosis is false?

A. It is endemic to New England, along the Northeastern Seaboard.
B. Most cases occur during the winter and the spring.
C. It can be transmitted by transfusion.
D. Infection is usually asymptomatic.

Review this! ❑

22. Which of the following individuals is not at increased risk for severe babesiosis?

A. A 76-year-old woman
B. A 32-year-old man with a previous splenectomy
C. A 56-year-old man with coronary artery disease

D. A 35-year-old woman with rheumatoid arthritis who is taking steroids continually

Review this! ❑

23. Which of the following is the preferred treatment for most patients who are moderately or seriously ill with babesiosis?

A. Atovaquone (Mepron)
B. Exchange transfusion
C. Quinine
D. Clindamycin plus quinine

Review this! ❑

24. Which of the following can be transmitted by poor handwashing after cleaning infected cat litter?

A. *Ascaris lumbricoides*
B. *Entamoeba histolytica*
C. *Enterobius vermicularis*
D. *Giardia lamblia*
E. *Toxoplasma gondii*

Review this! ❑

25. Which of the following statements about toxoplasmosis is false?

A. Toxoplasma infections are usually asymptomatic.
B. The most common clinical presentation is self-limited focal tender adenopathy in the head and neck region.
C. More than 80% of newborns infected during pregnancy will eventually develop chorioretinitis, learning disabilities, or mental retardation.
D. A positive immunoglobulin G test for toxoplasmosis distinguishes an acute infection from a past infection.

Review this! ❑

26. True or false: Most infections from toxoplasmosis in immunocompetent and nonpregnant patients require no antimicrobial therapy.

A. True
B. False

Review this! ❑

27. You are counseling a woman who recently became pregnant. To avoid toxoplasmosis, she should do all of the following, except:

A. Thoroughly cook all meat that is eaten until it is no longer pink.
B. Wear gloves when working in the garden.
C. Avoid swimming in public pools.
D. Avoid changing cat litter.

Review this! ❏

28. What is the best treatment for cercarial dermatitis?

   A. Antihistamines and/or topical or oral corticosteroids
   B. Mebendazole (Vermox)
   C. Ivermectin (Stromectol)
   D. Pyrantel (Antiminth)

Review this! ❏

29. Which of the following statements about scabies is false?

   A. Children in day care and primary school are the principal route of entry into the family.
   B. Direct contact is the primary means of transmission.
   C. Poor hygiene is a major risk factor for the development of disease.
   D. Institutionalized individuals are at risk for infection.

Review this! ❏

30. You are seeing a young man who complains of intense itching, especially at night. On examination, you notice erythematous papules in the web spaces of his fingers, the flexor aspect of his wrist, the axilla, and along the belt line. What is your most likely diagnosis?

   A. Pediculosis
   B. Toxoplasmosis
   C. Amebiasis
   D. Scabies
   E. Schistosomiasis

Review this! ❏

31. What is drug of choice for the treatment of scabies?

   A. Mebendazole (Vermox)
   B. Ivermectin (Stromectol)
   C. Gamma benzene hexachloride 1% (lindane, Kwell)
   D. Permethrin 5% (Elimite)

Review this! ❏

32. Which of the following statements about scabies is false?

   A. Symptoms may persist for several weeks after successful treatment.
   B. All clothing, bedding, cloth toys, and dolls that the patient has used during the prior 4 days should be washed with hot water and dried in a hot dryer for 10 minutes.
   C. Children need to wait for symptoms to resolve before they can return to day care or school.
   D. Reinfection may occur if one fails to treat all physical contacts and family members, even if they are asymptomatic.

Review this! ❏

33. Which of the following statements about pediculosis is false?

   A. Head lice are transmitted by direct head-to-head contact.
   B. Body lice are transmitted via contact with infested clothing, bedding, towels, or cloth-covered seats.
   C. Pubic lice are transmitted by physical and sexual contact.
   D. All three forms of lice can serve as vectors, carrying epidemic typhus.

Review this! ❏

28 Travel Medicine

George C. Wortley

1. Which of the following groups of overseas travelers would be the least likely to receive preventive medical services for travel-related medical problems?

   A. Peace Corps volunteers
   B. Military personnel
   C. Immigrants visiting friends and relatives
   D. Medical missionaries

   Review this! ❏

2. Which of the following is the most common health problem that affects travelers?

   A. Diarrhea
   B. Malaria
   C. Acquired immunodeficiency syndrome
   D. Febrile illness

   Review this! ❏

3. Which of the following is the most common cause of death among travelers?

   A. Infectious diseases
   B. Cardiovascular events
   C. Natural disasters
   D. Airplane crashes

   Review this! ❏

4. The goal of the pretravel consultation includes all of the following, except:

   A. Stabilizing current medical problems
   B. Giving appropriate immunizations
   C. Giving advice about disease prevention
   D. Screening for infectious diseases

   Review this! ❏

5. Which of the following is the ideal time for a pretravel consultation?

   A. 6 months before travel
   B. 6 weeks before travel
   C. 1 week before travel
   D. 1 day before travel

   Review this! ❏

6. An excellent and up-to-date source of health information for travelers may be obtained from which of the following?

   A. A travel agent
   B. A textbook of tropical medicine
   C. The Centers for Disease Control and Prevention (www.cdc.gov/travel)
   D. The tourism bureau of the destination country

   Review this! ❏

7. Pregnant patients should be discouraged from traveling after how many weeks' gestation?

   A. 12 weeks
   B. 24 weeks
   C. 32 weeks
   D. 36 weeks

   Review this! ❏

8. Altitude illnesses can be seen among travelers going to destinations with altitudes as low as which of the following?

   A. 4000 feet
   B. 8000 feet
   C. 12,000 feet
   D. 16,000 feet

   Review this! ❏

9. In addition to gradual acclimatization, effective measures to prevent altitude illness include which of the following?

   A. Acetazolamide (Diamox) begun 1 day before travel
   B. Furosemide (Lasix) begun the day of travel
   C. Alcohol
   D. Multivitamin with an iron supplement

   Review this! ❏

10. If symptoms of high-altitude cerebral edema occur, treatment may include all of the following, except:

Things to remember for the test.

Things to remember for the test.

A. A descent to a lower altitude.
B. Supplemental oxygen.
C. Dexamethasone.
D. Morphine.

Review this! ❏

11. Chloroquine is the drug of choice for malaria for which of the following situations?

   A. Patients who are allergic to mefloquine
   B. Patients with glucose-6-phosphate dehydrogenase (G6PD) deficiency
   C. Areas in which the malaria parasite is sensitive to chloroquine
   D. Patients with retinopathy

Review this! ❏

12. In areas with chloroquine-resistant *Plasmodium falciparum* malaria (CRPF), drugs effective as prophylaxis include all the following, except:

   A. Chloramphenicol.
   B. Doxycycline.
   C. Atovaquone/proguanil (Malarone).
   D. Mefloquine.

Review this! ❏

13. Which of the following antimalarials is started the day before travel and taken daily through 1 week after the return from the malarial area?

   A. Chloroquine
   B. Atovaquone/proguanil (Malarone)
   C. Mefloquine
   D. Doxycycline

Review this! ❏

14. Which of the following antimalarials requires that a G6PD level be obtained to prevent a fatal hemolysis?

   A. Chloroquine
   B. Atovaquone/proguanil (Malarone)
   C. Mefloquine
   D. Primaquine

Review this! ❏

15. Standby emergency treatment for malaria includes all of the following, except:

   A. Mefloquine.
   B. Atovaquone/proguanil (Malarone).
   C. Quinine-doxycycline.
   D. Pyrimethamine/sulfadoxine (Fansidar).

Review this! ❏

16. Which of the following is one of the most underused, safe, and effective means of preventing mosquito bites?

   A. DEET-based insect repellants
   B. Permethrin clothing spray
   C. DDT-based insecticides
   D. Screened or air-conditioned hotels

Review this! ❏

17. True or false: A single booster vaccine of poliomyelitis is currently recommended for adult travelers to countries in West Africa and South Asia, where wild-type polio transmission is still occurring.

   A. True
   B. False

Review this! ❏

18. With regard to the yellow fever vaccine, all of the following are true, except:

   A. It is safe for use during pregnancy.
   B. It can only be administered at certain official, registered centers.
   C. It is required for entry into many tropical countries.
   D. An intramuscular booster dose is needed every 10 years.

Review this! ❏

19. Which of the following statements about the hepatitis A vaccine is true?

   A. It is not generally recommended for travelers to third-world countries.
   B. It is only 50% effective after the first dose.
   C. It is given at least 2 weeks before travel.
   D. It is contraindicated during pregnancy.

Review this! ❏

20. Which of the following is the most common cause of traveler's diarrhea?

   A. Viruses
   B. Salmonella
   C. Preformed toxins
   D. Enterotoxigenic *Escherichia coli*

Review this! ❏

21. Recommended methods to prevent traveler's diarrhea include which of the following?

A. Antibiotic prophylaxis
B. Consuming only iced alcoholic drinks
C. Drinking purified water or bottled carbonated water
D. Consuming only fresh vegetables

Review this! ❏

22. Recommended self-treatment for persistent and distressing diarrhea includes loperamide plus which of the following?

A. Ciprofloxin for 3 days in adults
B. Ofloxin in children
C. Doxycycline in pregnant women
D. Metronidazole

Review this! ❏

23. The World Health Organization recommends screening for tropical diseases in which of the following groups?

A. All children who have spent more than 1 month in a developing country
B. Travelers with cardiovascular disease, diabetes, or chronic obstructive pulmonary disease
C. All women of childbearing age
D. Asymptomatic short-term travelers

Review this! ❏

24. Overseas health care workers should be screened on their return for which of the following?

A. Hepatitis C
B. Parasites
C. Tuberculosis
D. Human immunodeficiency virus

Review this! ❏

25. Fever in a traveler returning from the tropics should start an urgent work up for which of the following?

A. Intestinal parasites
B. Malaria
C. Ciguatera poisoning
D. Cutaneous leishmaniasis

Review this! ❏

26. Conjunctival suffusion may be seen in which of the following?

A. Leptospirosis
B. Dengue fever
C. Yellow fever
D. Malaria

Review this! ❏

27. For a recently returned traveler with persistent diarrhea, abdominal pain, cough, eosinophilia and repeatedly negative stool analysis, the work-up should include testing for which of the following?

A. Giardia
B. *Clostridium difficile*
C. *Helicobacter pylori*
D. Strongyloides

Review this! ❏

28. A nonhealing skin ulcer on the face, arms, or legs of a returned traveler should raise suspicion for which of the following?

A. Cutaneous leishmaniasis
B. Lyme disease
C. Scabies
D. Cutaneous larva migrans

Review this! ❏

29. Travel-related diseases that may be prevented with doxycycline prophylaxis include all the following, except:

A. Malaria.
B. Chagas disease.
C. Leptospirosis.
D. Cholera.

Review this! ❏

30. Which if the following vaccines may not be used during pregnancy?

A. Hepatitis A
B. Meningococcus
C. Measles
D. Tetanus and diphtheria

Review this! ❏

29 Obstetrics

Bill G. Gegas

1. Which of the following countries has the highest infant mortality rate?

   A. Japan
   B. Scandinavian countries
   C. Canada
   D. United States

   Review this! ❑

2. How much folic acid supplementation should be taken by women who are high risk for having a child with neural tube defects or who have had a previous child with a neural tube defect?

   A. 0.4 mg/day
   B. 400 mg/day
   C. 4 g/day
   D. 4 mg/day

   Review this! ❑

3. Prenatal screening for neural tube defects of the fetus and karyotypic abnormalities is best obtained at what time during the pregnancy?

   A. During the first trimester, at approximately 6 to 8 weeks' gestation
   B. During the second trimester, at approximately 16 to 18 weeks' gestation
   C. During the third trimester, at approximately 34 to 36 weeks' gestation
   D. During preconception counseling

   Review this! ❑

4. Which of the following is the most common reason for inconsistency between menstrual age and fundal height?

   A. Inaccurate menstrual age assignment and inaccurate measurements as a result of maternal obesity
   B. Uterine fibroids
   C. Multiple gestation
   D. Fetal demise

   Review this! ❑

5. In 2002, the Centers for Disease Control and Prevention recommended a strategy of vaginal-rectal cultures for group B streptococcal colonization that involves which of the following?

   A. Risk-based screening at 25 to 27 weeks' gestation
   B. Universal screening at 25 to 27 weeks' gestation
   C. Risk-based screening at 35 to 37 weeks' gestation
   D. Universal screening at 35 to 37 weeks' gestation

   Review this! ❑

6. The U.S. Food and Drug Administration has developed a risk factors index to help the practitioner classify a drug for use in pregnant women. According to this index, a drug classified as Category X indicates which of the following?

   A. There are no controlled studies in pregnant women or animals regarding the drug's effects.
   B. The drug should be given only if the potential benefit clearly justifies the potential risk to the fetus.
   C. There is positive evidence of human fetal risk, but the benefits of use may be acceptable.
   D. Studies in animals or human beings have demonstrated fetal abnormalities, or there is evidence of fetal risk based on human experience. The drug is contraindicated in women who are or who may become pregnant.

   Review this! ❑

7. Which of the following is the strongest predictor of the safety of vaginal birth after Cesarean delivery?

A. The location of the previous uterine scar
B. The use of oxytocin
C. Fetal macrosomia
D. Gestation beyond 40 weeks

Review this! ❏

8. Which of the following is the most serious consequence of human immunodeficiency virus (HIV) infection during pregnancy?

A. Congenital HIV syndrome abnormalities, including cataracts and chorioretinitis
B. Congenital hearing loss
C. Increases in miscarriages, hydrops fetalis, stillborn, and preterm deliveries
D. Transmission to the fetus

Review this! ❏

9. Which medication is contraindicated for the treatment of hypertension during pregnancy?

A. Alpha-methyldopa
B. Labetalol
C. Nifedipine
D. Diuretics

Review this! ❏

10. Screening for gestational diabetes is recommended at 26 to 28 weeks' gestation. The initial screening test is performed under which of the following circumstances?

A. In a fasting state using 50 g of glucose
B. In a non-fasting state using 50 g of glucose
C. In a fasting state using 100 g of glucose
D. In a non-fasting state using 100 g of glucose

Review this! ❏

11. What percentage of pregnant women will have asymptomatic bacteriuria?

A. 3%–5%
B. 15%–25%
C. 40%–50%
D. 75%–80%

Review this! ❏

12. Which of the following tests is not used for the identification and management of women with ectopic pregnancies?

A. Serum progesterone
B. Alpha-fetoprotein
C. Human chorionic gonadotropin
D. Vaginal ultrasound

Review this! ❏

13. The initial treatment of preterm labor may include all of the following, except:

A. Betamethasone.
B. Magnesium sulfate.
C. Calcium gluconate.
D. Ritodrine.

Review this! ❏

14. Which of the following is the most beneficial treatment modality for intrauterine growth restriction?

A. Long-term intravenous hydration
B. Prophylactic antibiotics
C. Bedrest in a lateral recumbent position
D. Genetic testing

Review this! ❏

15. Preeclampsia can progress to a HELLP syndrome, which involves all of the following, except:

A. Microangiopathic anemia.
B. Increases in transaminase and lactic dehydrogenase enzymes.
C. Lumbar puncture.
D. Decrements in the platelet count.

Review this! ❏

16. Which of the following statement about abruptio placenta is false?

A. Painful vaginal bleeding during the first trimester is characteristic.
B. Cocaine use is a risk factor.
C. Ultrasonography has a high false-negative rate.
D. Uterine or back pain is a common feature.

Review this! ❏

17. Which of the following statements about placenta previa is true?

A. It is most commonly the result of abnormalities in uterine anatomy, and it is usually diagnosed when the patient complains of painful vaginal bleeding.
B. It usually resolves spontaneously by term.
C. It is not usually seen by ultrasound until the third trimester.

Review this! ❏

Things to remember for the test.

Things to remember for the test.

18. Which of the following is the name given to a minimally invasive placenta that may be removed manually or by curettage?

    A. Placenta accreta
    B. Placenta increta
    C. Placenta percreta
    D. Low-lying placenta

    Review this! ❑

19. Women with a twin gestation are at higher risk for which of the following?

    A. Placenta previa
    B. Pyelonephritis
    C. Pregnancy-induced hypertension
    D. All of the above

    Review this! ❑

20. Which of the following is an assessment of fetal well-being used for antepartum fetal surveillance that includes ultrasound?

    A. Biophysical profile
    B. Nonstress test
    C. Contraction stress test
    D. Vibroacoustic stimulation test

    Review this! ❑

21. Which of the following medications should not be used in hypertensive women to control postpartum bleeding?

    A. Intramuscular oxytocin
    B. Intravenous oxytocin
    C. Intramuscular methylergonovine
    D. Intramuscular prostaglandin F_2-alpha

    Review this! ❑

22. Which of the following statements about cervical ripening and the induction of labor is false?

    A. With term premature rupture of membranes, labor may be induced with prostaglandins.
    B. In women with prior Cesarean section deliveries or uterine surgery, low-dose misoprostol should be used.
    C. Women in whom the induction of labor is indicated may be managed with either low- or high-dose oxytocin.
    D. Prostaglandin E analogues are effective for promoting cervical ripening and inducing labor.

    Review this! ❑

23. The prolonged latent phase of labor can be managed by which of the following?

    A. Avoidance of sedation
    B. Early amniotomy
    C. Oxytocin induction
    D. Cesarean section

    Review this! ❑

24. The interval between the complete dilatation of the cervix to the delivery of the infant is defined as which of the following?

    A. The first stage of labor
    B. The second stage of labor
    C. The third stage of labor
    D. The fourth stage of labor

    Review this! ❑

25. Which of the following statements about shoulder dystocia is true?

    A. Klumpke's palsy is the most common brachial plexus injury.
    B. Shoulder dystocia is defined as the impaction of the biparietal diameter of the fetal head against the pubic symphysis.
    C. Approximately one half of all shoulder dystocias occur in normal-weight fetuses and are unanticipated.
    D. Shoulder dystocia should be treated conservatively, including allowing maternal rest.

    Review this! ❑

26. All of the following maneuvers can be used during the management of shoulder dystocia, except:

    A. Flexion of the maternal thighs onto the abdomen.
    B. Suprapubic pressure.
    C. Fundal pressure.
    D. Cephalic replacement of the fetus.

    Review this! ❑

27. Which of the following statements about electronic fetal monitoring (EFM) is true?

    A. EFM is accurate and predictive of a bad outcome.
    B. EFM is not predictive of a good outcome.
    C. EFM has been recommended by the U.S. Preventative Services Task Force for routine use for the management of low-risk deliveries.
    D. EFM appears to have no inherent benefit over properly performed auscultation among low-risk women.

    Review this! ❑

28. Which of the following statements about fetal tachycardia of more than 200 bpm is true?

    A. It is seldom the result of fetal hypoxia.
    B. It is usually the result of fetal hypoxia.
    C. It is usually the result of maternal anxiety.
    D. It is usually the result of maternal fever.

    Review this! ❏

29. Which of the following statements about early fetal heart rate decelerations is true?

    A. They are considered reassuring, and they are associated with a good outcome.
    B. They have a variable relationship with contractions.
    C. They are usually associated with umbilical cord compression.
    D. They are characterized by an acute fall in the fetal heart rate with a rapid down slope and a variable recovery.

    Review this! ❏

30. Normal changes that occur in the mother during the postpartum period or the puerperium include all of the following, except:

    A. A drop in the pulse rate.
    B. An increase in temperature.
    C. A leukocytosis level of up to 20,000.
    D. Bleeding that results in hemodynamic instability.

    Review this! ❏

Things to remember for the test.

30 Care of the Newborn

David S. Gregory

Things to remember for the test.

1. Which of the following statements about perinatal group B streptococcus (GBS) recommendations is true?

   A. Routine maternal GBS screening significantly reduces early-onset neonatal GBS infections.
   B. Only women with a prior history of having a child with serious GBS disease should receive intrapartum antibiotics.
   C. GBS-exposed neonates do not need to be observed for 48 hours after discharge.
   D. The gestational age of a GBS-exposed neonate does not affect recommendations for neonatal evaluation.

   Review this! ❏

2. Preconceptual counseling recommendations include all of the following, except:

   A. Oral folic acid supplementation reduces the risk of neural tube defects.
   B. Women who have had a child with a neural tube defect should take 400 µg of folic acid per day.
   C. Women of childbearing age should be counseled about their risks for genetic diseases, such as cystic fibrosis.
   D. Substances of abuse, including tobacco and alcohol, should be eliminated.

   Review this! ❏

3. True or false: Routine endotracheal intubation with tracheal suctioning in vigorous neonates born with thick, meconium-stained amniotic fluid does not prevent meconium aspiration syndrome.

   A. True
   B. False

   Review this! ❏

4. Which of the following statements about the initial newborn examination is false?

   A. A comprehensive examination should be completed after the first 12 to 18 hours of life.
   B. The infant should be kept in a comfortable environment to observe activity, color, and respiratory effort.
   C. Maternal and prenatal histories should be obtained for every patient.
   D. A systematic examination of each system while the infant is calm is important.

   Review this! ❏

5. All of the following are examples of common benign findings from the newborn examination, except:

   A. Macular hemangiomas.
   B. Periodic breathing.
   C. Asymmetric limb movement.
   D. Fine pulmonary crackles.

   Review this! ❏

6. True or false: Infants should regain the weight they lose during the first few days by the time they are 2 weeks old.

   A. True
   B. False

   Review this! ❏

7. Which of the following interventions that can be made during neonatal resuscitation is the least commonly used?

   A. Positioning and clearing the airway
   B. Stimulating the infant to breathe
   C. Positive-pressure ventilation
   D. Epinephrine

   Review this! ❏

8. True or false: Apgar scoring helps to guide intervention during neonatal resuscitation.

   A. True
   B. False

   Review this! ❏

9. Which of the following statements about Apgar scores is true?

   A. Neonatal asphyxia is diagnosed with a 5-minute Apgar score of less than 7.
   B. Apgar scores of less than 7 at 5 minutes correlate with an increased risk of neonatal death.
   C. More than half of infants with 5-minute Apgar scores of less than 4 die within 28 days.
   D. One-minute Apgar scores are more predictive of outcomes than 5-minute Apgar scores.

   Review this! ❏

10. Ill neonates can present with all of the following signs or symptoms, except:

    A. Hypothermia.
    B. Grunting.
    C. Periodic breathing.
    D. Jaundice.
    E. Bradycardia.

    Review this! ❏

11. Which of the following statements about congenital hearing loss screening in the neonate is false?

    A. Universal screening programs are mandated in 35 states.
    B. The U.S. Preventive Services Task Force found sufficient evidence to recommend universal screening.
    C. Infants who fail a screening program should be promptly referred to a pediatric audiologist for further diagnostic testing.
    D. Currently, there are three screening tests available to detect congenital hearing loss.

    Review this! ❏

12. Which of the following statements about GBS sepsis is true?

    A. It presents with symptoms such as tachypnea, grunting, and poor feeding,
    B. It is an uncommon cause of neonatal mortality in the United States.
    C. An intervention for potential GBS sepsis involves a simple 2-day observation period to determine if treatment is needed.
    D. It is unpredictable and unpreventable.

    Review this! ❏

13. Which of the following would not explain tachypnea in a newborn?

    A. Respiratory distress syndrome
    B. Sepsis
    C. Transient tachypnea of the newborn
    D. Pneumonia
    E. Hyperbilirubinemia

    Review this! ❏

14. Which of the following statements about respiratory distress syndrome (sometimes called hyaline membrane disease) is true?

    A. It can be seen in infants of diabetic mothers delivered at 37 weeks' gestation.
    B. It presents immediately after birth with cyanosis.
    C. It cannot be easily distinguished from GBS sepsis in the preterm infant.
    D. It cannot be prevented.

    Review this! ❏

15. Which of the following statements about congenital pneumonia and meconium aspiration syndrome is false?

    A. They are associated with one another.
    B. Antibiotic treatment is unnecessary.
    C. Intubation may be required.
    D. Persistent pulmonary hypertension may subsequently develop.

    Review this! ❏

16. Which of the following statements about transient tachypnea of the newborn is true?

    A. It is the least common cause of tachypnea in the term newborn.
    B. It is caused by the newborn's nervous system slowly adjusting to breathing air.
    C. It starts up to 72 hours after birth.
    D. It is difficult to distinguish from other causes of tachypnea soon after birth.

    Review this! ❏

17. Which of the following statements about an infant with significant congenital heart disease is true?

    A. The infant will have an audible murmur.
    B. The infant will have an increase in pO_2 to more than 150 mm Hg on 100% oxygen.
    C. There is no need to transfer the infant to a neonatal intensive care unit.
    D. The infant will not require echocardiography.

    Review this! ❏

Things to remember for the test.

Things to remember for the test.

18. Which of the following statements about infantile hypoglycemia is true?

    A. Term infants do not develop hypoglycemia.
    B. Plasma glucose levels of less than 36 mg/dL are generally considered abnormal.
    C. Hypoglycemia is encountered within the first hour of life.
    D. Whole blood glucose testing using finger or heel sticks typically yields higher results than plasma levels.

    Review this! ❏

19. The following infants are at high risk for hypoglycemia, except:

    A. Infants of diabetic mothers.
    B. Small-for-gestational-age infants.
    C. Hypothermic infants.
    D. Large-for-gestational-age infants.

    Review this! ❏

20. Which of the following infants is least likely to develop hypoglycemia?

    A. A small-for-gestational-age infant delivered via Cesarean section as a result of nonreassuring fetal heart tracing
    B. A full-term, healthy, appropriate-for-gestational-age infant with concerns about "jitteriness"
    C. An actively breastfeeding, preterm, healthy, large-for-gestational-age infant with normal behavior and vital signs
    D. A septic infant with tachypnea

    Review this! ❏

21. Which of the following statements about treating hypoglycemia in newborns is true?

    A. Intravenous glucose is favored for all infants.
    B. Breastfed infants should be offered formula.
    C. The dosage of intravenous glucose depends on pretreatment serum glucose levels.
    D. The monitoring of post-treatment serum glucose levels is not required.

    Review this! ❏

22. Which of the following statements about newborn infants of diabetic mothers is true?

    A. They have perinatal mortality and morbidity rates similar to infants born to nondiabetic mothers.
    B. They may have a variety of birth-trauma–related injuries.
    C. They are rarely born smaller than gestational age.
    D. They tend to be anemic.

    Review this! ❏

23. Conditions that are of increased risk to an infant of a diabetic mother include all of the following, except:

    A. Respiratory distress syndrome.
    B. Congenital heart disease.
    C. Central nervous system anomalies.
    D. Hyperbilirubinemia.
    E. Umbilical hernia.

    Review this! ❏

24. Which of the following statements about neonatal hyperbilirubinemia is true?

    A. It can be caused by an increased clearance of blood pigment from the body.
    B. It is a common cause for readmission during the first week of life.
    C. It is not a particular concern for permanent neurologic disability.
    D. The determination of its severity does not require measuring serum or transcutaneous bilirubin.

    Review this! ❏

25. When neonatal hyperbilirubinemia is identified, the American Academy of Pediatrics recommends which of the following?

    A. Interpreting bilirubin levels on the basis of the infant's age in days
    B. Phototherapy if bilirubin levels exceed 15 mg/dL
    C. Determining the risk for severe hyperbilirubinemia before discharge based on risk factors
    D. Switching to bottle feeding for breastfed infants

    Review this! ❏

26. All of the following may explain asymmetric movement of the hands in a newborn, except:

    A. Clavicle fractures.
    B. Erb's palsy.
    C. Cervical spinal cord injury.
    D. Cephalohematoma.

    Review this! ❏

27. All of the following should be provided for the hospitalized breastfeeding mother, except:

    A. Assistance with holding the baby at the breast and establishing a good latch-on.
    B. Reassurance that normal newborns do not require supplementation unless there is a medical indication.
    C. Initial follow-up with the adequately breastfed infant at about 1 week of age.
    D. Trained observation to help correct breastfeeding problems before discharge.

    Review this! ❏

28. To reduce sudden infant death syndrome risk, caretakers of newborns should be instructed with regard to the following, except:

    A. "Back to sleep."
    B. Use a firm crib mattress without a quilt.
    C. Avoid pacifier use.
    D. Avoid co-bedding.

    Review this! ❏

29. Safety recommendations regarding infants discharged to their caretakers include all of the following, except:

    A. Insure proper car seat fit, installation, and location.
    B. A soaking bath in more than 3 inches of water is best.
    C. Never shake your baby.
    D. Return for immediate evaluation if fever occurs.

    Review this! ❏

30. When discussing the circumcision of infant males with their parents, it is important to explain which of the following?

    A. There are medical indications for neo-natal circumcision.
    B. The biggest risk of circumcision is bleeding.
    C. Uncircumcised newborn penises are more difficult to care for.
    D. No anesthesia is needed.

    Review this! ❏

Things to remember for the test.

119

31 Growth and Development

Daniel L. Stulberg

1. True or false: Growth in children after the embryonic phase is solely the result of increasing cell size.

   A. True
   B. False

   Review this! ❏

2. There has been a long debate regarding the effects of nature versus nurture. Which of the following influences a child's psychological and physiologic development?

   A. Nutrition
   B. Family
   C. Community
   D. All of the above

   Review this! ❏

3. Head circumference should be routinely obtained until what age?

   A. 1 year
   B. 18 months
   C. 2 years
   D. 3 years

   Review this! ❏

4. True or false: The fragile X syndrome is associated with microcephaly.

   A. True
   B. False

   Review this! ❏

5. Premature infants should have their growth parameters adjusted on the basis of gestational age until what age?

   A. 1 year
   B. 18 months
   C. 2 years
   D. 3 years

   Review this! ❏

6. True or false: Infant growth proceeds in a constant, continuous, gradual way.

   A. True
   B. False

   Review this! ❏

7. True or false: Children with genetic short stature usually have normal length and weight at birth.

   A. True
   B. False

   Review this! ❏

8. Of the following, which is the most useful test when short stature is a concern?

   A. Complete blood cell count
   B. Magnetic resonance imaging of the brain, with attention given to the pituitary
   C. Femur length for achondroplasia
   D. Bone-age radiograph of the hand

   Review this! ❏

9. Among patients with constitutional growth delay, which of the following is true?

   A. Bone age is more advanced than chronological age.
   B. Bone age is behind chronological age.
   C. The child's growth potential is better than if the bone age equals the chronological age.
   D. A and B
   E. B and C

   Review this! ❏

10. Which of the following are the correct general average ages for the onset of puberty in the United States?

    A. Girls, 8; Boys, 10
    B. Girls, 9; Boys, 13
    C. Girls, 10; Boys, 10
    D. Girls, 9; Boys, 11

    Review this! ❏

11. The clinician should evaluate for precocious puberty if onset occurs before which of the following ages?

    A. Girls, 8; Boys, 9
    B. Girls, 9; Boys, 11
    C. Girls, 10; Boys, 10
    D. Girls, 7; Boys, 11

    Review this! ❏

12. Which of the following is the average growth in height for girls after the onset of menarche?

    A. 2 cm
    B. 4 cm
    C. 6 cm
    D. 8 cm

    Review this! ❏

13. True or false: Infant formulas contain less protein than breast milk.

    A. True
    B. False

    Review this! ❏

14. Whole cow's milk is not appropriate for infants less than 12 months old for which of the following reasons?

    A. Higher renal solute load as compared with breast milk
    B. Lower concentration of iron as compared with breast milk
    C. Intestinal blood loss may occur
    D. All of the above

    Review this! ❏

15. Which of the following statements is incorrect?

    A. Solid foods may be introduced at the age of 4 to 6 months.
    B. When first introduced, foods should have only a single ingredient, and they should be tried for a week at a time.
    C. Honey may be introduced as a sweetener at the age of 6 months.
    D. Rice cereal can be a source of fortified iron.

    Review this! ❏

16. True or false: Vitamin deficiency is a concern among children who are following a strict vegetarian diet.

    A. True
    B. False

    Review this! ❏

17. True or false: Starting at the age of 8 years, all children should be screened for hypercholesterolemia.

    A. True
    B. False

    Review this! ❏

18. True or false: Temperament is a result of the resolution of a series of crises at discrete life stages (Erikson's psychosocial stages theory).

    A. True
    B. False

    Review this! ❏

19. Which of the following statements about "neurodevelopmental rules of thumb" is false?

    A. Children acquire developmental tasks in a predictable sequence.
    B. A delay in one developmental area should not prevent the astute practitioner from assessing delays in other areas.
    C. Children's responses progress from generalized reflex actions to discrete, cortically controlled actions.
    D. Development proceeds in a cephalocaudad and proximal-to-distal order.

    Review this! ❏

20. Which of the following statements about developmental screening is false?

    A. Clinical impression alone is a reasonable screening tool for developmental delay.
    B. All children with language delay should have a formal audiologic assessment to rule out hearing impairment.
    C. Parental report is a reliable way to identify children who are in need of further developmental assessment.
    D. It is a federal law that a physician refer children with suspected delays for further evaluation.

    Review this! ❏

21. All of the following are red flags for immediate evaluation for developmental delay, except:

    A. No babbling at 12 months.
    B. Loss of social skills at any age.
    C. No pointing at 12 months.
    D. Not walking at 13 months.

    Review this! ❏

Things to remember for the test.

Things to remember for the test.

22. Which of the following statements about developmental delay is true?

    A. The estimated prevalence is 2.5%, which is based on two standard deviations from the mean.
    B. The prevalence of autism is stable based on historical data and across cultures.
    C. Autistic children do not usually get diagnosed based on a presenting complaint of focusing on an aspect or portion of a toy or item instead of the entire item or its use.
    D. The diagnosis of global developmental delay requires significant delays in all aspects of development rather than just in a minimum of two areas.

    Review this! ❏

23. Which of the following statements about the Individuals with Disabilities Act is true?

    A. If a child is suspected of having a learning disability, then his or her school is required to evaluate the child free of charge upon request.
    B. The Multi-Factored Evaluation must be performed within a reasonable time-frame.
    C. If the child is eligible, special education services may be provided in the regular classroom.
    D. All of the above

    Review this! ❏

24. True or false: A child with a fever of 100.3°F should be advised to return at a later date for routine immunizations.

    A. True
    B. False

    Review this! ❏

25. True or false: Some families or clinicians are concerned about the number of injections that may occur at one time. There may be a problem with administering some of the routine vaccines at one visit and then having the child return in a week or two to get the other recommended vaccines.

    A. True
    B. False

    Review this! ❏

26. Which of the following statements about childhood immunizations is false?

    A. Most vaccines can be administered simultaneously at separate sites.
    B. Premature infants should receive their immunizations based on chronological age rather than adjusted age.
    C. A missed immunization visit does not require starting the series over.
    D. If a parent is concerned, the dose of a vaccine can be reduced as long as the total amount given over the series is the same.

    Review this! ❏

27. True or false: The safety levels of the oral polio vaccine and of the inactivated polio vaccine are equivalent, but the use of inactivated vaccine is more common as a result of the lower cost per dose.

    A. True
    B. False

    Review this! ❏

28. Which of the following statements about *Haemophilus influenza* type b (Hib) conjugate vaccine is false?

    A. Invasive Hib disease has only been modestly reduced; the real gain is in the reduction of otitis media.
    B. Healthy children between the ages of 15 and 59 months should have one dose of Hib vaccine.
    C. After the age of 60 months, healthy children are generally not vaccinated for Hib.
    D. Children with immune system defects or who are at higher risk of infection should be immunized for Hib, even if they present after 15 months without previous Hib vaccination.

    Review this! ❏

29. True or false: Pertussis vaccines confer life-long immunity, so no booster doses or vaccinations are recommended after the age of 5 years.

    A. True
    B. False

    Review this! ❏

30. A hepatitis vaccination should be given within how long of birth to the child of a mother who is known to have tested positive for hepatitis B surface antigen?

    A. 2 hours
    B. 6 hours
    C. 12 hours
    D. Before discharge

    Review this! ❏

31. Which of the following statements about the dosing of the pneumococcal conjugate vaccine, which is 90% effective for the prevention of invasive pneumococcal disease, is true?

    A. An 8-month-old child should get three doses.
    B. Starting at the age of 2 months, a child should receive four doses.
    C. A high-risk child who is 4 years old should receive two doses.
    D. All of the above

    Review this! ❏

32. Which of the following statements about the two meningococcal vaccines available in the United States (MCV4 and MPSV4) is false?

    A. The conjugate meningococcal vaccine should prevent almost all common types of meningitis.
    B. College students living in dormitories are at a higher risk for meningitis than those living off campus.
    C. Opportune times for administering the meningococcal vaccine are at a preadolescent visit or before high-school entry.
    D. The meningococcal vaccine should be given to travelers going to sub-Saharan Africa and to Mecca during the Hajj.

    Review this! ❏

Things to remember for the test.

32 Childhood and Adolescence

Ann M. Aring

1. Which of the following are the most common types of accidents that result in childhood fatalities?

   A. Falls from playground equipment
   B. Motor vehicle accidents
   C. Fires and burns
   D. Drowning

   Review this! ❏

2. Which method of birth control has the lowest likelihood of continued use among adolescent females?

   A. Oral contraceptive pills
   B. Condoms
   C. Diaphragm
   D. Injectable medroxyprogesterone acetate (Depo-Provera)

   Review this! ❏

3. Determine whether each statement below is true or false. Best evidence recommendations regarding screening for disease among healthy children include:

   (1) Only children with dietary risk factors need to be screened for iron-deficiency anemia.
   (2) Lead screening should only be performed for high-risk children at the ages of 9 months and 24 months.
   (3) Routine urinalysis may be used to screen for disease.
   (4) Children more than 2 years old with a family history of early heart disease should receive cholesterol screening.

   A. True
   B. False

   Review this! ❏

4. Which of the following is the most common viral agent associated with gastroenteritis in infants and young children?

   A. Norwalk virus
   B. Coxsackie virus
   C. Adenovirus
   D. Rotavirus

   Review this! ❏

5. All of the following are true about the diagnosis of failure to thrive, except:

   A. Children whose weight falls below the third or fifth percentile for age are more likely to receive this diagnosis.
   B. Children whose growth declines and crosses two major growth percentiles during a short period of time are more likely to receive this diagnosis.
   C. Failure to thrive is a common diagnosis in children over 12 months.
   D. Appropriate dietary changes should be suggested.

   Review this! ❏

Questions 6–8: For each numbered disease process below, match the physical examination finding that is most closely associated with it. Each choice may be used once, more than once, or not at all.

6. Croup
7. Bronchiolitis
8. Pneumonia

   A. Rales
   B. Expiratory wheezing
   C. Hoarseness

   Review this! ❏

9. All of the following are true about Osgood–Schlatter disease, except:

   A. Pain is aggravated by running and jumping activities.
   B. X-rays are not needed for the diagnosis.
   C. Ice applied to the area before and after activity may provide relief.
   D. Females are more commonly affected than males.

   Review this! ❏

10. Which one of the following medications should be used for the first-line treatment of chronic asthma in children?

    A. Inhaled corticosteroids
    B. Oral theophylline
    C. An oral β₂-agonist
    D. Inhaled ipratropium bromide (Atrovent)

    Review this! ❑

11. Which of the following is the first sign of puberty in a normal male?

    A. The appearance of facial hair
    B. The appearance of pubic hair
    C. Testicular enlargement
    D. A growth spurt

    Review this! ❑

12. A 6-month-old male is brought to your office by his mother for the evaluation of fever and poor feeding. The child has a rectal temperature of 39°C. His physical examination does not reveal the source of the fever. Reasonable diagnostic testing includes which of the following?

    A. A urine culture
    B. A complete blood cell count and a blood culture
    C. A chest x-ray
    D. All of the above

    Review this! ❑

13. Which of the following is the most common cause of cervicitis in a sexually active adolescent female?

    A. *Candida albicans*
    B. Chlamydia
    C. *Trichomonas vaginalis*
    D. Herpes simplex

    Review this! ❑

Questions 14–16: Match each of the following descriptions with the correct causative agent. Each choice may be used once, more than once, or not at all.
14. May be associated with bloody diarrhea
15. Most common bacterial cause of childhood diarrhea
16. Metronidazole used as first-line therapy

    A. Campylobacter
    B. Shigella
    C. Giardia
    D. Salmonella

    Review this! ❑

17. Determine whether each statement below is true or false. Appropriate anticipatory guidance for parents and their children includes:

    (1) Discouraging parents from using corporal punishment.
    (2) Encouraging children to get 30 minutes of exercise daily.
    (3) Reviewing appropriate car safety seats.
    (4) Direct supervision and monitoring of children's television viewing and access to the Internet.

    A. True
    B. False

    Review this! ❑

18. A 6-year-old girl was brought to your office for evaluation of 3-day history of fever (101.5°F oral), sore throat, headache, and swollen glands. She denies cough or rash. Physical examination is most notable for beefy red tonsils with white exudates and swollen tender cervical lymphadenopathy. The spleen tip is not palpable. Which of the following is the most likely diagnosis?

    A. Group A streptococcal pharyngitis
    B. Hand, foot, and mouth disease
    C. Herpangina
    D. Infectious mononucleosis

    Review this! ❑

19. A 14-month-old girl is seen in your office because of barky cough, fever, hoarseness, and inspiratory stridor. The diagnosis of croup is made. Which of the following is the most likely causative agent?

    A. Parainfluenza virus (types I and II)
    B. Streptococcus pneumonia
    C. Adenovirus
    D. Respiratory syncytial virus

    Review this! ❑

20. According to recent guidelines, the diagnosis of acute otitis media requires all of the following, except:

    A. The history of an acute onset of pain and fever.
    B. The presence of middle-ear effusion.
    C. A recent upper respiratory infection.
    D. Signs and symptoms of middle-ear inflammation, such as an erythematous tympanic membrane and distinct otalgia.

    Review this! ❑

Things to remember for the test.

125

21. Routine dental appointments should begin at what age?

    A. 1 year old
    B. 2–3 years
    C. 6–7 years
    D. 12–13 years

    Review this! ❏

22. A 5-year-old child comes to your office with his mother for a routine well-child checkup. His mother is concerned that he does not have all of the immunizations necessary to attend kindergarten. A review of his immunization record shows the following:

    - Birth: Hepatitis B #1
    - 2 Months: DTaP #1, IPV #1, Hepatitis B #2, Hib #1, Prevnar #1
    - 4 Months: DTaP #2, IPV #2, Hepatitis B #2, Hib #2, Prevnar #2
    - 6 Months: DTaP #3, IPV #3, Hepatitis B #3, Hib #3, Prevnar #3
    - 12 months: MMR #1, Varicella, Prevnar #4
    - 15 months: DTaP #4

    What immunization(s) does he need today?

    A. MMR
    B. DTaP
    C. IPV
    D. All of the above

    Review this! ❏

23. Determine whether each statement below is true or false. Certain patterns regarding substance use and abuse among adolescents include:

    (1) The use of alcohol or cigarettes is predictive of experimentation with other drugs.

    (2) Rates of substance abuse are declining among adolescent patients, according to nationally obtained data.
    (3) The critical time for drug experimentation is around the 9th and 10th grades.
    (4) Adolescents who regularly use illegal substances should be referred to a professional who is trained in adolescent substance abuse.

    A. True
    B. False

    Review this! ❏

For Questions 24–26: Match each of the following statements with the correct antibiotic choice. Each choice may be used once, more than once, or not at all.

24. Most common first-line treatment of acute otitis media in children
25. May be used as an option for penicillin-allergic patients
26. Parenteral single-dose therapy

    A. Amoxicillin (Amoxil)
    B. Azithromycin (Zithromax)
    C. Amoxicillin–clavulanate (Augmentin)
    D. Ceftriaxone (Rocephin)

    Review this! ❏

For Questions 27–30: Match each behavior with the correct stage of adolescence. Each choice may be used once, more than once, or not at all.
27. Peak of parental conflicts
28. Increased need for privacy
29. Conformity with peer values
30. Practical, realistic vocational goals

    A. Early adolescence
    B. Middle adolescence
    C. Late adolescence

    Review this! ❏

33 Behavioral Problems in Children and Adolescents

Katherine T. Balturshot

1. What percentage of children and adolescents have sleep problems that are of serious concern to both them and their families?

   A. 3%–5%
   B. 5%–10%
   C. 20%–30%
   D. 40%–50%

   Review this! ❑

2. Which of the following is true about night terrors?

   A. They usually occur during the early part of the night.
   B. Children experiencing them wake themselves up fully from sleep.
   C. Children are often unable to go back to sleep after they occur.
   D. Children's recall of the events is vivid.

   Review this! ❑

3. Obstructive sleep apnea in children is characterized by all of the following, except:

   A. Large tonsils or adenoids.
   B. More common among children with Down syndrome.
   C. Frequent brief awakenings.
   D. Drop in oxygen level similar to those seen among adults.

   Review this! ❑

4. Asperger's disorder differs from autism in which of the following ways?

   A. Impaired social interaction
   B. Delayed language and communication skills
   C. Repetitive movements
   D. Stereotyped behaviors

   Review this! ❑

5. True or false: Assertions that vaccines containing thimerosal contribute to the development of autism have been discounted.

   A. True
   B. False

   Review this! ❑

6. An 18-month-old girl presents to the office for a routine examination. She is growing well, with height and weight in the 75th percentile. She is walking on her own and meeting her motor-skill milestones. However, her mother is concerned because she isn't talking very much. What should you do?

   A. Reassure the mother that the child is fine, and follow up at 24 months.
   B. Tell the mother that the child is autistic, and refer for counseling.
   C. Get a detailed history, evaluate the child's hearing, and follow her closely.
   D. Use the Denver Developmental Screening Tool to reassure yourself and the mother that everything is fine.

   Review this! ❑

7. True or false: Anxiety problems affect 10% to 20% of school-aged children.

   A. True
   B. False

   Review this! ❑

8. Which of the following statements about encopresis is true?

   A. It is voluntary.
   B. It is never associated with organic disease.
   C. It is rarely accompanied by enuresis.
   D. It is associated with constipation.

   Review this! ❑

Things to remember for the test.

9. The best treatment for encopresis involves which of the following?

    A. Initial fiber supplementation
    B. Punishment for soiling clothes
    C. Intensive medical therapy plus behavioral management

    Review this! ❑

10. Which of the following statements about enuresis is true?

    A. As many as 15% to 20% of 5-year-old children have nocturnal enuresis.
    B. It is normal for a child who has attained continence to relapse.
    C. There is no increased incidence with a positive family history.
    D. Incontinence can happen at any time of the day.

    Review this! ❑

11. True or false: Asymptomatic children with primary enuresis with a normal examination and urine test can be treated without further workup.

    A. True
    B. False

    Review this! ❑

12. Which of the following statements about enuresis treatment is true?

    A. Alarms are an effective treatment.
    B. Medications are effective, and they have no serious side effects.
    C. Fluid restriction and scheduled voiding have no effect.
    D. Treating constipation does not affect incontinence rates.

    Review this! ❑

13. Which of the following statements about attention-deficit/hyperactivity disorder (ADHD) is true?

    A. Prevalence according to the Diagnostic and Statistical Manual of Mental Disorders, 4th Edition, Text Revision (DSM-IV-TR) classification is 20% to 30%.
    B. Boys and girls present equally with this condition.
    C. Three percent of behavior problems seen in a general pediatric practice are the result of ADHD.

    D. The diagnosis should be considered for a child who presents with academic underachievement.

    Review this! ❑

14. True or false: ADHD is not a chronic disorder.

    A. True
    B. False

    Review this! ❑

15. When making the diagnosis, it is most important to consider which of the following?

    A. Data about behavior from multiple sources in different contexts
    B. Only the child's perception of his or her behavior
    C. The child's performance in school
    D. The child's behavior in the doctor's office

    Review this! ❑

16. Which of the following is the first-line treatment for ADHD?

    A. Stimulant medication
    B. Counseling
    C. Behavior modification
    D. Neuropsychiatric testing

    Review this! ❑

17. True or false: If one stimulant medication does not work for the treatment of ADHD, there is no benefit to trying another one.

    A. True
    B. False

    Review this! ❑

18. Which of the following is the main benefit of Strattera?

    A. It works better than the stimulant medications.
    B. It works more quickly.
    C. It has no potential for abuse.
    D. It has a different side-effect profile.

    Review this! ❑

19. True or false: Parent training is an effective treatment for oppositional defiant disorder (ODD).

    A. True
    B. False

    Review this! ❑

20. "A pattern of negativistic, hostile, and defiant behavior lasting at least 6 months" best describes which of the following disorders?

    A. ADHD
    B. Depression
    C. Bipolar disorder
    D. ODD

    Review this! ❑

21. True or false: The mortality rate for seriously disturbed delinquents is 50 times higher than that seen among normal youths.

    A. True
    B. False

    Review this! ❑

22. The management of children with conduct disorder includes all of the following, except:

    A. Punishment for inappropriate behaviors.
    B. Family counseling.
    C. Social skills training.
    D. Assessment for proper school placement.

    Review this! ❑

23. "A repetitive and persistent pattern of behavior in which the basic rights of others or major age-appropriate societal norms or rules are violated" best defines which of the following disorders?

    A. Conduct disorder
    B. ODD
    C. ADHD
    D. Adjustment disorder

    Review this! ❑

24. What percentage of adolescents with depression will experience a manic episode within 5 years?

    A. 1%–3%
    B. 5%–10%
    C. 10%–20%
    D. 20%–40%

    Review this! ❑

25. True or false: The DSM-IV-TR uses the same diagnostic criteria to diagnose depression in both children and adults.

    A. True
    B. False

    Review this! ❑

26. Which of the following statements about the use of selective serotonin reuptake inhibitors among children and adolescents is true?

    A. They are the first-line treatment for depression.
    B. The side-effect profile is different for children than for adults.
    C. They are as effective as tricyclics for both children and adolescents.
    D. There is a causal link between their use and suicide.

    Review this! ❑

27. True or false: By the end of high school, 90% of students have tried alcohol, and 40% have tried an illicit drug.

    A. True
    B. False

    Review this! ❑

28. Which of the statements about drug tests is true?

    A. Tests for adulteration are available online.
    B. A negative test rules out abuse.
    C. A positive test equals a diagnosis of abuse.
    D. All substances can be tested for with a routine drug screen.

    Review this! ❑

29. Of cases involving the failure to thrive, what percentage has a psychosocial etiology?

    A. 5%
    B. 10%
    C. 25%
    D. 50%

    Review this! ❑

30. True or false: Among adolescent girls, eating disorders are the third leading chronic illness, after obesity and asthma.

    A. True
    B. False

    Review this! ❑

31. True or false: Anorexia is the most common eating disorder in the United States.

    A. True
    B. False

    Review this! ❑

Things to remember for the test.

34 Office Surgery

Ravi Balasubrahmanyan

1. Patients taking what popular herb are at increased risk of bleeding after a procedure?

   A. Ginkgo biloba
   B. Ginger
   C. Echinacea
   D. Ginseng

   Review this! ❑

2. The hepatitis B virus infection rate for a nonimmune person after a needlestick from a person who is positive for hepatitis B virus surface antigen is in which of the following ranges?

   A. 80%–90%
   B. 1%–2%
   C. 6%–30%
   D. 30%–50%

   Review this! ❑

3. Which of the following statements is true about level I office-based surgery?

   A. It includes minor surgery performed under topical or local anesthetic that does not involve a drug-induced alteration of consciousness.
   B. It involves procedures requiring deep sedation/analgesia.
   C. It involves procedures requiring moderate sedation anesthesia with postoperative monitoring.
   D. It is reserved for procedures that do not require anesthesia.

   Review this! ❑

4. True or false: When applied to abraded skin, most topical agents result in peak blood levels similar to those that result from local infiltration.

   A. True
   B. False

   Review this! ❑

5. The use of eutectic-mixture-of-local-anesthetics (EMLA) cream as a topical anesthetic is contraindicated in which of the following circumstances?

   A. Infants less than 3 months old
   B. Patients with anemia
   C. Patients with cardiopulmonary disease
   D. Glucose–6-phosphate dehydrogenase deficiency
   E. All of the above

   Review this! ❑

6. The maximal dose of lidocaine for cutaneous infiltration in adults and children should not exceed which of the following measurements?

   A. 10 ml
   B. 1 mg/kg
   C. 5 mg/kg
   D. 10 mg/kg

   Review this! ❑

7. Which of the following is the most common significant reaction from the use of infiltrative local anesthesia?

   A. Allergic reaction
   B. Catecholamine reaction
   C. Vasovagal reaction
   D. Infection

   Review this! ❑

8. The maximal oral dose of Valium for sedation before an office procedure is which of the following?

   A. 1 mg
   B. 2 mg
   C. 5 mg
   D. 10 mg

   Review this! ❑

9. The inflammatory phase of wound healing lasts from:

   A. Day 1 to 5.
   B. Day 5 to 14.
   C. 2 weeks to 2 months.
   D. 2 months to 2 years.

   Review this! ❑

10. Which of the following statements about keloids is false?

    A. They can occur in up to 15% of wounds.
    B. Scarring is excessive and remains within the original borders of the scar.
    C. They are seen 5 to 15 times more frequently among nonwhites.
    D. There is a familial predisposition.

    Review this! ❑

11. Factors associated with poor wound healing include which of the following?

    A. Diabetes mellitus
    B. Anemia
    C. Poor surgical technique
    D. Poor vascular supply
    E. All of the above

    Review this! ❑

12. Proper suture technique to minimize scar formation includes which of the following?

    A. Aligning the long axis of a wound perpendicular to the Langer lines
    B. Undermining of wounds to reduce skin tension being reserved for clean wounds
    C. Layering the closure of all wounds, regardless of the skin tension present
    D. Excising a lesion using a length of excision-to-lesion ratio of 2:1

    Review this! ❑

13. Which of the following statements about suture technique is false?

    A. Facial sutures should be removed in 10 to 14 days.
    B. Single-layered sutures should be placed through the entire thickness of the dermis and at right angles and the suture line approximately 2 to 3 mm apart and 2 to 3 mm from the wound edge.
    C. Sutures on hands, joints, the back, and the shoulders should be removed in 10 to 14 days.

    D. The distance between each suture should be approximately equal to the distance from the exit of the stitch from the wound.

    Review this! ❑

14. True or false: Tissue adhesives are effective and yield results that are comparable with those achieved by the conventional suturing of superficial, linear, and low-tension lacerations.

    A. True
    B. False

    Review this! ❑

15. Which of the following statements about complications of wound care is false?

    A. Wound infections usually occur within the first 24 hours of wound repair.
    B. A wound that has separated after suture removal should be left open to heal by secondary intention.
    C. Increasing and severe pain within 12 hours of wound repair can signify a clostridial or necrotizing infection.
    D. Wounds complicated by infection that require secondary intention to heal can be revised in the future.

    Review this! ❑

16. Which of the following statements about biopsy technique is false?

    A. Small, raised, noninflamed lesions that do not require the full thickness of the dermis can be removed by a shave biopsy.
    B. Punch biopsy is indicated for superficial inflammation as well as benign or malignant tumors.
    C. Suturing the wound is necessary for punch biopsies of less than 5 mm.
    D. A suspected malignant melanoma should be removed by excisional biopsy and include the removal of the entire lesion.

    Review this! ❑

17. True or false: The American Cancer Society's ABCDE criteria are a useful clinical prediction tool for the detection of malignant melanoma. This evaluation is considered positive if all of the criteria are met.

    A. True
    B. False

    Review this! ❑

Things to remember for the test.

18. Which of the following statements about laceration repair is false?

   A. A clean facial laceration can be closed primarily within 24 hours of injury.
   B. In general, uncomplicated clean puncture wounds can be cleaned and sutured primarily within 6 hours of injury.
   C. Cat bites require empiric coverage with β-lactam antibiotics that cover common contaminants such as *Pasteurella multocida*.
   D. Animal bites to the distal extremities should be closed primarily.

   Review this! ❏

19. Which of the following statements about cryosurgery is false?

   A. Cryosurgery is indicated for the treatment of benign, premalignant, and some malignant lesions, such as basal cell carcinoma.
   B. Cryosurgery can be used for all areas of the skin and for all age groups.
   C. There are no absolute contraindications to the use of cryosurgery.
   D. When treating a lesion, a margin of 1 mm to 3 mm beyond the border of the lesion is optimal.

   Review this! ❏

20. Which of the following statements about the incision and drainage of cutaneous abscesses is false?

   A. Fluctuance or the softening of the central area of infection is the easiest way to localize the area requiring drainage.
   B. If no fluctuance is present, drainage should be deferred and the patient given antibiotics.
   C. The incision and drainage of localized cutaneous abscesses in afebrile adults are unlikely to result in transient bacteremia; thus, no antibiotic prophylaxis is recommended.
   D. Local intradermal infiltration of lidocaine is very helpful to reduce the pain associated with the incision and drainage of a cutaneous abscess.

   Review this! ❏

21. Which of the following statements about office care of the nail is true?

   A. The optimal treatment of onychomycosis is pulse therapy using Lamisil.
   B. Subungual hematoma are best treated by melting a hole in the nail with a hand-held cautery device.
   C. Acute paronychia is best treated with antibiotics.
   D. Chronic paronychia is best treated with antibiotics and antifungals.

   Review this! ❏

22. Which of the following statements about anorectal disease is false?

   A. A patient with anorectal disease frequently presents with complaints of pain, itching, bleeding, discharge, or changes in bowel habits.
   B. Sigmoidoscopy detects a higher percentage of lesions in the anorectal region than anoscopy; it is the procedure of choice for the evaluation of rectal disease.
   C. Second-degree hemorrhoids cause mild discomfort and prolapse, but they spontaneously reduce themselves.
   D. Internal hemorrhoids are located above the pectinate line, and they are usually painless.

   Review this! ❏

23. Predisposing factors for the development of hemorrhoids include all of the following, except:

   A. Chronic constipation.
   B. Hypertension.
   C. Alcoholism.
   D. Pregnancy.

   Review this! ❏

24. True or false: Traditional rubber-band ligation is more effective, requires fewer additional treatments, and produces fewer complications than infrared coagulation and sclerotherapy for grade I, II, and III hemorrhoids.

   A. True
   B. False

   Review this! ❏

25. Which of the following statements about rubber-band ligation of the internal hemorrhoids is false?

A. The only absolute contraindication to banding is a patient's taking of anticoagulants.
B. Rubber rings cause tissue necrosis and generally fall off after 2 to 3 days.
C. Persistent bleeding beyond 5 days suggests a failed procedure.
D. The procedure is generally painless.
Review this! ❑

26. Which of the following statements about the treatment of thrombosed external hemorrhoids is true?

A. Rectal bleeding without pain is the most common manifestation of thrombosed external hemorrhoids.
B. Bleeding is usually severe, and it usually requires prompt treatment.
C. The incision of thrombosed hemorrhoids is the treatment of choice.
D. The excision of thrombosed hemorrhoids is the treatment of choice.
Review this! ❑

27. Which of the following statements about anorectal abscesses is false?

A. Anorectal abscesses are severely painful and disabling.
B. They occur three times more commonly among males than females.
C. Definitive treatment is broad-spectrum antibiotics.
D. Perianal and perirectal abscesses are the most common types.
Review this! ❑

28. Which of the following statements about colposcopy is false?

A. There are no absolute contraindications to endocervical curettage.
B. There are no absolute contraindications to colposcopy.
C. If the squamocolumnar zone is not entirely visualized, it is felt that the colposcopy was unsatisfactory.
D. The goals of colposcopy are to ensure that invasive disease is not missed and, if indicated, to biopsy the most appropriate site.
Review this! ❑

29. Which of the following statements about endometrial biopsy is true?

A. It is an accepted method of evaluating premenopausal and postmenopausal women for abnormal uterine bleeding.
B. It is useful for women with unexplained infertility to determine the presence of a luteal phase defect.
C. It is highly sensitive for detecting endometrial cancer.
D. It is highly specific for detecting intraluminal pathology in the uterus.
Review this! ❑

30. Which of the following statements about aspiration and injection of the knee joint is false?

A. It can be done up to five times over a 12-month period.
B. It is indicated for inflammatory exacerbations of osteoarthritis.
C. Intra-articular injections of hyaluronic acid (Synvisc) have been shown to provide clinical benefit.
D. It can be used diagnostically and therapeutically for large effusions, post-traumatic hemarthroses, and unexplained monarthritis.
Review this! ❑

31. Which of the following statements about neonatal circumcision is true?

A. EMLA cream is as effective as a dorsal penile nerve block for reducing the pain response during circumcision.
B. There are no strict medical indications for circumcision, and, generally, the decision to have a circumcision is based on the wishes of the parents or legal guardians.
C. Circumcisions should be delayed at least 48 hours to ensure that the infant is medically stable.
D. There are no medical contraindications to neonatal circumcisions.
Review this! ❑

Things to remember for the test.

133

35 Perioperative Care

Michael P. Rowane

1. Determine whether each of the following statements about general principles of perioperative care is true or false.

   (1) The preoperative risk is related to the proposed surgery.
   (2) Interventions to lower perioperative risk depend on the type of surgery.
   (3) It is essential to consider preoperatively what can be done before surgery to lessen or prevent complications postoperatively.
   (4) Perioperative outcomes are improved if there is good communication between the family physician, the surgeon, and the anesthesiologist.
   (5) The type of anesthesia has no bearing on the ultimate perioperative risk for the patient.

   A. True
   B. False

   Review this! ❑

2. Which of the following statements about the perioperative patient is true?

   A. Patients typically consider herbal preparations and over-the-counter preparations to be medications.
   B. Edema of the lower extremity is only caused by renal disease.
   C. A complete blood cell count should be performed for all surgical patients.
   D. Coagulation studies are a required preoperative test.
   E. A serum creatinine level is routinely ordered for patients who are 75 years old and older.

   Review this! ❑

3. Which of the following statements about preoperative cardiac testing is true?

   A. Pathologic Q-waves represent an extremely high risk for perioperative cardiac mortality.
   B. An electrocardiogram (EKG) is required before all surgical procedures.
   C. Stress imaging is performed before major vascular surgery.
   D. Diabetics do not require a preoperative EKG.
   E. All cardiac murmurs require an EKG and an echocardiogram.

   Review this! ❑

4. Which of the following is a major clinical predictor of increased perioperative cardiovascular risk?

   A. Advanced age
   B. Unstable coronary syndromes
   C. History of stroke
   D. Uncontrolled hypertension
   E. Rhythm other than sinus

   Review this! ❑

5. Which of the following is a minor clinical predictor of increased perioperative cardiovascular risk?

   A. A low functional capacity
   B. Severe valvular disease
   C. Significant arrhythmias
   D. Decompensated heart failure
   E. Unstable coronary syndromes

   Review this! ❑

6. Which of the following statements about cardiac status in a preoperative patient is true?

Things to remember for the test.

A. Patients with poor functional capacity are at low risk for perioperative cardiac morbidity and mortality.

B. Determining a patient's underlying cardiac function is the centerpiece of preoperative risk assessment.

C. Poor functional status is an indication for noninvasive cardiac testing before all surgeries.

D. Hypertrophic and dilated cardiomyopathy decreases the risk of perioperative heart failure.

E. Testing patients with prior heart failure or dyspnea of unknown origin is rarely indicated.

Review this! ❑

7. Determine whether each of the following statements about the perioperative patient is true or false.

(1) If valvular heart disease is suspected, more aggressive management is required for perioperative patients than for nonoperative patients.

(2) Tobacco use is not an absolute contra-indication to surgery.

(3) Patients with stable mild to moderate pulmonary disease can proceed directly to surgery after a thorough history and physical.

(4) Carbon dioxide retention can be improved by respiratory depressants used during the postoperative period.

(5) Surgery and anesthesia can often lead to an acute worsening of a restrictive defect.

A. True
B. False

Review this! ❑

8. Which of the following surgical conditions has the greatest perioperative ischemic stroke risk rate for general surgeries and clinical outcomes?

A. General surgery with carotid stenosis and bruit or prior symptoms

B. General surgery

C. General surgery after a prior stroke

D. Surgery with symptomatic vertebrobasilar stenosis

E. General surgery with or without carotid bruit

Review this! ❑

9. Which of the following medications must be stopped 1 week before surgery?

A. Ticlopidine (Ticlid)
B. Metformin (Glucophage)
C. Lisinopril (Zestril/Prinivil)
D. Digoxin (Lanoxin)
E. Insulin

Review this! ❑

10. Indications for perioperative β-blockers include which of the following?

A. A resting heat rate of less than 60 beats per minute

B. Known coronary artery disease

C. Second-degree heart block

D. Hypotension

E. Asthma

Review this! ❑

11. Which of the following statements about the perioperative patient is true?

A. Pulmonary function tests monitor the effectiveness of preoperative medical treatment for patients with severe pulmonary compromise.

B. Insulin is not used for type 2 diabetics who are controlled with oral agents preoperatively.

C. Autonomic dysfunction is rarely present among type 2 diabetics.

D. Diabetic patients with autonomic dysfunction and that have gastroparesis rarely develop orthostatic hypotension and diabetic diarrhea.

E. Patients with hypothyroidism should discontinue thyroid hormone during the perioperative period.

Review this! ❑

12. Which of the following statements about glycolic control among surgical patients is correct?

A. Glucose levels of more than 180 mg/dL typically involve excessive hydration.

B. There is no association between poor glycolic control and the risk of infection.

C. There is an association between poor glycolic control and wound healing.

D. Tight glycolic control does not alter survival.

E. Intermittent insulin is superior to continuous insulin drips for glycolic control among type 1 diabetics and among type 2 diabetics who use insulin.

Review this! ❑

13. Which of the following statements about the role of anesthetic techniques in the care of the operative patient is correct?

    A. The anesthetic technique makes little difference with regard to stress response.
    B. Epidural anesthesia has no effect on circulating glucose among nondiabetic patients.
    C. Regional techniques do not offer much patient feedback with regard to the quality of pain control.
    D. Regional techniques do offer an opportunity for a patient to report hypoglycemic symptoms.
    E. Circulating cortisol and norepinephrine are not blocked in nondiabetic patients with epidural anesthesia.

    Review this! ❏

14. Which of the following statements about the management of patients with thyroid disorders during the perioperative period is correct?

    A. Hypothyroid patients can tolerate high doses of sedative medications.
    B. Thyroid hormone in the severely hypothyroid surgical patient requires concomitant steroid replacement.
    C. The level of thyrotoxicosis has little correlation with the severity of the disease and the intraoperative risk.
    D. Avoid a euthyroid state among patients with hyperthyroidism.
    E. Avoid using β-blockers for hyperthyroid patients that are not euthyroid.

    Review this! ❏

15. Which of the following situations can precipitate an exacerbation in a patient with heart failure?

    A. Increased intravascular volume
    B. Stable blood pressure
    C. Increased stroke volume
    D. Total body water overload

    Review this! ❏

16. Which of the following clinical features of the Wells Clinical Prediction Rules for Pulmonary Embolism is the most concerning for the patient with a pulmonary embolism?

    A. Malignancy
    B. Another diagnosis less likely than pulmonary embolism

    C. Hemoptysis
    D. Previous deep venous thrombosis or pulmonary embolism
    E. Immobilization or surgery within the past 4 weeks

    Review this! ❏

17. Which of the following statements about wound infections of the surgical patient is true?

    A. Few of these patients are admitted to an intensive care unit.
    B. There is no significant difference in the number of patients with wound infections being readmitted to the hospital as compared with patients without wound infections.
    C. It is recommended to begin an antibiotic infusion within 1 hour of the surgical incision.
    D. Prophylactic antimicrobial agents should be discontinued 1 week after the surgical procedure.
    E. The addition of supplemental oxygen during the perioperative period has no effect on wound infections.

    Review this! ❏

18. Determine whether each of the following statements about adrenal insufficiency in the perioperative patient is true or false.

    (1) Major and minor surgery offer equal stress to the patient with adrenal insufficiency.
    (2) The use of chronic steroids is the most common cause of primary adrenal insufficiency.
    (3) The perioperative dose of corticosteroids can be immediately discontinued after surgery.
    (4) In cases of adrenal crisis, patients may require large-scale fluid resuscitation and pressors.
    (5) The doses of corticosteroids that are given for both adrenal insufficiency and adrenal crisis are equivalent.

    A. True
    B. False

    Review this! ❏

19. Which of the following risk factors is most consistently associated with perioperative ischemic stroke?

A. A history of stroke
B. A history of gout
C. Chronic obstructive pulmonary disease
D. Postoperative cardiac arrhythmia
E. Allergic rhinitis

Review this! ❏

20. Which of the following statements about pain management during the postoperative period is true?

   A. There is one method of postoperative pain relief that is clearly better.
   B. It is best to minimize activity level while minimizing and avoiding side effects.
   C. Postoperative epidural analgesia provides inferior pain relief as compared with intravenous narcotics.
   D. Intravenous narcotics are the standard against which all other pain control regimens are compared.
   E. Intravenous narcotics should not be supplemented with nonsteroidal anti-inflammatory drugs.

Review this! ❏

21. Which of the following statements about factors that can affect bleeding during the postoperative period is true?

   A. The prevention of postoperative bleeding can only begin after the surgical procedure is complete.
   B. Herbal medication has no effect on postoperative bleeding.
   C. Patients with liver disease are predisposed to postoperative bleeding complications.
   D. The best way to evaluate excessive bleeding is an urgent computed tomography scan.
   E. When postoperative bleeding is the result of a coagulopathy, the first stage of management for a bleeder is the exploration of the wound.

Review this! ❏

22. Determine whether each of the following statements about a pulmonary embolism is true or false.

   (1) Negative imaging studies of a pulmonary embolism do not warrant any further measures.
   (2) The diagnosis of a pulmonary embolism begins with a careful history and physical.

(3) Initial diagnostic test for a pulmonary embolism includes a computed tomography pulmonary angiogram or a ventilation-perfusion scan.
(4) When considering clinical prediction rules for pulmonary embolism, a physician's clinical judgment is nearly as good as the clinical prediction rule used.
(5) Patients with signs and symptoms of pulmonary embolism who are found to have a deep venous thrombosis should be treated for a pulmonary embolism even if they have negative imaging studies.

   A. True
   B. False

Review this! ❏

Things to remember for the test.

23. Which of the following statements about the management of a pulmonary embolism is true?

   A. Hospitalization is rarely required for patients with a pulmonary embolism.
   B. Warfarin is an acceptable alternative to using unfractionated heparin for treating a pulmonary embolism.
   C. Low-molecular-weight heparin is not an acceptable treatment for pulmonary embolism.
   D. A physician's clinical judgment is nearly as good as the clinical predicted role used.
   E. Thrombolysis is used to treat most cases of pulmonary embolism.

Review this! ❏

24. Determine whether each of the following statements about the perioperative adjustment of common medications is true or false.

   (1) Unless a medication is completely unnecessary or contraindicated, it should be continued through the morning of surgery.
   (2) It is unnecessary to check serum levels of medications before surgery.
   (3) β-Blockers can be stopped for several days without consequence.
   (4) Most antiarrhythmic medications can be held for a few days postoperatively until the patient is eating.
   (5) Most oral medications do not interfere with anesthesia and are well tolerated during surgery.

   A. True
   B. False

Review this! ❏

25. When comparing postoperative epidural analgesia to intravenous narcotics, which of the following statements about the patient who has a postoperative epidural is true?

    A. Extubation is delayed.
    B. There is a delay in ambulation.
    C. There is an increase in cardiac arrhythmias.
    D. The patients have longer hospital stays.
    E. There is a decrease in patients with ileus.

    Review this! ❏

26. Which of the following conditions is the most common cause of a postoperative fever?

    A. Seromas
    B. Hematomas
    C. Pneumonia
    D. Malignant hyperthermia
    E. Neuroleptic malignant syndrome

    Review this! ❏

27. Which of the following statements about postoperative fever is true?

    A. Postoperative fever is common during the first few days after a major surgery.
    B. A postoperative fever is defined as a temperature above 37°C (99°F).

C. The differential diagnosis is not related to the timing of the onset of postoperative fever.
D. Most late postoperative fevers are caused by the inflammation response to surgery.
E. Avoid treating postoperative fever, because this could mask the underlying etiology.

Review this! ❏

28. Determine whether each of the following statements about the general principles of nutrition in the perioperative patient is true or false.

    (1) Malnutrition is associated with an increase in surgical morbidity and mortality.
    (2) There is a higher mortality rate among cardiac patients with a normal serum albumin.
    (3) Patients will have no adverse outcomes with no nutritional intake for a week after surgery.
    (4) Postoperative oral intake requires a functioning digestive system.
    (5) Parenteral nutrition is the preferred route of feeding for postoperative patients.

    A. True
    B. False

    Review this! ❏

36 Gynecology

Patricia Pletke

1. An annual well-woman examination offers an opportunity to address screening and health-maintenance issues. Which of the following is an A-level recommendation of the U.S. Preventive Services Task Force?

   A. Screening for cervical cancer at age 18 or at the onset of sexual activity
   B. Screening all sexually active women 25 years old and younger for chlamydia
   C. Screening all women 35 years old and older for lipid disorders
   D. Screening all women 45 years old and older for thyroid disease

   Review this! ❏

2. Recommendations for screening for cervical cancer include all of the following, except:

   A. Annual screening for women with human immunodeficiency virus (HIV).
   B. Screening via Pap smears at 2- to 3-year intervals for those women with two or fewer lifetime partners and no other risk factors after they have had three consecutive negative Pap smears.
   C. Liquid-based cytology screening for high-risk women.
   D. Discontinuation of screening around the age of 65 to 70 years among women who have had regular screening and two to three normal Pap smears during the last 10 years.

   Review this! ❏

3. Which of the following is true about the collection of cervical cytology specimens?

   A. When both a spatula and a cytobrush are used, each is smeared on a separate and labeled slide.
   B. The most abnormal portion of the cervix should be sampled.
   C. The method of collecting the specimen is different when liquid-based testing is done.

   D. Reflex human papilloma virus (HPV) testing can be performed on liquid-based specimens.

   Review this! ❏

4. Colposcopy allows for visualization of the genital tract and, in particular, the cervix, under magnification. All of the following statements are true, except:

   A. Normal columnar epithelium has a "grape-like" appearance.
   B. Abnormal areas identified by colposcopy should be frozen to prevent progression to cervical cancer.
   C. Acetic acid (vinegar) is used to help identify abnormal areas.
   D. Adequate colposcopy requires visualization of the entire transformation zone.

   Review this! ❏

5. Atypical squamous cells of undetermined significance (ASCUS) may be managed by any of the following means, except:

   A. Testing and treating for infection.
   B. Repeat cytology in 3 to 6 months.
   C. Testing for high-risk HPV types.
   D. Colposcopy.

   Review this! ❏

6. Patients with glandular-cell abnormalities identified on Pap testing should have colposcopy as well as which one of the following?

   A. Testing for high-risk HPV
   B. Endometrial biopsy
   C. Ultrasound evaluation of the cervix and uterus
   D. Hysteroscopy

   Review this! ❏

7. Which of the following is true about testing for HPV?

Things to remember for the test.

Things to remember for the test.

A. It is recommended for all women with low-grade squamous intraepithelial lesion, atypical squamous cells—one cannot exclude high-grade squamous intraepithelial lesion, ASCUS, or high-grade squamous intraepithelial lesion.

B. Reflex testing can be performed with liquid-based cytology.

C. It is less sensitive than repeat cytology testing for women with ASCUS seen on Pap smears.

D. If it is positive, this indicates a need for treatment with cryotherapy, laser, cautery, or podophyllin.

Review this! ❑

8. Which of the following statements about menstruation is false?

A. The menstrual cycle is controlled by hormones from the hypothalamus, the pituitary gland, and the ovaries.

B. Flow typically lasts 3 to 7 days for each cycle.

C. Metrorrhagia is bleeding that is excessive in amount and duration of flow at regular intervals.

D. Oligomenorrhea is infrequent and irregular bleeding.

Review this! ❑

9. Which of the following statements about abnormal vaginal bleeding is false?

A. It is important to rule out pregnancy.

B. Breakthrough bleeding seen with combination oral contraceptive pills may be an indication to change pill formulations.

C. Bleeding associated with progestin-only contraception can be managed by reassurance, supplemental estrogen, or nonsteroidal anti-inflammatory drugs.

D. Blood dyscrasias, although an infrequent cause of abnormal uterine bleeding, need to be considered, especially among older patients.

Review this! ❑

10. In the evaluation of abnormal uterine bleeding, an endometrial biopsy should be performed for women who are at risk for endometrial hyperplasia. Risk factors include all of the following, except:

A. History of hormonal contraception.

B. Obesity.

C. Age of more than 35 years.

D. History of anovulatory cycles.

Review this! ❑

11. Which of the following statements about anovulation is true?

A. It leads to atrophic changes of the uterine lining and abnormal uterine bleeding.

B. It is a risk factor for ovarian cancer.

C. It may be treated with oral contraceptives or cyclic progestins to control abnormal bleeding.

D. A and C

Review this! ❑

12. True or false: Primary amenorrhea is diagnosed when an adolescent female has not had a menstrual period by age 16.

A. True

B. False

Review this! ❑

13. Which of the following statements about a progesterone challenge (10 mg medroxyprogesterone acetate daily for 10 days) is true?

A. It is the first step in the evaluation of secondary amenorrhea.

B. It is positive if the patient bleeds for 10 to 14 days after the last dose of medroxyprogesterone acetate.

C. It is usually negative if the cause of amenorrhea is polycystic ovarian syndrome.

D. If it is positive, this indicates that the uterus has been exposed to endogenous estrogen.

Review this! ❑

14. Which of the following statements about physiologic vaginal discharge is true?

A. It is consistent in amount and character.

B. It usually has a pH between 5 and 6.

C. It has a predominance of long, rod-shaped bacteria.

D. It adheres to the vaginal walls.

Review this! ❑

15. Which of the following is the most common cause of abnormal vaginal discharge in the adult heterosexual woman?

A. Chlamydia
B. Gonorrhea
C. Monilial vaginitis
D. Bacterial vaginosis

Review this! ❏

16. Which of the following statements about bacterial vaginosis is true?

    A. It is associated with a decrease in vaginal pH.
    B. It is associated with pelvic inflammatory disease, postpartum endometritis, and postabortion infection.
    C. It can be diagnosed by culture showing *Gardnerella vaginalis.*
    D. It is usually initiated by an overgrowth of lactobacilli.

    Review this! ❏

17. Which of the following statements about the treatment of bacterial vaginosis is true?

    A. It is indicated in asymptomatic women because of the condition's association with significant pelvic infections.
    B. It is indicated for the sexual partners of women with recurrent or difficult-to-eradicate cases.
    C. Even when it is effective, infection may recur in 20% to 30% of patients.
    D. It includes triple sulfa cream, erythromycin, or tetracycline in the metronidazole-allergic patient.

    Review this! ❏

18. All of the following statements about candidal vaginal infections are true, except:

    A. They are characterized by pruritic vaginal discharge.
    B. Oral contraceptives, steroids, HIV infection, and diabetes increase the risk for these infections.
    C. Topical, intravaginal medications are contraindicated during pregnancy.
    D. The presence of *Candida* species on culture may be found in 20% of asymptomatic women.

    Review this! ❏

19. Which of the following statements about Trichomonas vaginitis is true?

    A. It is usually transmitted by sexual contact.

B. It is characterized by a "strawberry" cervix.
C. It is treated with topical or oral metronidazole.
D. Treatment failure is usually the result of metronidazole resistance.

Review this! ❏

20. All of the following statements about atrophic vaginitis are true, except:

    A. It may occur among postpartum and lactating women as well as among women taking tamoxifen.
    B. It is characterized clinically by itching, vaginal soreness, spotting, dyspareunia, and urinary incontinence.
    C. It may be treated with topical or oral estrogen.
    D. The pH of the discharge is usually decreased.

    Review this! ❏

21. Which of the following statements about the evaluation of a woman with pelvic pain and a positive pregnancy test is true?

    A. A serum progesterone level of more than 25 usually indicates a normal pregnancy.
    B. A quantitative human chorionic gonadotropin level that doubles over 72 hours is suggestive of a normal pregnancy.
    C. An intrauterine gestational sac should be visible by transvaginal ultrasound if the human chorionic gonadotropin level is 1000 or greater.
    D. A history of bilateral tubal ligation decreases the probability that the pregnancy is ectopic.

    Review this! ❏

22. True or false: A woman who has had an ectopic pregnancy has a one in four chance of recurrence with a subsequent pregnancy.

    A. True
    B. False

    Review this! ❏

23. All of the following statements about the treatment of pelvic inflammatory disease are true, except:

A. Treatment should cover both sexually transmitted organisms as well as anaerobic organisms.
B. Inpatient treatment is indicated for pregnant women.
C. Patients receiving outpatient treatment should receive follow-up at the end of treatment to ensure resolution of the infection.
D. Failure to improve by 72 hours after treatment is started may indicate a tubo-ovarian abscess or another abdominal process.

Review this! ❏

24. Which of the following is the most common cause of chronic pelvic pain identified on laparoscopy?

A. Ovarian cysts
B. Fibroids
C. Infection
D. Endometriosis

Review this! ❏

25. Which of the following statements about the evaluation and treatment of endometriosis is true?

A. The physical examination usually reveals nodularity of the uterosacral ligaments or a fixed, retroverted uterus.
B. Magnetic resonance imaging is the imaging method of choice and the gold standard for diagnosis.
C. Surgical treatment may be effective for reducing pain, but, over time, pain recurs in about half of patients.
D. Treatment with nonsteroidal anti-inflammatory drugs or hormones may reduce pain and increase fertility.

Review this! ❏

26. All of the following statements about adenomyosis are true, except:

A. It is endometrial tissue growing with the muscle of the uterus.
B. It may present as an enlarged, tender uterus.
C. Definitive treatment is hysterectomy.
D. When the diagnosis is suspected, a pelvic ultrasound should be performed.

Review this! ❏

27. Which of the following statements about chronic pelvic pain is true?

A. Gynecologic causes may be distinguished from non-gynecologic causes based on the association of symptoms with the menstrual cycle.
B. Interstitial cystitis may be the most common cause found among women presenting to the family physician.
C. It may be the result of psychological issues relating to a previous history of sexual violence.
D. Mittelschmerz is recurrent pelvic pain that occurs during the middle of the menstrual period.

Review this! ❏

28. All of the following statements about fibroids are true, except:

A. They are more common among white women than black women.
B. They are associated with pregnancy complications such as preterm labor, placental abruption, Cesarean section, and breech presentation.
C. They can be treated medically with progesterone, danazol, or gonadotropin-releasing hormone agonists.
D. Presentation may be with back pain or with urinary or bowel symptoms.

Review this! ❏

29. All of the following statements about cysts are true, except:

A. Contraceptive pills should be stopped when a cyst is diagnosed.
B. Approximately 70% resolve within several months.
C. Further evaluation is indicated for cysts that are more than 5 cm in diameter.
D. Simple cysts are unlikely to be malignant.

Review this! ❏

30. Which of the following statements about ovarian cancer is true?

A. It is diagnosed by measuring blood levels of CA–125.
B. Its risk is increased among women who have used oral contraceptives for more than 5 years.
C. It has a 5-year survival rate of 35%.
D. It usually presents with pelvic pain or abnormal bleeding.

Review this! ❏

31. The appropriate management of vulvar lesions includes all of the following, except:

    A. Antibiotics covering common sexually transmitted diseases and warm heat for Bartholin's gland infections.
    B. The biopsy of white areas to rule out dysplasia or carcinoma.
    C. Trichloroacetic acid for condylomas.
    D. Topical steroids for lichen sclerosis.

    Review this! ❏

32. During the evaluation of infertility, which of the following is not considered an indication that ovulation is occurring?

    A. Premenstrual symptoms
    B. A positive home urinary luteinizing hormone detection test
    C. A progesterone level of 15 at mid-cycle
    D. An endometrial biopsy done 2 to 3 days before the expected menses showing histologic evidence of ovulation

    Review this! ❏

33. Which of the following statements about infertility evaluation is true?

    A. Semen analysis is performed when the workup of the female partner fails to reveal an etiology for the infertility.
    B. A hysterosalpingogram with an oil-based dye to identify tubal patency is associated with a higher rate of pregnancy than that done with a water-based dye.

    C. For all couples, it is appropriate to begin workup for infertility after 1 year of unprotected intercourse.
    D. In 5% of cases, both partners have some form of infertility.

    Review this! ❏

34. All of the following statements about menopause are true, except:

    A. Symptoms of vaginal dryness, sleep disturbances, and hot flashes can be relieved with estrogen therapy.
    B. Hormone therapy is indicated for high-risk women to help prevent heart disease and osteoporosis.
    C. Raloxifene is appropriate for women who are candidates for the prevention of osteoporosis or to prevent fractures among women who have established osteoporosis.
    D. History of deep venous thrombosis or pulmonary embolus is a contraindication to treatment with raloxifene or tamoxifen.

    Review this! ❏

35. Which of the following is the most common cause of incontinence in women?

    A. Urge incontinence
    B. Urinary tract infection
    C. Stress incontinence
    D. Estrogen deficiency

    Review this! ❏

37 Contraception

Christine D. Hudak

Things to remember for the test.

1. All of the following statements are true about contraception, except:

   A. Half of the pregnancies in the United States each year are unintended.
   B. Approximately 53% of women who experience an unintended pregnancy were using a contraceptive method at the time.
   C. Effective birth control can provide primary prevention of sexually transmitted infections (STIs).
   D. The role of the physician is to select the most effective form of contraception for each patient.
   E. Unintended pregnancies account for most of the 1.3 million abortions each year in the United States.
   Review this! ❏

2. Factors influencing a woman's choice of contraception include all of the following, except:

   A. Number of past pregnancies.
   B. Number of past/current sexual partners.
   C. Compliance with past/current methods.
   D. Methods of STI prevention.
   E. Personal beliefs about methods.
   Review this! ❏

3. Dosages of ethinyl estradiol available in today's combined oral contraceptives include all of the following, except:

   A. 20 μg.
   B. 25 μg.
   C. 35 μg.
   D. 50 μg.
   E. 80 μg.
   Review this! ❏

4. In addition to providing contraceptive benefits, combined oral contraceptives can also be effective for all of the following situations, except:

   A. Suppression of ovarian cyst formation.
   B. Decreasing dysmenorrhea.
   C. Decreasing menorrhagia and the subsequent iron-deficiency anemia.
   D. Reducing vasomotor symptoms in perimenopausal women.
   E. Decreasing STI transmission.
   Review this! ❏

5. Which of the following statements about the risks of combination oral contraceptives (COCs) is true?

   A. Women who use COCs have a much higher risk of breast cancer.
   B. The risk of deep venous thrombosis is higher with COC use than with pregnancy.
   C. The risk of myocardial infarction and stroke associated with COC use appears to be limited to women who are more than 35 years old and who have other risk factors, especially smoking and hypertension.
   D. The use of COCs increases the risk of cervical cancer.
   E. COC use causes gallbladder disease.
   Review this! ❏

6. Which of the following statements about breakthrough bleeding (BTB) with the use of COCs is true?

   A. If a patient experiences BTB on the first cycle of COCs, the type of pill should be changed.
   B. Smokers are more likely to experience BTB than nonsmokers.
   C. Women taking prolonged COCs, such as Seasonale, are at less risk of BTB than those taking the standard 28-day regimens.
   D. BTB is uncommon with the use of COCs.
   E. Lower-dose estrogen pills are associated with lower rates of BTB.
   Review this! ❏

7. Common side effects of COCs include all of the following, except:

   A. Amenorrhea.
   B. Breast tenderness.
   C. Headaches.
   D. Heart palpitations.
   E. Nausea.

   Review this! ❑

8. All of the following patients would be good candidates for progestin-only pills, except:

   A. Lactating women.
   B. Adolescent women.
   C. Hypertensive women.
   D. Women with nausea from taking COCs.
   E. Women who smoke and who are more than 35 years old.

   Review this! ❑

9. Which of the following statements about the contraceptive patch—as compared with COCs—is true?

   A. It is associated with a higher risk of venous thromboembolism.
   B. It is less likely to cause breast tenderness.
   C. It is a progestin-only form of contraception.
   D. It is associated with fewer contraceptive failures.
   E. It is not affected by the patient's weight.

   Review this! ❑

10. Regarding the vaginal contraceptive ring, all of the following are true, except:

    A. The ring is made out of latex; thus, it is contraindicated for those with latex allergies.
    B. The ring can be removed for a short time (less than 3 hours) and still maintain its efficacy.
    C. The ring does not need to be placed over the cervix, because it is not a barrier device.
    D. As compared with COCs, lower incidences of BTB and nausea are reported.
    E. Vaginitis, headache, and leukorrhea are the most common side effects.

    Review this! ❑

11. Which of the following statements about injectable depomedroxyprogesterone acetate (DMPA) is true?

    A. It is given once every 2 months.
    B. It does not suppress ovulation effectively.
    C. DMPA does not decrease pain from endometriosis.
    D. In 2004, the U.S. Food and Drug Administration added a black-box warning to DMPA, stating that it may result in a loss of bone density.
    E. There is typically a quick return to fertility after the discontinuation of DMPA.

    Review this! ❑

12. Which of the following statements about the contraceptive etonogestrel implant (Implanon) is true?

    A. This system has only two subcutaneous rods to insert.
    B. It provides 3 years of highly effective contraception.
    C. Special training is not necessary for the removal and insertion of Implanon.
    D. After removal, the return to fertility is prolonged.
    E. Irregular bleeding and amenorrhea do not occur with Implanon.

    Review this! ❑

13. Which of the following is a significant benefit of the levonorgestrel-secreting intrauterine device (IUD)?

    A. Users experience a 90% reduction in average menstrual blood loss.
    B. Users experience a 50% reduction in average menstrual blood loss.
    C. This device provides 10 years of effective contraception.
    D. This device decreases the risk of pelvic inflammatory disease.
    E. Ovulation suppression is the primary mechanism of action of this IUD, so it is helpful for women with symptomatic ovarian cysts.

    Review this! ❑

14. All of the following statements are true about the use of condoms for contraception, except:

Things to remember for the test.

A. Condoms can be made from latex, polyurethane, and lamb cecum (natural membrane condoms).

B. Natural membrane condoms offer similar protection from STIs as latex or polyurethane condoms.

C. The Reality condom (or female condom) is safe for those who are allergic to latex.

D. The Reality condom offers protection from viral and bacterial STIs.

E. The male condom use may be associated with decreased penile sensitivity.

Review this! ❏

15. The use of a diaphragm for contraception is associated with a decreased risk of transmission of all of the following STIs, except:

A. Gonorrhea.
B. Chlamydia.
C. Trichomoniasis.
D. Human immunodeficiency virus (HIV).
E. Pelvic inflammatory disease.

Review this! ❏

16. Which of the following statements about the use of spermicides containing nonoxynol-9 is true?

A. The spermicide sponge (the Today sponge) can only be left in the vagina for 6 hours after intercourse.

B. Pregnancy failure rates are 5% to 10% with typical use at 1 year.

C. Spermicides are only available in gel delivery systems in the United States.

D. Studies regarding STI and HIV transmission have yielded conflicting results.

E. A dose of spermicide remains effective for approximately 6 hours after insertion.

Review this! ❏

17. In contrast with the levonorgestrel-secreting IUD (Mirena), the copper-T 380A IUD (ParaGard) is more likely to cause which of the following?

A. Ectopic pregnancy
B. Prolonged return to fertility after removal
C. Abortions of established pregnancies
D. Shorter duration of contraception efficacy
E. Increased menstrual bleeding

Review this! ❏

18. Fertility-awareness–based contraceptive methods include all of the following, except:

A. The breast-sensitivity method.
B. The calendar-rhythm method.
C. The basal body-temperature method.
D. The ovulation (cervical mucus or Billings) method.
E. The symptothermal method.

Review this! ❏

19. Which of the following factors makes the lactation amenorrhea method of contraception highly effective (>98%) for the prevention of pregnancy?

A. The woman is less than 12 months postpartum.

B. The infant is exclusively or nearly exclusively breastfeeding.

C. The woman has not had more than two menstrual cycles postpartum.

D. Solid foods are introduced to the infant no sooner than 4 months of age.

E. Formula is given to the infant no more than twice daily.

Review this! ❏

20. All of the following surgical approaches can be used for tubal ligation, except:

A. Mini-laparotomy.
B. Laparoscopy.
C. Ultrasound-guided tubal ligation.
D. Hysteroscopy.
E. Laparotomy.

Review this! ❏

21. Which of the following statements about emergency contraception (EC) is true?

A. The Yuzpe method consists of taking two doses of levonorgestrel, 0.75 mg each, 12 hours apart.

B. The copper-T IUD is a form of EC.

C. Plan B is a combination estrogen and progestin EC regimen.

D. Current combination and progestin-only contraceptives cannot be used for EC.

E. The use of EC can terminate an established pregnancy.

Review this! ❏

22. Which of the following is the proper timing for use of EC?

A. The progestin-only method can be used up to 120 hours after intercourse.
B. It must be used within 24 hours of intercourse (hence the nickname "the morning-after pill").
C. The copper-T IUD can be placed up to 72 hours after intercourse.
D. The progestin-only regimen must include a 12-hour period between two doses of levonorgestrel.
E. The progestin-only method can be used up to 72 hours after intercourse.

Review this! ❑

23. All of the following statements about EC are true, except:

A. EC is extremely safe.
B. EC is 75% or more effective when used properly.
C. Nausea and vomiting are uncommon with the use of the Yuzpe regimen.
D. After providing EC, a plan for routine contraception should be discussed with the patient.
E. The advance prescription of EC is not associated with higher rates of promiscuity or sexually transmitted infections.

Review this! ❑

24. Which of the following statements about the use of abstinence as a form of contraception is true?

A. It is strictly defined as the avoidance of vaginal intercourse only.
B. It is uncommon.
C. It is not often associated with partner pressure.
D. It is a primary process only.
E. It is common, normal, and acceptable.

Review this! ❑

25. Without the use of any form of contraception, which of the following is the percentage of pregnancies during the first year of unprotected intercourse?

A. 15%
B. 30%
C. 50%
D. 70%
E. 85%

Review this! ❑

26. For a female smoker over the age of 35 years, all of the following contraception methods are acceptable, except:

A. The Ortho Evra patch.
B. A levonorgestrel-secreting IUD.
C. DMPA.
D. Progestin-only oral contraceptives
E. A diaphragm.

Review this! ❑

27. Male polyurethane condoms have all of the following advantages over latex condoms, except:

A. They are thinner than latex condoms.
B. They are less likely to slip or break as compared with latex condoms.
C. They are less likely to degrade when exposed to oil-based products.
D. They offer similar STI prevention as latex condoms.
E. They increase male penile sensitivity.

Review this! ❑

28. Which of the following statements about the cervical cap (Lea's Shield) is true?

A. It is made of latex; thus, it is unsafe for latex-allergic individuals.
B. It comes in a variety of sizes.
C. Efficacy is improved among women who are multiparous.
D. It is designed to be a "one-size-fits-all" device.
E. Concurrent use of a spermicide with the device does not improve efficacy.

Review this! ❑

29. All of the following statements are true about vasectomy, except:

A. It is more effective than female sterilization.
B. Complications of vasectomy include bleeding, hematomas, and infection.
C. "No-scalpel" vasectomy is most commonly performed in the operating room.
D. Risk factors for regret after a vasectomy include young age and unstable marriage.
E. There is no evidence to support an association between vasectomy and prostate cancer.

Review this! ❑

Things to remember for the test.

30. Contraception methods that are preferable for a woman who has difficulties being compliant include all of the following, except:

    A. DMPA.
    B. NuvaRing.
    C. The Ortho Evra patch.
    D. An IUD.
    E. Combination oral contraceptive pills.

    Review this! ❑

38 Interpretation of the Electrocardiogram

Cheyn Onarecker

1. All of the following are true about the electrocardiogram (ECG) during systole, except:

   A. The T wave is the result of the repolarization of the ventricles.
   B. Hyperkalemia produces a large U wave in practically all leads.
   C. Depolarization of the ventricles causes the QRS wave.
   D. The P wave is caused by the depolarization of the atria.
   E. The U wave is an afterwave of repolarization.

   Review this! ❏

2. True or false: The standard limb leads (I, II, III, AVL, AVR, and AVF) assess the horizontal plane of the heart's electrical field.

   A. True
   B. False

   Review this! ❏

3. With regard to the QRS axis, all of the following are true, except:

   A. The direction of QRS is normally between 0 and +90 degrees.
   B. A simple method of determining the axis can be performed by assessing leads I and AVF.
   C. Newborns usually exhibit left-axis deviation as a result of the relative preponderance of left ventricular forces.
   D. Extreme right-axis deviation occurs when the axis falls between 180 and −90 degrees.
   E. The mean QRS axis projects itself in all of the leads.

   Review this! ❏

4. True or false: It is unusual for the electrocardiogram of an elderly person to exhibit left-axis deviation.

   A. True
   B. False

   Review this! ❏

5. True statements about the precordial leads include all of the following, except:

   A. Chronic obstructive pulmonary disease causes decreased amplitudes in V_1, V_2, and V_6.
   B. High voltages in V_3, V_4, and V_5 may not necessarily indicate the presence of pathology.
   C. The electrode for V_1 is placed in the fourth intercostal space at the right sternal border.
   D. The precordial leads provide an accurate measurement of the amplitude and direction of the QRS axis.
   E. There is a gradual increase in the voltage of the R wave as it progresses from V_1 to V_5.

   Review this! ❏

6. Which of the following statements about the P wave is true?

   A. The amplitude is considered abnormal when it is less than 0.25 mV.
   B. When the P wave is very small, isoelectric, or negative in lead I, it is likely the result of left atrial enlargement.
   C. The P wave is usually negative in lead II.
   D. Practically all V leads show a positive P wave.
   E. All of the above

   Review this! ❏

7. True or false: Atrial repolarization is seldom detected on the ECG, because it is usually canceled out by the QRS complex.

   A. True
   B. False

   Review this! ❏

8. All of the following statements accurately describe the T wave, except:

A. Practically all V leads show a positive T wave.
B. Negative T waves in V_1 through V_3 can indicate strain in the anterior wall of the left ventricle.
C. Ventricular strain describes a condition in which the T is negative in the lead of highest QRS positivity or positive in the lead of highest QRS negativity.
D. The term "flipped Ts" refers to the appearance of negative T waves in leads in which the T waves are usually positive.
E. All of the above

Review this! ❑

9. True or false: When the negative portion of QRS in V_1 (S_1) added to the positive portion of QRS in V_5 (R_5) exceeds 35 mm, the diagnosis of left ventricular hypertrophy should be considered.

A. True
B. False

Review this! ❑

10. The condition referred to as left ventricular strain can occur with which of the following?

A. Hypertrophy
B. Bundle branch block

C. Ischemia
D. Digitalis
E. All of the above

Review this! ❑

11. The features of Figure 38-1 that indicate left bundle branch block include all of the following, except:

A. The duration of the QRS is greater than 0.12 sec.
B. Right-axis deviation is present.
C. The magnitude of the QRS is usually normal.
D. Slurring of the QRS in several leads is present.
E. Left ventricular strain is present.

Review this! ❑

12. Which of the following is true about left anterior hemiblock?

A. It is most often the result of mitral valve disease.
B. It usually causes right-axis deviation.
C. It occurs much more often than left posterior hemiblock.
D. It typically produces a QRS duration of more than 0.12 sec.
E. It causes an increased magnitude of the QRS.

Review this! ❑

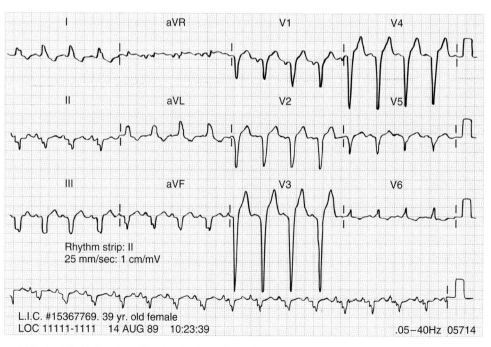

Figure 38-1 In Rakel RE, editor: *Textbook of family medicine,* ed 7, Philadelphia, WB Saunders, 2007.

13. All of the following statements are true about right atrial enlargement and its ECG findings, except:

    A. The magnitude of the P wave is greater than 0.25 mV in lead II, causing a peaked P wave.
    B. A small P wave is usually seen in lead I.
    C. Most cases are the result of chronic obstructive pulmonary disease, pulmonic valve disease, or pulmonary artery disease.
    D. The P wave in several of the standard limb leads shows a double-hump pattern.
    E. The duration of the P wave is usually less than 0.8 sec.

    Review this! ❏

14. Which of the following is true about left atrial enlargement?

    A. The term may be used interchangeably with the term *P-pulmonale.*
    B. It frequently results in peaked P waves in V_1.
    C. It is usually the result of atherosclerotic cardiovascular disease.
    D. It typically causes a P-wave duration of less than 0.8 sec.
    E. It exhibits ECG findings similar to those of left atrial abnormalities.

    Review this! ❏

15. ECG findings attributable to the effect of chronic obstructive pulmonary disease include which of the following?

    A. Poor R-wave progression
    B. P-mitrale
    C. An overall increase in the magnitude of the QRS in the standard limb leads
    D. Left atrial enlargement
    E. Normal transmission of electrical forces to the precordial leads

    Review this! ❏

16. One of the criteria used to make the diagnosis of an acute myocardial infarction is the presence of which of the following?

    A. Prominent ST displacement (up or down)
    B. A prominent negative T wave in the leads with a positive QRS (strain pattern)
    C. Slurring in S waves
    D. Small, narrow Q waves in leads that do not normally have Q waves

E. All of the above

Review this! ❏

Questions 17–20: Match the area of the myocardial infarction with the coronary artery that is most likely to be occluded:

17. The posterior segment of the right coronary artery
18. The dominant right coronary artery
19. The circumflex artery
20. The left anterior descending artery

    A. Anterior or anteroseptal wall infarction
    B. Anterolateral wall infarction
    C. Inferior wall infarction
    D. Posterior wall infarction

    Review this! ❏

21. Which of the following statements about Prinzmetal syndrome is true?

    A. The condition produces a transient depression in the ST segment.
    B. Brief periods of chest pain at rest are typical.
    C. It is usually seen among elderly women.
    D. The ST changes and chest pain are usually detected during exercise.
    E. All of the above

    Review this! ❏

22. In addition to myocardial infarction, ST segment elevation is also seen with which of the following conditions?

    A. Digitalis
    B. Pericarditis
    C. Left bundle branch block
    D. Left ventricular hypertrophy
    E. All of the above

    Review this! ❏

23. Findings that distinguish pericarditis from early repolarization include which of the following?

    A. Small elevations of the ST segment are seen in early repolarization.
    B. Pericarditis occurs among younger patients.
    C. ST-segment elevation in the anterior leads is seen in early repolarization.
    D. No significant Q waves appear in early repolarization.
    E. Pericarditis is associated with characteristic clinical signs and symptoms.

    Review this! ❏

Things to remember for the test.

Questions 24–27: Match the following electrocardiograms with the correct diagnosis.
24. Old inferior wall myocardial infarction
25. Subacute lateral wall myocardial infarction
26. Old posterior wall myocardial infarction
27. Acute anterior wall myocardial infarction

A. Tracing 34–19
B. Tracing 34–23
C. Tracing 34–24
D. Tracing 34–21

Review this! ❏

28. ECG changes consistent with a postmyocardial infarction ventricular aneurysm include which of the following?

A. Very small or nonexistent ST segment displacement in the standard limb leads
B. A QS pattern in leads V_1 through V_4
C. An elevated ST segment in the anterior leads
D. A history of anterior wall myocardial infarction
E. All of the above

Review this! ❏

29. A prolonged PR interval is caused by which of the following?

A. First-degree atrioventricular block as a result of coronary artery disease
B. Wolff–Parkinson–White syndrome
C. Wandering pacemaker

D. Nodal rhythm
E. Premature atrial contractions

Review this! ❏

30. All of the following are true about the QT interval, except:

A. It is inversely proportional to the heart rate.
B. Hypocalcemia, hypokalemia, and some psychotropic drugs can prolong the duration.
C. A QT_c value of more than 0.44 sec is considered abnormal in adults.
D. It is prolonged in two rare congenital syndromes that are associated with the occurrence of torsade de pointes.
E. Quinidine typically produces a shortened interval.

Review this! ❏

31. Criteria for the diagnosis of Lown–Ganong–Levine syndrome include which of the following?

A. The presence of supraventricular tachycardia
B. A normal QRS
C. A delta wave
D. A prolonged QT
E. An abnormal P wave

Review this! ❏

39 Cardiovascular Disease

Lance C. Brunner

1. Risk factors for the development and progression of atherosclerosis include all of the following, except:

   A. Dyslipidemia.
   B. Impairments in glycemic control.
   C. Low bone density.
   D. Family history.
   E. Systemic inflammation.

   Review this! ❏

2. Which of the following best describes endothelial dysfunction with regard to the development of atherosclerosis?

   A. It is a passive progress caused simply by the accumulation of lipids within the arterial wall.
   B. It is not related to oxidative insult.
   C. It is mediated, at least partially, by inflammatory processes.
   D. It is related to increased vasodilatory capacity.
   E. It is triggered by a downregulation of the VCAM-1 cell-adhesion molecule.

   Review this! ❏

3. True or false: In the majority of cases, atheromatous lesions giving rise to acute myocardial infarction (AMI) are flow-limiting in nature.

   A. True
   B. False

   Review this! ❏

4. Properties of high-density lipoprotein (HDL) particles include which of the following?

   A. The extraction of extracellular cholesterol from macrophages and subsequent delivery to the liver for elimination as bile salts
   B. Increased endothelial cell-adhesion molecule expression
   C. Increased endothelial nitric oxide and prostacyclin production

   D. Decreased platelet aggregation
   E. C and D

   Review this! ❏

5. The National Cholesterol Education Program Adult Treatment Panel III (ATP III) includes which of the following?

   A. An HDL level of <40 mg/dL is now defined as a categorical risk factor for coronary artery disease (CAD).
   B. The optimal low-density lipoprotein-cholesterol complex (LDL-C) level has now been lowered to <100 mg/dL, irrespective of race or gender.
   C. LDL-C reduction is the primary goal of therapy for patients with dyslipidemia.
   D. All of the above

   Review this! ❏

6. True or false: The Heart Protection Study has recommended that physicians consider treating LDL-C to <70 mg/dL in very high-risk patients (e.g., a patient with recent acute coronary syndrome [ACS] or a diabetic with multiple poorly controlled risk factors).

   A. True
   B. False

   Review this! ❏

7. A large number of recent, prospective, placebo-controlled trials have revealed the following risk reductions in relation to the drug class of statins, except:

   A. A reduction in myocardial infarction (MI) rates.
   B. A reduction in cerebrovascular accident rates.
   C. A reduction in stable and unstable angina rates.
   D. A lack of preliminary evidence suggesting plaque resorption.
   E. A reduction in atheromatous plaque progression.

   Review this! ❏

Things to remember for the test.

Things to remember for the test.

8. Adverse events associated with statin therapy include which of the following?

   A. An increased risk of liver failure
   B. Rhabdomyolysis
   C. Renal failure
   D. Elevated transaminase levels
   E. B, C, and D
   F. All of the above

   Review this! ❏

9. Complications of fibrate therapy can include which of the following?

   A. Myopathy
   B. Cholelithiasis
   C. Increased prothrombin time with concurrent warfarin use
   D. Elevated transaminase levels
   E. All of the above

   Review this! ❏

10. True or false: Fish oils enriched with omega-3 and omega-6 fatty acids have no effect on triglyceride levels, but they can reduce very-low-density lipoprotein levels and increase high-density lipoprotein-cholesterol complex (HDL-C) levels in a dose-dependent manner.

    A. True
    B. False

    Review this! ❏

11. Which of the following statements about hypertension is true?

    A. If you are normotensive at the age of 55 years, your risk of developing hypertension is low.
    B. For every 20/10 mm Hg increase in blood pressure above 140/90 mm Hg, the risk of cardiovascular disease increases twofold.
    C. Treatment of diastolic hypertension decreases the risk of cardiovascular disease more so than treating the systolic hypertension.
    D. Approximately one third of patients with hypertension in the United States are currently treated to their target level.
    E. All of the above

    Review this! ❏

12. Which of the following recommendations were made in "The Seventh Report of the Joint National Committee on Prevention,

Detection, Evaluation, and Treatment of High Blood Pressure"?

    A. Aggressive lifestyle modification is suggested for those with a systolic blood pressure of 120 to 139 mm Hg or a diastolic blood pressure of 80 to 89 mm Hg.
    B. Loop diuretics are generally the first-line choice for treatment of hypertension.
    C. If the baseline blood pressure is more than 20/10 mm Hg above the target level, then initial therapy should be a high dose of a single agent rather than a drug combination.
    D. The majority of patients will need one drug to get reach their hypertension goal.

    Review this! ❏

13. Which of the following statements about the management of hypertension is false?

    A. Congestive heart failure (CHF) is a compelling indication for the use of calcium-channel blocker in cases of complicated hypertension.
    B. An elevation of serum creatinine level of up to 35% above baseline is tolerable and not an indication for discontinuing an angiotensin-converting enzyme inhibitor (ACEI) or an angiotensin-II receptor blocker (ARB).
    C. α-Blockers have the added effect of increasing serum HDL levels.
    D. Patients with hypertension and arteriosclerotic heart disease should be placed on a β-blocker if there are no contraindications.

    Review this! ❏

14. ATP III criteria for diagnosing metabolic syndrome include all of the following, except:

    A. Abdominal obesity with a waist circumference of more than 40 inches in men.
    B. Hypertriglyceridemia with a level of more than 250 mg/dL.
    C. A fasting blood sugar level of 100 mg/dL or more.
    D. An HDL-C for women of less than 50 mg/dL.
    E. None of the above

    Review this! ❏

15. True or false: Visceral adipose tissue is highly metabolically active, and increases in quantity are correlated with insulin resistance, serum-free fatty acid level elevation, and nonalcoholic steatohepatitis development.

    A. True
    B. False

    Review this! ❑

16. True or false: Data from the Diabetes Prevention Project suggest that aggressive lifestyle modification in patients with metabolic syndrome can reduce the risk of the development of diabetes mellitus by around 58%.

    A. True
    B. False

    Review this! ❑

17. Which of the following statements about diabetes mellitus is true?

    A. Most patient with diabetes die of renal failure.
    B. Type 2 diabetes is decreasing in prevalence in the portion of the population that is less than 21 years old.
    C. Patients with type 2 diabetes are generally hypercoagulable and are at higher risk of thrombosis.
    D. A and C
    E. All of the above

    Review this! ❑

18. Which of the following statements about the aggressive management of patients with type 2 diabetes is false?

    A. The UK Prospective Diabetes Study suggests that, for every 1% drop in hemoglobin A1c, diabetics experience a 21% reduction in any diabetes-related endpoint.
    B. The UK Prospective Diabetes Study suggests that metformin therapy reduces the risk of acute cardiovascular events by about 38%.
    C. Data from the National Health and Nutrition Examination Survey III suggest that the vast majority of diabetics do eventually have controlled blood pressure.

    D. The Hypertension Optimal Treatment trial demonstrated that there was no confirmation of the "J-curve hypothesis," which is that cardiovascular events increased as diastolic pressure decreased.

    Review this! ❑

19. True or false: Both ACEIs and ARBs have been demonstrated to reduce the degree of microalbuminuria and to decrease the rate of progression to overt nephropathy.

    A. True
    B. False

    Review this! ❑

20. Which of the following statement about C-reactive protein (CRP) is true?

    A. In the Physicians Health Study, men in the highest quartile of CRP had a 10-fold higher risk for myocardial infarction over an 8-year period.
    B. The Women's Health Study data suggested that CRP levels were a better predictor of cardiovascular disease than serum LDL-C.
    C. Elevated CRP levels are not associated with a greater stroke risk.
    D. High-risk patients (i.e., those with a coronary artery disease risk equivalent or 10-year risk or more than 20%) should not be screened with an ultrasensitive CRP level.

    Review this! ❑

21. Which of the following is true about elevated homocysteine levels?

    A. They are an established risk factor for atherosclerotic disease.
    B. They are associated with an increased risk of CAD.
    C. In patients with CAD, they can be treated with vitamins B_6 and B_{12} and folate. This treatment has been demonstrated in all available studies to decrease the rate of plaque progression.
    D. They should be screened for in patients with a high risk of CAD.

    Review this! ❑

22. Which of the following statements about cigarette smoking is true?

Things to remember for the test.

A. Cigarette smoking is the single most preventable cause of mortality in the United States.
B. Smoking cessation results in a 36% reduction in the risk for both myocardial infarction and mortality.
C. Relapse rates are high in the absence of education, encouragement, and individualized courses of therapy and follow up.
D. Bupropion can reduce nicotine-withdrawal symptoms.
E. All of the above

Review this! ❏

23. Which of the following statements about cardiac physiology is true?

A. Most coronary blood flow occurs during diastole.
B. Myocardial ischemia can be silent in patients with diabetes.
C. Coronary supply is determined by oxygen transport capacity, nitric oxide, endothelin, the autonomic nervous system, metabolic activity, neural control, and perfusion pressure.
D. All of the above
E. B and C

Review this! ❏

24. Causes of a false-positive electrocardiogram include which of the following?

A. Digoxin use
B. Left bundle branch block
C. Left ventricular hypertrophy
D. All of the above

Review this! ❏

25. Which of the following statements about treadmill stress testing is true?

A. It has a fairly high sensitivity and specificity for all patients, irrespective of risk factors.
B. It has low diagnostic accuracy for many cases if the target heart rate is not achieved.
C. It has a low positive predictive value when patients have angina symptoms and 1-mm ST-segment depression during exercise.
D. It is not affected (from a sensitivity standpoint) by the concurrent use of nitrates or β-blockers.

Review this! ❏

26. Absolute contraindications to stress testing include all of the following, except:

A. Ongoing chest pain at rest.
B. An AMI within the previous week.
C. Compensated CHF.
D. Severe hypertension.
E. Intractable arrhythmia.

Review this! ❏

27. Which of the following statements about pharmacologic stress myocardial perfusion is false?

A. Adenosine is a vasodilator, and it stresses the heart by a "steal phenomenon."
B. Dipyridamole dilates normal coronary arteries, which serves to create a discrepancy in perfusion.
C. Adenosine injection rarely causes flushing and shortness of breath.
D. Dobutamine increases heart rate and contractility.

Review this! ❏

28. If there are no contraindications, the pharmacologic management of stable angina should include which of the following?

A. Nitrates, because they have been demonstrated to decrease mortality
B. β-blockers, because of their ability to prolong survival in most situations
C. Short-acting calcium-channel blockers, because of their antianginal properties
D. Aspirin
E. B and D

Review this! ❏

29. In general, patients with CAD benefit from coronary artery bypass grafting if they demonstrate all of the following, except:

A. Asymptomatic CAD.
B. Severe left main artery disease.
C. Unsuitable anatomy for coronary angioplasty.
D. Triple vessel disease in patients with diabetes and a low ejection fraction.
E. None of the above

Review this! ❏

30. Which of the following statements about ACS is true?

A. More than 60% of AMIs are induced by culprit lesions that initially obstruct less than 50% of the arterial lumen.
B. Angiographic and coronary ultrasounds always show the same amount of disease burden.
C. When an ACS occurs, there is usually only one lesion that is vulnerable at the time of the event.
D. All of the above are true.
E. All of the above are false.

Review this! ❏

31. Which of the following statements about the creatine kinase and the creatine kinase, myocardial-bound serum cardiac markers is true?

A. They are less sensitive than serum myoglobin for myocardial injury.
B. Creatine kinase reaches its peak at about 24 hours after injury.
C. They are only 50% accurate for diagnosing an AMI at 6 hours after symptom onset.
D. They usually return to normal after about 7 days after injury.

Review this! ❏

32. Acute therapy for unstable angina/non–ST-segment myocardial infarction should include all of the following, except:

A. Aspirin.
B. Plavix.
C. Unfractionated or low-molecular-weight heparin.
D. Fibrinolytics.
E. Glycoprotein IIb/IIIa inhibitors in certain clinical situations.

Review this! ❏

33. Which of the following statements about patients with an ST-elevation myocardial infarction is true?

A. They generally have an acute coronary plaque rupture.
B. They should receive thrombolytics within 30 minutes or angioplasty within 90 minutes of arriving in the emergency room.
C. They have a more favorable outcome from angioplasty as compared with thrombolytics in most situations, but especially for those patients with cardiogenic shock or CHF.
D. All of the above

Review this! ❏

34. Which of the following statements about the inappropriate remodeling of the heart and the subsequent development of CHF is true?

A. It can be mediated by angiotensin-II–related cellular proliferation.
B. It is associated with low levels of aldosterone.
C. It is often associated with elevated endothelin-1 production.
D. It is not affected by rising catecholamine levels.
E. None of the above

Review this! ❏

35. Aggressive risk-factor modification for patients with CHF includes which of the following?

A. Target blood pressure of less than 130/85 mm Hg for patients with diabetes
B. Dyslipidemia control
C. Aggressive diabetes management
D. Increasing exercise
E. B, C, and D
F. All of the above

Review this! ❏

36. Medications that improve survival in patients with CHF with left ventricular dysfunction under certain situations include all the following, except:

A. β-Blockers.
B. Digoxin.
C. ACEIs.
D. Spironolactone.

Review this! ❏

37. Which of the following statements about the development of aortic stenosis is true?

A. It is not associated with congenital bicuspid valves.
B. It never leads to the development of diastolic dysfunction and CHF.
C. It can lead to anginal symptoms, even in the presence of a normal coronary angiogram.
D. It is associated with a calcific aortic valve among younger patients.

Review this! ❏

38. True or false: In patients with aortic stenosis and syncope at rest, the syncope is usually associated primarily with aortic root and cerebral vascular hypoperfusion as a result of outflow obstruction.

    A. True
    B. False

    Review this! ❏

39. Which of the following statements about the surgical treatment of aortic stenosis (specifically valve replacement) is true?

    A. It should always be offered and completed in patients with asymptomatic severe aortic stenosis.
    B. It is associated with the same positive outcomes as valvuloplasty.
    C. It is often combined with coronary artery bypass grafting, should underlying CAD be present.
    D. It will usually require lifelong anticoagulation with warfarin if a bioprosthetic tissue valve is selected.

    Review this! ❏

40. Which of the following statements about mitral valve stenosis is true?

    A. It is more common among males.
    B. It is generally caused by primary valve degeneration.
    C. It is predominantly caused by rheumatic carditis.
    D. It is never associated with pulmonary hypertension.

    Review this! ❏

41. Which of the following statements about the management of mitral stenosis is true?

    A. It does not require antibiotic prophylaxis before genitourinary procedures.
    B. It can include the use of β-blockers to prolong diastole.
    C. It often includes oral anticoagulation as a result of an increased risk of intermittent or persistent atrial fibrillation.
    D. B and C
    E. All of the above

    Review this! ❏

42. Which of the following statements about mitral regurgitation is true?

    A. It is often associated with a loud, holo-diastolic murmur.

    B. It cannot lead to the development of cardiomegaly.
    C. It is not associated with a past history of rheumatic fever.
    D. It is associated with a lower surgical threshold relative to aortic regurgitation.

    Review this! ❏

43. Which of the following statements about mitral valve prolapse is true?

    A. It is currently felt that there is no increased stroke risk with this condition.
    B. A click is often heard in diastole.
    C. No treatment is generally necessary, unless patients have coexisting mitral regurgitation.
    D. A, B, and C
    E. A and B

    Review this! ❏

44. True or false: The presence of peripheral artery disease is an independent predictor of overall mortality.

    A. True
    B. False

    Review this! ❏

45. Which of the following statements about peripheral vascular disease (PVD) is true?

    A. The degree of claudication is proportional to the degree of arterial compromise.
    B. Approximately 50% of patients with this condition are asymptomatic.
    C. Above-the-knee amputees achieve greater long-term mobility as compared with below-the-knee amputees.
    D. All of the above

    Review this! ❏

46. Risk factors for PVD include which of the following?

    A. Age
    B. Smoking
    C. Type 2 diabetes
    D. Hyperlipidemia
    E. Hypertension
    F. All of the above

    Review this! ❏

47. All of the following statements about PVD are true, except:

A. Approximately 40% of patients with PVD manifest symptoms in other vascular beds.

B. The all-cause mortality rate among patients with PVD is higher for men.

C. The lower the ankle-brachial index (ABI), the higher the risk of cardiovascular events.

D. Patients with critical limb ischemia have an annual mortality rate of about 25%.

Review this! ❏

48. Patients with critical limb ischemia often have which of the following physical examination findings?

A. Pain is worse when allowing the leg to dangle over the side of the bed.

B. An absence or decrease of hair on the affected foot

C. Limb elevation produces increased rubor

D. All of the above

Review this! ❏

49. True or false: Patients with PVD may have an ABI that is normal at rest but that may be significantly decreased with exercise.

A. True

B. False

Review this! ❏

50. Which of the following statements about ABIs is true?

A. Calcified vessels can lead to a false-negative ABI.

B. A mildly depressed resting ABI does not indicate significant PVD.

C. Given that most epidemiological studies use a resting ABI to diagnose PVD, the true disease burden may be underestimated.

D. All of the above

Review this! ❏

51. Management of PVD should include which of the following?

A. Bedrest without aerobic exercise because of the increased risk of foot ulcers

B. Antiplatelet therapy, if there are no contraindications

C. Trental, because of the overwhelming randomized, controlled trial data that support its use

D. Revascularization for asymptomatic individuals without critical limb ischemia

Review this! ❏

52. Which of the following statements about cardiac anatomy is true?

A. The distal portion of the atrioventricular node becomes the bundle of His.

B. The atrioventricular node arises in the right atrium.

C. The sinoatrial node lies at the apex of the triangle of Koch.

D. All of the above

Review this! ❏

53. Which of the following statements about atrial-based arrhythmias is false?

A. Sinus bradycardia originates in the sinus node with a P wave that is different in morphology from the normal sinus beat.

B. A sinus pause is typically the result of changes in vagal tone, such as gagging, carotid sinus stimulation, and pain and as a consequence of neurocardiogenic activation.

C. Premature atrial contractions are often seen among patients without cardiac disease.

D. An ectopic atrial rhythm is said to occur when there is not an upright P wave visible in limb leads I, II, and III.

Review this! ❏

54. True or false: During atrial fibrillation, atria are depolarized from a single ectopic focus, which results in markedly elevated atrial rates that exceed several hundred beats per minute.

A. True

B. False

Review this! ❏

55. Which of the following statements about atrioventricular nodal conduction disorders is true?

A. First-degree atrioventricular block is defined as a PR interval of greater than 100 msec.

B. Type 2 second-degree atrioventricular block is characterized by a progressive prolongation of the PR interval followed by a dropped ventricular beat.

Things to remember for the test.

C. Type-2 second-degree atrioventricular block demonstrates regular PR intervals.

D. Third-degree atrioventricular block results from the failure of atrial impulses from the atrioventricular node to conduct down to the ventricle.

Review this! ❑

56. Which of the following statements about long QT syndrome is true?

A. It is a result of ion-channel abnormalities in the cell membranes.

B. It can be inherited in an autosomal-dominant fashion.

C. It can result in life-threatening ventricular arrhythmias.

D. It is often seen in families with a history of sudden cardiac death.

E. All of the above

Review this! ❑

57. Which of the following statements about the management of atrial fibrillation is true?

A. It includes improved hospitalization rates among patients who have rhythm control over rate control.

B. It should include, in most nonurgent situations of nonvalvular atrial fibrillation, anticoagulation with warfarin for at least 3 weeks before electrical cardioversion.

C. Direct cardioversion is an unsafe practice and has been supplanted by the use of intravenous chemical cardioversion drugs.

D. All of the above

Review this! ❑

58. For patients with refractory CHF, which of the following is true?

A. There is a 6- to 9-fold increase in the rate of sudden cardiac death.

B. Cardiac pacing resynchronization therapy has not been demonstrated to affect mortality.

C. An implantable defibrillator has been shown to reduce mortality.

D. A and C

E. All of the above

Review this! ❑

59. In which of the following situations has an implantable defibrillator been shown to provide a superior mortality benefit as compared with drug therapy for the management of primary lethal tachycardia events (i.e., ventricular tachycardia and ventricular fibrillation)?

A. Prior myocardial infarction and low ejection fraction

B. Class II/III CHF for more than 3 months and an ejection fraction of less than 35%

C. Asymptomatic ventricular ectopy and inducible ventricular tachycardia

D. All of the above

Review this! ❑

40 Emergency Medicine

Stephen E. Markovich

Things to remember for the test.

1. Which of the following is indicated for the early treatment of traumatic rhabdomyolysis resulting from a crush injury to muscular tissues or from prolonged extrication?

   A. Fluid restriction to prevent edema
   B. Alkalinization of the urine
   C. Serial urine examination for haptoglobin
   D. Fasciotomy

   Review this! ❑

2. Shock is best defined by which of the following?

   A. Hypotension as a result of massive blood loss
   B. Changes in mentation as a result of open or closed head injury
   C. Hypercarbia as a result of poor airway maintenance
   D. Hypoperfusion of tissues with resulting metabolic acidosis

   Review this! ❑

3. Which of the following best describes why diagnostic peritoneal lavage is useful during the management of trauma?

   A. It is superior to ultrasound for assessment of the retroperitoneum.
   B. It can be used to determine which patients should be transferred.
   C. It can be used to determine which patients need urgent laparotomy.
   D. It allows for rapid assessment when trained surgical teams are not available.

   Review this! ❑

4. Which of the following best describes why trauma in children requires special consideration?

   A. Children are able to maintain blood pressure despite significant acute blood loss.
   B. The small surface area of a child increases the risk of hyperthermia.
   C. Higher muscle tone increases the risk of multisystem injury.
   D. Cricothyroidotomy is the standard for airway management for children who are less than 12 years old.

   Review this! ❑

5. Which of the following is preferred for airway management in young children?

   A. Cuffed endotracheal tubes
   B. Cuffed nasotracheal tubes
   C. Uncuffed endotracheal tubes
   D. Uncuffed nasotracheal tubes

   Review this! ❑

6. In general, if a pregnant woman is involved in a trauma, which of the following is the best treatment plan for the fetus?

   A. Kleihauer–Betke testing
   B. Serial nonstress testing
   C. Cervical cerclage
   D. Proper resuscitation of the mother

   Review this! ❑

7. Which of the following statements about the impact of trauma on society is true?

   A. Most trauma occurs in the elderly.
   B. Today's advanced trauma life-support guidelines are based on World War II and Vietnam experiences.
   C. A lack of training and public awareness results in more deaths than disabilities.
   D. The death rate from trauma is approximately 150,000 annually.

   Review this! ❑

8. When approaching the seriously injured trauma patient with obvious mental status changes, long bone fractures, and bleeding, which of the following is the most important task to accomplish?

A. Immobilizing the cervical spine
B. Gaining control of the airway
C. Directing pressure to stop bleeding
D. Establishing two large-bore intravenous lines and providing vigorous fluid resuscitation

Review this! ❏

9. Initial emergency fetal assessment includes all of the following, except:

A. Sterile vaginal speculum examination.
B. Maternal abdominal examination.
C. Fetal heart rate determination.
D. Fetal ultrasound.

Review this! ❏

10. The management of high-pressure injection injuries generally involves which of the following?

A. Digital block to provide immediate pain relief
B. Radiologic studies to assess extent of injury
C. Observation with delayed open debridement
D. Close evaluation by a hand specialist in 1 to 3 days

Review this! ❏

11. During the assessment of a traumatic dislocation of the knee, in addition to plain radiographs, the physician should consider obtaining which of the following?

A. A computed tomography scan of the knee
B. A magnetic resonance image of the knee
C. Compartment pressures
D. Angiography

Review this! ❏

12. Which of the following statements about decompression sickness is false?

A. It can affect the gastrointestinal, pulmonary, ocular, and musculoskeletal systems.
B. All divers who experience vertigo or tinnitus should be considered for hyperbaric oxygen therapy.
C. Aspirin therapy should be considered.
D. Initial treatment is oxygen and placing the patient in the Trendelenburg position.

Review this! ❏

13. True or false: Cervical spine injury can be ruled out by a complete neurological examination

A. True
B. False

Review this! ❏

14. A patient with a closed head injury who was lucid on arrival suddenly begins to deteriorate neurologically. Which of the following would be the next appropriate step?

A. Ordering an immediate computed tomography scan of the head
B. Completing the secondary survey
C. Confirming a central cord injury by assessing rectal tone
D. Repeating the primary survey

Review this! ❏

15. Which of the following is not consistent with a patient presenting with hypotension, tachycardia, decreased urine output, and mental status changes?

A. Hemorrhagic shock
B. Major head trauma
C. Anaphylaxis
D. Sepsis

Review this! ❏

16. Which of the following is not consistent with cardiogenic shock?

A. Decreased systemic vascular resistance
B. Narrow pulse pressure
C. Elevated central venous pressure
D. Decreased cardiac output

Review this! ❏

17. Primary treatment of disseminated intravascular coagulation in septic shock should focus on which of the following?

A. Correction of the elevated prothrombin time and partial thromboplastin time
B. Prevention of significant thrombosis with heparin
C. Replacement of coagulation factors with cryoprecipitate
D. Treatment of the underlying infection with antibiotics, debridement, or drainage

Review this! ❏

18. Which of the following would be most helpful during the initial management of shock?

    A. Foley catheter
    B. Central venous catheter
    C. Swan-Ganz catheter
    D. Transcutaneous catheter

    Review this! ❏

19. Which of the following is the intravenous fluid of choice for the initial stabilization of the patient in shock?

    A. Type-specific, non-crossmatched blood
    B. Crystalloid
    C. Free water with glucose
    D. Albumin-containing solutions

    Review this! ❏

20. Which of the following sutures poses the lowest risk of infection?

    A. Synthetic monofilament
    B. Absorbable, synthetic, braided
    C. Natural gut
    D. Silk

    Review this! ❏

21. The initial management of patients who have been poisoned begins with which of the following?

    A. Arterial blood gas determination
    B. Anion gap determination
    C. Glucose level determination
    D. Airway stabilization

    Review this! ❏

22. Acetaminophen metabolism induces hepatic injury how long after ingestion?

    A. 30–60 minutes
    B. 12–24 hours
    C. 1–3 days
    D. 5–7 days

    Review this! ❏

23. The decision to treat with *N*-acetylcysteine (Mucomyst) is based on what two factors?

    A. Body weight in kilograms
    B. Milligrams ingested
    C. Acetaminophen level
    D. Time
    E. Salicylate level

    Review this! ❏

24. Which of the following is most closely associated with tricyclic antidepressant overdose?

    A. Hepatic abnormalities
    B. Renal failure
    C. Cardiac ischemia
    D. Cardiac arrhythmias

    Review this! ❏

25. When evaluating burn extent on adults using the body surface area technique, an individual's palmar surface represents what percentage of the body surface area?

    A. 1%
    B. 3%
    C. 5%
    D. 9%

    Review this! ❏

26. On the basis of the criteria of the American Burn Association, which of the following situations would require admission at a burn center?

    A. A circumferential burn of the forearm
    B. A sunburn of the dorsum of both feet
    C. A 5% partial-thickness burn of the thigh from grease
    D. An electrical burn of the fingertip

    Review this! ❏

27. Which of the following requires rabies prophylaxis?

    A. A domestic dog
    B. A raccoon
    C. A squirrel
    D. A rat

    Review this! ❏

28. Which of the following is the drug of choice for patients who are not allergic to penicillin and who have received an animal bite?

    A. Levaquin
    B. Gentamicin
    C. Vancomycin
    D. Augmentin

    Review this! ❏

41

Sports Medicine

Douglas DiOrio

1. Which of the following is one of the primary objectives of a pre-participation physical examination?

   A. To get adolescents to see their doctors
   B. To promote health and safety
   C. To detect potentially life-threatening or disabling medical conditions
   D. To get patients vaccinated appropriately

   Review this! ❏

2. Which of the following is not a major warning sign or "red flag" during the pre-participation physical examination?

   A. A murmur that increases during a Valsalva maneuver
   B. Syncope at rest
   C. Exertional chest pain
   D. A diastolic murmur

   Review this! ❏

3. True or false: Although echocardiograms have been found to detect many life-threatening cardiovascular problems, they are not recommended because of cost.

   A. True
   B. False

   Review this! ❏

4. Which of the following is true?

   A. A supraventricular tachyarrhythmia can be normal, and no workup is needed.
   B. Ventricular tachyarrhythmias are life threatening, and they occur in the presence of structural heart disease.
   C. Tachyarrhythmias never occur in structurally normal hearts.
   D. Atrial tachyarrhythmias require no workup.

   Review this! ❏

5. Which of the following is false?

   A. Among individuals who are more than 35 years old, the most common cause of sudden cardiac death is coronary artery disease.
   B. Commotio cordis is commonly seen among patients who are more than 17 years old, because these individuals can throw a ball much harder than younger individuals.
   C. Structural heart disease is the most common cause of sudden cardiac death among those who are less than 35 years old.
   D. Sudden cardiac death is a rare event, occurring at a rate of 1 in 100,000 to 1 in 300,000 among high school and college athletes.

   Review this! ❏

6. Which of the following statements about concussions is true?

   A. Unconsciousness marks the severity of the injury.
   B. A return-to-play decision depends on the parents' and coach's desire to have the athlete in the game.
   C. The assessment of the concussed individual can be performed without an evaluation of cognitive function or a cranial nerve examination.
   D. A concussion is a traumatically induced disturbance of neurologic function, with variable symptoms.

   Review this! ❏

7. Which of the following statements about stingers is true?

   A. They are not very common in American football.
   B. They are unilateral, and they usually resolve within minutes.
   C. A bilateral stinger can be managed on the field in the same way as a unilateral one.
   D. Stingers commonly cause axonotmesis, and they should be evaluated by magnetic resonance imaging.

   Review this! ❏

8. True or false: A history of transient neuropraxia in an athlete with functional or anatomic spinal stenosis is an absolute contraindication to return to a contact or collision sport.

   A. True
   B. False

   Review this! ❏

9. True or false: In an unconscious football player, the helmet should always be removed to establish airway control.

   A. True
   B. False

   Review this! ❏

10. Which of the following statements about heat illness is true?

    A. Heatstroke is not a common problem among high school athletes.
    B. Evaporation is the primary mechanism of cooling the body.
    C. Thirst is a good indicator of when someone needs a drink.
    D. About 1 L of water should be taken in every 15 minutes when an athlete is practicing on a hot day.

    Review this! ❏

11. Which of the following statements about exertional hyponatremia (i.e., serum sodium of less than 130 mmol/L) is true?

    A. Typical victims are inexperienced female marathoners who tend to be light sweaters and who finish the race in more than 4 hours.
    B. Individuals who suffer from exertional hyponatremia usually suffer water overload at rest.
    C. Sufferers usually have a very high core body temperature.
    D. Hyponatremia should be treated onsite at the marathon, and transportation to the hospital is rare.

    Review this! ❏

12. Which of the following statements about working out in the cold is true?

    A. The layer closest to the skin should be windproof to avoid windchill.

    B. The outer layer should wick the sweat from the body.
    C. Moisture is the most dangerous variable and should be controlled.
    D. Dehydration plays no role in frostbite.

    Review this! ❏

13. The treatment of hypothermia includes all of the following, except:

    A. Immediate warming before moving from subfreezing temperatures.
    B. Finding shelter from wind and moist areas.
    C. Removing wet layers.
    D. Administering warm intravenous fluids in the setting of severe hypothermia.

    Review this! ❏

14. Which of the following statements about altitude illness is true?

    A. A good level of physical fitness is protective.
    B. The speed of ascent does not play a role.
    C. A previous history of altitude sickness is predictive of recurring symptoms.
    D. An altitude of 3000 feet seems to be where acute mountain sickness starts.

    Review this! ❏

15. True or false: When a patient has high-altitude pulmonary edema, he or she should wait a day at that level before ascending further.

    A. True
    B. False

    Review this! ❏

16. Which of the following statements about tooth avulsion is true?

    A. Pulp involvement requires an urgent dental referral.
    B. Enamel fractures are an emergency, and the patient should be sent to the hospital.
    C. The avulsed tooth fragment should be kept dry to avoid dentin softening.
    D. Luxation without impaction should not be touched, and the individual should see a dentist immediately.

    Review this! ❏

17. True or false: After nasal trauma with epistaxis, anterior packing should be performed immediately to avoid septal hematoma, prolonged bleeding, and fracture displacement.

    A. True
    B. False

    Review this! ❑

18. True or false: Athletes with eye pain after trauma should be evaluated for visual acuity, globe rupture, extraocular movements, pupil reactivity, and hyphema. Any sign of globe rupture, orbital fracture, or hyphema requires an urgent ophthalmologic consultation.

    A. True
    B. False

    Review this! ❑

19. Which of the following statements about when an individual can return to playing a sport after being infected with mononucleosis is true?

    A. Mononucleosis is usually a 2-month illness that requires removal from collision sports.
    B. Splenomegaly is easy to assess, and, when the spleen tip is not palpable, the athlete may return.
    C. Splenic rupture associated with a sports activity almost always happens during the first 3 weeks of illness.
    D. A normal ultrasound of the spleen is required before return to contact and collision sports.

    Review this! ❑

20. Which of the following statements about *Herpes gladiatorum* is true?

    A. It is rare among college wrestlers, and it has no serious consequences.
    B. The rash is causes may be difficult to evaluate because of trauma.
    C. It usually occurs 1 to 2 weeks after exposure.
    D. Research has definitively shown that team prophylaxis will prevent all infections for a season.

    Review this! ❑

21. Which of the following statements about exercise-induced bronchospasm (EIB) is true?

    A. EIB should be confirmed by spirometry both before and after exercise.
    B. Among individuals with EIB, spirometry will demonstrate a 50% drop in forced expiratory volume after exercise.
    C. Inhaled corticosteroids before exercise are the mainstay of treatment.
    D. Athletes with EIB should be limited to sports with a short duration of physical activity and those that keep them out of the cold, such as sprint swimming.

    Review this! ❑

22. Which of the following statements about patients with sports anemia is true?

    A. They have a true pathology and should be treated.
    B. They have no need to be checked for iron deficiency.
    C. They have increased plasma volumes that dilute their hemoglobin levels by 0.5 g/dL.
    D. They should be tested only if their hemoglobin levels are below 10 g/dL.

    Review this! ❑

23. True or false: Sickle-cell trait occurs in 6% to 8% of blacks in the United States, but it poses no increased risk of sudden death.

    A. True
    B. False

    Review this! ❑

24. True or false: Hematuria is a symptom of endurance athletes that is common and that requires no workup.

    A. True
    B. False

    Review this! ❑

25. Which of the following statements about low back pain is true?

    A. It 90% of cases, it resolves in 6 to 12 weeks, so nothing needs to be done.
    B. Previous back pain is a predictor of subsequent pain.
    C. A patient with sudden onset of pain should obtain radiographs in an acute setting to rule out spondylolysis.
    D. Oral steroids help calm the inflammation of spondylolysis.

    Review this! ❑

26. Which of the following statements about muscle tendon injuries is true?

    A. They are commonly caused by eccentric forces placed on the muscle.
    B. With an acutely injured muscle, non-steroidal anti-inflammatory drugs have been shown to shorten the time of healing.
    C. Tendinosis plays no role in the pathology of tendon injuries.
    D. The immobilization of tendinopathy has been shown to increase the strength of muscle and to promote faster healing.
    Review this! ❑

27. The differential diagnosis of shin pain in runners should include all of the following, except:

    A. Medial tibial stress syndrome.
    B. Stress fracture.
    C. Compartment syndrome.
    D. Chondromalacia.
    Review this! ❑

28. All of the following are true about stress fractures, except:

    A. About half of all stress fractures in runners are tibial stress fractures.
    B. Stress fractures of the femoral neck, the navicular, and the anterior tibia should be non-weightbearing and referred to a sports specialist.
    C. Stress fractures never hurt at rest, which distinguishes them from shin splints.
    D. Treatment of stress fractures includes rest and activity modification.
    Review this! ❑

29. True or false: The open physes in long bones and the apophyses at tendon attachments to bones do not change overuse injury patterns among pediatric patients; they can be treated as adults.

    A. True
    B. False
    Review this! ❑

30. Which of the following statements about athletic amenorrhea is false?

    A. It is caused by hypothalamic pituitary axis suppression.
    B. Hormonal testing is not required for diagnosis in a marathon runner with weight loss.
    C. Strenuous exercise with adequate energy intake usually does not disrupt the menstrual cycle.
    D. Psychological stress can play a role in menstrual dysfunction.
    Review this! ❑

42 Orthopedics

Glenn Loomis and William J. Martin

1. Which of the following is *not* a function of the human bony skeleton?

   A. To serve as a chemical storehouse for calcium and phosphate
   B. To provide motor power
   C. To serve as a protective shell for underlying soft tissues
   D. To serve as a factory for blood production

   Review this! ❑

2. Which of the following statements about greenstick fractures is true?

   A. They commonly occur as a result of rotational forces applied to long bones.
   B. They are rarely seen among the pediatric population.
   C. They are commonly seen among the elderly.
   D. They frequently occur when angular force is applied to a long bone.

   Review this! ❑

3. A 35-year-old male patient presents to the emergency room with a chief complaint of a fall from a 12-foot ladder, from which he landed with his right arm extended. He is extremely tender around the distal radius and the ulna. There is marked swelling and what appears to be a small puncture site in the area of the swelling, with minimal active bleeding and no exposed bone. An x-ray reveals that the patient has complete, transverse fracture of the distal third of his ulna, with approximately 20 degrees of angulation. The area of interrupted skin appears to be overlying the fracture site. Which of the following is the most appropriate next step in the management of this patient?

   A. Set up an immediate surgical consultation for wound irrigation and debridement.
   B. Have the patient rest, ice, and elevate the arm. Place the arm in a short arm splint, and ask the patient to return in 2 weeks for casting.
   C. Prescribe 2 weeks of oral antibiotics along with splinting and pain medicine until the swelling subsides enough that the arm may be casted safely.
   D. Perform a closed reduction of the fracture with gentle traction. The arm should be placed in a short arm cast with slight radial deviation of the wrist to allow for correct healing of the ulnar fracture.

   Review this! ❑

4. True or false: The epiphyseal plate in growing bone is weaker than the ligaments and tendons that attach nearby.

   A. True
   B. False

   Review this! ❑

5. Which of the following joints does not contribute to the true functional shoulder joint?

   A. The glenohumeral joint
   B. The scapuloclavicular joint
   C. The acromioclavicular joint
   D. The sternoclavicular joint

   Review this! ❑

6. A patient has a single fracture line moving through the distal radial epiphyseal plate and extending into the metaphysis that is visible on x-ray. The periosteum is intact on the concave side of the injury, and there is no angulation or comminution. Classify the injury using the Salter–Harris classification system.

   A. Salter–Harris type I
   B. Salter–Harris type II
   C. Salter–Harris type III
   D. Salter–Harris type IV

   Review this! ❑

7. A mother brings her 8-year-old son to see you in the emergency room during the night. She states that she awoke to hear her son crying in his bedroom. It appeared that he had fallen from the top bunk of his new bunk bed set and landed on his right shoulder. The child was crying and holding his arm at his side, and he was reluctant to move it. Upon examination, you see an otherwise healthy 8-year-old male who is appropriately developed for his age and who is holding his right arm at his side. There is tenderness and swelling at about the middle third of his clavicle, with palpable crepitus. There is no pain directly over the AC or SC joints. The patient is reluctant to allow you to passively manipulate his arm. Neurovascular examination is intact, and the patient has symmetrical radial pulses. Select the most likely diagnosis and the appropriate management from the options below.

A. The patient likely has an AC joint separation, and he should have radiographs of the shoulder, including the AC joint.
B. The patient likely has a fracture of his clavicle, and he should have radiographs of the entire length of the clavicle and shoulder to rule out other bony pathology.
C. The patient likely has a torn rotator cuff, and he should have magnetic resonance imaging to rule out both bony and tendinous injury.
D. The patient likely has a shoulder contusion, and he requires no further imaging or workup.

Review this! ❏

8. On x-ray, you notice a superiorly displaced distal clavicle without fracture of either the clavicle or the acromion process. The width of the displacement is slightly less than the width of the clavicle itself, and there is no sign of overlying skin interruption. Which of the following is the appropriate grade for this type of AC joint separation?

A. Grade 0
B. Grade 1
C. Grade 2
D. Grade 3

Review this! ❏

9. During the physical examination of a 45-year-old male with complaints of chronic right shoulder pain, you notice that his right scapula has an asymmetrical appearance with respect to his left scapula and that it appears to "wing" outward during the active protraction of his arms against resistance. Entrapment of which nerve would account for these physical examination findings?

A. The spinal accessory nerve
B. The long thoracic nerve
C. The deltoid nerve
D. The median nerve

Review this! ❏

10. Which of the following groups of muscles comprise the rotator cuff?

A. Supraspinatus, infraspinatus, teres major, and biceps brachialis
B. Subscapularis, infraspinatus, teres minor, and brachioradialis
C. Supraspinatus, infraspinatus, teres minor, and subscapularis
D. Subscapularis, infraspinatus, brachioradialis, and biceps brachialis

Review this! ❏

11. In your office, you see a 21-year-old male pitcher for a local collegiate baseball team with a chief complaint of shoulder pain. The patient states that he has had pain in his shoulder exacerbated by repetitive throwing motions for some time. The pain has recently changed, and for the past 4 days, it has been constant. He states that the new pain began during the sixth inning of a game in which he was the starting pitcher. He cannot recall any specific mechanism of injury, but he states that, since that game, his pain has gotten worse and now wakes him from sleep routinely. He denies any numbness or tingling in his hand, but he does describe weakness about the shoulder that he has not noticed before. His examination is remarkable for marked unilateral weakness to resisted abduction of the shoulder as well as external rotation with the elbow flexed to 90 degrees. When the patient performs the "empty can" maneuver, his right arm falls to his side, and he complains of severe worsening of his pain. The rest of his physical examination is unremarkable. What is the most

appropriate next step in the management of this patient?

A. The patient likely has rotator cuff tendonitis, and he should be given oral nonsteroidal anti-inflammatory medications and instructions for cuff-strengthening exercises.

B. The patient likely has rotator cuff impingement, and he should be reassured that the condition will improve with rest and icing.

C. The patient likely has rotator cuff tendonitis, and he should be given a 5-day course of oral prednisone along with a referral to physical therapy.

D. The patient likely has a torn rotator cuff, and he should undergo magnetic resonance imaging of the shoulder. He should also be referred to an orthopedic surgeon for possible correction of the defect.

Review this! ❏

12. In your office, you see a 17-year-old female tennis player. She tells you that, during her most recent high school tournament 3 weeks ago, she dislocated her shoulder during a service swing and had to be taken by her assistant coach to the emergency room. She states that the emergency room physician was able to put her shoulder back in place, and her pain has resolved slowly since the incident. She and her parents were very frightened by the incident, and they would like to know about her chances of having the same thing happen again. You tell her that, among young patients with similar histories, the chance of recurrence after a first-time dislocation is which of the following?

A. 10%
B. 50%
C. 75%
D. 90%

Review this! ❏

13. Which of the following statements about lateral epicondylitis or "tennis elbow" is false?

A. It is thought to be primarily the result of inflammation surrounding the lateral epicondyle of the ulna.

B. It is often caused by repetitive overuse of the wrist extension and forearm supinator muscles.

C. Microtears, chronic granulation tissue, and scar-tissue formation are commonly seen in pathological specimens of surgical cases of "tennis elbow."

D. Patients may complain of pain worsened by gripping and lifting exercises, particularly with the palm down.

Review this! ❏

For Questions #14 and #15, refer to the following clinical scenario:

In your office, you see a 22-year-old male water polo player for a chief complaint of medial elbow pain. The patient states that his pain began during his most recent match, when he was attempting to throw the ball into the opposing team's goal. During his throwing motion, he noted pain in the medial aspect of his elbow, along with a loss of throwing velocity. Later that evening, he noted some tingling in his fourth and fifth fingers. He has never had problems of this nature before. On physical examination, the patient has a full range of both active and passive motion about the shoulder. His rotator cuff examination is unremarkable. He has marked tenderness on palpation of the medial aspect of his elbow, and he has tenderness with valgus stress of the elbow. No instability is appreciated, and his neurovascular examination is intact, with the exception of decreased sensation to light touch in the fourth and fifth digits.

14. Which of the following injuries best explains this patient's constellation of symptoms and his physical examination findings?

A. Medial epicondylitis
B. Lateral epicondylitis
C. Olecranon bursitis
D. Ulnar collateral ligament injury

Review this! ❏

15. In the above scenario, the patient asks you how long it will be before he can return to water polo competition. What do you tell him?

A. After 2 weeks of rest and nonsteroidal anti-inflammatory medication, he will be able to return to play.

B. When he is pain free on examination and after he has completed rehabilitation exercises, a slow reintroduction to throwing activities may begin.

C. There is no need for him to restrict his activities at all, because his condition is not related to water polo.

D. He has likely suffered a career-ending injury, and, even with surgical correction, his chances of returning to his previous level of sport are less than 10%.

Review this! ❏

16. In your office, you see a 42-year-old female patient with a chief complaint of elbow pain. On questioning, she states that she had taken her niece ice skating the previous day when she fell, landing on her outstretched right arm. She immediately noted pain and swelling in her elbow that was worsened by motion and localized to the lateral aspect of the elbow. You suspect that she may have fractured her radial head. Your clinical suspicion is confirmed when her elbow radiographs (Figure 42-1) demonstrate a single, nondisplaced fracture of the radial head. Her neurovascular examination is fully intact, and dual energy x-ray absorptiometry reveals T scores and Z scores within the normal range. Treatment of this patient's fracture should include which of the following?

A. Splinting for 14 days or until her swelling has subsided, followed by immobilization in a long arm cast for 4 to 6 weeks

B. Computed tomography scanning to delineate the fracture more completely, followed by orthopedic referral

C. Splinting and sling immobilization until pain is controlled, followed by early mobilization

D. Surgical consultation for complete excision of the radial head

Review this! ❏

17. In your office, you see a 38-year-old female patient with a chief complaint of elbow pain. She tells you that 2 days prior she was rollerblading with her 15-year-old daughter. While doing this, she lost her balance and fell backwards, landing on her right elbow. She was not wearing any protective gear. She immediately felt pain and swelling in the area of her elbow, which has gotten progressively worse. On physical examination, you note pain on palpation of the olecranon and a palpable step-off deformity. You obtain anteroposterior and lateral views of the elbow, which show a 5-mm displaced complete fracture of the olecranon. With flexion of the elbow to 90 degrees, the displacement increases to 6.5 mm. The neurovascular examination is fully intact, and the remainder of the patient's physical examination is unremarkable. What is the most appropriate management for the injury described in the case above?

A. A long-arm cast with the elbow at 45 to 90 degrees of flexion for 6 weeks

Things to remember for the test.

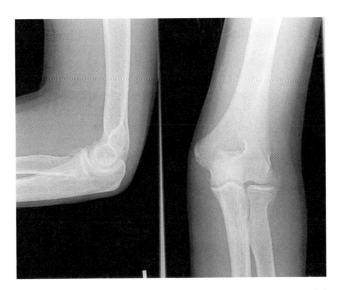

Figure 42-1 Copyright James L. Moeller, MD. In Rakel RE, editor: *Textbook of family medicine,* ed 7, Philadelphia, WB Saunders, 2007.

B. A long-arm cast with the elbow at 45 to 90 degrees of flexion for up to 3 weeks, followed by gentle range-of-motion activities to avoid excessive stiffness and potential long-term motion loss at the elbow

C. Referral to an orthopedic surgeon for open reduction and internal fixation or excision of the fracture fragment

D. Rest, ice, elevation, and pain management for 14 days or until the swelling subsides, followed by 3 weeks of casting and early mobilization

Review this! ❏

For Questions #18 and #19, refer to the following clinical scenario:

In your office, you see a 52-year-old male patient with a chief complaint of right wrist pain. The patient states that he is a computer programmer and that he noticed this pain beginning approximately 6 months ago and progressing to this point. Also, for the past 3 weeks, he has noted some pins-and-needles sensation throughout his fingers. On physical examination, you document slightly decreased sensation to light touch over the right thumb and first two digits. You also notice that, when asked to grasp your index and middle fingers in his hands and hold them tightly, the patient loses grip with his right hand and allows your fingers to slip away. This does not happen with his left hand.

18. Which test is not indicated for the patient's condition?

A. Tapping over the flexor retinaculum of the affected wrist to illicit a pain response

B. Magnetic resonance imaging of the patient's distal right extremity, with focus on the carpal tunnel

C. Having the patient flex his wrists to 90 degrees, holding the dorsal aspects of the hands back to back, and holding the position for 1 minute or until symptoms develop

Review this! ❏

19. Which of the following is the most appropriate initial management of this patient?

A. An injection of 2% lidocaine along with depot corticosteroids under sterile technique into the carpal tunnel

B. Oral nonsteroidal anti-inflammatory medications and return to previous activity

C. Surgical decompression of the flexor retinaculum by a qualified hand surgeon, followed by physical therapy

D. Oral analgesic therapy along with ergonomic changes to his computer station to minimize stress on the wrist

Review this! ❏

20. Pain when the thumb is flexed and abducted, the fingers are closed around the thumb, and the wrist is placed into ulnar deviation is known as _____, and it is indicative of _____.

A. Tinel's test; de Quervain's tenosynovitis

B. Phalen's sign; carpal tunnel syndrome

C. Finkelstein's test; de Quervain's tenosynovitis

D. Martin's sign; scaphoid fracture

Review this! ❏

For Questions #21 and #22, refer to the clinical scenario below:

In the emergency room, you see a 16-year-old female patient with a chief complaint of pain in her left wrist. The patient tells you that she is currently running track and that, during today's meet, she fell while running the hurdles. She tripped over one of the hurdles, and, in an attempt to catch herself, she fell on her outstretched left hand. She immediately noted pain and swelling of her left wrist, and she is actively guarding the injury with her right hand. She is extremely reluctant to allow you to examine her because of the severity of her pain. You decide to obtain radiographic images to rule out a fracture before examining the patient.

21. Figure 42-2 shows a three-view radiographic series of the patient's left wrist. Following a review of these images, you examine the patient and find that she is palpably tender over the distal radius and that her pain is worsened with movement. Which of the following should be your diagnosis?

A. Nondisplaced distal ulnar fracture

B. Salter–Harris type III fracture

C. Nondisplaced distal radial fracture

D. Wrist sprain without evidence of fracture

Review this! ❏

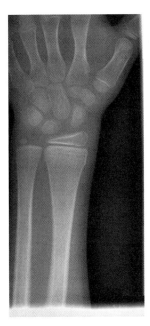
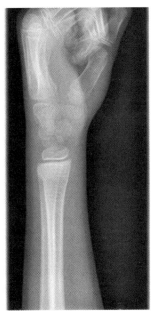
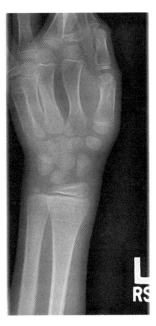

Figure 42-2 Copyright James L. Moeller, MD. In Rakel RE, editor: *Textbook of family medicine*, ed 7, Philadelphia, WB Saunders, 2007.

22. On further examination, you notice that the patient is also tender in the area of the anatomic snuff box. You order another image (Figure 42-3) to include a view of the scaphoid. It clearly shows a transverse fracture through the waist of the scaphoid bone. What is the proper management of this injury?

   A. An orthopedic consultation for percutaneous pinning of the fracture site
   B. Thumb spica casting with close radiographic evaluation to document proper healing of the fracture
   C. Short-arm casting for 3 weeks, followed by early mobilization
   D. Thumb spica splint to be worn at night, with daily mobilization exercises to prevent range-of-motion restriction from developing

   Review this! ❑

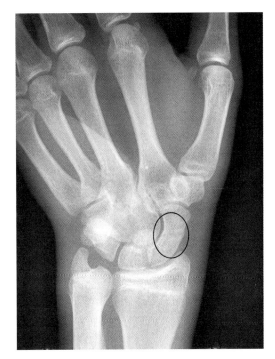

Figure 42-3 Copyright James L. Moeller, MD. In Rakel RE, editor: *Textbook of family medicine*, ed 7, Philadelphia, WB Saunders, 2007.

23. In the emergency room, you see a 63-year-old male patient with a chief complaint of right knee pain. He has never had pain of this nature before. The pain began with minimal swelling around his knee several days ago. Since that time, his knee has become more painful and more swollen. The patient states that he cannot remember any specific injury taking place or any other event that could explain his symptoms. He also notes that, when he awoke this morning, he felt warm; when his wife took his temperature, it was 100.3°F. On physical examination, the patient is a slightly obese male with a swollen and red right knee. The

patient will not move his knee actively at all, and he is very apprehensive about allowing you to move it. When you palpate the patient's knee, it is exquisitely tender, and it feels warm to your touch. The patient has a history of poorly controlled diabetes mellitus. What is the proper course of management for this patient?

A. Knee-joint aspiration under sterile technique with fluid analysis, including gram stain, cell count, culture, and crystal evaluation; immediate orthopedic referral

B. Knee-joint aspiration under sterile technique with fluid Gram stain and culture and 4 weeks of oral antibiotics directed at the suspected offending organism

C. Serial aspiration of the patient's knee for pain-control purposes and weekly radiographic evaluation

D. Knee-joint aspiration under sterile technique with fluid Gram stain and culture and 2 weeks of intravenous antibiotics followed by 2 weeks of oral antibiotics directed at the suspected offending organism

Review this! ❑

24. In your office, you see a 13-year-old boy who has been brought by his mother for a chief complaint of bilateral knee pain. She states that her son has constantly complained of pain in both of his knees for the past 3 months. He is a very active athlete, and she is concerned that he may have injured his knees. He has undergone a bit of a "growth spurt" over the past 6 months or so. The mother believes that her husband's mother had rheumatoid arthritis in her later years. On physical examination, the boy appears to be in generally good health, and he is appropriately developed for his age. The ligamentous examination of his knee is within normal limits and symmetrical. He has full range of motion about the knee, and his only significant clinical finding is palpable tenderness over the tibial tubercle. You tell the mother that her son has which of the following?

A. Apophysitis of the tibial tubercle, requiring straight-leg braces and 2 weeks of immobilization

B. Patellar tendons that have been avulsed from their attachment points on the anterior tibia, requiring surgical correction

C. Possibly an early presentation of juvenile rheumatoid arthritis; blood work can be done to rule this out

D. Osgood–Schlatter disease, which will most likely improve with rest, flexibility exercises, and gradual return to activity.

Review this! ❑

25. While you are performing the examination shown below, the patient grimaces and reaches for the knee that you are examining (Figure 42-4). This sign is known as _____, and it is indicative of _____ having taken place at some point in the past.

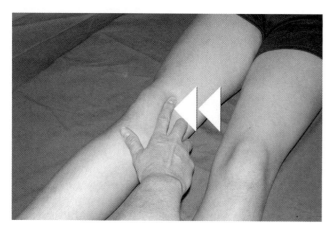

Figure 42-4 See Color Insert. Copyright Mark R. Hutchinson, MD. In Rakel RE, editor: *Textbook of family medicine,* ed 7, Philadelphia, WB Saunders, 2007.

A. Lachman's sign; medial collateral ligament injury
B. Apprehension sign; patellar dislocation
C. Posterior drawer sign; posterior cruciate ligament injury
D. Apprehension sign; septic arthritis

Review this! ❑

26. Which of the following structures is not associated with a twisting or valgus mechanism of injury to the knee?

A. Posterior cruciate ligament
B. Medial collateral ligament
C. Medial meniscus
D. Anterior cruciate ligament

Review this! ❑

27. In your office, you see a 34-year-old female patient who has had a chief complaint of knee pain for 2 weeks after a motor vehicle accident. During the accident, she suffered several injuries, including multiple fractured ribs, "whiplash," and a number of lacerations. After the accident, her right knee was swollen and tender, but she had attributed her symptoms to having struck her leg on her dashboard. Because she was recovering from her other injuries, her knee was not particularly debilitating to her. Since she has returned to walking, however, she has noticed some feelings of instability in her knee. On physical examination, she has firm endpoints with Lachman's testing, varus and valgus stress. On posterior drawer testing, the patient has posterior sagging of her distal lower extremity, no appreciable endpoint, and significant pain. During ambulatory examination, the patient has significant difficulty. Which of the following is the most appropriate course of treatment?

A. Straight-leg bracing for 4 to 6 weeks with appropriate pain control, followed by rehabilitation
B. Injection of 2% lidocaine and depot corticosteroids within the knee joint, followed by physical therapy and rehabilitation
C. Surgical reconstruction of the posterior cruciate ligament by an orthopedic surgeon
D. Conservative treatment with nonsteroidal anti-inflammatory medications and physical therapy with a focus on quadriceps rehabilitation

Review this! ❑

28. Which of the following ligaments of the ankle is the most commonly injured during an ankle sprain?

A. Anterior talofibular ligament
B. Calcaneofibular ligament
C. Posterior talofibular ligament
D. None of the above

Review this! ❑

29. In your office, you see a 17-year-old female who suffered an inversion injury to her ankle during a volleyball match the previous day. Immediately after the injury, she could bear weight for 5 to 6 steps, and she can bear weight for 10 steps with discomfort now in your office. She has experienced swelling and discoloration. On physical examination, she has mild anterior drawer laxity and swelling about the ankle, with no appreciable pain over the distal tip of the fibula. Which of the characteristics suggest that her ankle injury should be x-rayed according to the "Ottawa rules" for ankle injury?

A. The patient's age
B. The mechanism of her injury
C. Her inability to bear weight without pain 24 hours after an acute ankle injury
D. The laxity noted during the anterior drawer testing by the examiner

Review this! ❑

30. Figure 42-5 shows an example of heterotopic ossification. This adverse outcome occurs after 25% to 90% of cases of which of the following types of injury?

A. Grade 3 ankle sprain
B. Ankle sprain with syndesmosis sprain
C. Distal fibular fracture
D. Ankle mortise fracture

Review this! ❑

31. During the examination of a patient who you suspect may have an Achilles tendon injury, you perform the following examination. With the patient lying prone and with his knee flexed to 90 degrees and his ankle initially in the neutral position, you squeeze the right mid gastrocnemius, and you notice that the patient's foot plantarflexes. When repeating the examination on the left leg, the ankle remains in the neutral position. This is indicative of which of the following injuries?

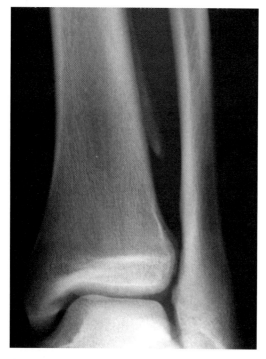

Figure 42-5 Copyright James L. Moeller, MD. In Rakel RE, editor: *Textbook of family medicine,* ed 7, Philadelphia, WB Saunders, 2007.

A. Chronic Achilles tendonitis on the right, with scarring of the tendon
B. Gastrocnemius strain on the right, with voluntary guarding
C. Probable Achilles tendon rupture on the left
D. Leg-length discrepancy causing right-sided Achilles tendonitis

Review this! ❏

32. For which of the following conditions is a cortisone injection typically not recommended?

A. Plantar fasciitis
B. Achilles tendonitis
C. Infrapatellar bursitis
D. Trochanteric bursitis

Review this! ❏

33. In your office, you see a 55-year-old female patient with a chief complaint of foot pain. The patient tells you that she runs 10 miles a week and that she has had this pain for several months, without resolution. She describes the pain as being sharp and stabbing in nature, and she says that it is located in her heel. She denies any specific injury that may have led to this problem. The pain seems to bother her more in the morning and then subsequently less throughout the day. As she rises from her chair to move to the examination table, she winces in pain with her first step and states, "That was the pain just then." Which of the following is your tentative diagnosis?

A. Calcaneal fracture
B. Achilles tendonitis
C. Plantar fasciitis
D. Avulsion fracture of the calcaneus

Review this! ❏

34. In which of the following patients is a normal-appearing x-ray not sufficient to rule out a fracture?

A. A 35-year-old female with a history of fall on an outstretched hand and tenderness in the anatomic snuff box
B. A 13-year-old male basketball player with a history of an inversion ankle injury and mild laxity on anterior drawer testing of the ankle
C. A 22-year-old female with a history of a fall landing on her flexed elbow and palpable tenderness over the olecranon process
D. A 45-year-old retired football player with chronic pain behind his right patella

Review this! ❏

35. Which rotator cuff muscle does the physical examination shown in Figure 42-6 isolate and test?

A. Supraspinatus
B. Teres minor
C. Subscapularis
D. Infraspinatus

Review this! ❏

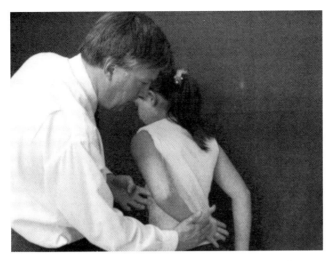

Figure 42-6 See Color Insert. Copyright Mark R. Hutchinson, MD. In Rakel RE, editor: *Textbook of family medicine,* ed 7, Philadelphia, WB Saunders, 2007.

36. Which of the following fractures would be least likely to require surgical correction?

    A. A Salter–Harris type IV fracture of the distal radial epiphysis
    B. A nondisplaced fracture through the proximal third of the fifth metatarsal
    C. A 0.5-cm superiorly displaced fracture of the middle third of the clavicle
    D. A distal fibular fracture with evidence of widening of the ankle mortise

    Review this! ❏

37. For which of the following fracture types is short-arm casting the most appropriate form of immobilization?

    A. Distal radial fracture
    B. Nondisplaced olecranon fracture
    C. Nondisplaced radial head fracture
    D. Scaphoid fracture

    Review this! ❏

38. Which of the following bones is the most commonly fractured in humans?

    A. Radius
    B. Scaphoid
    C. Clavicle
    D. Femur

    Review this! ❏

39. Digital flexor tendon tenosynovitis or "trigger finger" is commonly described by which of the following?

    A. The inability to relax a finger from the flexed position, resulting in the appearance of holding a pistol
    B. A nodular growth on the flexor tendon of one of the fingers in the area where the finger would make contact with a trigger
    C. A finger that sticks in a partially flexed position and that, with continued attempts at flexion, will finally complete the motion
    D. A loss of flexion motion in the index finger as a result of thickening and fibrosis of the flexor tendon

    Review this! ❏

40. In your office, you see a 14-year-old girl who has fractured her distal radius. The fracture is slightly angulated, and it will require closed reduction. In the area of the fracture, the patient has a tender, swollen, purple discoloration, which is not expanding in size. Before closed reduction of the fracture, you pass a needle under sterile conditions into the swollen area, and you aspirate what appears to be old blood. Without withdrawing the needle, you inject some 2% lidocaine and proceed with the reduction. This procedure is known as which of the following?

    A. Fracture block
    B. Hematoma block
    C. Reduction block
    D. Bone block

    Review this! ❏

43 Rheumatology and Musculoskeletal Problems

Darrin Bright

1. What percentage of patients with rheumatoid arthritis has a positive rheumatoid factor (RF)?

   A. 100%
   B. 80%
   C. 60%
   D. 40%

   Review this! ❏

2. What percentage of the healthy population has a positive RF?

   A. 20%–25%
   B. 10%–15%
   C. 2%–5%
   D. 0%

   Review this! ❏

3. What percentage of patients with lupus has a positive antinuclear antibody test?

   A. 100%
   B. 95%
   C. 85%
   D. 75%

   Review this! ❏

4. True or false: Urate crystals are shaped like needles, and they are weakly positively birefringent.

   A. True
   B. False

   Review this! ❏

5. The risk of iatrogenic infection associated with arthrocentesis is which of the following?

   A. 1 in 100,000
   B. 1 in 10,000
   C. 1 in 1000
   D. 1 in 100

   Review this! ❏

6. Arthritis affects what percentage of the population?

   A. 50%
   B. 40%
   C. 30%
   D. 20%

   Review this! ❏

7. Osteoarthritis is associated with all of the following deformities, except:

   A. Boutonniere deformity.
   B. Heberden's nodes.
   C. Bouchard's nodes.
   D. All of the above

   Review this! ❏

8. True or false: Osteoarthritis is a chronic noninflammatory type of arthritis.

   A. True
   B. False

   Review this! ❏

9. All of the following activities have been shown to cause osteoarthritis, except:

   A. Laying carpet.
   B. Working in a shipyard.
   C. Long-distance running.
   D. All of the above

   Review this! ❏

10. Osteoarthritis is typically associated with which of the following symptoms?

    A. Improvement as the day progresses
    B. Relief with activity
    C. Morning stiffness of less than 30 minutes
    D. Fatigue

    Review this! ❏

11. All of the following findings are typical radiographic abnormalities associated with osteoarthritis, except:

    A. Marginal erosions.
    B. Asymmetric joint-space narrowing.
    C. Subchondral sclerosis.
    D. Osteophyte formation.

    Review this! ❏

12. True or false: Nonsteroidal antiinflammatory drugs (NSAIDs) have been shown to alter the natural history of osteoarthritis through their effects on prostaglandin activity.

    A. True
    B. False

    Review this! ❏

13. True or false: Aerobic conditioning and walking programs have been shown to relieve symptoms associated with osteoarthritis.

    A. True
    B. False

    Review this! ❏

14. True or false: The American College of Rheumatology recommends NSAIDs as the initial drug of choice for osteoarthritis.

    A. True
    B. False

    Review this! ❏

15. Which of the following is the recommended dose of acetaminophen for symptom control of osteoarthritis?

    A. 1000 mg four times daily
    B. 750 mg four times daily
    C. 500 mg four times daily
    D. 325 mg four times daily

    Review this! ❏

16. Risk factors for upper gastrointestinal bleeding associated with NSAIDs use include all of the following, except:

    A. Age of more than 65 years.
    B. History of peptic ulcer disease.
    C. Concurrent use of prednisone.
    D. All of the above

    Review this! ❏

17. True or false: Cyclooxygenase-2 NSAIDs remain the treatment of choice for the prevention of NSAID-induced gastric ulcerations.

    A. True
    B. False

    Review this! ❏

18. All of the following have documented efficacy for the treatment of osteoarthritis, except:

    A. Glucosamine.
    B. Lycopene.
    C. SAMe.
    D. Avocado/soybean unsaponifiables.

    Review this! ❏

19. True or false: Rheumatoid arthritis is a chronic noninflammatory type of arthritis.

    A. True
    B. False

    Review this! ❏

20. Which of the following is the prevalence of rheumatoid arthritis in the segment of the population that is more than 65 years old?

    A. 1%
    B. 5%
    C. 10%
    D. 20%

    Review this! ❏

21. True or false: Morning stiffness that lasts for more than 1 hour is suggestive of rheumatoid arthritis.

    A. True
    B. False

    Review this! ❏

22. True or false: Cervical spine involvement in rheumatoid arthritis is rare.

    A. True
    B. False

    Review this! ❏

23. Rheumatoid arthritis typically involves all of the following joints, except:

    A. The distal interphalangeal joint.
    B. The proximal interphalangeal joint.
    C. The metacarpophalangeal joint.
    D. All of the above

    Review this! ❏

24. Felty's syndrome is associated with which of the following conditions?

    A. Rheumatoid arthritis
    B. Lupus
    C. Reiter's syndrome
    D. None of the above

    Review this! ❏

25. Periarticular osteoporosis is associated with which of the following conditions?

Things to remember for the test.

A. Lupus
B. Ankylosing spondylitis
C. Reiter's syndrome
D. None of the above

Review this! ❑

26. True or false: It is likely that a patient with rheumatoid arthritis will develop symptoms in multiple joints as the disease progresses over several years.

    A. True
    B. False

Review this! ❑

27. True or false: NSAIDs are considered a disease-modifying agent for patients with rheumatoid arthritis, and early initiation improves prognosis.

    A. True
    B. False

Review this! ❑

28. True or false: Methotrexate should be taken with folic acid to decrease the incidence of mouth sores.

    A. True
    B. False

Review this! ❑

29. Toxicities associated with methotrexate include which of the following?

    A. Hepatotoxicity
    B. Hodgkin's lymphoma
    C. Pulmonary nodules
    D. None of the above

Review this! ❑

30. Which of the following is the percentage of patients with rheumatoid arthritis who will be hospitalized or die from a gastrointestinal bleed?

    A. 5%
    B. 10%
    C. 25%
    D. 33%

Review this! ❑

31. True or false: Fries and colleagues (1991) studied the toxicities associated with traditional NSAIDs, and they found indomethacin (Indocin) to be the least toxic.

    A. True
    B. False

Review this! ❑

32. True or false: Indocin has been shown to be the most effective NSAID for patients with rheumatoid arthritis.

    A. True
    B. False

Review this! ❑

33. The periodic assessment of rheumatoid arthritis patients should include all of the following, except:

    A. RF.
    B. Erythrocyte sedimentation rate.
    C. C-reactive protein.
    D. Plain radiographs.

Review this! ❑

34. True or false: Asymptomatic hyperuricemia (>8 mg/dL) should be treated to prevent gout.

    A. True
    B. False

Review this! ❑

35. True or false: Ninety percent of individuals with gout are considered to underexcrete uric acid.

    A. True
    B. False

Review this! ❑

36. What percentage of patients with hyperuricemia will develop an attack of acute gouty arthritis?

    A. 0%
    B. 5%–10%
    C. 10%–20%
    D. 20%–30%

Review this! ❑

37. The most important risk factors for acute gouty arthritis include all of the following, except:

    A. Obesity.
    B. Purine-rich food.
    C. Alcohol.
    D. All of the above

Review this! ❑

38. All of the following medications are indicated during an acute attack of gouty arthritis, except:

A. Colchicine.
B. Indomethacin (Indocin).
C. Allopurinol.
D. Corticosteroids.

Review this! ❏

39. True or false: A positive test for human leukocyte antigen B27 is needed to confirm the diagnosis of ankylosing spondylitis.

A. True
B. False

Review this! ❏

40. Extra-articular manifestations of ankylosing spondylitis include all of the following, except:

A. Acute uveitis.
B. Aortitis.
C. C-spine fractures.
D. All of the above

Review this! ❏

41. True or false: Patients with ankylosing spondylitis should be started on disease-modifying antirheumatic drugs early in the course of the disease to prevent the progression of disease.

A. True
B. False

Review this! ❏

42. The classic triad of reactive arthritis (Reiter's syndrome) includes all of the following, except:

A. Urethritis.
B. Conjunctivitis.
C. Uveitis.
D. Arthritis.

Review this! ❏

43. Which of the following is the joint that is the most commonly affected by septic arthritis?

A. The knee joint
B. The hip joint
C. The shoulder joint
D. The first metatarsophalangeal joint

Review this! ❏

44. True or false: Patients with a septic joint will always have a fever with a red, swollen joint.

A. True
B. False

Review this! ❏

45. Erythema migrans is associated with which of the following conditions?

A. Enteropathic arthritis
B. Reiter's syndrome
C. Wegner's granulomatosis
D. Lyme disease

Review this! ❏

46. All of the following drugs are indicated as the first-line treatment of Lyme disease, except:

A. Azithromycin.
B. Doxycycline.
C. Amoxicillin.
D. All of the above

Review this! ❏

47. Which of the following percentages represents the likelihood of developing Lyme disease after attachment by an infected tick for less than 72 hours?

A. 0%
B. 1%
C. 5%
D. 20%

Review this! ❏

48. True or false: Group A streptococcal impetigo is associated with rheumatic fever, and it should be treated promptly with appropriate antibiotic therapy.

A. True
B. False

Review this! ❏

49. Sjögren's syndrome is characterized by all of the following, except:

A. Dry eyes.
B. Constipation.
C. Dry mouth.
D. All of the above

Review this! ❏

50. Which of the following diagnoses should be considered for a 70-year-old patient presenting with headache and an erythrocyte sedimentation rate of 110?

A. Giant cell arteritis (temporal arteritis)
B. Wegener's granulomatosis
C. Polyarteritis nodosa
D. Takayasu's arteritis

Review this! ❏

Things to remember for the test.

51. Which of the following is the leading cause of death among patients with diffuse cutaneous systemic sclerosis?

    A. Gastrointestinal obstruction
    B. Sepsis
    C. Cardiopulmonary disease
    D. Associated malignancies

    Review this! ❏

52. Which of the following diagnoses should be considered for a child presenting with purpura in the dependent areas of the buttocks and the lower extremities with associated abdominal pain?

    A. Kawasaki syndrome
    B. Juvenile rheumatoid arthritis
    C. Spondyloarthropathy of childhood
    D. Henoch–Schönlein purpura

    Review this! ❏

44 Dermatology

Quincy Scott

1. Which one of the following is used as a first-generation antihistamine for an urticarial itch?

   A. Fexofenadine (Allegra)
   B. Loratadine (Claritin)
   C. Cetirizine (Zyrtec)
   D. Hydroxyzine (Atarax)

   Review this! ❑

2. Which of the following statements about the use of a topical steroid is true?

   A. To achieve maximal penetration and efficacy, topical steroids should be applied to dry skin.
   B. Class VII agents should be used for severe dermatosis over nonfacial and nonintertriginous areas, especially the palms and soles.
   C. Class I topical steroids are known to be 10 times more potent than 1% hydrocortisone.
   D. Occlusive dressings are found to promote cutaneous hydration, which will increase absorption and which may possibly increase the potency of the steroid by as much as 100 times.

   Review this! ❑

3. Which of the following statements about papulosquamous diseases is true?

   A. Seborrheic dermatitis in infants (cradle cap) is usually not self-limited, and it usually requires that topical corticosteroids be applied to the scalp.
   B. The goal of the treatment of psoriasis is to maintain control of the lesions.
   C. Pityriasis rosea usually has a bacterial etiology, and it is easily treated with erythromycin.
   D. Miliaria (heat rash) is a condition that is mainly found in infants and that usually does not persist into adulthood.

   Review this! ❑

4. When considering treatment for the condition shown in Figure 44-1, which one of the following statements is true?

   A. Treatment usually involves oral antibiotics because of the bacterial etiology.
   B. Ultraviolet radiation is safe and has no known side effects.
   C. Persistence despite treatment beyond 12 weeks should be alarming, and reconsideration should be given by obtaining a more thorough history and possibly obtaining a biopsy.

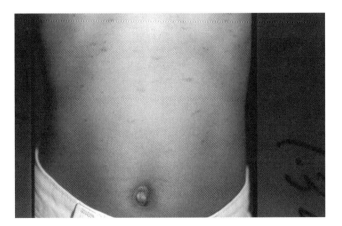

Figure 44-1 See Color Insert. In Rakel RE, editor: *Textbook of family medicine,* ed 7, Philadelphia, WB Saunders, 2007.

D. Pruritus is uncommon, and treatments such as calamine lotion, topical steroids, and antihistamines are usually not necessary.

Review this! ❑

5. Which one of the following is an autoimmune bullous disease that, if not treated with appropriate immunosuppressive agents, may be fatal?

A. Pemphigoid
B. Pemphigus vulgaris
C. Dyshidrotic eczema
D. Erythema multiforme minor

Review this! ❑

6. Which one of the following statements about dermatitis herpetiformis is true?

A. It is common among blacks and Asians.
B. It usually only occurs in the 45- to 65-year-old age group.
C. It commonly affects mucous membranes, and it usually occurs in an asymmetrical pattern on the flexor surfaces of the body.
D. It is usually found in most asymptomatic patients who have an underlying gluten-sensitive enteropathy.

Review this! ❑

7. Ninety percent of worker's compensation cases for skin conditions are due to which one of the following?

A. Atopic dermatitis
B. Nummular dermatitis
C. Stasis dermatitis
D. Contact dermatitis

Review this! ❑

8. Which one of the following statements best describes atopic dermatitis?

A. The most frequent symptom is pruritus, which can cause sleep disruption; it is known as "the itch that rashes."
B. It is rare among children, and it usually occurs after the age of 20 years.
C. Immunoglobulin A levels are often elevated.
D. Antihistamines and topical corticosteroids are usually not effective.

Review this! ❑

9. Which viral exanthema is described as having a "slapped cheek" appearance,

involves a reticular rash that may wax and wane for several weeks, and is associated with fetal hydrops and fetal death?

A. Rubella
B. Rubeola
C. Erythema infectiosum
D. Exanthema subitum

Review this! ❑

10. Which viral exanthema is distinguished by the presence of Koplik's spots in the oral mucosa?

A. Roseola, or exanthema subitum
B. Erythema infectiosum, or Fifth disease
C. Rubella
D. Rubeola

Review this! ❑

11. Which of the following treatment options is considered the mainstay of therapy for the disease shown in Figure 44-2?

A. Cold compresses or ice packs
B. Thermal pads
C. Aveeno baths
D. Avoidance of known triggering agents

Review this! ❑

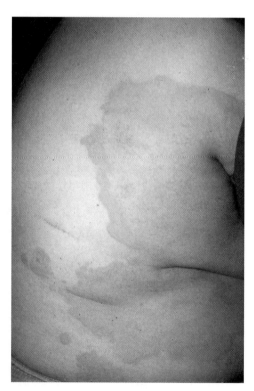

Figure 44-2 See Color Plate. In Rakel RE, editor: *Textbook of family medicine,* ed 7, Philadelphia, WB Saunders, 2007.

12. Which of the following statements about the nodules shown in Figure 44-3 is true?

    A. The condition is more common among men, and it is most commonly caused by a staphylococcal infection.
    B. Patients present with fever, malaise, and painless nodules.
    C. Sarcoidosis, tuberculosis, salmonella, and Campylobacter have been reported to be known causes.
    D. Spontaneous resolution usually does not occur, and nonsteroidal anti-inflammatory drugs offer no benefits.

    Review this! ❑

13. Which one of the following accurately describes the characteristics of sarcoidosis?

    A. The hallmark of the disease is a caseating granuloma.
    B. Lesions of cutaneous sarcoidosis are easy to treat with topical steroids, and they usually do not recur.
    C. Both papules and plaques usually take on a distinct orange color, and they are usually asymmetrical.

    D. Lesions on the alar rim of the nose, known as *lupus pernio,* are known to be associated with granulomatous infiltration of the upper airway.

    Review this! ❑

14. Which of the following statements about the lesions shown in Figure 44-4 is true?

    A. They are usually caused by *Pediculosis humanus capitis.*
    B. Patients usually present with a pruritic, papular rash with linear excoriations or burrows.
    C. In adults, the head and neck are frequently involved.
    D. These obligate human parasites are known to survive apart from their host for only 12 hours, which makes reinfestation unlikely.

    Review this! ❑

15. Which one of the following statements about pruritic conditions is true?

    A. Foods associated with pruritus ani include tea, coffee, chocolate, citrus fruits, and tomatoes.

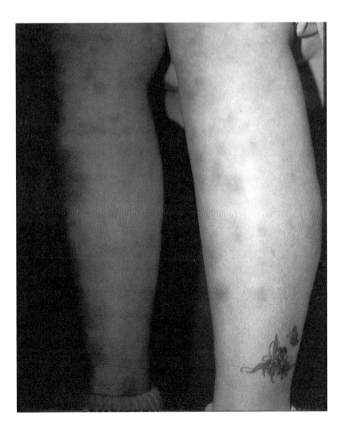

Figure 44-3 See Color Plate. In Rakel RE, editor: *Textbook of family medicine,* ed 7, Philadelphia, WB Saunders, 2007.

Things to remember for the test.

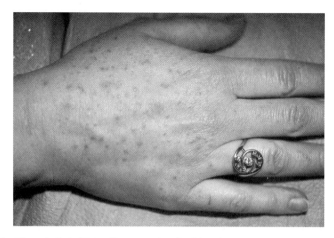

Figure 44-4 See Color Plate. In Rakel RE, editor: *Textbook of family medicine,* ed 7, Philadelphia, WB Saunders, 2007.

B. In cases of lichen simplex chronicus, pruritus is usually better during periods of inactivity, such as at bedtime and during the night.

C. Several live head lice that cause pruritus need to be visualized for the infestation to be diagnosed.

D. Lindane shampoo is used frequently after the pruritus, and the diagnosis is made because the shampoo has no known side effects and is very effective at killing the parasite.

Review this! ❑

16. Which of the following is the treatment of choice for the lesion shown in Figure 44-5?

A. Polymyxin B sulfate (Polysporin)
B. Mupirocin (Bactroban)
C. Povidone-iodine (Betadine)
D. Doxepin (Zonalon)

Review this! ❑

17. Which of the following is the treatment of choice for "hot tub folliculitis" caused by *Pseudomonas* species and that has persisted for more than 5 days?

A. Pen VK (Veetids)
B. Cephalexin (Keflex)
C. Azithromycin (Zithromax)
D. Ciprofloxin (Cipro)

Review this! ❑

18. Which of the following statements about bacterial cutaneous infections is true?

A. The treatment of a furuncle usually does not require drainage of the lesion.

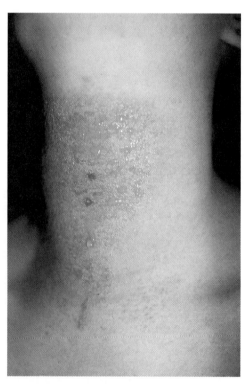

Figure 44-5 See Color Plate. In Rakel RE, editor: *Textbook of family medicine,* ed 7, Philadelphia, WB Saunders, 2007.

B. Staphylococci have been reported to be the cause of erysipelas in as many as 80% of cases.

C. The preferred treatment of erythrasma is a course of oral erythromycin plus daily cleansing.

D. Methicillin-resistant *Staphylococcus aureus* is not a known bacterial cause of impetigo.

Review this! ❑

19. Which of the following statements describing the lesion seen in Figure 44-6 is true?

    A. Both of the herpes simplex virus (HSV) serotypes cannot be present at oral and genital sites.
    B. Recurrent outbreaks are the same for HSV-1 and HSV-2.
    C. HSV infection is not related to the spread of human immunodeficiency virus.
    D. HSV infection can be characterized by episodes of latency, with asymptomatic viral shedding.

    Review this! ❏

20. Which of the following statements is the most important to consider when diagnosing the lesion shown in Figure 44-7?

    A. Analgesics are usually not required, because pain occurs before the lesions appear and then resolves.
    B. The incidence is lower among the elderly.
    C. The rash usually crosses the midline of the body.
    D. Corneal involvement should be suspected when lesions appear on the tip of the nose.

    Review this! ❏

21. Which subtypes of human papillomavirus are associated with the development of carcinoma?

    A. 4 and 6
    B. 8 and 10
    C. 12 and 14
    D. 16 and 18

    Review this! ❏

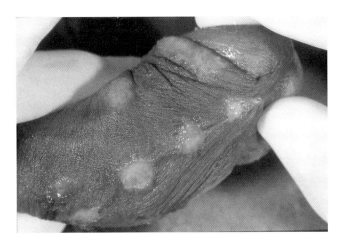

Figure 44-6 See Color Plate. In Rakel RE, editor: *Textbook of family medicine,* ed 7, Philadelphia, WB Saunders, 2007.

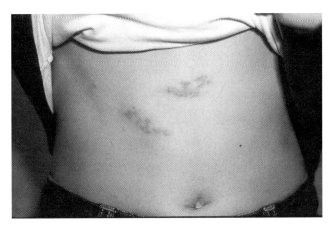

Figure 44-7 See Color Plate. In Rakel RE, editor: *Textbook of family medicine,* ed 7, Philadelphia, WB Saunders, 2007.

22. Which of the following requires treatment with oral antifungals?

    A. Tinea pedis
    B. Tinea corporis
    C. Tinea barbae
    D. Tinea curis

    Review this! ❑

23. Which of the following statements about Lyme disease is true?

    A. The tick is almost always of the genus *Borrelia.*
    B. The disease is a systemic infection caused by the spirochete *Ixodes.*
    C. Zithromax is one of the oral antibiotics used for treatment, and it should be given for 10 to 21 days.
    D. Patients with erythema migrans and history of a tick bite should have serologic testing, because the sensitivity of the testing is known to be high during the early stages of infection.

    Review this! ❑

24. Which of the following statements best describes the characteristics of Rocky Mountain spotted fever?

    A. The bright pink to red macular rash usually spares the soles and the palms, but it usually includes the face.
    B. Indirect fluorescent antibody testing is highly specific, but it is not sensitive, and antibodies appear within 1 to 2 days.
    C. Doxycycline is the drug of choice for the treatment of both adults and children.
    D. Nausea, vomiting, and diarrhea are rare, and they are not associated with the vascular injury of the pancreas and the gastrointestinal tract.

    Review this! ❑

25. Isotretinoin (Accutane) should be used in women of childbearing age only when which one of the following conditions is met?

    A. Contraception counseling has occurred and there is agreement among the counselor, the physician, and the patient that pregnancy will be avoided during treatment.
    B. There is documentation that a complete blood cell count has been performed in the past and is normal.
    C. An office pregnancy test is reported as negative on the day that treatment is initiated.
    D. After the initial criteria are met, pregnancy tests and required laboratory examinations are repeated monthly during treatment.

    Review this! ❑

26. The patient shown in Figure 44-8 presents with a complaint of intermittent central facial flushing and erythema. Which of the following is important to discuss with the patient at the time of the office visit?

    A. Sun exposure and cold weather are known to help the condition.
    B. Hot beverages, spicy foods, and alcohol have no effect on the condition.
    C. Nearly half of patients with acne rosacea develop ocular symptoms, some of which may be chronic and lead to corneal neovascularization and keratitis.

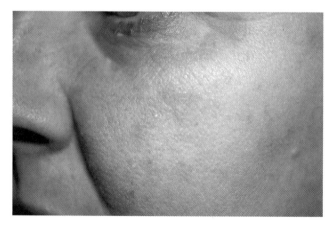

Figure 44-8   See Color Plate. In Rakel RE, editor: *Textbook of family medicine,* ed 7, Philadelphia, WB Saunders, 2007.

D. Most patients respond well to short-term topical antibiotic treatment but not to topical retinoid therapy.
Review this! ❏

27. Which of the following statements best describes the condition shown in Figure 44-9?

A. This condition is known to have a higher prevalence in Caucasians.
B. Genetic factors are known to not play a role.
C. It occurs at any age group, and it is known not to peak.
D. Repigmentation therapy includes the use of corticosteroids, ultraviolet light, and surgery.
Review this! ❏

28. When performing a physical examination on the patient shown in Figure 44-10, you notice the following lesions. Which of the following statements is true?

A. A biopsy must be performed, because there is a chance of malignancy.
B. A lipid profile must be performed, and, if needed, the cholesterol lowered, because this can help with the regression of the lesions.
C. Surgery, carbon dioxide laser, and trichloroacetic acid are contraindicated, and they are known to spread the lesions.
D. The lesions found in primary biliary cirrhosis are very distinct, and they do not resemble xanthelasma.
Review this! ❏

Things to remember for the test.

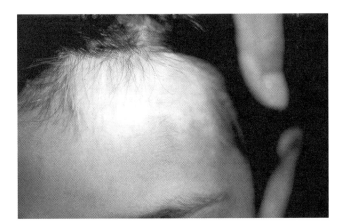

Figure 44-9 See Color Plate. In Rakel RE, editor: *Textbook of family medicine,* ed 7, Philadelphia, WB Saunders, 2007.

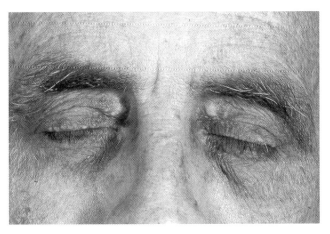

Figure 44-10 See Color Plate. In Rakel RE, editor: *Textbook of family medicine,* ed 7, Philadelphia, WB Saunders, 2007.

29. The common lesion shown in Figure 44-11 has which of the following characteristics?

    A. This "stuck-on" lesion is most commonly found on the trunk, and it is known as seborrheic keratosis.
    B. This lesion is known as actinic keratosis. It has the potential to become malignant, and it can transform into basal cell carcinoma.
    C. This lesion is known as squamous cell carcinoma, and it is the most common form of skin cancer.
    D. This lesion is known as basal cell carcinoma; it is fast growing, and it metastasizes quickly.

    Review this! ❑

30. Which of the following is the appropriate initial treatment for the condition shown in Figure 44-12?

    A. Topical antibiotics
    B. Oral antibiotics
    C. Oral antifungals
    D. Incision and drainage

    Review this! ❑

31. Which of the following techniques is a good initial choice for the removal of acrochordons, seborrheic keratoses, and some dermatofibromas but not for pigmented lesions?

    A. Punch biopsy
    B. Shave biopsy
    C. Electrosurgery
    D. Incision and drainage

    Review this! ❑

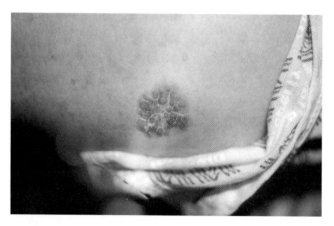

Figure 44-11 See Color Plate. In Rakel RE, editor: *Textbook of family medicine,* ed 7, Philadelphia, WB Saunders, 2007.

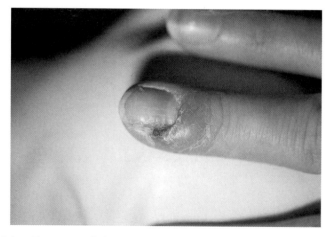

Figure 44-12 See Color Plate. In Rakel RE, editor: *Textbook of family medicine,* ed 7, Philadelphia, WB Saunders, 2007.

32. Which of the following is described as a circumscribed, elevated, fluid-containing lesion less than 0.5 cm in its greatest diameter that may be intraepidermal or sub-epidermal in origin?

    A. Macule
    B. Papule
    C. Pustule
    D. Vesicle

    Review this! ❏

Things to remember for the test.

45

Diabetes Mellitus

Alan R. Roth

Things to remember for the test.

1. Which of the following may not be used as diagnostic criteria for a patient with diabetes mellitus?

   A. More than two random serum glucose values of greater than 200 mg/dL
   B. A fasting blood glucose level of 126 mg/dL or greater
   C. A 2-hour glucose challenge level of greater than 200 mg/dL
   D. A hemoglobin A1c value of greater than 6.5%

   Review this! ❏

2. Which of the following serum glucose values have been designated as demonstrating prediabetes?

   A. 75–99 mg/dL
   B. 100–125 mg/dL
   C. 126–150 mg/dL
   D. 151–199 mg/dL
   E. >200 mg/dL

   Review this! ❏

3. The metabolic syndrome is a condition that is associated with all of the following, except:

   A. Dyslipidemia.
   B. A family history of diabetes mellitus.
   C. Insulin resistance.
   D. Hypertension.
   E. Abdominal obesity.

   Review this! ❏

4. Which of the following diagnostic tests may be useful for differentiating atypical presentations of type 1 diabetes from type 2 diabetes?

   A. Anti-glutamic acid decarboxylase
   B. Insulin level
   C. C-peptide
   D. Hemoglobin A1c
   E. Human leukocyte antigen genotypes

   Review this! ❏

5. The patient with new-onset type 2 diabetes mellitus is most often found to have which of the following?

   A. Polyuria
   B. Polydipsia
   C. A screening abnormal blood glucose
   D. Weight loss
   E. Peripheral neuropathy

   Review this! ❏

6. Which of the following is the daily insulin requirement for most patients with type 1 diabetes mellitus?

   A. 0.1–0.4 U/kg
   B. 0.5–1.0 U/kg
   C. 1.1–1.5 U/kg
   D. 1.6–2.0 U/kg
   E. 2.1–2.5 U/kg

   Review this! ❏

7. Which of the following regimens is most appropriate for the initial insulin management of a patient with type 1 diabetes mellitus?

   A. 100% short-acting insulin
   B. 75% short-acting insulin and 25% basal coverage with long-acting insulin
   C. 50% short-acting insulin and 50% long-acting insulin
   D. 25% short-acting insulin and 75% long-acting insulin
   E. 100% long-acting insulin

   Review this! ❏

8. Which of the following is the target fasting and prandial glucose level that is the current recommendation of the American Diabetes Association for the control of type 1 diabetes?

   A. <100 mg/dL
   B. <120 mg/dL
   C. <140 mg/dL
   D. <160 mg/dL
   E. <200 mg/dL

   Review this! ❏

9. The progression of microangiopathic complications of diabetes mellitus may be prevented with tight glycemic control and a near-normal hemoglobin A1c. Which of the following best describes this statement's level of evidence?

    A. Level A
    B. Level B
    C. Level C
    D. Level D
    E. There is no evidence for this statement.
       Review this! ❏

10. All of the following statements about dietary principles and weight loss for patients with diabetes are true, except:

    A. A comprehensive exercise plan is important to maintain glucose control.
    B. A meal plan that includes a variety of usual foods is recommended as long as the plan is a healthy one.
    C. A strict American Diabetes Association caloric-counted diabetic diet is recommended for all patients.
    D. The conscious control of carbohydrate intake is important for glucose regulation.
    E. Weight loss will improve glycemic control as well as blood-pressure regulation.
       Review this! ❏

11. The current American Diabetes Association and American Heart Association guidelines recommend which of the following dietary guidelines for the treatment of all patients at risk for diabetes and cardiovascular disease?

    A. 80% carbohydrate, 10% fat, 10% protein
    B. 60% carbohydrate, 30% fat, 10% protein
    C. 40% carbohydrate, 40% fat, 20% protein
    D. 25% carbohydrate, 30% fat, 45% protein
    E. It is not necessary to monitor the percentages of carbohydrate, fat, and protein content in food.
       Review this! ❏

12. Diabetic peripheral neuropathy is a significant source of morbidity, mortality, and potential limb loss. Which of the following findings is the most sensitive for the diagnosis of diabetic peripheral neuropathy?

    A. The loss of microfilament touch sensation
    B. A diminished Achilles reflex
    C. The loss of the proprioceptive sense
    D. A diminished dorsalis pedis pulse
    E. The presence of venous stasis dermatitis
       Review this! ❏

13. According to the most up-to-date data with a level of evidence of A as published by the Diabetes Control and Complications Trial Research Group, the management of type 1 and type 2 diabetes should be continually modified to find the optimal therapeutic regimen, which yields a hemoglobin A1c level of which of the following?

    A. <6%
    B. <7%
    C. <8%
    D. <9%
    E. <10%
       Review this! ❏

14. Most clinicians recommend which of the following drugs as the first-line therapy for patients with type 2 patients, especially those who are overweight?

    A. Metformin
    B. Glitazones
    C. Insulin
    D. Sulfonylureas
    E. α-Glucosidase inhibitors
       Review this! ❏

15. Which of the following medications is relatively contraindicated for diabetic patients with congestive heart failure?

    A. Metformin
    B. Glitazones
    C. Insulin
    D. Sulfonylureas
    E. α-Glucosidase inhibitors
       Review this! ❏

16. Which of the following medications is associated with the highest risk of hypoglycemia in the management of patients with non–insulin-dependent diabetes?

    A. Metformin
    B. Glitazones
    C. α-Glucosidase inhibitors
    D. Sulfonylureas
    E. Meglitinides
       Review this! ❏

Things to remember for the test.

Things to remember for the test.

17. The early initiation of insulin therapy for type 2 diabetics is becoming an increasingly effective management tool when behavioral therapy and combined oral agents have not achieved near normalization of the hemoglobin A1c and fasting glucose levels. Which of the following insulin preparations is best used as first-line therapy?

    A. Regular insulin in multiple doses
    B. N-insulin in multiple doses
    C. An insulin pump
    D. Ultra-short-acting insulin
    E. Glargine insulin (Lantus)
    Review this! ❑

18. Insulin pump therapy is becoming more readily available for routine use. This device is most suited for which of the following patients?

    A. Diabetic patients who are noncompliant with home glucose monitoring
    B. Well-controlled type 1 diabetic patients
    C. Motivated type I diabetics who have not attained glycemic control
    D. Type 2 diabetics
    E. Elderly diabetic patients
    Review this! ❑

19. Which of the following laboratory findings is not consistent with a diagnosis of diabetic ketoacidosis?

    A. A pH level of less than 7
    B. Elevated serum bicarbonate
    C. Hemoconcentration
    D. Hyperkalemia
    E. Hypokalemia
    Review this! ❑

20. Which of the following is the initial fluid of choice for hydrating the patient who presents in diabetic ketoacidosis?

    A. Lactated Ringer's solution
    B. 0.45% saline
    C. 0.9% saline
    D. Dextrose 5% in water
    E. Dextrose 5% in 0.45% saline
    Review this! ❑

21. Which one of the following abnormalities is not consistent with a diagnosis of nonketotic hyperosmolality syndrome?

    A. Mild ketoacidosis
    B. Azotemia

    C. Hyperosmolality
    D. Severe dehydration
    E. Marked hyperglycemia
    Review this! ❑

22. All of the following factors are associated with increased complications in pregnant diabetic patients, except:

    A. The degree of hyperglycemia.
    B. The duration of diabetes mellitus.
    C. The presence of nephropathy.
    D. Type 2 diabetes.
    E. An increased age at the time of conception.
    Review this! ❑

23. Which of the following diabetes medications is not approved for use in pregnant patients?

    A. Human R insulin
    B. Human N insulin
    C. Insulin pump therapy
    D. Metformin
    E. Glargine insulin (Lantus)
    Review this! ❑

24. What percentage of patients with gestational diabetes will go on to develop type 2 diabetes?

    A. <5%
    B. 15%
    C. 25%
    D. 50%
    E. 75%
    Review this! ❑

25. Screening for diabetes must be performed in all of the following pregnant patients, except:

    A. A 29-year-old black female of healthy weight.
    B. A 21-year-old white female of healthy weight.
    C. A 32-year-old Hispanic female whose mother has diabetes.
    D. A 30-year-old obese white female.
    E. A 31-year-old obese black female.
    Review this! ❑

26. Which of the following is the most appropriate management of a diabetic patient undergoing a surgical procedure?

A. Oral medications on the day of surgery
B. Short-acting insulin injection the morning of surgery
C. Long-acting insulin for basal coverage along with glucose intraoperatively
D. Oral medications until the day before surgery
E. Discontinuing oral medications 1 week before the procedure but continuing regular insulin coverage

Review this! ❏

27. Tight control of type 1 diabetes can reduce the incidence of the microangiopathic changes of diabetes by which of the following percentages?

A. 10%
B. 25%
C. 50%
D. 75%
E. 90%

Review this! ❏

28. Which of the following medications has been shown to be most effective for reducing and reversing the presence of microalbuminuria and slowing the onset of diabetic nephropathy?

A. β-Blockers
B. Calcium-channel blockers
C. Angiotensin-converting enzyme inhibitors or angiotensin receptor blockers
D. Diuretics
E. Aspirin

Review this! ❏

29. Which of the following is the most important part of the evaluation for signs of early diabetic foot disease?

A. Observing the foot immediately after stocking removal
B. Evaluating peripheral pulses

C. Touching the foot for temperature
D. Evaluating the Achilles reflex
E. Observing for the presence of the Charcot deformity

Review this! ❏

30. Which of the following presentations is the least consistent with the presence of diabetic peripheral neuropathy?

A. The presence of paresthesias perceived as numbness, burning, or a "pins and needles" sensation
B. Symptoms that are significantly worse in the morning
C. The alleviation of symptoms with foot massage
D. The loss of vibratory or position sense
E. The inability to perceive monofilament fine-touch testing

Review this! ❏

31. Which of the following medications is the least appropriate for the management of a patient with symptomatic diabetic peripheral neuropathy?

A. Gabapentin (Neurontin)
B. Amitriptyline (Elavil)
C. Duloxetine (Cymbalta)
D. Acetaminophen or nonsteroidal anti-inflammatory drugs
E. Narcotic analgesics

Review this! ❏

32. Which of the following is the target level of low-density lipoprotein cholesterol in a patient with diabetes mellitus?

A. 160 mg/dL
B. 130 mg/dL
C. 100 mg/dL
D. 70 mg/dL
E. 40 mg/dL

Review this! ❏

Things to remember for the test.

46

Endocrinology

Nikhil Hemady

1. Which one of the following statements about thyroid hormones is true?

   A. T3 is a major product of the thyroid gland.
   B. T4 is the biologically active thyroid hormone.
   C. Estrogen-containing oral contraceptives can increase total T4 levels.
   D. An elevated thyroglobulin level in a patient with a suppressed thyroid-stimulating hormone (TSH) level suggests factitious hyperthyroidism.

   Review this! ❏

2. Patients with subclinical hypothyroidism who have anti-tissue peroxidase are less likely to progress to overt hypothyroidism.

   A. True
   B. False

   Review this! ❏

3. A decreased tracer uptake on a radioiodine isotope scan is shown in patients with all of the following causes of hyperthyroidism, except:

   A. Postpartum thyroiditis.
   B. Subacute thyroiditis.
   C. Silent (lymphocytic) thyroiditis.
   D. Graves' disease.
   E. Factitious thyrotoxicosis.

   Review this! ❏

4. Determine whether each statement below is true or false. Radioiodine is the most common modality of treating hyperthyroidism in the United States. Regarding this form of treatment:

   (1) Pregnancy should be ruled out before therapy is started.
   (2) Graves' ophthalmopathy can worsen after such treatment.
   (3) Treatment efficacy is approximately 45% to 50% at 1 year after treatment.

   (4) Agranulocytosis is a feared complication of radioiodine therapy.

   A. True
   B. False

   Review this! ❏

5. Determine whether each statement below is true or false. A 22-year-old female is diagnosed with a thyroid nodule. She has no history of prior head and neck irradiation, and her family history is unremarkable. She is presently clinically euthyroid, and her TSH level is normal.

   (1) Chances of her thyroid nodule being malignant are higher because of her age.
   (2) The most cost-effective initial approach to evaluate her nodule is fine-needle aspiration.
   (3) Overall, approximately 25% of thyroid nodules are malignant.

   A. True
   B. False

   Review this! ❏

6. All of the following statements about thyroid cancers are true, except:

   A. Iodine-131 is used both for the diagnosis and treatment of thyroid adenocarcinomas.
   B. An elevated thyroglobulin level is a tumor marker for anaplastic carcinomas.
   C. Papillary carcinomas have the best prognosis.
   D. Follicular carcinomas are aggressive, and they are more likely to involve metastatic disease.

   Review this! ❏

7. Pregnant women with hypothyroidism require which of following adjustments to their thyroid hormone replacement therapy?

A. Decrease the thyroid hormone dose by 25% of the prepregnancy level.

B. Discontinue the thyroid hormone during pregnancy.

C. Leave the thyroid hormone dose unchanged.

D. Increase the thyroid hormone dose by 50% of the prepregnancy level.

Review this! ❑

8. Which of the following thyroid cancers is seen with increased frequency among patients with a long-standing history of Hashimoto's thyroiditis?

A. Papillary adenocarcinoma

B. Medullary carcinoma

C. Anaplastic carcinoma

D. Follicular adenocarcinoma

E. Lymphoma

Review this! ❑

9. Which of the following is the most common cause of hypercalcemia in an office setting?

A. Milk–alkali syndrome

B. Malignancy

C. Sarcoidosis

D. Lithium

E. Primary hyperparathyroidism

Review this! ❑

10. A 45-year-old black male with a history of well-controlled hypertension is found to have a mildly elevated serum calcium level. He is presently asymptomatic, and his laboratory tests, including a serum albumin level, are normal. Which of the following classes of antihypertensives is known to cause hypercalcemia?

A. Calcium channel blockers

B. Angiotensin receptor blockers

C. Loop diuretics

D. Thiazide diuretics

E. Angiotensin-converting enzyme inhibitors

Review this! ❑

11. All of the following drugs are effective for the reduction of vasomotor symptoms in postmenopausal women, except:

A. Gabapentin (Neurontin).

B. Venlafaxine (Effexor).

C. Raloxifene (Evista).

D. Clonidine (Catapress).

E. Sertraline (Zoloft).

Review this! ❑

12. All of the following statements about raloxifene are true, except:

A. It increases the risk of deep vein thrombosis.

B. It is less effective than bisphosphonates for the treatment of osteoporosis.

C. It increases the risk of endometrial cancer.

D. It decreases the risk of breast cancer.

E. Leg cramps are a common side effect.

Review this! ❑

13. All of the following statements about adrenal insufficiency are true, except:

A. The most common underlying cause of primary adrenal insufficiency is autoimmune.

B. Acute adrenal insufficiency should be suspected in a patient who presents with refractory uncontrolled hypertension.

C. A morning serum cortisol level greater than 19 µg/dL rules out adrenal insufficiency.

D. Intravenous dexamethasone is the preferred initial drug for the management of acute adrenal insufficiency.

Review this! ❑

14. Which of the following is the screening test of choice for a suspected case of hyperaldosteronism?

A. A serum potassium level of less than 3.5 mEq/L

B. An increased ratio of plasma aldosterone concentration to plasma renin activity

C. A 24-hour urinary sodium level of greater than 200 mg

D. A computed tomography scan of the adrenal glands

Review this! ❑

15. Which of the following is the most common cause of hypopituitarism in adults?

A. Sarcoidosis

B. Pituitary adenoma

C. Hemochromatosis

D. Craniopharyngioma

E. Sheehan's syndrome

Review this! ❑

16. True or false: Adults with growth-hormone deficiency have a reduced life expectancy compared with age-matched controls.

Things to remember for the test.

A. True
B. False

Review this! ❏

17. True or false: A 35-year-old female presents with secondary amenorrhea. There is an absence of withdrawal bleeding after the progesterone challenge test, and her serum follicle-stimulating hormone (FSH) level is elevated. Her workup is most suggestive of ovarian failure.

A. True
B. False

Review this! ❏

18. Recombinant human growth hormone is used to treat adults with growth-hormone deficiency. Which of the following tests is used to monitor the effectiveness of hormone replacement therapy?

A. Serum adrenocorticotropic hormone
B. Serum insulin-like growth factor 1 (IGF-1)
C. Serum growth hormone
D. Urinary calcium

Review this! ❏

19. A 32-year-old female presents with a 4-month history of bilateral milky nipple discharge. She denies any vision problems or headaches, and she is otherwise asymptomatic. She has a long-standing history of poorly controlled type 1 diabetes mellitus, and she has numerous diabetes-related complications. Her current medications include aspirin, insulin, enalapril, gabapentin, and metoclopramide. Her breast examination, along with the rest of her physical examination, is normal. What is the next best step in the management of this patient's galactorrhea?

A. Obtain an ultrasound of the breast.
B. Discontinue the aspirin.
C. Obtain a magnetic resonance image of the hypothalamus and the pituitary gland.
D. Discontinue the metoclopramide.
E. Check the serum TSH level.

Review this! ❏

20. All of the following statements about acromegaly are true, except:

A. There is an increased incidence of valvular heart disease among patients with this condition.
B. Medical management with the somatostatin analog octreotide is preferred over surgical management.
C. The serum IGF-1 level is the single best screening test.
D. Cardiovascular disease is a cause of increased mortality.
E. Hypogonadism is a common feature.

Review this! ❏

21. A 36-year-old female with a history of chronic headaches is found to have a pituitary adenoma on neuroimaging. On physical examination, she has truncal obesity, abdominal striae, and easy bruising. Other features of Cushing's disease caused by an adrenocorticotropic hormone producing pituitary adenoma include all of the following, except:

A. Hypercoagulability.
B. Postural hypotension.
C. Proximal muscle weakness.
D. Osteopenia.

Review this! ❏

22. True or false: A 24-hour urinary cortisol excretion is the first step in the evaluation of Cushing's syndrome.

A. True
B. False

Review this! ❏

23. All of the following can cause galactorrhea, except:

A. Excessive nipple manipulation.
B. Oral contraceptives.
C. Bromocriptine.
D. Chronic renal failure.
E. Risperidone (Risperdal).

Review this! ❏

24. Which of the following is the most common cause of hirsutism?

A. Androgenic drug intake
B. 21-hydroxylase–deficient nonclassic adrenal hyperplasia
C. Polycystic ovary syndrome (PCOS)
D. Androgen-secreting tumors

Review this! ❏

25. All of the following statements about PCOS are true, except:

    A. All patients with PCOS should be screened for impaired glucose tolerance with a 2-hour glucose tolerance test.
    B. Sulfonylureas are recommended to improve insulin sensitivity.
    C. Serum luteinizing hormone and FSH levels are not recommended as part of the initial evaluation.
    D. Patients have an increased risk of endometrial carcinoma.

    Review this! ❏

26. All of the following statements about Turner's syndrome are true, except:

    A. Thyroid disorders are common.
    B. The diagnosis is confirmed by karyotyping.
    C. These patients need to be evaluated for aortic root abnormalities.
    D. Hormone replacement therapy is contraindicated.

    Review this! ❏

27. Cryptorchidism is the most common endocrine disorder in the pediatric male. All of the following statements about this disorder are false, except:

    A. Hormonal therapy with human chorionic gonadotropin or gonadotropin-releasing hormone is unlikely to increase the rate of testicular descent.
    B. It is prudent to wait and watch for spontaneous testicular descent until the child is 2 years old.
    C. There is a lower incidence of the disorder among preterm males.
    D. Imaging studies such as computed tomography scanning and ultrasound have poor accuracy for locating undescended testes.

    Review this! ❏

28. True or false: The most common cause of male infertility is a varicocele.

    A. True
    B. False

    Review this! ❏

29. Hyponatremia can be associated with all of the following, except:

    A. Diabetic ketoacidosis.
    B. Diabetes insipidus.
    C. Hyperproteinemia.
    D. Hypertriglyceridemia.
    E. Syndrome of inappropriate secretion of antidiuretic hormone

    Review this! ❏

30. True or false: Demeclocycline is the primary treatment for central diabetes insipidus.

    A. True
    B. False

    Review this! ❏

47 Obesity

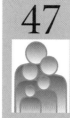

Julie S. Cantrell

1. Which of the following statements about the assessment for adult obesity is true?

    A. The body fat percentage is the most precise way to assess adiposity, and it can be performed easily and accurately in an office setting.
    B. Body mass index (BMI) can be misleadingly high in a tall, thin patient.
    C. The distribution of body fat is not of significance when evaluating for obesity-related complications.
    D. A normal waist circumference should be 35 inches or less for a woman and 40 inches or less for a man.

    Review this! ❑

2. Which of the following statements about assessing for obesity in children is true?

    A. Because obesity is defined by percentiles, the absolute values will increase as the population becomes heavier overall; this may become more significant, because there has been a marked increase in the prevalence of overweight and obese children in the pediatric population.
    B. Overweight is defined by the Centers for Disease Control and Prevention as a BMI greater than the 95th percentile for age from infancy to the age of 19 years.
    C. Obesity during infancy is clearly linked to the risk for adult obesity.
    D. An obese adolescent has a 40% chance of becoming an obese adult.

    Review this! ❑

3. Which of the following statements about the U.S. patient population is true?

    A. Obesity is more common among white women than black women.
    B. Immigrants to the United States continue to have a lower risk of obesity over their lifespan as compared with native-born Americans.

    C. Asians are at lower risk for being overweight, but they may see weight-related health complications at a lower BMI than other ethnic groups.
    D. Risk for obesity is greater among poor, less-educated, and urban-dwelling patients.

    Review this! ❑

4. Which of the following statements about the role of genetics in obesity is the most accurate?

    A. Chromosomal mapping has identified a handful of specific gene sites that control weight and that are determined by basic Mendelian genetics.
    B. A correlation is seen in the adult body weight of identical twins who have been raised apart.
    C. An excess of leptin, which is involved in appetite control, may be a genetic cause of obesity.
    D. Genetic factors are estimated to be responsible for 60% to 70% of variability in adult weight.

    Review this! ❑

5. Which of the following statements about central/visceral obesity is the most accurate?

    A. Central (or truncal) obesity is the result of increased estrogenic effects, and it is more often seen in women.
    B. Polycystic ovary syndrome (PCOS) is closely connected to "pear-shaped" obesity in women, either as a cause or as a consequence.
    C. Increased visceral fat may increase one's risk of metabolic syndrome.
    D. Computed tomography scanning of the abdomen has been proposed as a cost-effective means of assessing visceral fat deposits.

    Review this! ❑

6. Which of the following statements about biochemical modulators of appetite is the most accurate?

   A. Ghrelin is a gastrointestinal peptide that inhibits appetite.
   B. Central nervous system neurotransmitters, which modulate appetite, can be affected by weight-loss medications.
   C. Glucose level fluctuations do not play a significant role.
   D. Leptin is produced by the brain to stimulate hunger sensations in the gastrointestinal tract.

   Review this! ❑

7. Which of the following statements about energy expenditure is true?

   A. The basal metabolic rate (BMR) is chiefly determined by the BMI.
   B. Most of the decrease in energy expenditure in the United States over the past few decades is the result of less scheduled exercise.
   C. The most variable component of energy expenditure is the BMR.
   D. A person's total energy requirements are based on the BMR, the energy needed for physical activities, and the thermic effect of food.

   Review this! ❑

8. Which of the following statements about caloric intake is the most accurate?

   A. Portion size increase over the past few decades has been attributed to sales of bulk-size groceries at discount stores.
   B. Satiety is largely determined by the calorie content of the food eaten.
   C. A few larger meals per day leads to a greater insulin release than several smaller meals, and this possibly contributes to weight gain.
   D. Although the typical U.S. diet may be high in fat, there has been a gradual but consistent decline in sugar consumption.

   Review this! ❑

9. In which of the following ways may medications contribute to weight gain?

   A. Topiramate can lead to significant weight gain, whereas gabapentin may actually cause weight loss.
   B. Within the class, there is no significant difference between selective serotonin reuptake inhibitors with regard to the risk of weight gain.
   C. Newer neuroleptics, such as clozapine and olanzapine, are not associated with the risk of weight gain seen with older neuroleptics, such as haloperidol.
   D. Although insulin and most oral hypoglycemics can promote weight gain, metformin is associated with a modest weight loss.

   Review this! ❑

10. Which of the following statements about endocrine causes of obesity is true?

    A. Among children, hypothyroidism, Cushing's syndrome, and growth-hormone deficiency will all present not only with obesity but also with slow statural growth.
    B. Approximately 10% to 15% of patients with obesity will have an underlying endocrine disorder that can be diagnosed via clinical and laboratory evaluation.
    C. Unexplained weight gain is often the only presenting symptom of hypothyroidism in adults.
    D. Cushing's syndrome is characterized by a "buffalo hump," striae, hypotension, and glucose intolerance.

    Review this! ❑

11. Which of the following statements about PCOS is true?

    A. More than 80% of women with PCOS are obese.
    B. Insulin resistance, which is seen frequently among patients with PCOS, is always the result of obesity.
    C. Signs and symptoms of PCOS include central/truncal obesity, hirsutism, and irregular menses.
    D. Elevated testosterone and follicle-stimulating hormone levels are typically seen among patients with PCOS.

    Review this! ❑

12. Which of the following statements about patients with obesity-related hypertension is true?

A. Weight loss is the most effective lifestyle change for decreasing blood pressure.

B. Weight loss is more effective for reducing blood pressure among blacks as compared with whites.

C. The age-related increase in the frequency of hypertension diagnoses is independent of weight gain.

D. Obesity-related hypertension is associated with increased vascular resistance and sodium resorption but not with changes in insulin levels.

Review this! ❏

13. Which of the following statements about obesity's relationship to hyperlipidemia and heart disease is true?

A. The benefit of aerobic exercise for improving dyslipidemia is the same, regardless of whether the exercise results in weight loss.

B. Obesity, even without coexisting risk factors, may lead to cardiomyopathy and congestive heart failure.

C. Obesity has consistently been found to be an independent risk factor for coronary artery disease.

D. Of the various cholesterol subtypes, weight loss will most greatly improve low-density lipoprotein cholesterol levels.

Review this! ❏

14. Which of the following statements describing the relationship of obesity to type 2 diabetes mellitus is true?

A. The risk of type 2 diabetes among men with a BMI of greater than 35 kg/m^2 is 40-fold greater than it is among men of normal weight; among women with a BMI of greater than 35 kg/m^2, the risk is 60-fold greater than it is among women of normal weight.

B. As weight increases, insulin resistance and serum insulin levels increase as well.

C. There is an approximately 20-year delay between the onset of weight gain and the development of type 2 diabetes.

D. After a patient is diagnosed with type 2 diabetes, weight loss will not improve blood glucose levels, because insulin resistance is already established.

Review this! ❏

15. Which of the following statements most accurately applies to metabolic syndrome?

A. According to NCEP-III, to diagnose metabolic syndrome, a blood pressure elevation of 130/85 mm Hg must be present.

B. It is estimated that 20% of individuals over the age of 50 years meet the criteria for metabolic syndrome.

C. Metabolic syndrome is thought to primarily be the result of insulin resistance.

D. The presence of metabolic syndrome increases the risk for the development of type 2 diabetes, but it is not clearly linked to cerebrovascular or cardiovascular disease.

Review this! ❏

16. Which of the following statements about the relationship of obesity to cancer is correct?

A. Obesity is the largest avoidable cause of cancer.

B. An increased risk of death from stomach cancer, Hodgkin's disease, and melanoma is seen among the obese.

C. The mechanism by which obesity increases the risk for breast and endometrial cancer is most likely an increase in estrogen levels.

D. Breast cancer is most often seen among women with "pear-shaped" obesity.

Review this! ❏

17. Which of the following statements about obstructive sleep apnea (OSA) is true?

A. The increased risk of OSA among the obese is most likely the result of an increase in chest circumference and abdominal pressure.

B. A person with mild OSA who has a 10% gain in body weight may have a twofold increased risk of progressing to more severe OSA.

C. The primary health concerns of untreated OSA are daytime somnolence and the increased risk for motor vehicle accidents.

D. OSA is associated with right ventricular dysfunction, systemic hypertension, pulmonary hypertension, and erectile dysfunction.

Review this! ❏

18. Obesity may lead to liver and/or gallbladder disease in which of the following ways?

    A. Nonalcoholic steatohepatitis is associated with insulin resistance.
    B. Fatty liver is second only to alcoholic cirrhosis as a cause of elevated liver enzymes.
    C. Nonalcoholic steatohepatitis and nonalcoholic fatty liver disease are relatively benign processes that do not typically lead to liver inflammation or fibrosis.
    D. An increased risk of symptomatic gallstones can be seen with weight gain, but the risk significantly decreases with rapid weight loss.

    Review this! ❑

19. Which of the following statements about other obesity-related medical problems is true?

    A. Among adults, obesity increases the risk of degenerative joint disease symmetrically in all joints that are typically affected by the disease.
    B. Slipped capital femoral epiphysis and genu varum are increased among obese children.
    C. Obesity is associated with depression equally in both sexes.
    D. Obesity can affect lung function by worsening asthma, by reducing residual lung volume and leading to a restrictive lung disease pattern, and by causing the obesity-hypoventilation syndrome in severe cases.

    Review this! ❑

20. Which of the following statements about screening for and managing childhood obesity is the most accurate?

    A. Risk factors for childhood obesity include maternal alcohol use during pregnancy and excessive milk consumption during the toddler years.
    B. The BMI will normally decrease until a period of "adiposity rebound" at around the ages of 5 to 7 years.
    C. The goal of treatment should be a reduction in BMI to less than the 75th percentile for age.
    D. A lipid panel and a fasting blood glucose level should be a part of routine preventive screening for all adolescents.

    Review this! ❑

21. Which of the following statements about the approach to the treatment of childhood/adolescent obesity is true?

    A. A reasonable goal of treatment is a weight loss of 1 kg per week.
    B. Sedentary activities should be limited to 4 hours per day.
    C. A diet that is too restrictive can adversely effect growth rate, bone mineralization, and menstruation.
    D. Sibutramine has been found to be safe and effective for children who are 6 years old and older.

    Review this! ❑

22. Which of the following statements about the evaluation and treatment of obesity in adults is the most accurate?

    A. The U.S. Preventive Services Task Force recommends neither for nor against screening for obesity among adults.
    B. Initial evaluation should include measuring the BMI and the waist circumference and identifying comorbidities.
    C. Calorie restriction without exercise will produce similar changes in total adiposity and lean body mass as the combination of the two; a longer period of dieting will be required.
    D. Weight-loss medication should only be used for patients with a BMI of more than 30 kg/m^2.

    Review this! ❑

23. Which of the following statements about setting weight loss goals for adults is true?

    A. A weekly weight loss of 4 to 5 lb can be achieved with a daily calorie deficit of 500 to 1000 kcal.
    B. A goal weight should be set to achieve a BMI of 25 kg/m^2; looking at the "big picture" will help to keep the patient motivated.
    C. Using a process-oriented target may be less frustrating for some patients than an outcome-oriented target.
    D. Lifestyle changes that lead to weight loss should be maintained for approximately 3 months until a new "setpoint" is achieved.

    Review this! ❑

24. Factors to consider when choosing a weight-loss diet include which of the following?

    A. A low-calorie diet guideline would be 1000 to 1200 kcal per day for women and 1200 to 1600 kcal per day for men.
    B. Low-carbohydrate diets have been shown to be superior to other types of diets in long-term weight loss studies.
    C. "Very-low-calorie diets," which restrict calorie intake to 400 to 800 kcal per day, produce significantly greater weight loss over time.
    D. To achieve weight loss, the overall volume of food eaten daily must decrease.

    Review this! ❑

25. Which of the following statements about behavioral methods and lifestyle changes to help with weight loss is true?

    A. Thirty minutes of moderate physical activity most days of the week is adequate to achieve and maintain weight loss.
    B. The use of a pedometer with a goal of 10,000 steps per day, along with limiting sedentary activity time, may be helpful.
    C. Behavioral approaches as a whole have not been found to be effective for helping with weight loss.
    D. Depression among obese patients is most often the result of poor self-image; it should be addressed if it is persistent after weight loss is achieved.

    Review this! ❑

26. When prescribing sibutramine to assist with weight loss, it is important to remember which of the following?

    A. Sibutramine works to increase satiety by increasing the levels of serotonin without affecting other neurotransmitter levels.
    B. Because sibutramine has the potential to increase heart rate and blood pressure, the diagnoses of hypertension or coronary artery disease are absolute contraindications to its use.
    C. As compared with placebo, patients will lose an additional 10 kg in 1 year while taking sibutramine.

    D. The serotonin syndrome, which may occur if combining sibutramine with other serotonergic drugs such as selective serotonin reuptake inhibitors, presents as confusion, hypomania, hyperthermia, diaphoresis, tachycardia, and emesis.

    Review this! ❑

27. Which of the following statements about the use of orlistat to assist with weight loss is true?

    A. Gastrointestinal side effects occur in 50% of patients taking this drug, and they continue for the duration of its use.
    B. Because of concern about B-vitamin deficiency among patients taking orlistat, a daily multivitamin is recommended.
    C. Patients should follow a very-low-fat, calorie-restricted diet while taking orlistat.
    D. Orlistat acts by inhibiting gastric and pancreatic lipase.

    Review this! ❑

28. Which of the following statements about alternative medicines or herbal compounds that may help with weight loss is true?

    A. Green tea, although it is free of caffeine, contains catechin, which may stimulate weight loss.
    B. Ephedra, or ma huang, was removed from the market because of the associated risk of stroke, arrhythmias, seizure, and death.
    C. An increase in dietary soluble fiber can lead to water retention and, therefore, an increase in total body weight.
    D. *Guarana* and *gotu kola* are other herbal names for ephedra.

    Review this! ❑

29. Which of the following statements about surgical options for the treatment of obesity is true?

    A. Candidates for bariatric surgery should have a BMI of 40 kg/m^2 of more or weight-related health complications.
    B. Gastric banding has the advantage of being the only bariatric surgical procedure that can be done laparoscopically.

C. Roux-en-Y gastric bypass is more effective than gastroplasty for weight loss.
D. Vitamin and mineral deficiencies may occur during the immediate postoperative period (6–8 weeks) after gastric bypass, and they should be prevented with supplementation during this period.

Review this! ❏

30. Which of the following is the correct formula for calculating BMI?

A. Weight (kg)/Height (m)^2
B. Weight (lb) × 450/Height (in)^2
C. Weight (kg)^2/Height (m)
D. Weight (lb)^2/Height (in) × 450

Review this! ❏

48 Nutrition

Ann Riehl

1. The U.S. Department of Agriculture and the U.S. Department of Health and Human Services recently released the 2005 Dietary Guidelines. You decide to use this as a guideline for health education for your family medicine patient population, because the clinical medicine interest in nutrition applies to treating diseases with nutritional therapies. The public health dietary guidance program MyPyramid Food Guidance System (www.MyPyramid.gov) works best as an interactive interface. Limitations would include which of the following?

   A. The need for internet access
   B. The ability to navigate the Web site
   C. The Web site being geared toward professionals
   D. The program being too individualized
   E. The recommendation of physical activity

   Review this! ❑

2. A 30-year-old male who just recently moved to the area has an appointment today to establish himself as a new patient. The personal health history form that he will complete includes questions that can be used as a brief screen of his nutritional status. Your initial nutritional assessment should include which of the following?

   A. Changes in weight and appetite
   B. Medical history, including illnesses and medications
   C. General clinical appearance
   D. Special diet
   E. All of the above

   Review this! ❑

3. A 20-year-old female college student who is well known to the family medicine center presents with recurrent complaints of irritable bowel syndrome: fatigue, cessation of menses, and recent episodes of diarrhea. She reports that it its finals week; in addition, she is working part time and training for a 5-km run. You suspect some mild malnutrition. On physical examination, which of the following indicators would confirm your diagnosis?

   A. 10% weight loss since fall quarter
   B. Patient reports thinning hair
   C. Temporal wasting
   D. Complete blood cell count

   Review this! ❑

4. As a community service, you are volunteering at the high school to do physicals for a sports team. The students will need blood pressure and pulse readings, height and weight determinations, and—new this year—random drug testing. What questions can be asked to provide information for a brief nutrition assessment during the limited amount of time available with each student?

   A. Number of meals eaten in each day
   B. Daily servings of dairy
   C. Weight gain/loss since last season
   D. Multivitamin use
   E. Alcohol consumption
   F. The sniff test (i.e., does he or she smell like smoke?)
   G. All of the above

   Review this! ❑

5. A 45-year-old female patient comes to your office for evaluation after a recent hospital stay for surgery related to diverticulitis. You are concerned about her nutritional status. Because physiologic changes related to adequacy of nutrition occur slowly, what laboratory test would you need to evaluate her nutritional status?

   A. Complete blood cell count
   B. Prealbumin
   C. Thyroid-stimulating hormone
   D. Weight
   E. Iron, folic acid

   Review this! ❑

6. Nutrition counseling 2 to 3 months before conception can have a positive influence on the outcome of pregnancy. The family medicine doctor is in a perfect position to counsel female patients. Increased nutritional needs before conception and through the first trimester include which of the following?

   A. Protein
   B. Iron
   C. Calories
   D. Calcium and iodine
   E. Folic acid

   Review this! ❏

7. A new parent can become quite frustrated trying to introduce new foods or even just feeding his or her new baby. What advice can you give?

   A. Children have the innate ability to self-regulate intake.
   B. New foods should be introduced eight different times before a child shows true acceptance or rejection.
   C. Children have reserve stores of most nutrients from birth to 4 years of age.
   D. Offer meals at a separate time from the family meal time so that the child does not get distracted.
   E. Provide the parent with tips about age-appropriate foods and textures.

   Review this! ❏

8. Calories and nutrient needs in the adult population are not mutually inclusive. Obesity is often the direct result of excess nonnutritive calories and sedentary life. What body mass index (BMI) defines obesity?

   A. <18.5
   B. 18.5 to 24.9
   C. 25 to 29.9
   D. >30

   Review this! ❏

9. Nutritional status can be assessed by routine laboratory evaluation as part of a patient's yearly checkup. All of the following can be included, except:

   A. A complete blood cell count.
   B. C-reactive protein level.
   C. Lipid levels.
   D. A determination of fasting blood glucose.

   Review this! ❏

10. A 30-year-old menopausal woman comes to establish herself as a patient, stating that she has had no routine checkups since the birth of her second and last child at the age of 20 years. What nutritional concern should be addressed with a preventative disease focus in mind?

    A. Bone density
    B. Blood glucose
    C. Fasting lipids
    D. Blood pressure
    E. BMI

    Review this! ❏

11. Dehydration is a result of not drinking enough fluid, losing too much fluid, or both. Which of the following major nutrients has been associated with this condition?

    A. Protein
    B. Water
    C. Carbohydrate
    D. Fat

    Review this! ❏

12. An elderly female patient who is new to you but who is established at your family medicine practice is brought to the office by her daughter. Reviewing and updating her nutritional assessment more in depth can reveal nutrient needs that are unique to a patient in this stage of the life cycle. A reliable nutritional assessment tool should include which of the following?

    A. Psychosocial components
    B. Functional status
    C. Mental status
    D. All of the above

    Review this! ❏

13. In 2003, the Seventh Report of the Joint National Committee on Prevention, Detection, Evaluation, and Treatment of High Blood Pressure established the following blood pressure designations:

    - Prehypertension: systolic blood pressure (SBP), 130 to 139 mm Hg; diastolic blood pressure (DBP), 85 to 89 mm Hg;
    - Stage I hypertension: SBP, 140 to 159 mm Hg; DBP, 90 to 99 mm Hg;
    - Stage II hypertension: SBP, 160 to 179 mm Hg; DBP, 100 to 199 mm Hg; and

Things to remember for the test.

- Stage III hypertension: SBP, >180 mm Hg; DBP, 110 mm Hg. The recommendation to lower sodium intake to 2 to 4 g per day would be sufficient management for which level?

  A. Prehypertension
  B. Stage I hypertension
  C. Stage II hypertension
  D. Stage III hypertension
  E. All of the above

  Review this! ❑

14. Dyslipidemia can be characterized as one of a group of metabolic risk factors for metabolic syndrome. Dietary therapeutic lifestyle changes recommended by the National Cholesterol Education Program include all of the following, except:

  A. Less than 200 mg of cholesterol a day.
  B. Less than 7% saturated fat in the diet.
  C. 25% to 35% total fat in the diet.
  D. Less than 10% trans fat in the diet.
  E. 50% to 60% carbohydrates in the diet.
  F. 15% protein in the diet.

  Review this! ❑

15. Dietary therapy for mild and moderate hyperlipidemia is always recommended, and it should be accompanied by weight reduction and exercise. What other metabolic risk factors would benefit?

  A. Elevated triglyceride level
  B. Low high-density lipoprotein cholesterol level
  C. High blood pressure
  D. Impaired glucose tolerance
  E. All of the above

  Review this! ❑

16. The MyPyramid Food Guidance System recommends increasing consumption of a variety of whole grains, fruits, vegetables, legumes, and nuts. More fiber in the diet would benefit which of the following?

  A. Hypertension
  B. Hypercholesterolemia
  C. Type 2 diabetes
  D. Cardiovascular disease
  E. Elevated triglyceride level
  F. Insulin resistance
  G. All of the above

  Review this! ❑

17. The secondary prevention of cardiovascular and cerebrovascular disease can be managed with diet intervention. Best-evidence recommendations for the prevention of further events in people with existing cardiovascular disease include all of the following, except:

  A. Increasing omega-3 fat intake.
  B. Following the Mediterranean diet.
  C. Taking a folate supplement.
  D. Lowering saturated fat levels in the diet.

  Review this! ❑

18. A 42-year-old truck driver with a BMI of 34 was referred to you after a health-fair screening revealed a random blood glucose level of 175 mg/dL. You suspect and confirm type 2 diabetes with a hemoglobin A_{1c} level of 8%. Best-evidence recommendations suggest which of the following?

  A. Consuming carbohydrates from fruits, whole grains, vegetables, and low-fat milk
  B. Avoiding foods high in glycemic index
  C. A reduction in weight and insulin resistance by reducing calorie intake
  D. Increasing physical activity by making lifestyle modifications

  Review this! ❑

19. A new-onset diabetic may be surprised to be told that his or her total cholesterol level of 200 mg/dL and low-density lipoprotein cholesterol level of 120 mg/dL that are not currently being treated pharmacologically are now too high. Initiating behavioral interventions to lower the low-density lipoprotein cholesterol level would include which of the following?

  A. 7% or less calories from saturated fat
  B. 200 mg cholesterol
  C. 5%–7% weight reduction
  D. None of the above

  Review this! ❑

20. The Subjective Global Assessment is a tool that is used to assess the nutritional status in the hospitalized patient. The findings would rate the patient as well nourished, mildly malnourished, or severely malnourished. Of the history and physical examination findings, what is the most significant finding to determine appropriate nutritional support to heal wounds and recover from illness?

*Things to
remember for
the test.*

A. Prealbumin level of 10 mg/dL
B. Weight loss
C. Edema and ascites
D. Chronic gastrointestinal symptoms

Review this! ❑

21. Nutritional support should be considered
for a hospitalized patient in which of the
following situations?

A. On a case-by-case basis
B. If calorie counts show low total calorie
and protein intake
C. If a patient is hospitalized for surgery
D. When a patient admitted to the hospital
is malnourished
E. All of the above

Review this! ❑

22. Your patient requires nutritional support.
Protein is a macronutrient of concern for
patients with protein-calorie malnutrition,
especially for surgery and trauma patients.
How much protein should be delivered in
an enteral or parenteral formula?

A. 0.8 g of protein per kilogram per day,
calculated by body weight
B. 1.5–2.0 g of protein/kg/day of the
calculated resting energy expenditure
calorie requirement
C. Check with the hospital formulary.
D. Wait 48 hours after surgery or trauma to
calculate the needs if the patient is not
consuming enough protein at meals.
E. Consult a dietitian for nutritional
support.

Review this! ❑

23. Counseling patients about dietary changes
requires educating the patient not just about
dietary modifications but also about the
behavioral management necessary to accomplish them. You have a prehypertensive
patient in the office. Knowing that lowering
sodium intake is recognized as sufficient
treatment for this condition, what behaviors
would you concentrate on with your patient?

A. Advise the patient to check nutrition
fact labels.
B. Advise the patient to remove the salt
shaker from the table.
C. Advise the patient to not add salt when
cooking food.
D. All of the above

Review this! ❑

24. A 55-year-old postmenopausal patient
presents to your office with nondescript
symptoms. Finally, she admits to just not
"feeling well." It has been years since she has
received medical attention. Your initial full
workup reveals that she is suffering from
the metabolic syndrome. She is refusing
medication at this time, but she is asking
about making lifestyle modifications.
Behavioral change requires which of the
following elements?

A. Readiness to change
B. Goal setting and tracking
C. Relapse prevention
D. Support
E. All of the above

Review this! ❑

25. Your office has a system established to
identify patients who require dietary
changes. What elements are needed to assist
patients with making diet-related health
behavior changes?

A. Assessing their readiness to change.
B. Assisting with their changes in the office.
C. Referring them to related programs.
E. Providing them with handouts about
diet modifications for different disease
states.

Review this! ❑

26. The future holds promise for the emerging
field of nutritional genomics. The family
medicine physician is able to do a form of
this every day in the office. What is the best
genomic tool—albeit an old-fashioned
one—to predict individual risks for diseases?

A. The family history
B. The thorough workup
C. Research of like patient populations
D. Clinical observations

Review this! ❑

27. You are providing care for a 42-year-old
pregnant woman. What pregnancy outcomes
are linked to inappropriate weight gain?

A. Increased risk of gestational diabetes
B. Increased risk for a low-birthweight
infant
C. Increased risk for a large-for-gestational-
age infant
D. All of the above

Review this! ❑

28. The role of nutrients has expanded greatly since the original reference for nutritional adequacy was adopted almost 20 years ago. The new generic term *dietary reference intake* replaces which of the following?

    A. Daily nutrient needs
    B. Estimated energy requirement
    C. Adequate intake
    D. Recommended daily intake

    Review this! ❑

29. Only three of the four macronutrients supply calories, and the amount of each that is needed is usually stated in Kcal/kg. Which of the following macronutrients is the most calorically dense?

    A. Carbohydrates
    B. Fat
    C. Protein
    D. Water

    Review this! ❑

30. Educating a patient about the nutritional management of diabetes and the associated behavioral changes can be challenging. A female patient who has been recently diagnosed with type 2 diabetes returns to the office for follow-up; however, her blood sugar log reveals that her blood sugar levels are unchanged. She reports eating no sugar and reading food nutrition labels, but she has not started exercising, and she cannot understand why her blood sugar levels are still high. Your next plan to lower this patient's blood sugar levels and control her diabetes would include which of the following?

    A. Giving the patient additional in-depth information about diabetes management
    B. Referring the patient to a certified diabetes educator
    C. Prescribing oral diabetes medication
    D. Asking the patient to return to the office for an expanded visit to provide diabetes education

    Review this! ❑

49 Gastroenterology

Gina M. Basello

1. When evaluating and managing the patient with acute abdominal pain in the office setting, physicians should do which of the following?

   A. Formulate a differential diagnosis on the basis of the location of the pain.
   B. Use serial abdominal examinations over several hours when the etiology of pain is unclear.
   C. Differentiate surgical from medical causes of abdominal pain by the presence or absence of fever.
   D. Avoid the use of narcotic analgesia for patients with abdominal pain until a diagnosis is made.
   E. Perform occult blood stool testing only for elderly male patients.

   Review this! ❏

2. Which of the following is the most important imaging modality for evaluating the patient who presents with abdominal pain and fever?

   A. Ultrasound
   B. Magnetic resonance imaging
   C. Plain films
   D. Computed tomography scanning
   E. None have been shown to be superior

   Review this! ❏

3. Which of the following principles is incorrect for the management of an infant or child with acute gastroenteritis?

   A. The early administration of oral rehydration solutions has been proven to be effective for reducing mortality.
   B. During rehydration therapy, breastfeeding should be continued on demand.
   C. Early refeeding has not been shown to improve nutritional outcomes.
   D. The BRAT (*b*ananas, *r*ice, *a*pples, and *t*ea) diet, although commonly recommended, is unnecessarily restrictive, and it can provide suboptimal nutrition for the recovering gut.
   E. Foods high in simple sugars should be avoided, because the osmotic load may worsen the diarrhea.

   Review this! ❏

4. Which of the following statements best describes the appropriate pharmacological treatment of diarrhea?

   A. Oral metronidazole is superior to oral vancomycin for the treatment of *Clostridium-difficile*–associated diarrhea.
   B. Antidiarrheal medications are recommended for use in infants and children.
   C. In adult cases of traveler's diarrhea, prompt treatment with a fluoroquinolone has been shown to reduce the duration of illness.
   D. Antibiotics should be used prophylactically to reduce the likelihood of the secondary transmission of a diarrheal illness.
   E. Antimotility agents are recommended for the treatment of Shiga-toxin–producing *Escherichia coli* infections.

   Review this! ❏

5. Most patients with achalasia present with all of the following, except:

   A. Dysphagia.
   B. Weight loss.
   C. Regurgitation.
   D. Odynophagia.
   E. Chest pain.

   Review this! ❏

6. Which of the following is an evidence-based standard of care for the detection and management of *Helicobacter pylori* infection?

A. Patients less than 45 years old with dyspepsia and no alarm symptoms should be tested for *H. pylori* and treated if positive.

B. Patients more than 45 years old with dyspepsia should be referred for endoscopy only if *H. pylori* testing is positive.

C. Empiric treatment for functional dyspepsia is not recommended.

D. Serologic testing for *H. pylori* is more accurate than urea breath tests.

E. The prevalence of *H. pylori* and its association with peptic ulcer disease are highest in wealthier nations.

Review this! ❑

7. Which of the following is the most common cause of peptic ulcer disease in *H.-pylori*–negative patients?

A. Noncompliance with proton-pump inhibitors

B. False-negative *H. pylori* serologic testing

C. Nonsteroidal antiinflammatory drug (NSAID) use

D. Acetaminophen use

E. Cigarette smoking

Review this! ❑

8. The eradication of *H. pylori* requires a 14-day course of treatment. Which of the following pharmacological regimens is not appropriate?

A. A proton-pump inhibitor, clarithromycin 500 mg twice daily, and amoxicillin 1000 mg twice daily

B. A proton-pump inhibitor and clarithromycin 500 mg twice daily

C. A proton-pump inhibitor, clarithromycin 500 mg twice daily, and metronidazole 500 mg twice daily

D. Ranitidine 150 mg twice daily, bismuth subsalicylate 525 mg four times daily, metronidazole 250 mg four times daily, and tetracycline 500 mg four times daily

E. A proton-pump inhibitor, bismuth subsalicylate 525 mg four times daily, metronidazole 250 mg four times daily, tetracycline 500 mg four times daily

Review this! ❑

9. Gastroesophageal reflux disease (GERD) is a chronic, relapsing condition that is often diagnosed clinically, with a high risk for morbidity and potential complications. Which of the following patients with GERD warrants further diagnostic testing?

A. A 32-year-old male with an improvement of symptoms after 4 weeks of treatment with omeprazole (Prilosec)

B. A 46-year-old female with concomitant hypertension who is taking an angiotensin-converting enzyme inhibitor and who complains of chronic cough

C. A 62-year-old male diabetic complaining of early satiety and odynophagia

D. A 50-year-old female who has an improvement of symptoms on a maximal dose of lansoprazole (Prevacid)

E. A 49-year-old male who has experienced GERD symptoms twice monthly for the past year and who takes a proton-pump inhibitor on an as-needed basis, with relief

Review this! ❑

10. All of the following are risk factors for the development of upper gastrointestinal bleeding, except:

A. *H. pylori* infection

B. NSAID use

C. Admission to an intensive care unit

D. Obesity

E. Prior history of upper gastrointestinal bleeding

Review this! ❑

11. Stress ulceration, which is a form of hemorrhagic gastritis, is most likely to occur in all of the following patients, except:

A. A 42-year-old female with a past medical history of hypertension who was admitted with left-lower-lobe pneumonia

B. A 91-year-old male with multi-organ failure

C. A 72-year-old female nursing-home resident admitted with urosepsis

D. A 49-year-old male involved in a motor vehicle accident with multiple fractures

E. A 56-year-old female in the surgical intensive care unit after a craniotomy

Review this! ❑

12. Gastroparesis, which involves impaired and delayed gastric emptying, is primarily treated with dietary management along with antiemetics and prokinetic agents. Which of the following is a recommended dietary guideline for patients with this condition?

    A. A high-fiber diet
    B. Frequent, small meals
    C. Increased solid foods and fewer liquids
    D. Two larger meals per day
    E. Increased fat content

    Review this! ❏

13. Which of the following laboratory findings is expected in cases of acute cholecystitis?

    A. Elevated serum amylase
    B. An aspartate aminotransferase (AST) level that is greater than the alanine aminotransferase (ALT) level
    C. Leukocytosis
    D. Hyperbilirubinemia
    E. Elevated alkaline phosphatase

    Review this! ❏

14. Which of the following is the best screening modality for the evaluation of gallstones?

    A. Computed tomography scanning
    B. Plain films
    C. Ultrasound
    D. Endoscopic retrograde cholangiopan-creatography
    E. Cholescintigraphy

    Review this! ❏

15. All of the following are indications for cholecystectomy, except:

    A. Persisting or worsening pain.
    B. Persistent fever.
    C. Increasing leukocytosis.
    D. Asymptomatic cholelithiasis.
    E. Worsening of physical examination.

    Review this! ❏

16. Which of the following is the most common etiology of asymptomatic jaundice?

    A. Acute hepatitis
    B. Chronic pancreatitis
    C. Pancreatic carcinoma

    D. Acute cholecystitis
    E. Acetaminophen overdose

    Review this! ❏

17. Which of the following laboratory findings best represents a patient who is a chronic carrier of hepatitis B virus?

    A. Positive hepatitis B surface antigen (HBsAg), negative antibody to hepatitis B surface antigen (anti-HBs), negative hepatitis B e antigen (HBeAg), positive antibody to hepatitis B e antigen (anti-HBe)
    B. Positive HBsAg, positive anti-HBs, negative HBeAg, negative anti-HBe
    C. Negative HBsAg, positive anti-HBs
    D. Positive HBsAg, negative anti-HBs, positive HBeAg

    Review this! ❏

18. Alarm symptoms of severe hepatic parenchymal destruction include all of the following, except:

    A. Mental status changes.
    B. Asterixis.
    C. Ascites.
    D. Prolonged elevation of prothrombin time.
    E. Marked elevation of transaminases.

    Review this! ❏

19. Which of the following is most consistent with a laboratory diagnosis of alcoholic hepatitis?

    A. Proportionate elevation of AST and ALT
    B. AST greater than ALT, with normal gamma-glutamyl transpeptidase
    C. AST greater than ALT, with elevated gamma-glutamyl transpeptidase
    D. Elevation of serum amylase
    E. Elevation of alkaline phosphatase

    Review this! ❏

20. Which of the following is the incubation period of viral hepatitis A?

    A. Less than 2 weeks
    B. 2–6 weeks
    C. 7–12 weeks
    D. 13–18 weeks
    E. 19–24 weeks

    Review this! ❏

Things to remember for the test.

Things to remember for the test.

21. The most effective therapy for the management of patients with chronic hepatitis C includes which of the following?

    A. Immunoglobulin therapy
    B. Pegylated interferon
    C. Ribavirin
    D. Pegylated interferon and ribavirin
    E. Acyclovir

    Review this! ❑

22. All of the following are associated with cirrhosis-related morbidity and mortality in the United States, except:

    A. Excessive alcohol consumption.
    B. Overuse of acetaminophen.
    C. Hepatitis B.
    D. Hepatitis C.
    E. Obesity.

    Review this! ❑

23. All of the following accurately describe the pain that is often associated with acute pancreatitis, except:

    A. Gnawing, epigastric pain.
    B. Pain that radiates to the back.
    C. Pain that lasts from hours to days.
    D. Pain that is intermittent and colicky.
    E. Pain that may be worsened by food.

    Review this! ❑

24. Which of the following statements most accurately reflects the use of laboratory studies in the evaluation of acute pancreatitis?

    A. Serum markers can reliably predict the severity of disease.
    B. Serum amylase is only elevated in acute pancreatitis.
    C. Elevated serum lipase has a sensitivity of 10% for acute pancreatitis.
    D. A C-reactive protein value of greater than 150 mg/L indicates severe disease.
    E. Amylase and lipase are cleared from the blood at the same rates.

    Review this! ❑

25. All of the following agents are used for the management of inflammatory bowel disease, except:

    A. Mesalamine.
    B. Sulfasalazine.
    C. Steroids.
    D. Methotrexate.
    E. Ribavirin.

    Review this! ❑

26. Which of the following statements is least consistent with a diagnosis of irritable bowel syndrome?

    A. It is characterized by the presence of abdominal pain, bloating, and disturbed defecation.
    B. It is more prevalent among men than among women.
    C. It is associated with the absence of a known structural or biochemical abnormality.
    D. It is associated with a high frequency of concomitant anxiety disorders, somatoform disorders, and/or sexual abuse.
    E. It involves an unremarkable evaluation including laboratory, radiologic, and endoscopic testing.

    Review this! ❑

27. Which of the following is the most appropriate diagnostic study for the initial evaluation of a patient presenting with a probable lower gastrointestinal bleed?

    A. Radiographic angiography
    B. A technetium-99m pertechnetate-labeled red blood cell scan
    C. A computed tomography scan with intravenous contrast
    D. A colonoscopy
    E. An air-contrast barium enema

    Review this! ❑

28. Which of the following is not indicated during the initial assessment of a patient who presents with a suspected diagnosis of diverticulitis?

    A. A comprehensive history and physical examination, including rectal and pelvic examinations
    B. A complete blood cell count, urinalysis, and flat and upright abdominal radiographs
    C. A colonoscopy
    D. Abdominal and pelvic computed tomography scanning with oral and intravenous contrast
    E. Abdominal and pelvic ultrasonography

    Review this! ❑

29. Which of the following is the gold standard for colorectal carcinoma screening?

    A. Annual screening with fecal occult blood testing and digital rectal examination beginning at the age of 50 years
    B. Colonoscopy at the age of 50 years
    C. Virtual colonoscopy or computed tomography colonoscopy
    D. Flexible sigmoidoscopy with digital rectal examination and fecal occult blood testing

    E. Double-contrast barium enema

    Review this! ❏

30. Which of the following is the most common presentation of hemorrhoids?

    A. Asymptomatic bleeding
    B. Diarrhea
    C. Pain on defecation
    D. Perianal itching
    E. Bloody rectal discharge

    Review this! ❏

Things to remember for the test.

Chapter

50 Oncology

William C. Crow

1. Which of the following is the leading cause of cancer death overall for both men and women?

   A. Lung and bronchus cancer
   B. Colorectal cancer
   C. Pancreatic cancer
   D. Renal cell cancer
   E. Bladder cancer

   Review this! ❑

2. All of the following are examples of primary prevention, except:

   A. Wearing sunscreen and a broad-brimmed hat when exposed to the sun
   B. Avoiding smoking
   C. Using condoms
   D. Using tamoxifen in women with estrogen-receptor–positive breast tumors to prevent recurrent disease

   Review this! ❑

3. Which one of the following is the best dietary source of lycopene?

   A. Bananas
   B. Nuts
   C. Tomatoes
   D. Yogurt
   E. Green vegetables

   Review this! ❑

4. Which of the following has the potential to progress to colon cancer?

   A. Hyperplastic polyp
   B. Adenomatous polyp
   C. Diverticulum
   D. Melanosis coli

   Review this! ❑

5. A woman presents with a malignant mass in her breast that is too large to remove with lumpectomy. She undergoes chemotherapy before surgery to shrink the tumor and to allow her to have a lumpectomy rather than a mastectomy. This an example of which of the following?

   A. Neoadjuvant chemotherapy
   B. Adjuvant chemotherapy
   C. Chemoprevention
   D. Palliative chemotherapy

   Review this! ❑

6. Examples of biological therapy include all of the following, except:

   A. Interferons.
   B. Monoclonal antibodies.
   C. Interleukins.
   D. Tumor vaccines.
   E. Flutamide and tamoxifen.

   Review this! ❑

7. Which of the following is the average survival time after the diagnosis of extensive small-cell lung cancer?

   A. 2–4 months
   B. 9 months
   C. 15 months
   D. 18 months
   E. 2 years

   Review this! ❑

8. Contraindications to lumpectomy include all of the following, except:

   A. Prior radiation therapy to the affected breast.
   B. Having two or more cancers widely separated in the same breast.
   C. A 2-cm tumor.
   D. Pregnancy in women who would require radiation therapy while still pregnant.
   E. Tumors that are larger than 5 cm.
   F. Tumors that are relatively large as compared with breast size.

   Review this! ❑

9. Risk factors for prostate cancer include which of the following?

A. Increasing age
B. High-fat diet
C. Black race
D. Physical inactivity
E. Obesity
F. All of the above

Review this! ❏

10. Regarding prostate cancer, the Gleason score is based on which of the following?

A. The two most prevalent differentiation patterns seen in the tissue examined
B. The number of involved lymph nodes
C. The percentage of free prostate-specific antigen (PSA)
D. The total PSA
E. The PSA velocity

Review this! ❏

11. The United States Preventive Services Task Force recommends screening for cervical cancer in all of the following, except:

A. Those who have been sexually active within 3 years of the onset of sexual activity or all women at the age of 21 years, whichever comes first.
B. Atleast every 3 years.
C. Those who have had a hysterectomy for benign disease.

Review this! ❏

12. The 5-year survival rate for all cervical cancer is approximately which of the following?

A. 30%
B. 50%
C. 70%
D. 90%

Review this! ❏

13. Screening for patients who are not at increased risk for colon cancer should begin at which of the following ages?

A. 35 years
B. 40 years
C. 50 years
D. 60 years
E. Routine screening is not recommended.

Review this! ❏

14. A patient is found to have an adenomatous polyp on flexible sigmoidoscopy. The next step in the evaluation should be which of the following?

A. Colonoscopy
B. Air contrast barium enema
C. Abdominal and pelvic computed tomography scanning
D. Magnetic resonance imaging

Review this! ❏

15. Poor prognosis in colon cancer is associated with which of the following?

A. Recurrent disease
B. Extension into the bowel wall
C. Bowel obstruction
D. Bowel perforation
E. An elevated carcinoembryonic antigen level before treatment
F. All of the above

Review this! ❏

16. Women with advanced ovarian cancer may present with which of the following?

A. Abdominal bloating
B. Pain
C. Gas
D. Indigestion
E. Nausea
F. Unexplained weight gain or loss
G. Any of the above

Review this! ❏

17. Which of the following is the tumor marker that is most commonly associated with ovarian cancer?

A. CA 125
B. CA 19–9
C. CEA
D. PSA

Review this! ❏

18. Which of the following is the most common form of cancer in men between ages 15 and 44 years?

A. Hodgkin's disease
B. Testicular cancer
C. Renal cell cancer
D. Thyroid cancer

Review this! ❏

19. Useful tumor markers for testicular cancer include all of the following, except:

A. Alpha-fetoprotein.
B. Lactate dehydrogenase.
C. Beta human chorionic gonadotropin.
D. CA 19–9.

Review this! ❏

Things to remember for the test.

20. Good prognostic factors in testicular cancer include all of the following, except:

    A. The tumor is a seminoma.
    B. Metastases, if they are present, are in the lung only.
    C. If the tumor is a seminoma, all hormone levels are normal.
    D. For non-seminomas, tumor markers are no greater than 1.5 times the normal level.
    E. The tumor is a non-seminoma that started in the mediastinum.

    Review this! ❏

21. For the evaluation of breast-cancer survivors, the American Cancer Society recommends all of the following, except:

    A. History and physical every 3 to 6 months during the first 3 years after initial therapy
    B. After 3 years, history and physical every 6 to 12 months for the next 2 years
    C. Mammogram 6 months after treatment, then annual mammograms
    D. Routine periodic bone scans

    Review this! ❏

22. Which of the following statements about breast cancer during pregnancy is true?

    A. Ultrasound may be required to evaluate a breast mass.
    B. Women with stage I and II disease should wait 3 years after radiation before conceiving.
    C. Women with stage III and IV disease should allow a 5-year interval after radiation before conception.
    D. All of the above

    Review this! ❏

23. A living will deals with all of the following issues, except:

    A. Which specific medical treatments are desired or not desired.
    B. Whether to continue life support.
    C. Whether to continue or discontinue feeding.
    D. The appointment of specific a person(s) chosen by the patient to make health-care decisions for him or her

    Review this! ❏

24. When assessing breast-cancer risk, all of the following factors should be considered, except:

    A. Age at menarche.
    B. First-degree relatives with breast cancer.
    C. Any breast biopsy that is consistent with atypical hyperplasia.
    D. The consumption of more than two alcoholic drinks per day.
    E. Coffee consumption.

    Review this! ❏

25. Factors to be considered when assessing cervical-cancer risk include which of the following?

    A. Age at first sexual encounter
    B. History of genital warts, human immunodeficiency virus, herpes, or chlamydia
    C. History of abnormal vaginal or uterine bleeding
    D. Cigarette smoking
    E. All of the above

    Review this! ❏

26. All of the following are risk factors for endometrial cancer, except:

    A. Age of more than 50 years.
    B. History of estrogen-only replacement therapy.
    C. Diabetes and hypertension.
    D. History of colon, rectal, or breast cancer.
    E. Asian ethnicity.

    Review this! ❏

27. The American Cancer Society guidelines for prostate cancer screening include which of the following?

    A. Offering annual PSA and digital rectal examinations to men beginning at age 50 if they have a life expectancy of more than 10 years
    B. Beginning screening at age 45 for black men and for men with a first-degree relative with prostate cancer
    C. Discussing with male patients the benefits and limitations of the screening for, testing for, and treatment of early stage prostate cancer
    D. All of the above

    Review this! ❏

28. The American Cancer Society Guidelines for breast cancer screening include all of the following, except:

A. Mammograms starting at the age of 40 years and continuing annually as long as the woman is in good health.

B. Clinical breast examinations every 3 years for women between the ages of 20 and 39 and annually for women who are more than 40 years old.

C. Women who are at increased risk as a result of family history, previous diagnosis of breast cancer, or genetic tendency should ask their providers about earlier testing.

D. Thermography may be substituted for mammography.

Review this! ❏

29. Which of the following is the one primary treatment for stage IB non–small-cell lung cancer (tumor that is 3 cm or larger, with some invasion into local areas)?

A. Surgery
B. Radiotherapy
C. Intensive chemotherapy
D. High-dose interferon

Review this! ❏

30. In children, which of the following is the malignancy that is most likely to present with pain in the bones and joints, weakness, bleeding, and fever?

A. Neuroblastoma
B. Hodgkin's lymphoma
C. Wilms' tumor
D. Leukemia

Review this! ❏

Things to remember for the test.

51 Hematology

Charles E. Driscoll

1. Bone marrow recovery and regrowth after severe suppression from chemotherapy or radiation therapy is supported by which of the following?

   A. T cells
   B. Stem cells
   C. Monocytes/macrophages
   D. Natural killer cells

   Review this! ❏

2. According to the 1999 and 2000 National Health and Nutrition Examination Surveys, iron deficiency has the highest prevalence among which of the following groups?

   A. Whites
   B. Blacks
   C. Mexican Americans
   D. Asian Americans

   Review this! ❏

3. The amount of oxygen available in the red cells of the body is "sensed" by special cells lining the capillaries that are located in which of the following areas?

   A. The brain
   B. The lungs
   C. The carotid artery
   D. The kidneys

   Review this! ❏

4. True or false: Of all hematologic disorders, anemia is the most frequent seen in a family medicine practice.

   A. True
   B. False

   Review this! ❏

5. All of the following disorders are examples of hypoproliferative anemias, except:

   A. Aplastic anemia.
   B. Anemia of inflammation.
   C. Myelodysplasia.

   D. Anemia associated with hypothyroidism.

   Review this! ❏

6. Which of the following is the most common form of anemia seen in the hospitalized patient?

   A. Aplastic anemia
   B. Anemia of chronic renal insufficiency
   C. Hypothyroidism
   D. Anemia of inflammation

   Review this! ❏

7. Which of the following is the best laboratory test to use to distinguish anemia caused by iron deficiency from anemia caused by inflammation?

   A. Serum iron
   B. Total iron-binding capacity
   C. serum ferritin
   D. Red blood cell protoporphyrin level

   Review this! ❏

8. A two-step Schilling test is performed to assess an anemic patient for suspected pernicious anemia. The first step (a small oral dose of radioactively labeled vitamin B_{12} along with a very large flushing dose of B_{12} given parenterally) and the second step (an oral dose of radioactively labeled B_{12} given with intrinsic factor along with a very large flushing dose of B_{12} given parenterally) are both reported as positive. Tagged B_{12} is absent from the urine. This confirms which of the following conditions?

   A. Pernicious anemia
   B. Disease of the terminal ileum
   C. Iron-deficiency anemia
   D. Folate deficiency

   Review this! ❏

9. Three iron tablets (ferrous sulfate) per day will supply 150 mg of elemental iron and result in reticulocytosis within which of the following time frames?

A. 1 day
B. 1 week
C. 1 month
D. 2–4 months

Review this! ❏

10. A 28-year-old Asian woman who is the mother of two young children is found to be mildly anemic (hemoglobin level, 10.4), and a 2-month trial of iron replacement therapy is given. Despite the patient's insistence that she took three iron pills per day, her hemoglobin recheck shows only a small increase to 10.8. Which of the following should you suspect?

A. Patient noncompliance with therapy
B. Malabsorption syndrome or interference by foods in the diet
C. Homozygous alpha thalassemia
D. Hemoglobin Constant Spring

Review this! ❏

11. Which of the following is the most common inborn error of red-cell metabolism in the world, affecting nearly half a billion members of the world's population?

A. Thalassemia
B. Sickle cell anemia
C. Glucose-6-phosphate dehydrogenase deficiency
D. Hereditary spherocytosis

Review this! ❏

12. True or false: Most patients with extravascular hemolysis resulting from pyruvate kinase deficiency have a mild anemia, and they generally do not require transfusions.

A. True
B. False

Review this! ❏

13. Which of the following statements about people with hemoglobin AS and SS is true?

A. They are somewhat protected against malaria.
B. They are equally distributed among the black population.
C. They are affected by an inherited, sex-linked, recessive gene.
D. They are more prevalent among the Mediterranean and Indian populations than among the black population.

Review this! ❏

14. Howell–Jolly bodies in the blood of adult patients with sickle cell disorder indicate which of the following?

A. An acute microvascular occlusive crisis is occurring.
B. Autoinfarction of the spleen has occurred.
C. The patient has experienced avascular necrosis of the bone.
D. The patient has sickle cell trait AS and not sickle cell trait SS.

Review this! ❏

15. Splenectomized patients with sickle cell anemia should receive which of the following?

A. Salmonella vaccine
B. Pneumococcal vaccine
C. Mild acidification of the blood
D. Sodium metabisulfite tablets at the onset of an acute crisis

Review this! ❏

16. A 10-year-old child with a history of severe sickle cell disease is noted to be performing poorly in school, to be inattentive, and to have reading difficulties, and he is felt by his teachers to have attention-deficit/hyperactivity disorder. What should you do?

A. Refer him to a child psychiatrist for evaluation for depression and for counseling.
B. Image his hips for the presence of avascular necrosis.
C. Order hearing and vision evaluations.
D. Rule out cerebral infarctions with magnetic resonance imaging of the brain.

Review this! ❏

17. Which of the following is the diagnostic test for autoimmune hemolytic anemia?

A. Serum protein electrophoresis
B. Serum complement
C. Coombs antiglobulin test
D. Bone marrow examination

Review this! ❏

18. A 52-year-old man has a confirmed hemoglobin measurement of 21 gm/dL, and he is suspected of having polycythemia. Before labeling him with that diagnosis, you wish to run a confirmatory test. Which of the following tests is the best to use to establish the fact that there is a true increase in red cell mass?

A. Isotope dilution techniques for direct measurement
B. Bone marrow biopsy
C. Serum carboxyhemoglobin
D. Circulating erythropoietin serum level

Review this! ❏

19. Phagocytes in the white blood cell series are responsible for the ingestion and killing of bacteria. Which of the following is not a phagocytic cell?

A. Neutrophil
B. Lymphocyte
C. Eosinophil
D. Monocyte
E. Macrophage

Review this! ❏

20. Hyperlobulated neutrophils suggest a deficiency state of which one of the following?

A. Folate
B. Protein (e.g., protein-calorie malnutrition)
C. B_{12}
D. Reticuloendothelial factor

Review this! ❏

21. In nodular sclerosing type of Hodgkin's disease, Reed–Sternberg cells produce interleukin-5, which increases which of the following?

A. Kupffer cells
B. Monocytes
C. Platelet activation factor
D. Eosinophils

Review this! ❏

22. A patient presents to the emergency department with confusion and a neutrophilia level of 12,000, with 22% bands. Dohle bodies, toxic granulations, and cytoplasmic vacuoles are reported on the peripheral smear examination. Which of the following is the most likely diagnosis?

A. Acute infection
B. Cryoglobulinemia
C. Central nervous system intoxication with a benign inflammatory reaction
D. Bone marrow stress reaction

Review this! ❏

23. When severe neutropenia occurs, patients are at risk for serious infection from breaks in cutaneous or mucosal barriers in areas such as the gastrointestinal tract or the oropharynx. What absolute neutrophil count is the cutoff for outpatient therapy as compared with hospitalization for febrile patients?

A. 1500
B. 1000
C. 500
D. 200

Review this! ❏

24. A 43-year-old female patient reports gingival bleeding with toothbrushing that has occurred during the previous 4 months. She takes thyroid medication for hypothyroidism that began 6 years ago after thyroiditis. The physical examination is negative, except for petechiae over the lower extremities. You make a diagnosis of idiopathic thrombocytopenic purpura. Which of the following statements is true?

A. Treatment should be reserved until the platelet count falls below 100,000.
B. All patients with platelet counts of less than 20,000 should be hospitalized.
C. Treatment is indicated for patients with platelet counts in the 20,000 to 30,000 range.
D. When treatment is initiated with prednisone, it should be continued for 6 months and then tapered.

Review this! ❏

25. Von Willebrand's disease is an example of which of the following?

A. Thrombocytosis
B. An inherited impairment of platelet adhesion
C. An acquired platelet dysfunction
D. A myeloproliferative disorder

Review this! ❏

26. An 18-year-old male patient has the following results reported on a complete blood cell count:

Total white blood cells	13,500
Neutrophils	53%
Band neutrophils	0
Lymphocytes	40%
Monocytes	3%
Eosinophils	3%
Basophils	1%

True or false: The absolute lymphocyte count is within normal limits for this patient's age.

A. True
B. False

Review this! ❏

27. A 4-year-old child has gray, exudative pharyngitis, a severe cough, and a temperature of 104°F. His white blood cell count reveals an absolute lymphocytosis of 55,000. Which of the following is the most likely diagnosis?

A. Acute lymphocytic leukemia
B. Infectious mononucleosis
C. Human immunodeficiency virus
D. Pertussis

Review this! ❏

28. An enlarged, firm, nontender, left supraclavicular node (Virchow's node) is suspicious for malignancy in which of the following locations?

A. The submandibular region
B. The paratracheal structures
C. The lung parenchyma
D. Below the diaphragm

Review this! ❏

29. Which of the following statements about acute myeloid leukemia (AML) is true?

A. AML is seen predominantly in adults.
B. AML arises from precursor cells of the B and T cell lymphocyte lines.
C. The peak age for the diagnosis of AML is between 3 to 5 years.
D. AML is more common among blacks than whites.

Review this! ❏

30. True or false: The cumulative exposure to radiation from diagnostic x-ray imaging is a risk factor for leukemia.

A. True
B. False

Review this! ❏

31. Chronic lymphocytic leukemia is diagnosed in a 72-year-old woman by the chance finding of white cell count that is elevated to 30,000. The patient is asymptomatic, and the physical examination is normal. What should be done next?

A. Nothing
B. A splenectomy
C. Monoclonal antibody therapy
D. Cytoreduction chemotherapy

Review this! ❏

Things to remember for the test.

52 Urinary Tract Disorders

Bruce T. Vanderhoff

1. Which of the following statements about routine urinalysis is true?

   A. Annual screening is recommended for asymptomatic adults between the ages of 18 and 45 years.
   B. Routine microalbuminuria screening is recommended for all diabetic adults.
   C. Although false-negative results are quite rare, false-positive results are common.
   D. There is nearly universal agreement that screening urinalysis is an important component of pediatric preventive care.

   Review this! ❑

2. Which of the following statements about the urine culture is true?

   A. It can be reliably obtained from a catheter bag, because this is a sterile, sealed system.
   B. In women with typical urinary tract infection (UTI) symptoms, colony counts as low as 10^2 signify infection if Enterobacteriaceae are isolated.
   C. The culture results do not signify infection in men unless the colony count is 10^5.
   D. It has been clearly demonstrated to be reliable only when it is obtained from a midstream, clean-catch specimen.

   Review this! ❑

3. Which of the following statements about ultrasound is true?

   A. It is the method of choice for evaluating the renal parenchyma, but it is a poor diagnostic modality for imaging renal cysts.
   B. It is a better choice than computed tomography for evaluating solid renal masses.
   C. It is nearly 100% sensitive for testicular tumors.

   D. It is the test of choice for renal calculi.

   Review this! ❑

4. Which of the following statements about microscopic hematuria is true?

   A. It is rarely an incidental finding on urinalysis, and it generally indicates significant pathology.
   B. It is generally defined as 10 or more red blood cells per high-powered field.
   C. It is nearly always present on samples that are collected from patients receiving warfarin (Coumadin).
   D. It is initially evaluated with urinalysis, urine culture (if indicated), and serum creatinine.

   Review this! ❑

5. Risk factors for urologic malignancy include all of the following, except:

   A. A history of UTIs.
   B. A history of tobacco use.
   C. Age of more than 25 years.
   D. Analgesic abuse.
   E. Irritative voiding symptoms.

   Review this! ❑

6. All of the following statements about nocturia are true, except:

   A. It is more common among the elderly.
   B. It increases the risk of falling.
   C. It is common among both men and women.
   D. It is uncommon among men without prostatic obstruction.
   E. Treating obstructive sleep apnea may help alleviate symptoms.

   Review this! ❑

7. Which of the following statements about proteinuria is true?

A. It is a marker of kidney disease in adults.
B. It may contribute to renal impairment.
C. Benign orthostatic proteinuria is common among adults, adolescents, and children.
D. It is considered transient in children unless it is confirmed by two out of three weekly urine samples.

Review this! ❏

8. All of the following statements about infants with fetal hydronephrosis are true, except:

A. They require an ultrasound during the first 6 weeks of life.
B. They should, upon diagnosis confirmation, have a urinalysis, a urine culture, a basic metabolic panel (if the condition is bilateral), and a voiding cystourethrogram.
C. They should receive a furosemide renogram to evaluate possible obstruction if the voiding cystourethrogram is normal.
D. They can be managed conservatively in the absence of severe obstruction or high-grade vesicoureteral reflux.

Review this! ❏

9. Which of the following statements about hypospadias is true?

A. It is seen commonly.
B. It should be recognized within the first year of life.
C. It need not delay circumcision, provided that the urethral opening does not extend more than 5 mm beyond the corona.
D. It can occur with or without chordee.

Review this! ❏

10. Which of the following statements about labial adhesions, phimosis, and paraphimosis is true?

A. Labial adhesions are not believed to contribute to urinary tract infections.
B. Retrospective data do not support the treatment of labial adhesions with estrogen cream.
C. Phimosis and paraphimosis are commonly seen among circumcised males.
D. Acute paraphimosis requires urgent medical attention.

Review this! ❏

11. Which of the following statements about testicular torsion is true?

A. It is a condition that is most commonly observed in middle-aged men.
B. It can usually be managed expectantly.
C. It generally cannot be diagnosed by physical examination.
D. It can occur in cases involving systemic illnesses, such as Henoch–Schönlein purpura.

Review this! ❏

12. All of the following statements are true, except:

A. Peyronie's disease is most often self-limited.
B. Infants with hydroceles should be routinely referred for urologic evaluation and surgical correction.
C. Torsion of the appendix testis can be managed with supportive care.
D. Undescended testicles increase the risk for cancer in both the undescended and the contralateral testicle.

Review this! ❏

13. Approximately how many persons in the United States have chronic kidney disease?

A. 20 million
B. 12 million
C. 60 million
D. 2 million
E. 160 million

Review this! ❏

14. Conditions that increase the risk for chronic kidney disease include all of the following, except:

A. Diabetes.
B. Hypertension.
C. Hypercholesterolemia.
D. Autoimmune disorders.
E. Renal calculi.

Review this! ❏

15. True statements about angiotensin-converting enzyme (ACE) inhibitors and angiotensin receptor blockers (ARBs) include all of the following, except:

Things to remember for the test.

A. Patients with type 2 diabetes and nephropathy clearly benefit from treatment with either ACE inhibitors or ARBs.

B. The evidence for preventing end-stage renal failure in patients with advanced nephropathy is stronger for ACE inhibitors than it is for ARBs.

C. There is scant evidence to support either ACE inhibitors or ARBs as superior for the treatment of patients with isolated diabetes or isolated nephropathy.

D. ACE inhibitors are less expensive than ARBs, and they have more proven benefits for other comorbidities, such as chronic heart failure.

Review this! ❏

16. Recommendable interventions for a child with nocturnal enuresis include all of the following, except:

A. Bed-wetting alarms followed with immediate punishment.

B. Desmopressin plus an alarm.

C. Tricyclic medications.

D. Reassurance.

Review this! ❏

17. Which of the following statements about erectile dysfunction is true?

A. Sexual function declines with age.

B. Erectile dysfunction before age 30 is almost unheard of.

C. Erectile dysfunction occurs in approximately 50% of men with diabetes.

D. Approximately 10 million men are estimated to have erectile dysfunction.

Review this! ❏

18. Which of the following statements about interstitial cystitis is true?

A. It is usually associated with an infectious etiology.

B. It is more common in middle-aged men than women.

C. It may mimic the symptoms of a urinary tract infection.

D. It has no available treatments that have been approved by the U.S. Food and Drug Administration.

E. It has been shown by prospective data to respond to a variety of dietary interventions.

Review this! ❏

19. True or false: There are important differences in the effectiveness of various anticholinergic drugs for the treatment of overactive bladder.

A. True

B. False

Review this! ❏

20. Which of the following statements about renal calculi is true?

A. Black men have the highest risk.

B. Intravenous urography is the test of choice for diagnosing renal calculi.

C. Stones that are less than 10 mm will likely pass without intervention.

D. Stones that have not passed within 4 weeks are unlikely to do so.

Review this! ❏

21. True or false: *Chlamydia trachomatis* and *Neisseria gonorrhoeae* are the most common causes of epididymitis in men under the age of 35 years.

A. True

B. False

Review this! ❏

22. Which of the following statements about acute bacterial prostatitis is true?

A. It should be suspected in men who present with symptoms of UTI.

B. Unlike UTI, it is rarely associated with *Escherichia coli*.

C. It should prompt physicians to perform prostate massage to speed healing and provide symptom relief.

D. It is rarely associated with a urine culture that is positive for the causative organism.

Review this! ❏

23. All of the following statements about sexually transmitted infections are true, except:

A. Chancroid should be suspected in a patient with painful genital ulcers and adenopathy with negative testing for herpes and syphilis.

B. Patients with gonorrhea who are not ruled out for chlamydia should be treated for both infections.

C. Most visible genital warts are caused by human papillomavirus types 6 and 11.

D. Primary syphilis is treated with a single dose of penicillin.

E. Syphilis infection is typically associated with a painful genital ulcer known as a *chancre*.

Review this! ❑

24. All of the following statements about bacteriuria and UTI are true, except:

A. Identifying and treating asymptomatic bacteriuria are only important for pregnant women.

B. Women with dysuria and frequency without vaginal symptoms have a 90% chance of having a UTI.

C. Few women treated with trimethoprim-sulfamethoxazole who have a resistant organism on culture achieve clinical cure.

D. Cranberry juice can prevent recurrent UTI.

Review this! ❑

25. All of the following statements are true, except:

A. Smoking is the most prominent risk factor for bladder cancer.

B. Prostate cancer is the most common cancer among men.

C. Black men have a 60% higher incidence of prostate cancer as compared with white men, and they experience a disproportionate share of deaths from prostate cancer.

D. When ordering a prostate-specific antigen test, clinicians should discuss the risks, benefits, and uncertainties with patients and make a shared decision about screening.

E. Renal cancers are twice as common among women as they are among men.

Review this! ❑

Things to remember for the test.

53 Ophthalmology

Jennifer J. Mitchell and Kelly Mitchell

1. Causes of a red eye that should force a family physician to consider an immediate referral to an ophthalmologist for further evaluation include all of the following, except:

   A. Iritis.
   B. Acute angle closure glaucoma.
   C. Subconjunctival hemorrhage.
   D. Ophthalmia neonatorum.

   Review this! ❏

2. Which of the following associated symptoms should a patient be asked about when he or she calls the office complaining of a red eye?

   A. Purulent discharge
   B. Eye pain
   C. Photophobia
   D. Diminished visual acuity
   E. All of the above

   Review this! ❏

3. Of the following possible causes of red eye in an infant, all should be referred to an ophthalmologist, except:

   A. Ophthalmia neonatorum.
   B. Acute dacryocystitis.
   C. Congenital glaucoma.
   D. Chronic dacryocystitis or nasal lacrimal duct obstruction.

   Review this! ❏

4. Topical steroids are very effective for the treatment of which of the following?

   A. Ophthalmia neonatorum
   B. Glaucoma
   C. Viral conjunctivitis
   D. Iritis

   Review this! ❏

5. A chemical injury to the eye is a true ocular emergency. When a patient calls with the complaint of a chemical ocular injury, what should that patient be told?

   A. Come to the office immediately.
   B. Go to the nearest emergency room immediately.
   C. Call the eye doctor immediately.
   D. Immediately irrigate the eye by placing the face with the eyelids open under a gently flowing stream of water from a sink, spigot, or shower for 15 minutes.

   Review this! ❏

6. Hyphema can be associated with serious complications, including all of the following, except:

   A. A trigger for a systemic sickle cell crisis.
   B. Corneal blood staining.
   C. Optic nerve atrophy.
   D. Anterior and posterior synechiae (scarring of the iris to the lens or of the anterior chamber angle, respectively).

   Review this! ❏

7. Which of the following ocular injuries should be routinely referred to an ophthalmologist?

   A. Corneal abrasion
   B. Eyelid contusion (black eye)
   C. Foreign body in the conjunctival sac
   D. Corneal laceration

   Review this! ❏

8. True or false: Vision screening of infants and children can detect strabismus, amblyopia, ocular disease, and refractive errors.

   A. True
   B. False

   Review this! ❏

9. Which of the following is the most worrisome cause of asymmetrical red reflex or leukocoria?

A. Congenital cataract
B. Ocular infection caused by *Toxocara canis*
C. Persistent hyperplastic primary vitreous
D. Retinoblastoma

Review this! ❑

10. True or false: Myopia and farsightedness are the same thing.

A. True
B. False

Review this! ❑

11. True or false: Crossed eyes and esotropia are the same thing.

A. True
B. False

Review this! ❑

12. True or false: Amblyopia and strabismus are the same thing.

A. True
B. False

Review this! ❑

13. True or false: Laser in situ keratomileusis (LASIK) and photorefractive keratectomy (PRK) are surgical techniques that are used to correct refractive errors.

A. True
B. False

Review this! ❑

14. Which of the following ocular medications is paired with an accurate list of its side effects?

A. β-Blockers: bradycardia, problems with breathing, and erectile dysfunction
B. Carbonic anhydrase inhibitors: malaise, kidney stones, and hypokalemia
C. α-Agonists: low blood pressure, dry mouth, and fatigue
D. Prostaglandins: an increase in iris and/ or eyelid or lash pigmentation
E. All of the above

Review this! ❑

15. True or false: Adult patients who are more than 65 years old should have routine eye examinations at least every 3 to 5 years.

A. True
B. False

Review this! ❑

16. True or false: Presbyopia is the age-related loss of near vision and the required use of reading glasses by most adults in their 40s and 50s.

A. True
B. False

Review this! ❑

17. True or false: Currently, during cataract surgery, the cataract is removed with phacoemulsification.

A. True
B. False

Review this! ❑

18. What is the most common cause of permanent vision loss among black patients?

A. Cataracts
B. Retinal detachment
C. Diabetic retinopathy
D. Glaucoma

Review this! ❑

19. The treatment for glaucoma includes which of the following?

A. Laser eye surgery
B. Ocular medications
C. Oral medications
D. Incisional eye surgery
E. All of the above

Review this! ❑

20. Which of the following retinal diseases in the most common cause of the loss of reading vision among white adults?

A. Macular degeneration
B. Diabetic retinopathy
C. Retinal detachment
D. Temporal arteritis

Review this! ❑

21. Which of the following statements is true?

A. Dry or nonexudative macular degeneration is more common than wet or exudative macular degeneration.
B. Wet or exudative macular degeneration causes more severe vision loss than dry or nonexudative macular degeneration.
C. A and B

Review this! ❑

22. True or false: Currently, there is no cure for macular degeneration.

A. True
B. False

Review this! ❏

23. True or false: Diabetic retinopathy is the most common cause of blindness among Americans who are more than 20 years old.

A. True
B. False

Review this! ❏

24. True or false: Flashers, floaters, and a veil over the patient's vision could signify a posterior vitreous detachment or retinal detachment.

A. True
B. False

Review this! ❏

25. A sudden and painless loss of vision that returns over the course of a few minutes is most likely caused by which of the following?

A. Amaurosis fugax
B. Optic neuritis
C. Temporal arteritis
D. Retinal detachment

Review this! ❏

26. According to the Age-Related Eye Disease Study, which vitamin and mineral supplements, used in combination, produced a 25% reduction in the progression of age-related macular degeneration?

A. Vitamin C, 500 mg
B. Beta-carotene, 15 mg
C. Vitamin E, 400 IU
D. Zinc oxide, 80 mg
E. All of the above

Review this! ❏

27. A patient with optic neuritis and a magnetic resonance imaging scan that shows multiple plaques should be considered for treatment with any of the following, except:

A. Systemic intravenous methylpredniso-lone (1 g/day) for 3 days followed by 11 days of oral prednisone (1 mg/kg/day), for a total of 14 days of treatment.
B. Oral steroids for 3 days only.
C. Avonex (interferon β-1a).
D. Copaxone (Betaseron).

Review this! ❏

28. A 65-year-old woman with left-sided scalp and jaw pain complains about sudden, severe, and painless vision loss in her left eye. Her visual acuity has dropped to 20/400 in the left eye, and she has a left-sided afferent pupil defect. The direct ophthalmoscopic examination shows a swollen optic nerve in the left eye. The sedimentation rate and the C-reactive protein level are markedly elevated, and the CBC is normal. What should be done next?

A. Start steroid therapy immediately, with 100 mg of prednisone given intravenously for the first 48 hours. After steroid therapy is underway, plan for a temporal artery biopsy.
B. Arrange for magnetic resonance imaging of the brain to look for signs of multiple sclerosis, and arrange a neurology consult.
C. Because tissue diagnosis is important, before prescribing long-term steroid treatment, arrange for a temporal artery biopsy.

Review this! ❏

29. True or false: Dermatochalasis and ptosis are the same thing.

A. True
B. False

Review this! ❏

30. A child has significant strabismus (eyes that are misaligned) that requires surgery. Which of the following is important to discuss with this patient's parents?

A. During the surgery, the eye is never removed from the orbit.
B. Even if only one eye is misaligned, both eyes may require surgery.
C. The surgery is safe and effective, but more than one surgery may be required to get the best long-term alignment.
D. The long-term goals of strabismus surgery are to maintain equal vision in both eyes, to enable the eyes to work together, and to improve depth perception whenever possible.
E. All of the above

Review this! ❏

C h a p t e r

54 Neurology

Joseph M. Ginty

1. Which of the following statements about aphasia is true?

   A. Patients with Wernicke's aphasia have nonfluent speech, but their comprehension is preserved.
   B. Patients with Broca's aphasia have poor comprehension but fluent speech.
   C. Reading and writing are impaired among patients with both Wernicke's and Broca's aphasias.
   D. Aphasia results from damage to the nondominant hemisphere of the brain.

   Review this! ❏

2. Deep tendon reflexes are graded on a 5-point scale. Which of following examples of that scale is false?

   A. 0 = Absent reflex
   B. 3 = Normal reflex but brisker than average
   C. 2 = Normal
   D. 1 = Present without reinforcement

   Review this! ❏

3. All of the following features warn of an ominous cause of headache, except:

   A. A patient claiming that it is the worst headache that he or she has ever had.
   B. An early age of onset of new headache (before the age of 40 years).
   C. A progressively worsening headache.
   D. A headache associated with neurologic signs and symptoms other than aura.

   Review this! ❏

4. To establish a diagnosis of migraine without aura, there must have been at least five attacks fulfilling all of the following criteria, except:

   A. Headache attacks lasting more than 72 hours.
   B. Headache with unilateral location.

   C. During the headache, the patient experiences nausea and vomiting.
   D. Headache has a pulsating quality.

   Review this! ❏

5. For the treatment of mild migraine headaches, which of the following is a grade A recommendation?

   A. Triptans
   B. Dihydroergotamine mesylate
   C. Aspirin/acetaminophen/caffeine preparations
   D. Aqueous lidocaine

   Review this! ❏

6. The criteria for the diagnosis of cluster headaches includes all of the following, except:

   A. Bilateral orbital or supraorbital pain.
   B. Headache associated with lacrimation.
   C. A sense of restlessness or agitation.
   D. Eye edema.

   Review this! ❏

7. Characteristics of rebound headaches include which of the following?

   A. Well localized
   B. Unilateral
   C. Improved by mild physical or mental exertion
   D. Frequently present upon awakening

   Review this! ❏

8. The major risk after a transient ischemic attack (TIA) or a minor stroke is the subsequent occurrence of which of the following?

   A. Myocardial infarction
   B. Recurrent TIA
   C. Stroke
   D. Pulmonary embolism

   Review this! ❏

9. A patient goes to sleep at 10 PM and awakens from sleep at 6 AM the following day with a neurologic deficit. The stroke is assumed to have had its onset at which of the following times?

    A. 6 AM
    B. 10 PM
    C. Unknown
    D. 2 AM

    Review this! ❑

10. During the first 2 days after an ischemic stroke, elevated blood pressure should not be treated, unless which of the following is present?

    A. Systolic blood pressure consistently greater than 160 mm Hg
    B. Diastolic blood pressure consistently greater than 100 mm Hg
    C. Systolic blood pressure greater than 185 mm Hg in a patient who has received tissue plasminogen activator
    D. Elevated blood pressure should never be treated during the first 2 days after an ischemic stroke.

    Review this! ❑

11. Which of following statements about delirium is true?

    A. Delirium is a transient, global disorder of cognition and consciousness.
    B. It develops over a prolonged period of time.
    C. It remains stable during the course of the day.
    D. It cannot be diagnosed in patients with a previous history of dementia.

    Review this! ❑

12. Haloperidol is preferred over thioridazine for elderly patients for the treatment of delirium for which of the following reasons?

    A. It is more anticholinergic.
    B. It is more sedating.
    C. It is less likely to cause hypotension.
    D. It is less likely to cause hypertension.

    Review this! ❑

13. Which of the following statements about the use of feeding tubes in patients with end-stage dementia is true?

    A. Feeding tubes prolong life.
    B. Feeding tubes cause discomfort.
    C. Feeding tubes are strongly recommended for patients during the final stages of dementia.
    D. There are no medical complications associated with the use of feeding tubes.

    Review this! ❑

14. Which of the following definitions is false?

    A. *Lethargy* is a state of diminished arousal that can be maintained spontaneously or by light, repeated stimulation.
    B. *Delirium* is a state of alertness with impaired cognition.
    C. *Coma* is a state of sustained unresponsiveness.
    D. *Stupor* is the state of a patient who is unable to be aroused with repeated stimuli.

    Review this! ❑

15. For patients with coma, the odor of the breath may provide a valuable clue about the cause of the condition. Which of the following combinations of a smell and a cause of coma is incorrect?

    A. Garlic: arsenic poisoning
    B. Musty fetter: uremia
    C. Almond: cyanide poisoning
    D. Fruity odor: diabetic ketoacidosis

    Review this! ❑

16. The "coma cocktail" consists of all of the following, except:

    A. Naloxone.
    B. Thiamine.
    C. Flumazenil.
    D. Glucose.

    Review this! ❑

17. All of the following are associated with narcolepsy, except:

    A. Non-rapid-eye-movement (non-REM) sleep.
    B. Cataplexy.
    C. Hypnagogic hallucinations.
    D. Sleep paralysis.

    Review this! ❑

18. Which of the following statements is true?

    A. Apnea is obstructive if there is airflow but no respiratory effort.
    B. Hypopnea is a 50% reduction in airflow.
    C. Central apnea is characterized by the presence of airflow but no respiratory effort.
    D. The respiratory distress index is a measure of the frequency of events.
       Review this! ❏

19. All of the following statements about febrile seizures are true, except:

    A. Half of children who experience a first febrile seizure will experience at least one more.
    B. The younger the child when the first febrile seizure occurs, the more likely that child is to have another febrile seizure.
    C. Most recurrences of febrile seizures are within 1 year of the first seizure.
    D. A family history of febrile seizure is associated with an increased likelihood of recurrence.
       Review this! ❏

20. All of the following findings and characteristics seem to increase the likelihood of recurrence after a first nonfebrile seizure, except:

    A. Electroencephalogram abnormalities.
    B. Partial seizures.
    C. Family history of seizures.
    D. Prior neurological injury.
       Review this! ❏

21. The classic triad presentation for bacterial meningitis includes all of the following, except:

    A. Fever.
    B. Vision changes.
    C. Headache.
    D. Neck stiffness.
       Review this! ❏

22. The most common pathogens for community-acquired bacterial meningitis include all of the following, except:

    A. *Neisseria meningitidis*
    B. *Streptococcus pneumoniae*
    C. *Escherichia coli*
    D. *Haemophilus influenzae*
       Review this! ❏

23. Which of the following statements about the use of corticosteroids in patients with meningitis is true?

    A. Corticosteroids should be used for infants and children with *E. coli* meningitis who have not received antibiotics.
    B. Corticosteroids should be used for infants and children with *H. influenzae* type B meningitis who have not received antibiotics.
    C. Corticosteroid should be used for adults with pneumococcal meningitis who have received antibiotics.
    D. Corticosteroids have no role in the treatment of adults who have meningitis.
       Review this! ❏

24. Which of the following is the most common cause of peripheral neuropathy worldwide?

    A. Alcoholism
    B. Diabetes
    C. Human immunodeficiency virus
    D. Leprosy
       Review this! ❏

25. All of the following statements about Guillain-Barré syndrome are false, except:

    A. The presentation is one of the gradual progression of an ascending, symmetric weakness.
    B. Treatment usually consists of either plasmapheresis or intravenous human immunoglobulin.
    C. Treatment usually consists of high doses of steroids.
    D. The illness is never fatal.
       Review this! ❏

26. All of the following statements about Bell's palsy are false, except:

    A. The forehead is involved.
    B. It affects cranial nerve 5.
    D. Corticosteroids should not be used for the treatment of Bell's palsy.
    D. Bilateral Bell's palsy is common.
       Review this! ❏

27. All of the following statements about Duchenne's muscular dystrophy are true, except:

A. Pelvic girdle and thigh weakness force children to rise from the floor by placing their hands on their knees and walking up their thighs (Grower's sign).
B. Firm pseudohypertrophy of the calves results from the replacement of muscle with fibrous and fatty tissue.
C. Cardiac muscle is not affected.
D. It is an X-linked, recessive disorder.

Review this! ❏

28. All the following statements about myotonic dystrophy are true, except:

   A. *Myotonia* refers to the quick relaxation of a normal muscle contraction.
   B. In the early stages, there is more distal as opposed to proximal weakness and atrophy.
   C. It is associated with frontal balding.
   D. It is associated with testicular atrophy.

   Review this! ❏

29. The hallmark clinical features of Parkinson's disease include all of the following, except:

   A. Tremor.
   B. Good postural reflexes.
   C. Rigidity.
   D. Bradykinesia.

   Review this! ❏

30. All of the following statements about the treatment of Parkinson's disease are true, except:

A. After a few years of carbidopa-levodopa use, some patients develop dyskinesias as an unpredictable on-off response.
B. Monoamine oxidase type B inhibitors are relatively contraindicated for patients with peptic ulcer disease or cardiovascular disease.
C. Several different surgical procedures can be performed to decrease the symptoms of Parkinson's disease.
D. The best initial treatment for Parkinson's disease is the use of dopamine-agonist drugs.

Review this! ❏

31. Symptoms that are highly suggestive of multiple sclerosis include all of the following, except:

   A. Lhermitte's sign.
   B. Nystagmus.
   C. Weakness.
   D. Optic neuritis.

   Review this! ❏

32. The diagnosis of amyotrophic lateral sclerosis is based on the characteristic clinical signs, which include all of the following, except:

   A. Hyporeflexia.
   D. Progressive weakness.
   C. Fasciculations.
   D. Atrophy.

   Review this! ❏

55 Sexual Health Care

Christine D. Hudak

1. All of the following statements about the doctor–patient discussion of issues surrounding sexuality are true, except:

   A. Only a small portion of adults with a sexual problem seek medical assistance.
   B. Even if patients meet the criteria for sexual disorders, physicians have a very low rate of addressing and documenting this in the medical record.
   C. Most patients are embarrassed about inquiries regarding their sexual health, so it is best for physicians to avoid this topic if possible.
   D. Interviewing techniques such as inclusion, normalization, and universalization are helpful when taking a sexual history.
   E. The primary focus of sexual medicine should be the patient and/or the patient's partner's goals and expectations rather than the personal beliefs of the physician.

   Review this! ❏

2. Common factors that may contribute to sexual dysfunction include all of the following, except:

   A. Medical illness.
   B. Medications.
   C. Relationship issues.
   D. History of sexual abuse.
   E. Birth order in the family.

   Review this! ❏

3. Which of the following sexual disorders is characterized by the avoidance of all or nearly all sexual contact with a partner, thereby causing the patient distress or difficulty?

   A. Hypoactive sexual desire disorder
   B. Dyspareunia
   C. Sexual aversion disorder
   D. Orgasmic disorder
   E. Transvestic fetishism

   Review this! ❏

4. Which of the following statements about erectile dysfunction (ED) is true?

   A. Phosphodiesterase inhibitors can be used to treat ED, regardless of the etiology.
   B. Comorbid medical conditions do not typically contribute to ED.
   C. Psychological factors are rarely involved as a cause of ED.
   D. Approximately 26% of men between the ages of 60 and 69 years experience ED.
   E. Laboratory testing is unnecessary in the workup of ED.

   Review this! ❏

5. Which of the following is the most important component of the initial assessment of premature ejaculation?

   A. Performing a genital examination
   B. Ordering laboratory testing for hormone levels
   C. Taking a thorough history
   D. Referral for psychological testing
   E. Prompt referral to a urologist

   Review this! ❏

6. Treatment options for premature ejaculation include all of the following, except:

   A. Employing the squeeze technique.
   B. Use of selective serotonin reuptake inhibitors (SSRIs).
   C. Employing the stop-and-start technique.
   D. Masturbation training to improve ejaculatory control.
   E. Renewed focus for the couple on achieving simultaneous orgasm with intercourse.

   Review this! ❏

7. Which of the following statements about dyspareunia is false?

Things to remember for the test.

A. Dyspareunia is a gender-neutral term that can be applied to both men and women.

B. Dyspareunia always indicates a history of past sexual abuse.

C. Anal dyspareunia is usually the result of insufficient lubrication or spasm of the anal musculature.

D. Deep dyspareunia is often caused by over-vigorous penetration or excess cervical pressure.

E. Current evidence about the use of perineal ultrasound to treat postpartum dyspareunia is inconclusive.

Review this! ❑

8. Which of the following is the percentage of women who can reach orgasm with vaginal intercourse alone?

A. 10%
B. 25%
C. 50%
D. 75%
E. 95%

Review this! ❑

9. Which of the following statements about female orgasmic disorder is true?

A. *Primary inhibited orgasm* indicates that the patient has never been able to achieve orgasm.

B. *Secondary inhibited orgasm* indicates that the patient has never been able to achieve orgasm because of a secondary cause.

C. Religious and cultural beliefs rarely influence the ability to orgasm.

D. Female orgasmic disorder resolves after a woman gets married.

E. The inability to orgasm is most likely an irreversible phenomenon.

Review this! ❑

10. Which of the following statements about vaginismus is false?

A. Vaginismus is often idiopathic.

B. Vaginismus can be complete, partial, or situational.

C. Pelvic trauma and/or sexual abuse often precede vaginismus.

D. Vaginismus is under conscious control of the sufferer.

E. Sex therapy, vaginal dilators, and pelvic floor biofeedback are treatments that can be used for vaginismus.

Review this! ❑

11. Which of the following statements about teenage sexual practices in the United States is true?

A. Virginity pledges have been associated with a marked decrease in delaying sexual intercourse until marriage.

B. Nearly half of all high-school-aged teenagers have experienced sexual intercourse.

C. Adolescents prefer that their family doctors not inquire about their sexual knowledge and practices.

D. Family physicians should assume that adolescent sexual experiences are consensual and desired.

E. Ninety percent of teenagers report condom use with last sexual intercourse.

Review this! ❑

12. As compared with heterosexual youth, nonheterosexual youth are more likely to experience all of the following, except:

A. Earlier age of onset of tobacco, alcohol, and illegal drug use.

B. Dropping out of high school.

C. Becoming homeless.

D. Being subjected to harassment and violence.

E. Acceptance and support from family of origin.

Review this! ❑

13. Factors that influence participation in sexual relationships among older adults include all of the following, except:

A. Natural and inevitable loss of sexual interest as a result of aging.

B. Lack of an available partner.

C. Systemic side effects from medication that may inhibit sexual functioning.

D. Sexual disability from comorbid medical illness.

E. Physiologic changes that may influence erection, lubrication, and libido.

Review this! ❑

14. Which of the following statements about hypogonadism among older men is true?

A. Testosterone levels gradually decline with age, reaching about 20% of young adult levels.

B. Checking a serum testosterone level in an older male with complaints of decreased libido is not necessary; empiric testosterone replacement can be started and monitored clinically.

C. Transdermal preparations are the preferred form of testosterone replacement.

D. Periodic labs to monitor liver function and lipids are not necessary when treating a patient with testosterone replacement.

E. Oral testosterone preparations are a safe and effective alternative to transdermal therapy.

Review this! ❑

15. Which of the following statements about homosexual and bisexual sexual orientations is true?

A. They are most likely determined by a combination of genetic and social factors.

B. They are considered mental illnesses.

C. They are rare among nonhuman species.

D. They are caused by developmental impairment.

E. They are a phenomenon of the 20th century.

Review this! ❑

16. Examples of gender-neutral questions that should be used by physicians when taking a social and sexual history from patients include all of the following, except:

A. "Are you in a partnered relationship?"

B. "What kind of birth control do you use?"

C. "Who lives at home with you?"

D. "What are your plans regarding pregnancy?"

E. "Do you have sex with men, women, or both?"

Review this! ❑

17. Which of the following statements about gay, lesbian, and bisexual (GLB) persons is false?

A. The American Psychiatric Association has endorsed the legal recognition of same-gender unions and marriages.

B. GLB persons are a target group for hate crimes and violence.

C. Psychotherapy to change sexual orientation is no longer recommended.

D. Persons in same-sex couples are often eligible for spousal health insurance benefits.

E. Past efforts to change someone's sexual orientation resulted in feelings of shame and guilt and interfered with self-acceptance.

Review this! ❑

18. Which of the following statements about the health care of GLB patients is true?

A. Female–female transmission of human immunodeficiency virus is much less efficient than female–male transmission.

B. Lesbians do not need the same screening as heterosexual women for cervical or breast cancer.

C. Gay men are less likely to exercise regularly and more likely to be obese than heterosexual men.

D. When a male patient presents with urethritis, it is impolite to inquire about specific sexual behaviors.

E. GLB patients do not report experiences of provider prejudice.

Review this! ❑

19. All of the following statements about the concept of gender identity are true, except:

A. Anatomic genital sex is often—but not always—concordant with gender.

B. Gender is an internal, psychological self-perception of maleness or femaleness.

C. Transsexual persons usually desire full transition and sex-reassignment surgery.

D. *Cross-dresser* is another term for *transsexual.*

E. Many non-Western cultures recognize the existence of more than two genders.

Review this! ❑

20. Which of the following organizations publishes the standards of care for hormonal therapy and sex-reassignment surgery for transsexuals?

A. National Coalition for LGBT Health

B. Gay and Lesbian Medical Society

C. Human Rights Campaign

D. Harry Benjamin International Gender Dysphoria Association

E. Gender Education and Advocacy

Review this! ❑

21. For a patient who is experiencing sexual dysfunction, brief education about sexuality and sexual functioning can be very useful at all of the following times, except:

    A. College graduation.
    B. Puberty.
    C. Pregnancy.
    D. Menopause.
    E. Elder years.

    Review this! ❏

22. All of the following commonly contribute to male orgasmic disorder, except:

    A. Alcohol.
    B. SSRIs.
    C. Relationship issues.
    D. Diabetes.
    E. History of urinary tract infections.

    Review this! ❏

23. Which of the following statements about vulvar vestibulitis is false?

    A. It is characterized by severe pain on vestibular touch or attempted vaginal entry.
    B. It is characterized by tenderness to pressure localized within the vulvar vestibule.
    C. The only physical finding is vestibular erythema.
    D. The etiology of vulvar vestibulitis is currently unknown.
    E. The use of soothing creams, topical or oral antibiotics, laser treatments, and vestibulectomy are standard and well-accepted treatment options.

    Review this! ❏

24. The Kinsey Scale for the classification of sexual orientation asserts which of the following?

    A. Sexual orientation is either exclusively heterosexual or exclusively homosexual.
    B. There are three values on the Kinsey Scale: (1) heterosexual; (2) bisexual; and (3) homosexual.
    C. There seven values on the scale, representing the continuum of sexual orientation from exclusive heterosexuality to exclusive homosexuality.

    D. There is no value on the scale for those who only have an incidental experience with homosexuality.
    E. Only overt sexual experiences define where someone is on the scale.

    Review this! ❏

25. The normal physiology of the male orgasm includes all of the following, except:

    A. General loss of voluntary motor control.
    B. Descent of the testicles.
    C. Peak heart rate, respiratory rate, and sex flush.
    D. Contractions of the testes, penis, and anal sphincter.
    E. Ejaculation.

    Review this! ❏

26. When using phosphodiesterase E5 (PDE5) inhibitors for the treatment of erectile dysfunction, it is important to remember which of the following?

    A. The currently available formulations (sildenafil, vardenafil, and tadalafil) are renally metabolized.
    B. All of the currently available medications in this class have a length of effect of 6 hours or less.
    C. Ketoconazole and other potent cytochrome P450 3A4 inhibitors do not affect plasma levels of PDE5 inhibitors.
    D. Coadministration with nitrates or α-adrenergic blockers can cause significant hypotension.
    E. Dose reduction based on age or on hepatic or renal function is unnecessary.

    Review this! ❏

27. Other treatment modalities for ED include all of the following, except:

    A. Siberian ginseng.
    B. Intraurethral alprostadil (medicated urethral system for erection).
    C. Yohimbine.
    D. Intracavernous self-injections of alprostadil (Caverject, Edex).
    E. Vacuum therapy.

    Review this! ❏

28. Which of the following statements about providing care for transsexual persons is true?

A. Hormone therapy is necessary for the entire lifespan, even after sex-reassignment surgery.

B. Male-to-female transsexuals do not require prostate cancer screening.

C. Female-to-male patients who have had chest reconstruction surgery do not require any further breast cancer screening.

D. If a legal name change has not been finalized, the physician and staff should only refer to the patient by his or her legal name.

E. Female-to-male transsexuals who have not had a hysterectomy do not need cervical cancer screening if they are on testosterone therapy.

Review this! ❏

Things to remember for the test.

56 Clinical Genetics (Genomics)

Abbie Jacobs

1. True or false: The difference between genetics and genomics is that genetics looks at the factors that affect the expression of genetic mutations, whereas genomics considers the social and ethical issues that relate genetics to improved health.

   A. True
   B. False

   Review this! ❏

2. The human genome contains which of the following numbers of genes?

   A. 100,000 genes
   B. 30,000 genes
   C. 600,000 genes
   D. 78,000 genes

   Review this! ❏

3. All of the following are positive aspects of new genomic information, except:

   A. It provides information about the increased risk of a particular disease.
   B. It provides information about disease onset and severity.
   C. It helps target treatment, screening, and prevention.
   D. It illuminates the causes of disorders.

   Review this! ❏

4. True or false: Family physicians see mostly multifactorial genetic conditions, whereas geneticists see single-gene disorders.

   A. True
   B. False

   Review this! ❏

5. Which of the following is the least common genetic condition?

   A. Factor V Leiden (heterozygote)
   B. Klinefelter's syndrome (males)
   C. Cystic fibrosis (at birth)
   D. Huntington's disease

   Review this! ❏

6. A family physician's approach to counseling patients about genetic issues usually includes which of the following?

   A. Nondirective counseling
   B. Shared decision-making
   C. Single consultative services
   D. All of the above

   Review this! ❏

7. Which of the following statements about family history is false?

   A. The family history is the single best tool for recognizing genetic components of disease.
   B. No evidence exists for or against the usefulness of the routine family history for improving clinical outcomes.
   C. *FamilyGENES* identifies a series of family history questions that will reveal genetic implications.
   D. A complete genetic pedigree includes a history of at least three generations with all diseases, age at diagnosis, and age at death recorded for each person.

   Review this! ❏

8. True or false: The new genomic information confirms that most common chronic diseases are polygenic and multifactorial.

   A. True
   B. False

   Review this! ❏

9. Which of the following is not a single-gene disease?

   A. Venous thromboembolism
   B. Breast cancer
   C. Cystic fibrosis
   D. Early onset Alzheimer's disease

   Review this! ❏

Things to remember for the test.

10. Of the following diseases, which one is autosomal dominant in its mode of transmission?

    A. β-Thalassemia
    B. Adult hemochromatosis
    C. Cystic fibrosis
    D. Early-onset Alzheimer's disease

    Review this! ❏

11. Ashkenazi Jews are not considered a high-risk population for which of the following conditions?

    A. Cystic fibrosis
    B. Tay-Sachs disease
    C. Alzheimer's disease
    D. Breast cancer

    Review this! ❏

12. The gene involved and the gene frequency are both unknown for all of the following conditions, except:

    A. Diabetes.
    B. Hyperlipidemia.
    C. Depression.
    D. Coronary artery disease.

    Review this! ❏

13. Which of the following is the carrier rate for cystic fibrosis in the white population?

    A. 1 in 25
    B. 1 in 100
    C. 1 in 250
    D. 1 in 1000

    Review this! ❏

14. Cardiomyopathy, arthropathy, cirrhosis, diabetes, and skin pigmentation are characteristic of which of the following autosomal recessive diseases?

    A. Sickle cell disease
    B. Adult hemochromatosis
    C. β-Thalassemia
    D. Down syndrome

    Review this! ❏

15. True or false: The current approach to multifactorial diseases includes genetic testing and global risk assessment to identify high-risk individuals.

    A. True
    B. False

    Review this! ❏

16. All of the following statements about breast cancer are true, except:

    A. A family history of premenopausal breast cancer in a first-degree relative doubles the personal risk of breast cancer.
    B. One of every 40 people of Ashkenazi Jewish descent has BRCA mutations.
    C. An autosomal-dominant pattern of inheritance is seen in 20% of women with breast cancer.
    D. The tests for BRCA mutations can be ordered by any physician.

    Review this! ❏

17. Which of the following is recommended for women regarding genetic testing for breast cancer?

    A. All women with a first-degree relative with premenopausal breast cancer should be tested for BRCA mutations.
    B. Family physicians should always do testing for BRCA mutations for women with an autosomal-dominant pattern of inheritance of breast cancer.
    C. Counseling should always be done before testing for BRCA mutations.
    D. None of the above

    Review this! ❏

18. A patient of yours tests positive for the BRCA mutation. What does this mean?

    A. She has an 80% lifetime risk of breast cancer and a 50% risk of ovarian cancer.
    B. She should undergo chemoprevention strategies with tamoxifen or surgical prophylaxis.
    C. She should have yearly mammograms and breast magnetic resonance imaging if she does not opt for surgical prophylaxis.
    D. All of the above

    Review this! ❏

19. Which of the following statements about colorectal cancer is false?

A. Most groups recommend early screening at the age of 40 years for individuals with a first-degree relative with colorectal cancer.

B. A family history of multiple relatives with colorectal cancer with an onset before the age of 50 years suggests an autosomal-recessive pattern of inheritance.

C. Individuals with familial adenomatous polyposis have a 100% lifetime risk of colorectal cancer.

D. Hereditary nonpolyposis colon cancer mutations confer a 80% lifetime risk of colorectal cancer.

Review this! ❑

20. Which of the following is an advantage of early screening and genetic testing for colorectal cancer?

A. The early detection and removal of adenomatous polyps has made determining family history easier.

B. If a specific mutation is identified and a patient tests negative for that mutation, then early screening can be stopped.

C. Without a known mutation, all family members can be screened; if no polyps are found, then regularly screening intervals can be resumed.

D. None of the above

Review this! ❑

21. Which of the following statements about Alzheimer's disease is correct?

A. The genetic transmission of early onset Alzheimer's disease is autosomal dominant.

B. The most common presenting clinical scenario is dementia.

C. Patients with multiple family members with Alzheimer's disease occurring before the age of 70 years are at higher risk.

D. All of the above

Review this! ❑

22. A patient states that her mother had Alzheimer's disease, and she requests genetic testing for herself. What should you tell her?

A. Based on current recommendations, she should have testing for APOE4.

B. Current consensus panels have recommended against APOE4 testing as a predictive genetic test for Alzheimer's disease.

C. Less than 10% of normal, late-onset Alzheimer's disease cases are familial.

D. There are good treatments available, and testing may be useful for her.

Review this! ❑

23. Which of the following statements about iron overload is true?

A. It is the same thing as hemochromatosis.

B. It is an X-linked disease.

C. It is treated with phlebotomy at regular intervals.

D. It is only present in populations with HFE mutations.

Review this! ❑

24. Which of the following statements about hemochromatosis is true?

A. The Centers for Disease Control and Prevention recommends routine screening for hemochromatosis.

B. Iron overload inevitably leads to hemochromatosis.

C. Hemochromatosis is associated with mutations in the HFE gene.

D. B and C

Review this! ❑

25. A patient comes to you asking for serum iron testing, because her sibling has hemochromatosis. What should you tell her?

A. This is a good idea, because you may detect the disease early.

B. It would be good to do mutation testing for HFE.

C. There is no indication for her to have serum iron testing.

D. A and B

Review this! ❑

26. Research in the area of genetics and psychiatric illness has shown which of the following?

A. Family history increases the risk for a broad spectrum of psychiatric disorders.

B. Twin studies suggest the presence of genes with incomplete penetrance.

C. Serious psychiatric illness is usually multifactorial and polygenic in origin.

D. All of the above

Review this! ❑

27. A 25-year-old black woman comes to your office with questions about cystic fibrosis. She wants to get pregnant, but she is concerned because a family member has cystic fibrosis. What do you tell her?

    A. The common prenatal testing panels for carrier states cover the mutations found in almost all ethnic groups.
    B. It is important to test the family member for a mutation first.
    C. There are only two mutations of the gene, and you need two copies to get cystic fibrosis.
    D. B and C

    Review this! ❑

28. All of the following statements about newborn screening for cystic fibrosis are true, except:

    A. As a result of newborn screening, we know that many patients only have mild disease.
    B. Different mutations cause variable disease severity, and the same mutation can cause different disease severity in siblings.
    C. Newborn testing identifies at-risk siblings who have no apparent illness.
    D. Newborn screening is helpful because diagnosis before the onset of symptoms improves outcomes.

    Review this! ❑

29. All of the following statements about hemoglobinopathies are true, except:

    A. Sickle cell disease was the first genetic disorder with a known molecular basis.
    B. Sickle cell disease is believed to be common, because carriers have a natural resistance to malaria.
    C. In Southeast Asia and Africa, 10% of the population has α-thalassemia.
    D. There are four possible genotypes of α-thalassemia, each of which results in a different clinical syndrome.

    Review this! ❑

30. An asymptomatic patient shows you the result of a laboratory test done at her office, and it reveals microcytosis on her blood count. Because of this, you note that she could not have which of the following conditions?

    A. β-Thalassemia major
    B. Mutations in two α-globin genes

    C. Iron-deficiency anemia
    D. An autosomal-recessive hemoglobinopathy

    Review this! ❑

31. Which of the following gene variants does not increase the risk of venous thromboembolism?

    A. Factor V Leiden
    B. Factor VIII deficiency
    C. Protein C deficiency
    D. Antithrombin deficiency

    Review this! ❑

32. When considering genetic testing, it is important to think about which of the following?

    A. Testing the patient is just as good as a first step as testing the affected family member.
    B. Testing usually does not have any important psychological implications.
    C. Patients who test negative may feel a survivor's guilt.
    D. Most patients prefer to have testing even if there is no treatment for a disease.

    Review this! ❑

33. A patient comes to your office and requests a genetic test. When counseling the patient, it is important to remember which of the following?

    A. The presence of a known disease-causing mutation can predict disease onset but not severity.
    B. Very few diseases have 100% penetrance; other genetic and environmental factors are important.
    C. The absence of a mutation can change the baseline population risk of the disease.
    D. All of the above

    Review this! ❑

34. Tests that are routinely used for the prenatal diagnosis of potential genetic abnormalities include all of the following, except:

    A. Quadruple serum test.
    B. Cystic fibrosis testing.
    C. Hemoglobin electrophoresis.
    D. Chorionic villous sampling.

    Review this! ❑

35. Pharmacogenetics may allow us to better individualize medications for patients. Which of the following statements about pharmacogenetics is true?

    A. The cytochrome 450 system metabolizes many medications.
    B. Individuals can be rapid, intermediate, or slow metabolizers.
    C. Both ketoconazole and macrolide anti-biotics inhibit the cytochrome P450 3A4 pathway.
    D. All of the above

    Review this! ❑

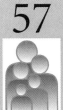

Chapter

57 Anxiety Disorders

Daniel A. Knight

Things to remember for the test.

1. Anxiety disorders have a lifetime prevalence in the general population of which of the following?

   A. 5%
   B. 12%
   C. 3%
   D. 25%
   E. 33%

   Review this! ❏

2. True or false: Anxiety is always related to the perception of an external threat.

   A. True
   B. False

   Review this! ❏

3. Anxiety disorders only occur among those patients with few psychological strengths and poor social support systems.

   A. True
   B. False

   Review this! ❏

4. Which of the following does not describe manifestations of a panic attack?

   A. Palpitations, chest pain, or chest discomfort
   B. Dizziness or faintness
   C. Feeling of unreality or being detached from one's self
   D. Gradual onset, with progression to a full-blown attack
   E. Nausea or abdominal distress

   Review this! ❏

5. To meet the *Diagnostic and Statistical Manual of Mental Disorders IV* (DSM-IV) criteria for panic disorder, which of the following must be present?

   A. No significant change in behavior after the attack has subsided.
   B. At least a 24-hour concern that another will occur.

   C. Worry about the implications of the attack or its consequences.
   D. At least two attacks must occur before the diagnosis can be made.
   E. All other causes of symptoms of panic must be ruled out.

   Review this! ❏

6. The onset of panic disorder generally occurs between which of the following ages?

   A. 12–18 years
   B. 6–15 years
   C. 25–42 years
   D. 30–60 years
   E. 17–30 years

   Review this! ❏

7. True or false: Anticipatory anxiety always occurs before the first panic attack.

   A. True
   B. False

   Review this! ❏

8. Which of the following statements about patients with agoraphobia and panic attacks is true?

   A. They are totally unable to leave the house.
   B. They gradually become more distant and detached from their family members.
   C. They have agoraphobia that occurs immediately after the first or second panic attack.
   D. They wish to be alone most of the time.
   E. They often cling regressively to significant others and require their presence to leave the house.

   Review this! ❏

9. Which of the following is the percentage of patients with chest pain with negative cardiac workups who have panic disorder?

A. Nearly 50%
B. Nearly 10%
C. Nearly 45%
D. Nearly 20%
E. Nearly 65%

Review this! ❑

10. True or false: Almost all patients with agoraphobia have panic attacks.

A. True
B. False

Review this! ❑

11. Patients with specific phobias and social phobias have all of the following characteristics, except:

A. They have considerable anticipatory anxiety when they know they will be exposed to the phobic stimulus.
B. They do not have panic attacks when they are not exposed to a phobic stimulus.
C. They often develop phobias without a precipitating stimulus.
D. Those with social phobias have a persistent fear and avoidance of situations in which unfamiliar people are present.
E. They recognize that the fear is excessive or unreasonable.

Review this! ❑

12. Persons with average-severity social phobias often have the same achievement levels as those without social phobias.

A. True
B. False

Review this! ❑

13. In addition to anxiety and worry, all of the following may be associated with generalized anxiety disorder (GAD), except:

A. Difficulty concentrating or the mind going blank.
B. Delusional ideation.
C. Muscle tension.
D. Irritability.
E. Sleep disturbance.

Review this! ❑

14. True or false: GAD is nearly always a primary disorder (i.e., it is not caused by another disorder).

A. True
B. False

Review this! ❑

15. Patients with post-traumatic stress disorder (PTSD) in primary care have which of the following symptoms?

A. Difficulty falling or staying asleep
B. Irritability or outbursts of anger
C. Difficulty concentrating
D. Hypervigilance
E. All of the above

Review this! ❑

16. Patients with PTSD persistently avoid stimuli associated with prior trauma as indicated by all of the following, except:

A. Inhibited range of affect.
B. Markedly diminished interest or participation in significant activities.
C. Heightened ability to recall all important aspects of the trauma.
D. Feelings of detachment or estrangement from others.
E. Efforts to avoid activities, places, or people who arouse recollection of the trauma.

Review this! ❑

17. Which of the following percentages of patients with major depression have a concurrent anxiety disorder?

A. 45%
B. 20%
C. 30%
D. 60%
E. 90%

Review this! ❑

18. Which of the following is a common physical finding in a patient with anxiety?

A. A handshake that frequently reveals a dry, hot palm
B. Breathing that is often deep and slow
C. A patient who sits rigidly, without movement
D. Facial muscles that may show twitching or tics
E. A patient who has pinpoint pupils

Review this! ❑

19. Which of the following medical illnesses may mimic symptoms of anxiety?

A. Heart disease
B. Adrenal insufficiency
C. Anemia
D. Cerebral atherosclerosis
E. All of the above

Review this! ❑

20. True or false: An anxious patient usually perceives his or her problem as psychological.

A. True
B. False

Review this! ❑

21. For the medical workup and management of an anxious patient, it is very important that which of the following be done?

A. The physician should confront the patient early with the probable diagnosis of an anxiety disorder.
B. The physician should exclude his or her own feelings and reactions to patients with this kind of problem.
C. Reassurance or advice should be given early during the workup.
D. After the diagnosis of anxiety has been made, follow-up visits can become much less frequent.
E. The physician should not continue to order laboratory or radiographic tests after the patient has been ensured of the absence of organic disease.

Review this! ❑

22. For the treatment of a patient with anxiety, all of the following are important, except:

A. The physician should seek out the patient's explanatory beliefs about what is going on.
B. The physician should tell the patient early on that nothing is wrong with him or her.
C. The physician should explain to the patient that there is often a genetic predisposition to anxiety disorders that can be provoked or expressed during periods of life stress.
D. The physician should identify the patient's support system.
E. The physician should introduce stress-reduction techniques.

Review this! ❑

23. For the treatment of panic disorder, which of the following guidelines should be used?

A. The patient should be told to avoid all situations that may initiate a panic attack.
B. Medication should be avoided if at all possible.
C. Cognitive-behavioral therapy is not useful for the treatment of panic disorder.
D. Education by the family physician about anxiety and relaxation techniques is often helpful.
E. Avoidance and phobic behavior do not often develop for many years.

Review this! ❑

24. Which of the following drugs are indicated for the pharmacologic therapy of panic disorder?

A. Tricyclic antidepressants
B. Serotonin reuptake inhibitors (SSRIs)
C. Monoamine oxidase inhibitors
D. High-potency benzodiazepines
E. All of the above

Review this! ❑

25. When treating patients with panic disorder with SSRIs, it is important to do which of the following?

A. Start at the highest tolerated dose and remain at that same dose for a significant period of time.
B. Realize that the panic attacks will probably not be totally alleviated.
C. Explain to the patients that they may have side effects of nausea, jitteriness, and headache that will not resolve.
D. Explain to the patients that anorgasmia occurs in 20% to 35% of patients taking SSRIs.
E. Explain to the patients that these drugs work fast and that they should feel better immediately.

Review this! ❑

26. Patient characteristics correlating with a successful outcome for counseling for anxiety disorders by family physicians include all of the following, except:

A. Faith that counseling can be helpful.
B. A lack of awareness of how counseling works.
C. Relative youth, attractiveness, and intelligence.
D. A high motivation to change the self.
E. A personal resource system that is supportive of the aims of counseling.

Review this! ❑

Things to remember for the test.

27. Which of the following are the major concerns about using benzodiazepines to treat GAD?

    A. The higher potential for dependence and abuse
    B. The higher lethality rate
    C. The higher frequency of side effects and allergic reactions
    D. The activation of liver microsomal enzymes
    E. The difficulty that many patients with anxiety disorders may have with stopping these medications

    Review this! ❏

28. True or false: For the treatment of phobic disorders, desensitization by imagery is less effective than in vivo exposure to the phobic stimulus.

    A. True
    B. False

    Review this! ❏

29. Which of the following statements about the treatment of PTSD is true?

    A. Recurrent and intrusive images and feelings of intense autonomic arousal are similar to those seen among patients with panic disorder.
    B. Medications with a dampening effect on the sympathetic nervous system have been found to be effective.
    C. Many patients with PTSD have major depression.
    D. Many patients with PTSD have panic disorder.
    E. All of the above

    Review this! ❏

30. All of the following drugs are useful for the treatment of PTSD in veterans, except:

    A. Imipramine.
    B. Monoamine oxidase inhibitors.
    C. SSRIs.
    D. Prazosin.
    E. Clonidine.

    Review this! ❏

58 Depression

Paul Moglia and Samuel A. Sandowski

1. Which of the following statements about the treatment of depression in the United States is false?

   A. There are about 18 million annual office visits for its treatment.
   B. A majority of patients receiving antidepressant therapy also receive psychiatric treatment.
   C. The cost of treating depression, including time lost from work, is more than $40 billion annually.
   D. About 10% to 15% of patients hospitalized for nonpsychiatric conditions are also suffering from a diagnosable form of depression.
   E. Depression increases the morbidity and mortality of several major diseases.

   Review this! ❏

2. Which of the following is the prevalence of depression in the general population?

   A. 2%–4%
   B. 1%–2%
   C. 10%–12%
   D. 15%
   E. 20%–25%

   Review this! ❏

3. Depression has been shown to increase the morbidity and mortality of all of the following conditions diseases, except:

   A. Fibromyalgia.
   B. Migraine headache.
   C. Cardiovascular disease.
   D. Diabetes.
   E. Osteoporosis.

   Review this! ❏

4. Depression is underdiagnosed and undertreated for all of the following reasons, except:

   A. Research shows that its prevalence is less than was believed.

   B. Family medicine residency training in psychiatry is usually not germane to typical family practice settings.
   C. Patients often present with somatic complaints rather than complaints related to mood.
   D. Family practitioners often do not consider affective disorders as part of the differential diagnosis when appropriate.
   E. Patients suffering with depression are often inclined to not recognize symptoms.

   Review this! ❏

5. Which of the following is not a risk factor for depression?

   A. Gender
   B. Pregnancy
   C. Nutritional status
   D. Family history
   E. Age

   Review this! ❏

6. Depression is more easily diagnosed among women than among children, adolescents, and men for all of the following reasons, except:

   A. As compared with the other groups, women are more likely to identify their prevailing emotional state and to report it during a medical visit.
   B. Depressive symptoms, such as positive neurovegetative signs, are typically more severe among women and thus more easily detected.
   C. Many depressed men believe it is not socially appropriate for them to report depressive symptoms and to seek help.
   D. Typical depressive signs and symptoms in children and adolescents are often atypical in adults and thus missed.
   E. Males are more likely than females to mask a depressed mood and outlook with chemical abuse.

   Review this! ❏

Things to remember for the test.

7. Which of the following statements about postpartum depression is true?

   A. About 1 in 100 pregnant women will develop postpartum depression.
   B. In general, antidepressants are not safe to use during pregnancy.
   C. Postpartum depression is typically milder than outright major depressive disorder.
   D. After a woman has had postpartum depression, she is at greater risk for developing it again if she has another child.
   E. None of the above

   Review this! ❑

8. Genetics play a significant role in depression as evidenced by all of the following statements, except:

   A. Monozygotic twins show a 90% concordance rate.
   B. Dizygotic twins show about a 20% concordance rate as compared with monozygotic twins.
   C. The children of two parents, one of which had a major depressive episode, have a relative risk that is up to 10 times greater than that of the general population.
   D. Adoption studies show a greater prevalence among biologic relatives than adoptive relatives.
   E. All of the above

   Review this! ❑

9. Suicidal potential is a result of many interacting factors that include all of the following, except:

   A. Chronic illness.
   B. Family or social disruption.
   C. Chemical abuse.
   D. Early life experiences.
   E. Severe depressive symptoms.

   Review this! ❑

10. Which of the following statements about suicide is false?

    A. In 2001, suicide was the eleventh leading cause of death in the United States.
    B. Women have more completed suicide attempts than men.
    C. About 1% of all suicide-attempt survivors will complete another suicide attempt within a year.

    D. Physical illness causes less mortality than suicide among 15- to 24-year-old individuals.
    E. Of those who complete suicide, about two thirds had been to see a physician within the previous 30 days.

    Review this! ❑

11. Physician-assisted suicide is illegal in all of the following states, except:

    A. Oregon.
    B. Alaska.
    C. Vermont.
    D. Hawaii.
    E. North Dakota.

    Review this! ❑

12. All of the following conditions preclude making a diagnosis of major depressive disorder, except:

    A. Symptoms caused by hypothyroidism.
    B. Feeling guilty about being sick.
    C. Observable psychomotor agitation or retardation.
    D. Bereavement.
    E. Mania or hypomania.

    Review this! ❑

13. Which of the following statements about the assessment of depression in the family practice setting is true?

    A. Case-finding depression questionnaires are administered every 1 to 2 years during the regularly scheduled general medical examination.
    B. Patients with depression are more likely than not to spontaneously describe emotional difficulties and negative affect or outlook.
    C. Self-reporting measures can be quickly completed and scored even when patients are cognitively impaired.
    D. All screening instruments abide by the same statistical cutoff for determining that depressive symptoms are significant.
    E. A positive depression screen must be followed by an interview, because depression screening measures do not diagnose depression.

    Review this! ❑

14. Identifying depression in children and adolescents is often difficult in the family practice office for all of the following reasons, except:

A. There are no screening instruments available for use, and variation in parent-reported and child-reported symptoms is common.
B. Changes in behavior and declining school and extracurricular performance are often not recognized as potential signs of depression.
C. Depressed adolescents are more likely to exhibit irritability, social withdrawal, and substance abuse than to exhibit sadness and depressed mood.
D. Depressed children report internalizing symptoms like feeling like a failure, not being able to succeed anymore, or always being in a bad mood.
E. Parents and teachers are more likely to attribute observed irritability, oppositional attitudes, and generalized moodiness as willful and voluntary.
Review this! ❏

15. Which of the following statements about interventions for the Counseling and Behavioral Interventions Work Group of the U.S. Preventive Services Task Force (USPSTF) is true?

A. Counseling sessions should be at least a half hour long to be effective.
B. Counseling should only be performed by health professionals certified in counseling, such as psychologists and psychiatrists.
C. Brief interventions designed to fit into everyday family practice have been found to produce clinically meaningful changes.
D. There is little evidence that supports interventions or counseling for the treatment of depression.
E. Behavioral interventions and counseling are a required part of the treatment of depression.
Review this! ❏

16. When is the BATHE technique best used?

A. After the patient is diagnosed with depression
B. To make a diagnosis of depression
C. When the clinician has concerns about the patient and approximately 20 minutes to administer the technique
D. When the clinician has concerns about the patient but only a few minutes to administer the technique

E. After the SPEAK technique has been used
Review this! ❏

17. When is the SPEAK technique best used?

A. In conjunction with the BATHE technique
B. To make a diagnosis of depression
C. Instead of the BATHE technique
D. To help assess the patient's concerns
E. After 1 month of antidepressant medications
Review this! ❏

18. Which of the following best describes the purpose of the DIG technique?

A. Identifying patients who are at risk for depression
B. Diagnosing patients with depression
C. Screening adolescents for depression
D. Creating solutions for problems for patients with depression
E. Replacing the BATHE technique
Review this! ❏

19. Which of the following statements about medications for the treatment of depression is true?

A. Medications are generally more effective than behavioral therapy for the treatment of depression in the outpatient setting.
B. Behavioral therapy is generally more effective than medications for the treatment of depression in the outpatient setting.
C. Behavioral therapy is generally as effective as medications for the treatment of depression in the outpatient setting.
D. Medications will usually reduce the risk of relapse, even if they are subsequently withdrawn.
E. Behavioral therapy usually provides a quicker response than medications for the treatment of depression in the outpatient setting.
Review this! ❏

20. Which of the following statements about family physicians and primary care providers treating depression is true?

Things to remember for the test.

Things to remember for the test.

A. Family physicians and other primary care providers should never treat depression.
B. Family physicians should always treat depression together with the assistance of a mental health provider.
C. Family physicians should always prescribe medications when they identify patients with depression.
D. Family physicians should be hesitant about prescribing medications without the consultation of a mental health provider.
E. Family physicians and other primary care providers prescribe the majority of antidepressant medications in the United States.

Review this! ❏

21. Which of the following statements best describes cognitive behavioral therapy?

A. It is based mostly on expert opinion, but there are few studies that actually document its success.
B. It usually takes years to complete.
C. It must be used in combination with medication.
D. It attempts to change dysfunctional thinking about life stressors.
E. It is synonymous with psychotherapy.

Review this! ❏

22. A response to antidepressant therapy is usually seen within which of the following timeframes?

A. 3–4 hours
B. 3–4 days
C. 3–4 weeks
D. 3–4 months
E. It is quite variable.

Review this! ❏

23. Which of the following is a side effect of selective serotonin reuptake inhibitors (SSRIs)?

A. Neuropathy
B. Sexual dysfunction
C. Arrhythmias
D. Urinary retention
E. Interaction with tyramine

Review this! ❏

24. What percentage of patients will have some response to medications for the treatment of depression?

A. 5%–15%
B. 20%–25%
C. 40%–50%
D. 60%–70%
E. 80%–90%

Review this! ❏

25. Which of the following tricyclic antidepressants (TCAs) generally has the fewest side effects?

A. Nortriptyline
B. Amitriptyline
C. Imipramine
D. Fluoxetine
E. Bupropion

Review this! ❏

26. During the month of June, a 44-year-old male who has been taking fluoxetine for the past 4 months has been feeling much improved. He decided he no longer needed his medication, so he stopped it of his own accord. He presents to your office with flu-like symptoms 4 days after stopping the medication. What do you tell him?

A. He probably has the flu.
B. It is probably the result of withdrawal of the fluoxetine.
C. He is fortunate that he stopped the fluoxetine, because he would likely have had worse symptoms if he were to have continued the medication.
D. His symptoms would have been worse if he were also taking buspirone.
E. He should not restart the medication, because this would likely exacerbate the symptoms.

Review this! ❏

27. Which of the following herbs has been used to treat depression?

A. Echinacea
B. Phytoestrogens
C. Saw palmetto
D. Hypericum extract
E. Garlic

Review this! ❏

28. Which of the following statements about exercise and depression is true?

    A. Exercise has no effect of the symptoms of depression.
    B. Exercise can be used instead of behavioral therapy or medications to treat depression.
    C. Exercise is generally contraindicated during depression, because depressed patients have little motivation, and requiring them to do more tends to make them more depressed.
    D. Exercise is only beneficial if it is performed daily for at least 60 minutes.
    E. Exercise has been shown to be as effective as behavioral therapy for the treatment of depression.

    Review this! ❏

29. Electroconvulsive therapy (ECT) should be used in which of the following situations?

    A. As standard first-line therapy for depression
    B. For patients with medication treatment failure
    C. For patients with lobotomy failure
    D. ECT is inhumane and should never be used.
    E. For patients who have contraindications to SSRIs

    Review this! ❏

Things to remember for the test.

59 Crisis Intervention

Gina M. Basello and Alan R. Roth

1. Which of the following percentages of patients are likely to experience a traumatic event during their lifetime?

   A. <10%
   B. 25%
   C. 40%–50%
   D. 60%–70%
   E. 75%

   Review this! ❑

2. The comprehensive evaluation of a crisis, trauma, or disaster involves an understanding of all of the following, except:

   A. The personal meaning of the event to the individual.
   B. Any preexisting psychiatric conditions.
   C. Current medications.
   D. The precipitant or stressor.
   E. A selective past history.

   Review this! ❑

3. Which of the following is one of the five domains that encompass the top external life stressors on the social readjustment scale?

   A. Love stress
   B. Friendship stress
   C. Sex stress
   D. Family stress
   E. Personal appearance stress

   Review this! ❑

4. Which of the following terms is best defined as "a brief psychological upheaval producing inner turmoil that overwhelms an individual's coping mechanisms"?

   A. Stress response
   B. Anxiety
   C. Crisis state
   D. Trauma
   E. Grief reaction

   Review this! ❑

5. Which of the following is part of the description of an acute stress disorder as classified by the *Diagnostic and Statistical Manual of Mental Disorders IV*?

   A. Impairment of occupational functioning
   B. May last less than 2 days
   C. Patients unable to return to baseline functioning
   D. Usually lasts longer than 6 weeks
   E. Poor adaptation does not predispose to future episodes

   Review this! ❑

6. Pretraumatic factors that affect the prognosis of a patient suffering from a significant crisis include all of the following, except:

   A. Prior psychiatric illness.
   B. Genetics.
   C. Typical coping styles.
   D. Culture or gender.
   E. Capacity for problem solving.

   Review this! ❑

7. Which of the following aspects of the past medical history is the least helpful when trying to understand a suicide attempt?

   A. History of depression
   B. Coping style
   C. Severe medical illness
   D. Alcoholism
   E. Family history of suicide

   Review this! ❑

8. Which of the following is most likely to contribute to an individual decompensating as a result of a crisis event?

   A. Comorbid medical conditions
   B. Economic status
   C. Gender
   D. Event that threatens the immediate social environment
   E. Educational level

   Review this! ❑

9. The basic comprehensive approach to the assessment of a patient in crisis includes all of the following, except:

   A. An evaluation of the precipitants of the crisis.
   B. The patient's personal meaning of the events.
   C. The crisis state itself.
   D. The patient's support network.
   E. The formulation of the crisis etiology.
   Review this! ❏

10. A pictorial representation of a patient's entire support network is known as which of the following?

    A. Timeline
    B. Eco map
    C. Genogram
    D. Family photo
    E. Life tree
    Review this! ❏

11. Which of the following is the most appropriate immediate treatment for the patient in crisis?

    A. Psychotherapy
    B. Medication
    C. Addressing the patient's major concern
    D. Safety issues
    E. Isolation
    Review this! ❏

12. Which of the following plans is not useful for the management of a patient in crisis?

    A. A problem-focused or symptom-oriented plan
    B. The formation of crisis-resolution strategies
    C. Fostering coping skills and adaptive problem solving
    D. Medication for symptoms or psychiatric disorders
    E. Cognitive therapy
    Review this! ❏

13. Which of the following coping styles is the least successful during crisis resolution?

    A. Intuitive
    B. Impulsive
    C. Trial and error
    D. Contemplative
    E. Controlling
    Review this! ❏

14. All of the following are recommended crisis resolution strategies, except:

    A. Recognizing early warning signs.
    B. Setting expectations for recovery.
    C. Avoiding the discussion of painful feelings and emotions.
    D. Normalizing the patient's symptoms.
    E. Prioritizing the patient's problem list.
    Review this! ❏

15. What is the preferred treatment for a patient suffering from a crisis who has not experienced a disruption in social or occupational functioning?

    A. Psychotherapy
    B. Group therapy
    C. Medication
    D. No treatment
    E. Cognitive behavioral therapy
    Review this! ❏

16. Which of the following is the therapeutic modality of choice for the treatment of the symptoms associated with a crisis event or mass trauma?

    A. Psychotherapeutic techniques
    B. Benzodiazepines
    C. Selective serotonin reuptake inhibitor antidepressants
    D. Hypnotherapy
    E. Biofeedback
    Review this! ❏

17. Which of the following is the medication of choice for the treatment of insomnia resulting from acute crisis or the immediate posttraumatic state?

    A. Diphenhydramine
    B. Zolpidem
    C. Alprazolam
    D. Amitriptyline
    E. Haloperidol
    Review this! ❏

18. Which of the following is the drug of choice for the treatment of post-traumatic stress disorder?

    A. Sertraline
    B. Amitriptyline
    C. Buspirone
    D. Benzodiazepines
    E. Atypical antipsychotics
    Review this! ❏

Things to remember for the test.

60 Personality Disorders

Kristen B. Rundell and Edward T. Bope

Things to remember for the test.

1. Patients with personality disorders often have clusters of symptoms, which makes choosing the right medication very important. For patients with psychotic symptoms, which of the following would be the best drug to use?

    A. Divalproex
    B. Risperidone
    C. Sertraline
    D. Lithium

    Review this! ❏

2. Amitriptyline could be used for a patient with a personality disorder with which of the following symptoms?

    A. Mood symptoms
    B. Psychotic symptoms
    C. Irritability
    D. Impulsivity

    Review this! ❏

3. Which of the following patient defenses would be found in the borderline patient but not in the narcissistic patient?

    A. Splitting
    B. Projection
    C. Acting out
    D. Projective identification
    E. Mini-psychotic experiences

    Review this! ❏

4. Which of the following is not a feature of the patient with paranoid personality disorder?

    A. Projection
    B. Projective identification
    C. Acting out
    D. Denial
    E. Splitting

    Review this! ❏

5. True or false: Patients with personality disorders are a source of dissatisfaction for physicians.

    A. True
    B. False

    Review this! ❏

6. Which of the following is true about personality disorders as compared with personality style?

    A. They are difficult to modify.
    B. They are stable over time.
    C. They are genetically determined.
    D. They can be modified to adapt to the environment.

    Review this! ❏

7. Which of the following is not a cluster of personality disorders?

    A. Odd and eccentric
    B. Dramatic, emotional, and erratic
    C. Anxious and fearful
    D. Suspicious

    Review this! ❏

8. Which of the following best describes patient-generated countertransference?

    A. It involves blaming the physician for the problem.
    B. It is usually therapeutic and helpful.
    C. It is the cause of atypical physician behavior.
    D. It reflects the negative feelings that the patient gets from the doctor.
    E. It involves feedback about the success of therapy.

    Review this! ❏

9. Cognitive-behavioral therapy is based on which of the following theories?

A. Thinking is as important as doing when it comes to achieving goals for behavioral change.

B. Core beliefs, a world view, and personality-specific fears can be directly influenced by conscious awareness.

C. Therapy should be directed toward changing the way individuals behave in times of stress or a changing environment.

D. Individuals are part of a nuclear group that has some innate cognitive connection.

Review this! ❑

10. Mary is a 54-year-old patient with borderline personality. She finds out that you will be gone on vacation next week, and she tells you that perhaps you should just quit being a doctor because you seem to care very little about your patients. Which of the following is the best response that you can give?

A. Tell her that you are hurt by her cutting remark.

B. Tell her that you do not understand why she would say such a thing after all that you have done for her.

C. Tell her that you empathize with her feelings of abandonment.

D. Tell her that you think patients like her make you take more vacations.

E. Tell her that she should see your partner for a check up while you are away.

Review this! ❑

11. In primary care, up to 24% of patients seen have a personality disorder. Which of the following is the major reason that these patients go unrecognized?

A. Most persons with personality disorders avoid health care.

B. Physicians are often too stressed to recognize common personality disorders.

C. Many of these patients do not demonstrate typical psychiatric symptoms.

D. Family and friends ignore the patient's signs and symptoms.

Review this! ❑

12. Behaviors associated with personality disorders may affect a patient's compliance with medical recommendations. Which

cluster type is most likely to adhere to medical recommendations?

A. Type A
B. Type B
C. Type C
D. Type D

Review this! ❑

13. Patients with personality disorders often respond to stressful situations with certain defense mechanisms or levels of behavior. Kernberg describes these three levels as neurotic, borderline, and psychotic. Of these three, which one uses the higher level of defense called repression?

A. Neurotic personality organization
B. Borderline personality organization
C. Psychotic personality organization
D. Psychosomatic personality organization

Review this! ❑

14. Psychotherapeutic techniques recommended to empathize and acknowledge patients' fears include all of the following, except:

A. Confrontation.
B. Contradiction.
C. Clarification.
D. Interpretation.

Review this! ❑

15. Along with psychotherapeutic techniques, additional interventions are suggested to empathize and decrease patient fears. These interventions include all of the following, except:

A. Modifying the patient's surroundings.
B. Empathizing with the patient's core beliefs.
C. Setting reasonable limits.
D. Suggesting ways of effective coping.
E. Challenging the patient's delusions.

Review this! ❑

16. Physicians often feel manipulated, angry, exhausted, and emotionally drained when dealing with which of the following personality types?

A. Borderline personality disorder
B. Histrionic personality disorder
C. Antisocial personality disorder
D. Schizoid and schizotypal personality

Review this! ❑

Things to remember for the test.

17. True or false: The primary evidence-based treatment for borderline personality is psychotherapy alone.

   A. True
   B. False

   Review this! ❑

18. A female patient presents to your clinic weekly with various somatic complaints. After each complaint is addressed, new complaints arise. You suspect that she fears recovery and improvement. This behavior is often associated with which of the following personality disorders?

   A. Narcissistic personality disorder
   B. Avoidant personality disorder
   C. Obsessive-compulsive personality disorder
   D. Self-defeating personality disorder

   Review this! ❑

19. Which of the following statements about dealing with patients with personality disorders is false?

   A. Physicians may have fantasies or thoughts that are uncharacteristic for them.
   B. Physicians may engage in behaviors that are atypical.
   C. Physician reactions should not be used as diagnostic tools when dealing with patients with personality disorders.
   D. Physicians often have intense feelings that are called "patient-generated countertransferences."

   Review this! ❑

20. Which of the following drugs would not be indicated for psychotic symptoms in a patient with personality disorder?

   A. Amitriptyline
   B. Olanzapine
   C. Haloperidol
   D. Clozapine

   Review this! ❑

61

Somatic Patient

Trish Palmer

1. A symptom is defined as which of the following?

   A. A subjective complaint
   B. An objective statement
   C. An observation
   D. A physical complaint

   Review this! ❏

2. Impairment is most often associated with which of the following?

   A. Depression
   B. Anxiety
   C. Somatization
   D. Panic disorder

   Review this! ❏

3. Physicians rate patients with which of the following conditions as the most difficult to work with?

   A. Depression
   B. Anxiety
   C. Multisomatoform disorder
   D. Panic disorder

   Review this! ❏

4. Somatization in families is related to which of the following?

   A. Male sex
   B. Sexual abuse as an adult
   C. Physical abuse as a child
   D. Female substance abuse

   Review this! ❏

5. A patient who is suspected of having somatization disorder should be prescribed a trial of which of the following?

   A. An anxiolytic
   B. An antidepressant
   C. A mood stabilizer
   D. A serotonin reuptake inhibitor

   Review this! ❏

6. Which of the following is the most effective plan for office visits for patients with somatoform disorders?

   A. Setting distinct limits
   B. Preplanned and frequent visits
   C. Patient-determined scheduling
   D. Family involvement

   Review this! ❏

7. Which of the following is the most effective workup for a patient with frequent visits for multiple complaints?

   A. A focused physical examination
   B. A thorough history
   C. Blood tests
   D. Imaging
   E. Hospitalization

   Review this! ❏

8. Most somatic patients would likely benefit from hearing which of the following?

   A. "Your symptom is all in your head."
   B. "Your symptom will resolve."
   C. "Your symptom appears to be quite mild."
   D. "Your symptom may not have an explanation."

   Review this! ❏

9. Specific, effective therapies for somatization disorder include all of the following, except:

   A. Group therapy.
   B. Cognitive-behavioral therapy.
   C. Dynamic therapy.
   D. Massage therapy.
   E. Family therapy.

   Review this! ❏

10. Effective medications for somatization patients includes which of the following?

A. Tricyclic antidepressants
B. St. John's wort
C. Selective serotonin and norepinephrine reuptake inhibitors
D. Benzodiazepines

Review this! ❏

11. A patient has low back pain with no physical findings or mechanism of injury, and it has lasted for 4 months. This condition is most likely the result of which of the following?

    A. Multiple myeloma
    B. Somatization disorder
    C. Spinal stenosis
    D. Herniated disk

    Review this! ❏

12. Patients with somatoform disorder are most likely to present with which of the following complaints?

    A. Back pain
    B. Blurred vision
    C. Leg weakness
    D. Insomnia

    Review this! ❏

13. Patients with somatization disorder and multiple complaints should have appointments that are focused on which of the following?

    A. The resolution of one symptom
    B. Time
    C. Blood testing
    D. Imaging

    Review this! ❏

14. A 15-year-old patient who has had recurrent headaches since the age of 10 years and who has normal physical examination, imaging, and laboratory results is likely to have which of the following?

    A. An undiagnosed brain malignancy
    B. Undiagnosed diabetes
    C. An undiagnosed somatization disorder
    D. Undiagnosed myopia

    Review this! ❏

15. A 9-year-old girl with recurrent year-round abdominal pain for the past 2 years and a negative laboratory workup is unlikely to be diagnosed with which of the following?

A. Somatization disorder
B. School phobia
C. Depression
D. Anxiety

Review this! ❏

16. A patient with somatization disorder is most likely to do which of the following?

    A. Avoid medical appointments as a result of dissatisfaction
    B. Seek psychological therapy for comorbid depression
    C. Miss appointments as a result of a lack of organization
    D. Have appointments with multiple specialists for multiple complaints

    Review this! ❏

17. Parallel diagnostic inquiry is a strategy by which the physician explains which of the following?

    A. That all symptoms are produced by both physical and psychosocial factors
    B. That all symptoms are produced by physical factors
    C. That all symptoms are produced by psychosocial factors
    D. That all symptoms are independent

    Review this! ❏

18. The formal diagnosis of somatization disorder may be assisted with the use of which of the following

    A. The PHQ-15 questionnaire
    B. Hormone levels
    C. Magnetic resonance imaging
    D. The response to medication

    Review this! ❏

19. Which of the following is the most effective interviewing technique for use with patients with somatization disorder?

    A. Role playing
    B. Confrontational
    C. Emotion-focused
    D. Paternalistic

    Review this! ❏

20. Emotion-focused interviewing involves which of the following?

A. Exploring charged situations and observing the patient's response
B. Confronting the patient
C. Observing family interaction
D. Making the patient cry

Review this! ❏

21. Emotion-focused interviewing allows for which of the following to be category directed?

A. The resolution of symptoms
B. The medication choice
C. Short-term psychotherapy
D. Research

Review this! ❏

22. The main patterns of somatization include all of the following, except:

A. Striated muscle tension.
B. Smooth muscle tension.
C. Cognitive perceptual disruption.
D. Conversion.
E. Emotion.

Review this! ❏

23. A 65-year-old male patient who is otherwise healthy but who has been diagnosed with somatization disorder sees you for the evaluation of new substernal chest pain. The physical examination is normal. What should you do?

A. Obtain an electrocardiogram
B. Obtain a chest x-ray
C. Change the patient's medication
D. Reassure the patient

Review this! ❏

24. Scheduled frequent visits with somatization patients have been shown to do which of the following?

A. Resolve symptoms
B. Anger the patient
C. Reduce health care costs
D. Increase drug use

Review this! ❏

25. Which of the following patients most likely has a diagnosis of somatization disorder?

A. A man with acute low back pain with no injury
B. A man with low back, left shoulder, and neck pain after a motor vehicle accident
C. A man with chronic shoulder pain with no injury
D. A man with low back, left shoulder, and neck pain with no injury

Review this! ❏

26. True or false: An experienced physician's clinical judgment about whether an explanation will be found for the patient's complaints is usually accurate.

A. True
B. False

Review this! ❏

27. True or false: A patient with multiple drug sensitivities suggests somatization.

A. True
B. False

Review this! ❏

28. A patient with multiple complaints that are difficult to explain physically would not be likely to benefit from which of the following?

A. Antidepressant therapy
B. Frequent scheduled visits
C. Shockwave therapy
D. Cognitive-behavioral therapy

Review this! ❏

Things to remember for the test.

62 Dementia

Jonathan D. Hollister

1. All of the following features are typical of dementia (as opposed to normal memory decline), except:

   A. Forgetting where you last put the car keys.
   B. Using the wrong word in a sentence.
   C. Being unable to comb your hair.
   D. Not recognizing a wristwatch.

   Review this! ❑

2. All of the following are recommended laboratory studies for the initial workup of dementia, except:

   A. A complete blood cell count.
   B. Thyroid-stimulating hormone level.
   C. Vitamin B$_{12}$ level.
   D. Serum electrophoresis.
   E. Syphilis serology.

   Review this! ❑

3. Dementia and delirium share multiple clinical features. Which of the following features helps distinguish dementia from delirium?

   A. Visual hallucination
   B. Preserved attention
   C. Fluctuating course
   D. Confusion

   Review this! ❑

4. A 72-year-old male is brought to your office by his daughter. She relates that the family is very concerned about the patient's memory. He is a retired college professor who had been very active traveling with his wife during retirement. He was widowed 3 years ago, but he seems to take everything in stride. However, the family noted that around 6 months ago he exhibited decreasing memory, repetitive conversations, social withdrawal, and declining hygiene. His Mini Mental State Examination result today is 0/30. Which of the following is the most likely diagnosis?

   A. Alzheimer's disease (AD)
   B. Depression
   C. Metastatic cancer
   D. Lewy body dementia

   Review this! ❑

5. True or false: Routine screening using apolipoprotein E genotyping of the first-degree relatives of patients with AD can help those family members make informed decisions about their future health care.

   A. True
   B. False

   Review this! ❑

6. Risk factors for developing AD include which of the following?

   A. Female gender
   B. History of head injury with loss of consciousness
   C. Exposure to neurotoxic chemicals
   D. All of the above

   Review this! ❑

7. Which of the following is not a symptom of Lewy body dementia?

   A. Early hallucinations
   B. Response to acetylcholine-esterase inhibitors
   C. Stairstep-like progression
   D. Fluctuation in cognitive symptoms

   Review this! ❑

8. You are examining the head computed tomography scan of a cognitively impaired patient. You note shrinking gyri, widening sulci (particularly frontotemporally), and hydrocephalus ex vacuo. What is your diagnosis?

   A. AD
   B. Pick's disease
   C. Central pontine myelinolysis
   D. More clinical information is needed

   Review this! ❑

9. Why do the choline acetyltransferase medications work?

   A. Increased acetylcholine levels negatively impact norepinephrine.
   B. Acetylcholine is the most prominent neurotransmitter deficit in most dementias.
   C. Acetylcholine in increased concentrations is neurotoxic.
   D. These medications help regulate dopamine.

   Review this! ❑

10. Which herbal product is undergoing further trials at the National Institute of Aging for the possible delay of the progression of AD?

    A. Ginkgo biloba
    B. Saw palmetto
    C. Ginseng
    D. Black cohosh

    Review this! ❑

11. Which of the following is not local coverage determinations (LCD) criteria for determining the terminal phase of AD?

    A. No unassisted activities of daily living
    B. Urinary and fecal incontinence
    C. Calling out
    D. No meaningful verbal communication

    Review this! ❑

12. Which of the following clinical features helps distinguish Parkinson's disease from Lewy body dementia?

    A. Pill-rolling tremor
    B. Bradykinesia
    C. Late-onset dementia
    D. Masked facies

    Review this! ❑

13. Which of the following types of dementia is associated with gait disturbance, urinary incontinence, and dementia?

    A. AD
    B. Frontotemporal dementia
    C. Creutzfeldt-Jakob disease
    D. Normal-pressure hydrocephalus

    Review this! ❑

14. Which of the following is the most common form of Creutzfeldt-Jakob disease?

    A. Sporadic
    B. Infectious
    C. Genetic
    D. New variant
    E. None of the above

    Review this! ❑

15. The U.S. Preventive Services Task Force recommends screening for dementia in which of the following clinical situations?

    A. Any patient over the age of 75 years
    B. A patient with a recent cerebral vascular accident without memory complaints and with no family concerns about memory
    C. A patient with a compliant of memory loss or a family concern about memory loss
    D. As part of a routine geriatric history

    Review this! ❑

16. You are seeing a 78-year-old female patient for the first time. She is very pleasant and conversant. Her dress, mannerisms, and hygiene are all appropriate. She lives alone, and she is still driving. Her biggest concern is that her daughter is constantly stealing her things. She rarely sees her daughter in the house, but she says that she knows her daughter has been there, because she cannot find her everyday items. She is convinced that it is her daughter behind this. She also says that lately a little girl has been coming into her house and leaving piles of papers on the dining room table. Although she has tried to talk with this girl, she has been unable to catch her. What is the mostly likely diagnosis based on the information provided?

    A. Psychotic depression
    B. Personality disorder
    C. Manic episode
    D. AD

    Review this! ❑

17. You are seeing a self-referred 75-year-old male patient who claims to have memory problems. He is accompanied by his son, who corroborates his concerns. He has become increasingly forgetful, and he is repeating conversations. He has lost numerous items around the house. He graduated college, and he is a retired plant manager. He scores a 25/30 on an Mini Mental State Examination performed by your staff at this visit. He is appropriate throughout the interview, with only occasional anosmia noted. A review of his social

history and geriatric syndromes shows independence with regard to all activities of daily living and instrumental activities of daily living, no falls, and no difficulty with executive functioning, such as balancing his checkbook or paying bills. Which of the following is the most likely diagnosis?

A. Early AD
B. Mild cognitive impairment
C. Creutzfeldt-Jakob disease
D. Vascular dementia

Review this! ❏

18. The daughter of a new 74-year-old female patient brings in her mother for a second opinion after a recent diagnosis of AD. After confirming the diagnosis, the daughter wants to know how far along her mother is in the course of the disease. Her current symptoms include aphasia, apraxia, impaired new learning, and disorientation for date and place. She is still continent, and she recognizes family members.

A. Mild impairment
B. Moderate impairment
C. Severe impairment
D. Terminal phase

Review this! ❏

19. You are seeing a very pleasant 82-year-old female. She comes to you with a diagnosis of dementia. She also has a history of hypertension, peripheral vascular disease, age-related macular degeneration, and chronic obstructive pulmonary disease. When you question family members about her dementia, they relate that her memory problems began 4 years ago and that they have progressed in spurts, with rapid decline at times and followed by a stable baseline. Her initial laboratory workup was negative. Her head computed tomography scan did not show any previous strokes, but it did show periventricular white matter changes and extensive ischemic changes in the basal ganglion and the cortical region. The patient is having trouble recognizing family members; she is somewhat paranoid, and she is incontinent of urine. Which of the following is the most likely cause of her dementia?

A. AD
B. Lewy body dementia

C. Vascular dementia
D. Frontotemporal dementia
E. Dementia of Parkinson's disease

Review this! ❏

20. Which of the following is a validated method of screening appropriately selected patients for dementia?

A. Mini Mental State Examination
B. Clock draw
C. Katz Index
D. A and C
E. A and B
F. All of the above

Review this! ❏

21. Which of the following is the most prevalent type of dementia in the United States?

A. Vascular dementia
B. Lewy body dementia
C. AD
D. Pick's disease

Review this! ❏

22. A 71-year-old man is brought to your office for an initial visit by his distraught daughter. He is a retired bank executive, and he has been widowed for 10 years. He has been living independently and traveling quite extensively. However, for the last 6 months, his behavior has been very out of character for him. His daughter relates her concern for his memory and his increasingly outrageous social behavior. It seems that he has gotten into several oral altercations at the local country club that almost resulted in physical fights. No one knows what the arguments were about, but the patient has been put on "parole" by the country club. He was also almost arrested during the previous week for fondling a woman's breast in a public restaurant. His daughter suspects that he either has AD or that he has had a stroke. What is the most likely diagnosis?

A. AD
B. Vascular dementia
C. Lewy body dementia
D. Frontotemporal dementia

Review this! ❏

23. What is the primary pharmacologic treatment of dementia caused by human immunodeficiency virus?

A. Atypical antipsychotics
B. Cholinesterase inhibitors
C. Highly active antiretroviral therapy
D. Mainly supportive care

Review this! ❏

24. Which of the following is an underlying cause of vascular dementia?

A. Systemic hypotensive episodes
B. Head injury
C. Lewy bodies
D. Tau phosphorylation

Review this! ❏

25. Which medications have been associated with adverse outcomes when they are used to treat psychotic symptoms of dementia?

A. Atypical antipsychotics
B. Major tranquilizers
C. Benzodiazepines
D. All the above
E. None of the above

Review this! ❏

Things to remember for the test.

Chapter

63

Alcohol Abuse

Penelope K. Tippy

Things to remember for the test.

1. As compared with the general population, alcohol abusers are high users of which of the following?

   A. Trauma-related services
   B. Transfusions
   C. Diagnostic procedures
   D. Psychiatric services
   E. All of the above

   Review this! ❑

2. True or false: Genetic markers are the causative factor for patients with alcoholism.

   A. True
   B. False

   Review this! ❑

3. *Diagnostic and Statistical Manual of Mental Disorders* (DSM)-III and DSM-IV criteria for the diagnosis of alcohol dependence include which of the following?

   A. Tolerance
   B. Withdrawal avoidance
   C. Withdrawal
   D. Ingestion of alcohol on a daily basis
   E. A, B, and C
   F. All of the above

   Review this! ❑

4. True or false: There is good evidence to support screening for alcohol dependency and alcohol-use disorders using screening tools such as the CAGE and MAST assessments.

   A. True
   B. False

   Review this! ❑

5. Physical findings suggestive of alcohol abuse include which of the following?

   A. The smell of alcohol on the breath
   B. Palmar erythema
   C. Rhinophyma
   D. Tachycardia

   E. A, B, and C
   F. All of the above

   Review this! ❑

6. Which of the following contribute to the etiology of alcoholism?

   A. Reward pathways, including GABA
   B. Hot spots on chromosomes 1, 2, 5, and 7
   C. Alcoholic parent
   D. Hot spots on chromosomes 1, 2, and 7
   E. A, B, and C
   F. A, C, and D
   G. All of the above

   Review this! ❑

7. Which of the following statements about the prevalence of alcoholism is true?

   A. It is second only to tranquilizers.
   B. It is more frequent among men than women.
   C. It exceeds that of hypertension and type 2 diabetes.
   D. The prevalence of binge drinking is greater than 10%.
   E. A and C
   F. B and D
   G. All of the above

   Review this! ❑

8. Alcohol abuse during pregnancy and during the periconception period may result in which of the following?

   A. Fetal alcohol syndrome
   B. Alcohol-related neurodevelopmental disorder
   C. Alcohol-related birth defects
   D. A and C
   E. All of the above

   Review this! ❑

9. The effect of alcohol on the fetus is dependent on which of the following?

A. The amount of alcohol consumed at one time during pregnancy
B. The timing of the alcohol ingestion
C. The duration of alcohol abuse during the pregnancy
D. A family history of alcoholism
E. The father's alcohol consumption at the time of conception
F. A, B, and C
G. All of the above

Review this! ❏

10. The adolescent who is suspected of alcohol abuse should be screened with which of the following?

A. Family history
B. Personal alcohol history
C. CAGE
D. Urine drug screen
E. A, B, and C
F. All of the above

Review this! ❏

11. Screening tools for alcoholism include which of the following?

A. A history of an arrest for driving under the influence
B. Pancreatitis
C. New-onset hypertension
D. A history of domestic violence
E. A, B, and D
F. All of the above

Review this! ❏

12. Diagnostic clues from the laboratory include which of the following?

A. An alanine aminotransferase level that is greater than the aspartate aminotransferase level
B. An elevated gamma-glutamyl transpeptidase level
C. An elevated platelet level
D. Unexplained leukopenia
E. A and C
F. B and D
G. All of the above

Review this! ❏

13. Which of the following is the generally accepted alcohol level that is considered unsafe for motor vehicle operation?

A. 100 mg /dL
B. 80 mg/dL
C. 50 mg/dL

D. 150 mg/dL

Review this! ❏

14. Which of the following is the evidence level for using benzodiazepines as the treatment of choice for alcohol withdrawal?

A. Level A
B. Level B
C. Level C

Review this! ❏

15. Characteristics of delirium tremens include which of the following?

A. Mild withdrawal symptoms initially
B. Symptoms generally occurring 1 to 2 days after the last drink
C. Tachycardia, hypertension, diaphoresis, and a low-grade fever
D. Somnolence
E. A and C
F. B and D

Review this! ❏

16. Screening tests for alcohol abuse or dependency include which of the following?

A. CAGE
B. MAST
C. TWEAK
D. AUDIT
E. All of the above

Review this! ❏

17. Gastric emptying may be considered in which of the following situations?

A. Any time the patient presents with alcohol intoxication
B. If the patient presents within 30 minutes of alcohol ingestion
C. If the patient presents within 60 minutes of alcohol ingestion
D. If the patient presents within 90 minutes of alcohol ingestion

Review this! ❏

18. The treatment of alcohol-induced coma includes all but which of the following?

A. Protection of the airway
B. Vitamin B_{12}
C. Thiamine
D. Glucose
E. Fructose

Review this! ❏

Things to remember for the test.

19. True or false: Best evidence demonstrates that patients with mild to moderate alcohol withdrawal symptoms and no serious psychiatric or medical comorbidities can be safely treated in the outpatient setting.

    A. True
    B. False

    Review this! ❏

20. Which of the following statements about seizures during alcohol withdrawal is true?

    A. They tend to occur frequently and over a long period of time.
    B. They should be treated with Dilantin.
    C. They most often occur 72 to 96 hours after alcohol cessation.
    D. They are usually generalized, grand mal, and self-limited.

    Review this! ❏

21. The best-evidence recommendations for withdrawal include which of the following?

    A. The revised Clinical Institute Withdrawal Assessment for Alcohol (CIWA-Ar) should be used.
    B. Only patients with severe withdrawal should be medicated.
    C. Benzodiazepines are the drug of choice, with an evidence level of A.
    D. A and C
    E. All of the above

    Review this! ❏

22. Which of the following statements about delirium tremens is true?

    A. It occurs in about 15% of alcoholics during withdrawal.
    B. The risk is increased in the patient who has previously experienced it.
    C. It usually begins 1–3 days after the last drink.
    D. It is usually preceded by a marked change in sensorium.
    E. A and C
    F. B and D

    Review this! ❏

23. Which of the following medications is generally accepted as a treatment option for withdrawal?

    A. Diazepam
    B. Chlordiazepoxide
    C. Atenolol
    D. All of the above

    Review this! ❏

24. True or false: Brief interventions for alcohol abuse during primary care can be very successful.

    A. True
    B. False

    Review this! ❏

25. Making personal habit changes involves progressing through which of the following states?

    A. Contemplative
    B. Preparation
    C. Action
    D. Maintenance
    E. All of the above

    Review this! ❏

26. Brief interventions include all of the following, except:

    A. Clear and direct advice to change.
    B. Confrontation.
    C. Emphasis on patient responsibility.
    D. Physician assessment and feedback.

    Review this! ❏

27. True or false: Patients with alcohol problems and anxiety or depression should be treated for the anxiety or depression first.

    A. True
    B. False

    Review this! ❏

28. Which of the following drugs receives a B recommendation from the UK Scottish National Guidelines for always alcoholism treatment?

    A. Naltrexone
    B. Antabuse
    C. Acamprosate
    D. A and C
    E. All of the above

    Review this! ❏

29. Which of the following statements about naltrexone is true?

A. It is an opioid antagonist.
B. It is an aversive agent.
C. It is hepatotoxic.
D. A and C
E. All of the above

Review this! ❏

30. Which of the following statements about female alcoholics is true?

A. They do more hidden drinking than men do.
B. The CAGE assessment is the most reliable screening tool.
C. They have lower rates of alcohol abuse than men.
D. A and C
E. All of the above

Review this! ❏

Things to remember for the test.

64 Nicotine Addiction

Dennis F. Ruppel

1. True or false: The *Diagnostic and Statistical Manual of Mental Disorders* (DSM)-IV[1] classifies tobacco dependence as an addiction.

   A. True
   B. False

   Review this! ❏

2. Which of the following kills more Americans in a year?

   A. Alcohol
   B. Car accidents
   C. Acquired immunodeficiency syndrome
   D. Tobacco

   Review this! ❏

3. What percentage of cancer deaths are the result of smoking?

   A. 20%
   B. 30%
   C. 40%
   D. 50%

   Review this! ❏

4. In what year did lung cancer surpass breast cancer as the leading cause of cancer death among women?

   A. 1981
   B. 1986
   C. 1991
   D. 1996

   Review this! ❏

5. True or false: Seventy percent of smokers say they would like to quit, but less than 5% succeed each year.

   A. True
   B. False

   Review this! ❏

6. True or false: There is not a clear dose–response relationship between lung cancer risk and daily cigarette smoking.

   A. True
   B. False

   Review this! ❏

7. What percentage of people with lung cancer die within 5 years?

   A. 55%
   B. 65%
   C. 75%
   D. 85%

   Review this! ❏

8. True or false: Smoking low-tar cigarettes decreases the risk of lung cancer.

   A. True
   B. False

   Review this! ❏

9. True or false: The effects of smoking and drinking appear to be synergistic and multiplicative for the risk of laryngeal cancer.

   A. True
   B. False

   Review this! ❏

10. What percentage of bladder cancers are caused by smoking?

    A. 20%
    B. 40%
    C. 60%
    D. 80%

    Review this! ❏

11. True or false: Cigarette smoking has no effect on leukemia.

    A. True
    B. False

    Review this! ❏

---

1. American Psychiatric Association: *Diagnostic and Statistical Manual of Mental Disorders*, 4th ed, text revision. Washington, DC, American Psychiatric Association, 2000.

12. True or false: Chronic obstructive pulmonary disease is the leading cause of disability in the United States.

    A. True
    B. False

    Review this! ❏

13. True or false: When a person quits smoking, he or she immediately reduces his or her risk of sudden death.

    A. True
    B. False

    Review this! ❏

14. What percentage of myocardial infarctions among women who are less than 50 years old have been attributed to cigarette smoking?

    A. 33%
    B. 50%
    C. 66%
    D. 75%

    Review this! ❏

15. True or false: Cigarette smoking is the greatest risk factor for stroke.

    A. True
    B. False

    Review this! ❏

16. True or false: Because they are addicted to nicotine, people who smoke low-nicotine cigarettes undergo "compensatory smoking."

    A. True
    B. False

    Review this! ❏

17. True or false: Health warnings are required for cigars, cigarettes, and smokeless tobacco.

    A. True
    B. False

    Review this! ❏

18. Long-term users of snuff increase the risk for cancer of the cheek and gum by which of the following amount?

    A. 20×
    B. 30×
    C. 40×
    D. 50×

    Review this! ❏

19. What percentage of the smoke from a burning cigarette never reaches the smoker's lungs?

    A. 33%
    B. 50%
    C. 66%
    D. 75%

    Review this! ❏

20. What percentage of lung cancers occur among nonsmokers who live with smokers?

    A. 10%
    B. 15%
    C. 25%
    D. 33%

    Review this! ❏

21. Which of the following is the third leading preventable cause of death in the United States?

    A. Direct smoking
    B. Passive smoking
    C. Alcohol use
    D. Auto accidents

    Review this! ❏

22. True or false: Children of a smoking parent are less likely to become smokers as adults.

    A. True
    B. False

    Review this! ❏

23. The risk of respiratory infections is increased by how many times among children who are exposed to their parents' smoke?

    A. Two times
    B. Four times
    C. Six times
    D. Eight times

    Review this! ❏

24. True or false: The average weight of babies born to women who smoke during pregnancy is 200 gm lighter than that of babies born to nonsmokers.

    A. True
    B. False

    Review this! ❏

25. What is the increased risk of spontaneous abortion among heavy smokers as compared with nonsmokers?

A. Two times
B. Three times
C. Four times
D. Five times

Review this! ❑

26. True or false: Cigarette smoking increases the fertility of women.

A. True
B. False

Review this! ❑

27. True or false: The tobacco companies are spending less today on the advertising of cigarettes.

A. True
B. False

Review this! ❑

28. True or false: Even when physicians do only minimal counseling (less than 3 minutes) about smoking cessation, it results in a quit rate of 13%.

A. True
B. False

Review this! ❑

29. Which of the following products that are recommended as first-line medications by *Treating Tobacco Use and Dependence*[2] is available exclusively as an over-the-counter medication?

A. Sustained-release bupropion
B. Nicotine inhaler
C. Nicotine nasal spray
D. Nicotine gum

Review this! ❑

30. True or false: Cigarette smoking relieves stress.

A. True
B. False

Review this! ❑

31. An adolescent who is a nonsmoker at 18 years of age has what chance of starting to smoke?

A. 10%
B. 20%
C. 30%
D. 40%

Review this! ❑

2. Fiore MC, Bailey WC, Cohen SJ, et al: Treating Tobacco Use and Dependence.Quick Reference Guide for Clinicians. Rockville, MD, U.S. Department of Health and Human Services, Public Health Service, October, 2000.

Chapter

65 Abuse of Controlled Substances

James R. Little

1. Approximately what percentage of Americans who are more than 12 years old will report using illicit drugs within the previous month?

   A. 4%
   B. 8%
   C. 12%
   D. 20%

   Review this! ❑

2. Which of the following is the most commonly used illicit drug?

   A. Cocaine
   B. Illicit use of prescription pain relievers
   C. Marijuana
   D. Methamphetamine

   Review this! ❑

3. *Abuse* is defined as which of the following?

   A. The use of a drug for pleasure or enjoyment
   B. The need for increased amounts of substance to achieve the desired effect or a diminished effect with continued use of the same amount
   C. A reversible syndrome caused by a specific substance that affects mental, behavioral, social, and occupational functioning
   D. The use of a drug in a manner that deviates from approved social or medical patterns

   Review this! ❑

4. All of the following statements about heroin abuse are true, except:

   A. Heroin must be injected intravenously for the user to get a good high.
   B. Heroin is an opioid that is derived from poppies.

C. Because of the drug's short half-life, heroin addicts must use the drug two to four times per day to avoid withdrawal.
D. Noninjectable methods of heroin abuse such as snorting and smoking are increasing in popularity.

   Review this! ❑

5. All of the following statements about nonmedical uses of prescription opioids are true, except:

   A. Short-acting pain medications like Vicodin and Percocet are the most commonly abused prescription pain medications.
   B. Long-acting pain medications like OxyContin may be broken or crushed and then snorted or injected to enhance their high.
   C. OxyContin abuse has surpassed heroine use in some areas.
   D. The appropriate use of opioids for cancer pain is likely to result in addiction.

   Review this! ❑

6. Which of the following statements about methamphetamine is true?

   A. Methamphetamine abuse is growing most rapidly in rural areas and among minority populations.
   B. Methamphetamine can be easily produced using over-the-counter pseudoephedrine and household chemicals.
   C. Methamphetamine must be injected for the user to get high.
   D. The effects of methamphetamine intoxication last only a few hours.

   Review this! ❑

7. All of the following statements about benzodiazepine use are true, except:

Things to remember for the test.

A. It is important to screen patients for a history of drug or alcohol abuse before prescribing benzodiazepines to them.
B. Many benzodiazepine abusers are initially prescribed the medications for legitimate indications by physicians.
C. Withdrawal from benzodiazepines is mild and not dangerous.
D. Benzodiazepines may be taken by some drug abusers to counteract the negative side effects of other drugs of abuse.

Review this! ❑

8. Common findings of drug abuse on the physical examination include all of the following, except:

A. Good dentition as a result of the protective effects of methamphetamine
B. Tachycardia and hypertension, which are often associated with withdrawal syndromes or acute intoxication
C. Anxiety and acute psychosis
D. Skin abscesses or track marks

Review this! ❑

9. Which of the following statements about drug use in adolescents is true?

A. As a result of the "War on Drugs," the incidence of steroid use in teens decreased slightly between 1991 and 2003.
B. Approximately 11% of teenagers between the ages of 12 and 17 years report current use of illicit drugs.
C. The abuse of prescription medications is uncommon among teenagers.
D. Teens who smoke cigarettes are twice as likely as nonsmokers to use drugs.

Review this! ❑

10. All of the following statements about the use of opioids for the treatment of pain are true, except:

A. Patients with a history of drug abuse are at increased risk of becoming addicted to prescription pain medications.
B. Red flags for the abuse of prescription drugs include requests for early refills and multiple lost prescriptions.
C. Pain medication contracts can be useful tools for both providers and patients.
D. Physicians often underestimate the risk of patients becoming addicted to pain medications.

Review this! ❑

11. The *Diagnostic and Statistical Manual of Mental Disorders* (DSM)-IV criteria for substance abuse include all of the following, except:

A. *Tolerance* is defined as the need for more of a substance to obtain the same effect or the diminished effect of the use of the same quantity of a substance.
B. To meet the criteria for substance abuse, the abuser must experience physiologic withdrawal when he or she stops using the substance.
C. Large amounts of time are spent trying to obtain or use the substance.
D. The substance use continues despite adverse effects of the substance.

Review this! ❑

12. All of the following statements about methadone maintenance therapy for opioid addiction are true, except:

A. Primary care physicians can prescribe methadone for maintenance therapy.
B. Methadone acts at μ-receptors to prevent the symptoms of withdrawal from opioids and to partially block the effects of heroin.
C. Typical doses of methadone used for maintenance therapy are 60 to 100 mg.
D. Methadone can reduce the risk of opioid abuse, including needle sharing, high-risk sexual activity, and criminal activity associated with illegal drug use.

Review this! ❑

13. All of the following statements about buprenorphine are true, except:

A. Buprenorphine is a partial opioid antagonist that is useful for the treatment of withdrawal symptoms and for maintenance therapy.
B. Buprenorphine can only be prescribed by physicians who have undergone special training and certification.
C. A Cochrane database review found evidence to support the effectiveness of buprenorphine for the treatment of opioid dependence.
D. Buprenorphine must be administered as a part of special drug treatment programs or at clinics.

Review this! ❑

14. Medications used to treat the symptoms of opioid withdrawal during detoxification programs include all of the following, except:

    A. Clonidine.
    B. Selective serotonin reuptake inhibitor antidepressants.
    C. Tapering doses of other narcotics (e.g., methadone).
    D. Nonsteroidal anti-inflammatory drugs for muscle aches.
    E. Antiemetics for nausea.

    Review this! ❑

15. Methadone maintenance therapy for opioid addicts has been shown to do all of the following, except:

    A. Reduce the incidence of criminal activity.
    B. Reduce use of illicit opioids.
    C. Reduce risk of needle sharing and other human immunodeficiency virus risk activities.
    D. Control cravings for opioids.
    E. Allow primary care physicians to easily supervise methadone therapy.

    Review this! ❑

16. Urine drug screens can be used for monitoring compliance with drug treatment programs or for patients who are taking chronic pain medications. Common medications that can cause false-positive drug screen results include all of the following, except:

    A. Pseudoephedrine, which can cause false-positive amphetamine results.
    B. Fluoroquinolones, which can cause false-positive opioid results.
    C. Benadryl, which can cause false-positive benzodiazepine results.
    D. Ibuprofen and naproxen, which can cause false-positive marijuana results.
    E. Dextromethorphan, which can cause false-positive phencyclidine results.

    Review this! ❑

17. All of the following statements about the typical duration of positive drug screens after the ingestion of illicit substances are true, except:

    A. With heavy use, marijuana may be positive for up to 30 days.
    B. Amphetamines are typically detectable for 2 to 3 weeks.
    C. Benzodiazepine detection is dependent on the half-life of the medication, which varies between 3 and 30 days.
    D. Cocaine is typically detectable for 2 to 3 days.
    E. Phencyclidine may be detected for up to 2 weeks.

    Review this! ❑

18. The CRAFFT questionnaire is an effective screening tool for drug abuse in teenagers. All of the following are questions from the CRAFFT questionnaire, except:

    A. Have you ever driven or ridden in a CAR driven by someone who was intoxicated?
    B. Do you ever use alcohol or drugs to RELAX or fit in?
    C. Do you ever use alcohol or drugs when ALONE?
    D. Do you ever FORGET things you did while using drugs or alcohol?
    E. Do your FAMILY or FRIENDS tell you to cut down on drinking or drug use?
    F. Do you find you need to TAKE MORE of a drug to get the same effect?

    Review this! ❑

19. Brief interventions with the repeated delivery of short motivational messages have been shown to be effective tools in drug treatment programs that can be incorporated into primary care settings. *FRAMES* is a pneumonic for one of these techniques. All of the following are part of the FRAMES method, except:

    A. Feedback.
    B. Remove substance.
    C. Menu.
    D. Empathy.
    E. Self-efficacy.

    Review this! ❑

20. The DSM-IV criteria for substance abuse include all of the following, except:

A. The substance is often taken in large amounts over a longer period than was intended.

B. There is a persistent desire or unsuccessful effort to cut down or control substance use.

C. A great deal of time is spent performing activities that are necessary to obtain the substance (e.g., visiting multiple doctors, driving long distances).

D. Important social, occupational, or recreational activities are given up or reduced because of substance use.

E. Use of the substance is stopped intermittently when the patient recognizes the harm that comes from using it, but it is eventually resumed, despite the adverse consequences.

Review this! ❑

66 Interpreting Laboratory Tests

Peter Nalin

1. Which of the following is the most frequent reference value?

   A. Confidence interval
   B. Positive predictive value
   C. Reference interval
   D. Laboratory directive
   E. Odds ratio

   Review this! ❏

2. True or false: Biologic variability is the variation of a test result in different persons at the same time.

   A. True
   B. False

   Review this! ❏

3. Which of the following does not cause biologic variability?

   A. Physiologic processes
   B. Analytic variation
   C. Constitutional factors
   D. Extrinsic factors

   Review this! ❏

4. True or false: Using current technology, analytic variation contributes more to the variability of results than biologic variation.

   A. True
   B. False

   Review this! ❏

5. The reference interval is most frequently defined by results chosen between which of the following percentiles?

   A. 25th to 75th
   B. 5th to 95th
   C. 2.5th to 97.5th
   D. 1st to 99th

   Review this! ❏

6. The Clinical Laboratory Improvement Act of 1998 (CLIA 1998) defined all of the following requirements for reference values, except:

   A. The reference ranges must be reported in a different color than the result.
   B. The reference ranges must be available to the clinician.
   C. The reference ranges must be included in the laboratory manual.
   D. The laboratory must establish specifications for performance characteristics.

   Review this! ❏

7. Which of the following statements best describes the relationship between amylase and lipase levels at their peak after the onset of acute pancreatitis?

   A. Amylase peaks before lipase.
   B. Lipase peaks before amylase.
   C. Lipase and amylase both peak at 12 hours.
   D. Lipase and amylase both peak at 24 hours.

   Review this! ❏

8. A normal amylase level does not exclude a diagnosis of pancreatitis, especially if the episode is induced by which of the following?

   A. Alcohol
   B. Medications
   C. Obstruction
   D. Hypertriglyceridemia

   Review this! ❏

9. The anti-DNA test is highly specific for which of the following?

   A. Rheumatoid arthritis
   B. Systemic lupus erythematosus
   C. Gilbert's disease
   D. Erythema multiforme

   Review this! ❏

Things to remember for the test.

10. A lupus-like syndrome can result from which of the following drugs?

    A. Hydrochlorothiazide
    B. Diphenhydramine
    C. Hydralazine
    D. Cyclobenzaprine

    Review this! ❏

11. With normal hepatic function, hemolysis is associated with a bilirubin level that is usually not higher than which of the following?

    A. 5 mg/dL
    B. 10 mg/dL
    C. 15 mg/dL
    D. 20 mg/dL
    E. 25 mg/dL

    Review this! ❏

12. Blood urea nitrogen (BUN) is produced by which of the following?

    A. The arterial circulation
    B. The brain
    C. The cardiac muscle
    D. The kidneys
    E. The liver

    Review this! ❏

13. Which of the following etiologies would explain a BUN-to-creatinine ratio of 10:1?

    A. Adrenal
    B. Prerenal
    C. Postrenal
    D. Intrinsic renal
    E. Eurenal

    Review this! ❏

14. Which of the following is the most common cause of a low total calcium level?

    A. Low albumin
    B. Malignancy
    C. Hyperparathyroidism
    D. Familial hypocalciuric hypercalcemia

    Review this! ❏

15. Which of the following is the physiologically active portion of calcium?

    A. Albumin-bound calcium
    B. Total blood calcium
    C. Chelated fraction of calcium
    D. Free or ionized calcium

    Review this! ❏

16. Carcinoembryonic antigen is an oncofetal glycoprotein antigen, the specificity of which can be best described as which of the following?

    A. Colonic
    B. Hepatic
    C. Ovarian
    D. Nonspecific

    Review this! ❏

17. The partial thromboplastin (PTT) time is significantly shortened by which of the following?

    A. Lupus anticoagulant
    B. Vitamin K deficiency
    C. Hemolysis
    D. Thrombocytopenia

    Review this! ❏

18. The Schilling test to confirm the diagnosis of pernicious anemia has been replaced by testing for which of the following?

    A. Antibodies to intrinsic factor
    B. Biopsy for atrophic gastritis
    C. Homocysteine level
    D. *Helicobacter pylori* antibodies

    Review this! ❏

19. The carbon dioxide content of the blood is mainly comprised of which of the following?

    A. Dissolved carbon dioxide
    B. Bicarbonate ion
    C. Carbonic acid
    D. Lactate

    Review this! ❏

20. Which of the following can cause a low anion gap?

    A. Lactic acidosis
    B. Ketoacidosis
    C. Multiple myeloma
    D. Ethylene glycol

    Review this! ❏

21. Which of the following is part of the five-part white blood cell differential?

    A. Thrombocytopenia
    B. Hemolysis
    C. Mean corpuscular volume
    D. Red cell distribution width
    E. Eosinophilia, if present

    Review this! ❏

22. Which of the following is the most common abnormality found by the complete blood cell count?

    A. Polycythemia
    B. Band forms
    C. Anemia
    D. Leukocytosis
    E. Thrombocytopenia

    Review this! ❑

23. Band forms are a subset of which of the following cell types?

    A. Lymphocytes
    B. Basophils
    C. Monocytes
    D. Neutrophils
    E. Eosinophils

    Review this! ❑

24. Which of the following can lead to thrombocytopenia by decreasing the production of platelets?

    A. Valproic acid
    B. Vitamin B_{12} deficiency
    C. Heparin
    D. Disseminated intravascular coagulation
    E. Sulfa drugs

    Review this! ❑

25. Which of the following can decrease the erythrocyte sedimentation rate (ESR)?

    A. Anemia
    B. Aspirin
    C. Sickle cell disease
    D. Hypoalbuminemia
    E. Nonfasting (or recent meal)

    Review this! ❑

26. Which of the following is associated with elevated homocysteine levels?

    A. Female gender
    B. Niacin
    C. Hyperthyroidism
    D. Sulfamethoxazole

    Review this! ❑

27. Which of the following can affect C-reactive protein levels?

    A. Aspirin
    B. Bacterial infection
    C. Circadian variation

    D. Diet
    E. Age

    Review this! ❑

28. The American Diabetic Association defines prediabetes as a fasting plasma glucose level of which of the following?

    A. Less than 50 mg/dL
    B. 50–69 mg/dL
    C. 70–99 mg/dL
    D. 100–125 mg/dL
    E. 126–135 mg/dL

    Review this! ❑

29. Which of the following is the test that is recommended for the diagnosis of diabetes mellitus?

    A. Glycosylated hemoglobin A1c
    B. Serum insulin level
    C. Fasting plasma glucose
    D. Glucose tolerance test
    E. Lipase

    Review this! ❑

30. *H. pylori* is associated with nearly 90% of ulcers of which of the following areas?

    A. The oral mucosa
    B. The esophagus
    C. The stomach
    D. The duodenum
    E. The jejunum

    Review this! ❑

31. Previous vaccination for hepatitis B should only produce a positive titer for which of the following?

    A. Hepatitis B surface antigen
    B. Hepatitis B virus e antigen
    C. Antibody to hepatitis B core antigen
    D. Antibody to hepatitis B surface antigen
    E. Antibody to hepatitis C virus

    Review this! ❑

32. An increased mortality rate from hepatitis B can be expected from which coexisting marker?

    A. Hepatitis A virus
    B. Antibody to hepatitis B core antigen
    C. Hepatitis C virus
    D. Hepatitis delta virus
    E. Hepatitis B virus e antigen

    Review this! ❑

Things to remember for the test.

Things to remember for the test.

33. Among neonates born to mothers with human immunodeficiency virus (HIV) infection, HIV infection can be identified early and accurately using which of the following tests?

    A. New rapid oral test for HIV
    B. Quantitative RNA polymerase chain reaction
    C. HIV-2 tests
    D. HIV-1 DNA polymerase chain reaction
    E. White blood cell count

    Review this! ❏

34. Physiologic variations in lipid measurements can be best described by which of the following?

    A. Negligible
    B. Less than analytic variation
    C. ± 3%
    D. ± 13%
    E. ± 33%

    Review this! ❏

35. The normal population carries which of the following false-positive rates for antibodies to Lyme disease?

    A. 0%
    B. 1%
    C. 5%
    D. 10%
    E. 15%

    Review this! ❏

36. Which of the following is the second most prevalent intracellular cation?

    A. Calcium
    B. Magnesium
    C. Potassium
    D. Sodium

    Review this! ❏

37. Which of the following is one cause of hyperkalemia?

    A. Alkalosis
    B. Hypomagnesemia
    C. Adrenal insufficiency
    D. Diuresis
    E. Periodic paralysis

    Review this! ❏

38. Which of the following is the best test to confirm or exclude thyroid disease in an ambulatory patient?

    A. Triiodothyronine
    B. Circulating thyroxine
    C. Thyroid-stimulating hormone
    D. Free t4
    E. Triiodothyronine resin uptake

    Review this! ❏

39. Negative results on most codeine immunoassays can be expected from urine drug testing for which of the following?

    A. Codeine
    B. Oxycodone
    C. Heroin
    D. Morphine

    Review this! ❏

40. Patients testing positive for which of the following tests are more likely to develop the radiologic progression of rheumatoid arthritis?

    A. Elevated ESR
    B. C-reactive protein
    C. Anticyclic citrullinated peptide
    D. Immunoglobulin M rheumatoid factor
    E. Rapid plasma reagent

    Review this! ❏

Question #1

Answer: B

Rationale: Several recent studies have identified the attributes that lead to patient satisfaction, and "Listening to me" makes every list. The style of the office, available services (like x-ray), and hospital affiliation may be important to some individuals, but they pale in comparison with the larger list of behavioral attributes. Patients consistently say that they do not want their doctor to be judgmental.

Page: 3

Question #2

Answer: A

Rationale: Family medicine is the specialty that has physicians who are the most likely to be satisfied with their careers; all of the other listed are more likely to describe themselves as dissatisfied.

Page: 4

Question #3

Answer: D

Rationale: More important than malpractice costs and decreasing income as causes for dissatisfaction is the loss of clinical autonomy. The inability to control time spent with patients is an aspect of this loss, but long work hours are not listed as an independent factor.

Page: 4

Question #4

Answer: D

Rationale: The ABFM, which was formed in 1969, was the first board of the American Board of Medical Specialties (ABMS) to require recertification (now called *maintenance of certification* [MOC]). The CME requirement is 50 hours each year. All diplomats have been required to pass a written examination.

Page: 5

Question #5

Answer: B

Rationale: Sixty-two percent of Americans in 1996 named a family physician as their usual source of care. Sixteen percent named an internist, and 15% named a pediatrician.

Page: 5

Question #6

Answer: C

Rationale: "Comprehensive care," "continuity of care," and "coordination of care" are typical descriptions of family medicine care. "Cost effective" has not been used, although many suspect that a less technological approach saves money for all involved.

Page: 5

Question #7

Answer: B

Rationale: Continuity of care is a core attribute of family medicine. The other statements are incorrect. Because continuity of case has been shown to improve quality of care, it can be of benefit for patients with emotional problems, and it can be used to serve pediatric patients as well as adults, particularly as they make the transition from adolescence to adulthood.

Pages: 6, 7

Question #8

Answer: D

Rationale: Families with continuity of care spend less money on their health care. They also have fewer hospitalizations and fewer operations, and they visit a physician less often.

Page: 7

Question #9

Answer: A

Rationale: Ninety percent of diabetics receive their care from a primary care physician. In addition, it has been noted that these patients have lower HbA1c levels than others who are cared for by non-primary care physicians.

Page: 7

Question #10

Answer: D

Rationale: Although the quality of care provided to the hospitalized pneumonia patient is equal, the patient cared for by a family physician will have a shorter and less expensive stay, with fewer resources used.

Page: 8

Question #11

Answer: A

Rationale: Starfield and colleagues[1] showed a worsening of health care outcomes in all 50 American states when the number of specialty physicians increased. They also noted that mortality is lower where there are more primary care doctors.

Page: 8

Question #12

Answer: C

Rationale: Family physicians and obstetricians have equal neonatal outcomes for low-risk pregnancies. However, family physicians have a lower Cesarean section rate and fewer episiotomies, and they are less likely to use epidural anesthesia.

Page: 8

Question #13

Answer: A

Rationale: The cost of health as expressed as a percentage of the gross national product is projected to reach 18% by the year 2012.

Page: 8

---

1. Starfield B, Shi L, Grover A, et al: The effects of specialist supply on populations' health: Assessing the evidence. Health Affairs 2005;0:W5-97-W5-107 (Web exclusive).

Question #14

Answer: A

Rationale: The underinsured population of the United States is growing rapidly, and it can currently be counted at about 50 million. These individuals are not unemployed and often are not even poor, with more than half of them having annual salaries of more than $75,000 per year.

Page: 9

Question #15

Answer: A

Rationale: It is sad to say that the United States stands alone among developed nations in not providing universal health coverage to all of its citizens.

Page: 9

Question #16

Answer: C

Rationale: The IOM has called for health care that is universal, continuous, affordable, and of high quality. They did not call for specialty care, because data do not support its use for meeting any of the other goals.

Page: 9

Question #17

Answer: B

Rationale: Despite being a relatively small specialty, family physicians provide more office visits than any other specialty.

Page: 9

Question #18

Answer: D

Rationale: Surgical specialists received 45.4% of the referrals that family physicians made, whereas medical specialists received 31%, obstetricians/gynecologists received 4.6%, and psychiatrists received the least number.

Page: 11

Question #19

Answer: B

Rationale: A primary care physician will manage an average of 1.65 problems during each visit.

Page: 12

Question #20

Answer: B

Rationale: Several factors have caused the recent increase in house calls, one of which is the increase in the number of homebound elderly patients. The financial incentive is still meager as compared with other home services, like repairs. It is unlikely that there will be an increase in the number of home visits to children who are acutely ill. The low rate of reimbursement by Medicare does not encourage house calls.

Page: 12

2   Answers

Question #1

Answer: B

Rationale: The first of the OHE ingredients is relationship-centered care: the existence of a human—albeit professional—relationship between the doctor and the patient. This is illustrated by the vignette, which establishes a relationship between the patient and the doctor.

Pages: 17, 19

Question #2

Answer: C

Rationale: The second ingredient of an OHE is healing space. The vignette points out the importance of the physical layout of a physician's office and the environment that it affords. Intuitively, one appreciates that this environment may be essential for establishing an optimal healing environment.

Pages: 18, 19

Question #3

Answer: D

Rationale: The third ingredient is self-care, which refers to the fact that the doctor must practice what he or she preaches and not shrink from openly displaying this. A smoking doctor, for example, is a weak role model for a patient who is contemplating quitting smoking.

Page: 19

Question #4

Answer: E

Rationale: The ingredient of intention and awareness refers to the doctor focusing fully on the patient when they are both in the examination room or the consultation room.

Page: 19

Question #5

Answer: A

Rationale: The ingredient of OHE called "wholism" refers to a holistic approach to the patient in the best way. In other words, the physician should not develop "tunnel vision" when evaluating and treating a patient for a specific set of problems; he or she must not think of a patient strictly as "a diabetic" or "a hypertensive." This is always a danger, but, over time, the physician must remember to approach and manage the patient as a whole person.

Page: 19

Question #6

Answer: B

Rationale: The sixth ingredient of an OHE is collaborative care, which is illustrated in the vignette by the close cooperation with the clinical psychologist for the treatment of the reactive depression that has evolved into endogenous depression. More typical examples in today's physician practices include the development of close working relationships with physical therapists, nutritionists, and podiatrists.

Page: 19

Question #7

Answer: C

Rationale: The seventh ingredient an OHE is lifestyle and empowerment. The vignette describes a patient lifestyle that is typically encountered and that needs to be addressed in primary care practice. Others include smoking, alcohol consumption, and amounts of time being spent with family or in meeting the requirements of the patient's job.

Page: 19

Question #8

Answer: E

Rationale: The spiritual meaning and purpose ingredient of an OHE involves more than understanding the patient's lifestyle; it means that the physician must understand the patient's personality, his or her strengths and weaknesses, and his or her vocation, avocations, talents, and wishes.

Page: 19

Question #9

Answer: D

Rationale: An OHE tends to minimize the use of resources, such as hospitalization and extra laboratory and other ancillary studies. Therefore, cost-effectiveness is enhanced by OHE.

Page: 19

Question #10

Answer: C

Rationale: The occurrences listed in the body of the question all refer to engagement in self-care practices by the team of healers. Each of the other characteristics is necessary for the provision of an OHE, but they are not exemplified by the occurrences listed.

Page: 20

Question #11

Answer: A

Rationale: All of the occurrences listed in the body of the question describe the ideal characteristics of a practice in which the healing team provides a process for facilitating access to the community and its services. The other choices are valid characteristics that should be present in an OHE, but they are not exemplified by the items listed.

Page: 17

Question #12

Answer: D

Rationale: Serum serotonin reuptake inhibiting agents are excellent pharmacologic agents for addressing the chemical aspects of depression, but they do not address or enhance a connection between the mind and the body.

Page: 16

Question #13

Answer: C

Rationale: Although mental health and self-awareness probably have beneficial effects for virtually any illness, of the conditions listed, there is general agreement that the connective tissue (autoimmune) diseases are the least affected by mind-body integration (or lack thereof).

Page: 16

Question #14

Answer: B

Rationale: Meditation is cited by Jonas and Rakel as an example of mindfulness. It is one of an array of self-directed techniques that may be taught to the patient. Other examples mentioned in the text are focused breathing, journaling, and dream work. All of the other choices listed for this question are examples of creating a positive expectancy (including the gentle confrontation of the alcoholic to start him on a path of healing) as initiated by the physician.

Pages: 15, 16

Question #15

Answer: E

Rationale: Negativity in a person's life in the forms of alienation, loneliness, and lack of social connectedness is associated with lowered life expectancy. This decreased longevity is not proven by prospective randomized studies. If there is causation of that association, it may well be that the decrement is mediated through any of the other choices given (cardiac dysrhythmias, dyslipidemia, hypertension, peptic ulcer disease). Moreover, studies have not been carried out to prove such cause-and-effect relationships among the social factors listed and any of the other risk factors listed.

Page: 20

Question #1

Answer: D

Rationale: "The National Institute of Mental Health defined family as a 'network of mutual commitment' and includes any group of people related either biologically, emotionally or legally."[1]

Page: 25

Question #2

Answer: A

Rationale: Many epidemiological studies have demonstrated the association between social support and health. The cumulative evidence showing that social support and social relationships affect morbidity and mortality are as strong as the evidence in the 1964 Surgeon General's report that established cigarette smoking as a risk factor for all-cause morbidity and mortality. Social support—particularly from family—is associated with improved health, whereas a lack of family and social support is associated with increased morbidity and mortality.

Page: 25

Question #3

Answer: A

Rationale: A substantial body of research demonstrates that, even when other factors are controlled for, marital status affects morbidity, overall mortality, and mortality from specific diseases. Married people are healthier, and the death of a spouse, separation, and divorce are all associated with increased mortality.

Page: 25

Question #4

Answer: B

Rationale: Many large studies have shown that, particularly for women, the quality of a patient's marital relationship affects the outcome of his or her chronic disease. For women, a poor marital relationship is associated with worsened coronary artery disease and congestive heart failure, higher risk of recurrence of breast cancer, and shortened survival from end-stage renal disease.

Pages: 25, 26

Question #5

Answer: B

Rationale: Research shows that supportive partner behaviors are associated with successful smoking cessation, whereas negative or critical partner behaviors are associated with relapse and failure to quit smoking. The Agency for Healthcare Quality and Research does recommend that social support interventions be required components of an effective smoking cessation program. A meta-analysis of nine randomized, controlled trials in which a social support intervention was added to a smoking cessation program confirmed that positive partner support predicts successful smoking cessation. However, the meta-analysis of these studies also showed that the social support interventions were not able to alter or influence partner support. These results indicate that it is not easy to alter partner behaviors or to increase partner support for smoking cessation; this is likely because partner behaviors are part of complex marital dynamics and thus strongly influenced by the history and quality of the marital relationship.

Page: 26

Question #6

Answer: C

Rationale: A meta-analysis of ten randomized, controlled trials of partner involvement and couples interventions in obesity treatment programs showed a small but significant improvement in weight loss at the end of the program but no apparent difference at 2- and 3-year follow-up evaluations. The couples interventions in these studies were not able to increase partner support. However, these studies did show an association between negative or critical partner behaviors and failure to lose weight. Dubbert and Wilson[2] report that patients with higher marital satisfaction lost more weight.

Page: 26

1. Pequegnat W, Bray JH: Families and HIV/AIDS. *J Fam Psychol* 11:3-10, 1997.

2. Dubbert PM, Wilson GT: Goal-setting and spouse involvement in the treatment of obesity. *Behav Res Ther* 22:227-242, 1984.

Question #7

Answer: B

Rationale: Multiple studies, including a recent Cochrane review, have shown that parental involvement in pediatric obesity treatment programs results in improved weight loss outcomes for both children and their parents.

Pages: 26, 27

Question #8

Answer: B

Rationale: Caregiving places a heavy burden on family members, and they have higher morbidity and mortality rates than age-matched controls. Family caregivers have more physical illnesses, depression, and anxiety, and those more than 65 years old who experience emotional strain are 63% more likely to die within 4 years than their age-matched controls.

Page: 27

Question #9

Answer: A

Rationale: Most families are affected by chronic disease. Family members deal with most of the daily physical demands of chronic illness; they provide direct care, clinical observation, case management, and a range of other services. Family caregivers are integral members of the health care team.

Page: 27

Question #10

Answer: C

Rationale: Mittelman developed and studied a family psychoeducational intervention for caregivers of patients with Alzheimer's disease that provided individual and group instruction and problem-solving sessions for managing the difficult behaviors of these patients. Families also attended support groups and had crisis intervention services available to them. Caregivers who received the intervention were less depressed and physically healthier. The patients with Alzheimer's disease whose caregivers received the intervention were able to live at home for a year longer than the control patients; this resulted in an overall savings in nursing-home costs that exceeded several times the cost of the intervention.

Page: 27

Question #11

Answer: A

Rationale: Research is beginning to explore the ways in which family relationships and dynamics influence the course of chronic illness positively and negatively. Family physicians must assess family relationships, support, and coping mechanisms. Negative behaviors and family relationships can adversely affect the outcome of chronic illness. Family physicians can provide early assessment and intervention, including referrals for family therapy to help families cope better. Family physicians can also help families mobilize their strengths and resources to provide care and cope with chronic illness.

Page: 27

Question #12

Answer: D

Rationale: Stress may refer to any of the three components of the stress process: (1) the stressors, (2) the physiologic response to the stressors, or (3) the health consequences of the stressors.

Pages: 27, 28

Question #13

Answer: C

Rationale: Studies by Blake in 1987 showed that life events that are perceived negatively or that are not under the individual's control have the most adverse effects on health. Many studies have shown that an increase in stressful life events does precede the development of disease. Ten of the 15 most stressful events on the Holmes and Rahe scale occur within the family.

Pages: 27, 28

Question #14

Answer: B

Rationale: A study of more than 1000 preschoolers found a strong association between family life events and subsequent physician visits and hospitalizations.

Another study showed that children in families that had more than 12 life events in 4 years had six times more hospital admissions.

Page: 28

Question #15

Answer: A

Rationale: Transitions in the family life cycle are key sources of stress that strongly influence physical and mental health. Physicians should always ask about family events and life-cycle transitions that may have occurred since the last visit. Family physicians can also anticipate changes in the family life cycle and offer help and support to families as they experience these transitions.

Page: 28

Question #16

Answer: B

Rationale: Individual family members may have very different experiences of a divorce, and the family physician must understand these differences to help each individual and the family through the transition.

Page: 28

Question #17

Answer: B

Rationale: Research shows that a conflicted, destructive home is far more harmful for family members—especially children—than a stable divorced home.

Page: 29

Question #18

Answer: D

Rationale: When a couple presents with marital discord and separation and divorce are being considered, the physician's role is to decrease the psychological risk to patients, to promote healthy methods of coping with stress, to teach parents ways of relating to their children to maximize their coping, and to make appropriate referrals. Early assessment and intervention—including a referral for marriage therapy—may facilitate reconciliation. Even if reconciliation does not occur, early

counseling or therapy can help reduce the stress and deleterious effects of separation and divorce for the family.

Pages: 21, 22

Question #19

Answer: A

Rationale: Studies show that, even after controlling for age, race, and income, divorced individuals have the highest rates of acute and chronic medical problems and disability.

Page: 29

Question #20

Answer: B

Rationale: Divorced men and women have reduced qualitative and quantitative immune functioning compared with married controls. Divorced men also have increased rates of suicide, mental hospital admissions, and physical illness, and they have an increased risk of being a victim of violence.

Page: 29

Question #21

Answer: C

Rationale: Studies show that, within 2 years after a divorce, most adults recover feelings of well-being and develop a more satisfied and stable life. Studies also show that adults expect that they will recover much more quickly after divorce, and physicians can help patients adjust their expectations and establish realistic goals for recovery.

Page: 29

Question #22

Answer: A

Rationale: Many studies have shown that boys experience more traumatic, severe, and long-lasting reactions to divorce than girls. Boys have been shown to develop more problems with behavior, sex-role adjustment, and school, and their problems often persist for 4 to 7 years after the divorce.

Page: 29

Question #23

Answer: A

Rationale: Individual children may display a wide range of reactions. Typical reactions by age are shown in Table 5-1. Children 3 years old or younger also display intensified separation anxiety when separated from their primary caretaker. Children up to the age of 6 years may show a regression in behavior and some developmental delay. Children between the ages of 6 and 11 years are likely to respond with sadness and upset and to report reconciliation fantasies; they are also less able to separate themselves psychologically from their parents, and they may blame themselves for the divorce. Children between the ages of 12 and 18 years are better able to separate themselves from their parents, and they do not blame themselves for the divorce. However, adolescents often react with anger, resentment, and hostility.

Page: 30

Question #24

Answer: C

Rationale: The first year after divorce is a crisis period during which structures and routines are disrupted as the family undergoes restructuring. Parents are less effective, because children respond differently to their parents and are less compliant. Parents also have trouble coping with their own feelings; they may feel guilt about the divorce and experience role overload. After the first 2 years, the family stabilizes. New structures and roles develop, parenting improves, and children become more responsive.

Page: 29

Question #25

Answer: B

Rationale: Remarriage creates both positive and negative stressors for the family. Children in stepfamilies have more difficulties and behavior problems than those in nuclear families, and girls tend to have more difficulty adjusting to remarriage than boys. Within 2 years after the remarriage, however, children tend to adjust, and these behavior problems decrease.

Page: 30

Question #26

Answer: B

Rationale: Health risk factors, like smoking excess, alcohol use, high cholesterol, obesity, and hypertension, tend to run in families, so every member should be screened. In addition, education and interventions should be aimed at the entire family.

Page: 31

Question #27

Answer: C

Rationale: Studies have shown that less than 10% of children had an adult talk with them about the divorce. Physicians need to understand how the divorce has been presented to the child, and they also need to be familiar with both the child's and the parents' feelings about and perceptions of the divorce. The physician should encourage and help parents to deal with their children's emotions and concerns during and after the divorce. Physicians should also act as the child's advocate with regard to helping the parents interpret the divorce appropriately to the child. The physician needs to identify early warning signs that a child may be at risk for serious problems and to refer such children for professional intervention. Both parents should be urged to monitor and support the child's well-being.

Page: 31

Question #28

Answer: A

Rationale: Family physicians should anticipate and assess for family life cycle transitions and provide support and encouragement. Physicians should provide psychoeducation to help families mobilize their resources and supportive roles. Physicians should assess the adaptation and functioning of individual family members and refer patients to mental health professionals when appropriate. Family-oriented care recognizes that the family is the primary source of health beliefs, health-related behaviors, stress, and emotional support.

Page: 31

4 Answers

Question #1

Answer: D

Rationale: To provide care that is appropriately responsive to psychosocial issues, the physician should keep in mind the following three imperatives:

1. The physician *sees the person first*, conceptualizing his or her symptoms and behaviors in both social and psychological contexts and responding with sensitivity to the patient's experience and priorities.
2. The physician *evaluates the dynamic nature of multiple biopsychosocial variables* to respond in a timely manner that optimizes positive results.
3. The physician *fosters a supportive and empathic doctor-patient relationship* to provide the foundation for gathering information and for intervening effectively.

Biomedical factors are but a small part of what patients bring to their physicians. Although the biomedical model—based on the assumptions of mind-body dualism, biologic reductionism, and linear causality—has resulted in miraculous achievements of high-technology medicine, primary care physicians who restrict their attention to purely "medical" considerations are of limited use to their patients. Nevertheless, the transformation of thinking from a purely biomedical model to a biopsychosocial paradigm has been a major challenge to modern medicine.

Page: 35

Question #2

Answer: B

Rationale: In 1977, psychiatrist George Engel proposed the biopsychosocial model, which included social and psychological variables as crucial determinants of disease and illness.

Page: 36

Question #3

Answer: B

Rationale: The following is a list of conceptual models cited that emphasize different dimensions of psychosocial influence on health:

- The life-span perspective,
- The ethnomedical cultural model,
- The systems approach,
- The biopsychosocial model, and
- The stress and coping model.

Page: 36

Question #4

Answer: D

Rationale: The life-span perspective emphasizes the importance of where an individual is on his or her personal developmental trajectory. Past development, current status, and anticipated developmental changes and challenges are taken into account.

Page: 35

Question #5

Answer: C

Rationale: The LEARN acronym is broken down as follows:

- *Listen* with empathy and understanding to a patient's perception of his or her problem by eliciting the patient's explanatory model for the illness.
- *Explain* your perceptions or explanatory model in language that the patient can understand.
- *Acknowledge* the differences and similarities between your explanatory model and that of the patient, and discuss any significant discrepancies between the two.
- *Recommend* treatment that you decide is optimal within your explanatory model.
- *Negotiate* treatment with the patient, seeking a compromise that is acceptable to the patient, that is consistent with your ethical standards, and that makes use of the patient's social network, when necessary.

Page: 36

Question #6

Answer: B

Rationale: The LEARN acronym was developed in 1983 by Berlin and Fowkes as part of the ethnomedical cultural model.

Page: 36

Question #7

Answer: B

Rationale: The systems approach has been very influential with regard to conceptualizations of family functioning. Smilkstein[1] developed one of the first applications of family systems thinking for family medicine. He suggested the importance of physician attention to the systemic interactions of family members and the impact of crisis, coping styles, and resources on family functioning. He incorporated these components into the family APGAR (Adaptation, Partnership, Growth, Affection, and Resolve), a simple instrument and mnemonic device for assessing the functioning of a family system in health and illness.

Page: 36

Question #8

Answer: A

Rationale: The biopsychosocial model was proposed as a scientific paradigm by Engel,[2] who encouraged the clinician to observe biochemical and morphologic changes in relation to a patient's emotional patterns, life goals, attitudes toward illness, and social environment. Engel proposed that the brain and the peripheral organs were linked in complex, mutually adjusting relationships that were affected by changes in social as well as physical stimuli.

Page: 36

Question #9

Answer: A

Rationale: The biopsychosocial model is based on three assumptions. First, clinical care needs to go beyond biomedicine, because illness can be fully understood only in the context of psychologic and social factors. Second, these three domains—biologic, psychological, and social—are interrelated. Third, as Engel noted, effective treatment requires attention to these complex interactions and to the integration of the biopsychosocial factors.

Page: 36

Question #10

Answer: E

Rationale: Burrell-Carrio and colleagues[3] proposed "a biopsychosocially oriented clinical practice whose pillars include (1) self-awareness; (2) active cultivation of trust; (3) an emotional style characterized by empathic curiosity; (4) self-calibration as a way to reduce bias; (5) educating the emotions to assist with diagnosis and forming therapeutic relationships; (6) using informed intuition; and (7) communicating clinical evidence to foster dialogue, not just the mechanical application of protocol."

Page: 36

Question #11

Answer: D

Rationale: Sarafino[4] classified personal control into the following five types:

1. Behavioral control
2. Cognitive control
3. Decisional control
4. Informational control
5. Retrospective control

Pages: 37, 38

Question #12

Answer: A

Rationale: Sarafino[4] defines cognitive control as involving the ability to use thought processes or strategies to modify the impact of a stressor. For example, focusing on a pleasant thought during the suturing of a laceration may decrease the pain sensation.

Page: 37

Question #13

Answer: B

Rationale: Kobasa and colleagues[5] demonstrated that people high in the "three Cs" of control, commitment,

1. Smilkstein G: The family APGAR: A proposal for a family function test and its use by physicians. *J Fam Pract* 6:1231-1239, 1978.
2. Engel GL: The need for medical model: A challenge for biomedicine. *Science* 196:129-136, 1977.
3. Borrell-Carrio F, Suchman AL, Epstein RM: The biopsychosocial model 25 years later: Principles, practice and scientific inquiry. *Ann Fam Med* 2:576582, 2004.
4. Sarafino EP: Health Psychology: *Biopsychosocial Interactions*. New York, John Wiley & Sons, 1990.
5. Kobasa SC, Maddi SR, Pucceti MC: Personality and exercise as buffers in the stress-illness relationship. *J Behav Med* 5:391-404, 1982.

and challenge tended to remain healthier than their less hardy counterparts. Studies show that illness increased with stress and decreased with greater hardiness and exercise. A physician's knowledge of a patient's degree of hardiness may help with the assessment of a patient's response to stressors.

Page: 38

Question #14

Answer: C

Rationale: According to Sarafino,[4] social support may be of several varieties. *Emotional support* involves the expression of caring, concern, and empathy toward the person. *Esteem support* involves the expression of positive regard for the person, and it counteracts feelings of inadequacy during stressful life events. *Tangible* or *instrumental support* involves direct assistance during the time when it is needed. *Information support* involves giving advice, suggestions, or feedback about how the person is doing.

Page: 38

Question #15

Answer: B

Rationale: Two hypotheses, called "buffering" and "direct effects," have been proffered to explain how social support affects health. The "buffering" hypothesis suggests that social support affects health by protecting the person against negative effects of stress, perhaps by affecting the cognitive appraisal of stress. When people encounter a strong stressor, such as a major financial crisis, those individuals with high levels of social support may appraise the situation as less stressful than will those with low levels of support. The second way that social support may buffer the stress by modifying the response to a stressor is that people can turn to their friends and family for advice, reassurance, or material aid. The "direct effects" hypothesis asserts that social support is beneficial to health and well-being by enhancing self-esteem and by fostering positive health behaviors among people who believe that others count on them.

Page: 38

Question #16

Answer: E

Rationale: The key points of the psychosocial database are as follows:

- Age, gender, and sexual orientation
- Religious, ethnic, and cultural group
- Family composition, structure, and functioning
- Work and/or school status
- Social support network and significant others
- Financial resources, including health insurance status
- Personal and family history of major loss, trauma, or illness
- Psychological functioning, including personality, defensive style, and current mental status
- Physical environment, including home, neighborhood, and environmental hazards
- Recent stressors and changes

Page: 38

Question #17

Answer: E

Rationale: Information gathered from dialogue with the patient can be supplemented by a variety of means, including the following: (1) the use of standard measures, such as health questionnaires (e.g., SF 36); screening inventories (e.g., Beck Depression Inventory); and measures of stress, coping, and social support; (2) interviews with family members, including structured assessments (e.g., family APGAR), (3) the review of existing records (e.g., school records), (4) consultation with multidisciplinary colleagues (e.g., psychologists, occupational therapists), (5) the observation of the patient environment through home visits, and (6) consultation with cultural informants and translators in cases in which patients are members of unfamiliar cultures.

Page: 39

Question #18

Answer: C

Rationale: Consideration of this model suggests several interventions that should be part of the standard repertoire for family physicians: interventions that tend to do no harm, that usually help, and that use skills that family physicians should have. Specifically, physicians can work with patients to directly reduce stress, to enhance or mobilize social support resources, and to reinforce or model positive stress appraisal and coping. For the provision of care within a biopsychosocial model, interdisciplinary teams—rather than solo practitioners—have the advantage, and physicians can have more positive impact on their patients' lives when they harness the wisdom of colleagues from other fields through referral or consultation.

Page: 39

Question #19

Answer: E

Rationale: There are certain times in the provision of medical care when interventions that attend to psychosocial issues are especially important.

Natural transitions in the family life cycle, such as the birth of a child or the death of a spouse, call on the physician to provide empathic support, to assess the patient's support system, to normalize emotional reactions, and to provide anticipatory guidance as patients confront changing family roles and functioning.

When compliance or lifestyle issues impinge on health, interventions that focus on biologic mechanisms alone are likely to be ineffective. The health effects of substance abuse, domestic violence, and poverty are best addressed through attention to social environment and psychological concerns.

A dramatic change in patient symptoms should also evoke the consideration of psychosocial factors. A psychosocial crisis can provoke an exacerbation of a chronic condition (e.g., rheumatoid arthritis), a new manifestation of illness (e.g., myocardial infarction), or emotional-psychiatric symptoms (e.g., anxiety, trouble sleeping) that are best treated through stress reduction as well as symptomatic care.

A significant medical diagnosis often precipitates a psychosocial crisis, and it requires the physician to attend to the patient's psychosocial environment. Effective physician intervention may involve anticipating the nature of the potential family crisis, including family members in discussions with the patient, and addressing family needs for support. The timely provision of accurate information can enhance a patient's sense of control. Direct support by the physician during the initial adjustment phase can minimize more serious emotional disruption.

Patients living with chronic illness require sensitive psychosocial care. These patients typically deal with a predictable set of issues in highly idiosyncratic ways. Adequate attention to these issues can make medical management easier and more successful. These issues can often be effectively addressed within the doctor-patient relationship and through judicious referral to support groups for the chronically ill.

Page: 39

Question #20

Answer: C

Rationale: Pollin[6] identified eight emotionally charged issues that people with chronic illnesses inevitably confront:

1. Control
2. Self-image
3. Dependency
4. Stigma
5. Abandonment
6. Anger
7. Isolation
8. Death

Page: 39

Question #21

Answer: A

Rationale: Managed care has introduced new challenges to the doctor-patient relationship, which provides the foundation for comprehensive care. Establishing and maintaining rapport is frequently challenged by forced discontinuity of care related to insurance coverage. Cost-containment pressures on physicians introduce an adversarial element in the doctor-patient relationship that may negatively affect this relationship. In terms of treatment, time constraints combined with the fragmentation of families across providers make it very difficult for any one provider to understand complex family dynamics or to intervene comprehensively within families. Under managed care, the focus of treatment is on crisis resolution, amelioration of commonly observed symptoms, and shortening of the length of treatment.

Page: 40

6. Pollin I. *Medical Crisis Counseling: Short-Term Therapy for Long-Term Illness.* New York: WW Norton, 1995.

5   Answers

Question #1

Answer: B

Rationale: Before 1910, physicians in America were trained almost exclusively in an apprenticeship experience. After 1910—and spurred on by the famous Flexner Report—the American medical education community adopted the university model, thereby bringing medical schools into the more traditional higher education graduate school format.

Page: 42

Question #2

Answer: A

Rationale: In the university model, medical investigators began performing scholarly inquiry as dictated by the tenets of the scientific method. In many ways, this led to the standardization of the body of medical knowledge, with an emphasis on science and on the use of reductionistic methodology in areas of scholarly exploration. This approach to medical education and medical inquiry led to extremely productive research findings in the biomedical sciences, pushing back the frontiers of our understanding of physiology and pathology.

Page: 42

Question #3

Answer: A

Rationale: Although the traditional reductionistic approach is ideally suited for scientific investigation, it has created a rather dichotomous situation with regard to patients. This scientific model creates a dichotomous structure for examining, classifying, and treating disease, and it classifies people as either having or not having a particular condition. Diseases are treated as independent entities that are amenable to categorization and that are presumed to have a specific cause. However, this process ignores many of those human qualities that comprise the patient's total being.

Page: 42

Question #4

Answer: C

Rationale: On a micro level, physicians deal with patients and biomedical problems. However, on a macro level, they also deal with patients and their complex relationships with others, with their communities, and with the world community. A failure to comprehend this dualistic role has the potential to fatally flaw any practitioner's best clinical efforts. It derives from the notion that physicians have multiple responsibilities, including the need to understand the biomedical condition and its associated behavioral, social, and cultural factors and to integrate them into the comprehensive management of patients.

Pages: 42–43

Question #5

Answer: A

Rationale: Regardless of the origin of a patient's dysfunction (whether a mechanical or chemical failure of the biomedical manifestation of some other problem), a patient presents to a primary care physician with symptoms and a diminished ability to deal with the "hand fate has dealt." A consistent companion of the patient in this process is stress; this stress may be generated by a biomedical dysfunction, or it may in fact be generating the biomedical dysfunction itself, which the patient then brings to the physician. How that patient responds to the stress associated with his or her problem will, in many ways, determine that patient's ultimate outcome.

Page: 43

Question #6

Answer: B

Rationale: Many physicians are unaware of their considerable capability to influence the thinking and behavior of their patients, and they do not always use it to full advantage to promote their patients' best interest. Five of the most predominate powers that are regularly attributed to physicians and that singularly qualify them to influence their patients are as follows:

1. Reward power,
2. Coercive power,
3. Expert power,
4. Referent power, and
5. Legitimate power.

Page: 43

Question #7

Answer: C

Rationale: Physicians are uniquely positioned to assist their patients with coping, regardless of the nature of the patients' problems. Five major, common components from schools of psychotherapy are as follows:

1. *The expectation of receiving help*: The helplessness, hopelessness, and other attributes that accompany the patient to the physician's office are carried by a patient who is frequently desperate to have that physician help him or her deal with this burden.
2. *The therapeutic relationship*: Physicians and patients bond for purposes of fostering the well-being of the patient. This bonding produces a contract for caring and concern that is at the core of any therapy.
3. *Obtaining an external perspective*: Patients expect a wise and knowledgeable physician to assist them in formulating their thought processes and their problem-resolution skills.
4. *Encouraging a corrective experience*: The physician provides the external motivation for patients to change the way in which they function, react, and/or respond. This is a positive attribute of the psychotherapeutic relationship, which will help patients translate insights into actions that are more productive and beneficial.
5. *The opportunity to test reality repeatedly*: In this capacity, the physician is the patient's "port in a storm." Patients may have to "dock" frequently as they attempt to wade through uncharted and stormy seas. It is the physician's responsibility to provide that perspective for the patient and to assist the patient with his or her voyage. In all of these activities, the physician is the supporting listener and the occasional commentator as the patient works through the process resolution and self-actualization.

Pages: 43, 44

Question #8

Answer: A

Rationale: To succinctly and expediently get to the core of psychosocial problems in the context of a busy office practice, a systemic assessment exemplified by the acronym *BATHE* (Stuart and Lieberman[1]) ideally investigates the history of the present illness and then allows the physician to react accordingly. BATHE stands for the following:

Background: A simple question such as "What's going on in your life?" will elicit the context of the patient's visit.
Affect (the feeling state): Questions such as "How do you feel about that?" and "What is your mood?" allow the patient to report his or her current feeling state.
Trouble: The question "What about the situation troubles you the most?" helps both the physician and the patient focus on the situation's subjective meaning.
Handling: The answer to the question "How are you handling that?" gives an assessment of functioning.
Empathy: The statement "That must be very difficult for you" legitimizes the patient's reaction.

Page: 44

Question #9

Answer: B

Rationale: The physician's inquiry into the patient's psychosocial status is designed to produce an enhanced comprehension on the part of the physician of the overall dimensions of a patient's problem. However, it is not designed so that the physician will assume responsibility for the patient's situation; rather, the physician will make therapeutic suggestions that may enable the patient to deal with his or her problem more effectively. The patient continues to own his or her problem, but the physician is better able to assist that patient with the resolution of the problem, because the physician has a complete and comprehensive understanding of the derivation of the problem.

Page: 44

Question #10

Answer: B

Rationale: Although patients may ask for advice, focusing them on their own resources and providing

---

1. Stuart MR, Lieberman JA: *The Fifteen Minute Hour, Practical Therapeutic Interventions in Primary Care*, 3rd ed. Philadelphia, WB Saunders, 2002.

them with some guidance for developing alternatives is always more effective. When the physician gives advice or directly solves a problem, this does not empower the patient. It is better to make patients aware of their own strengths and their abilities to assess and exercise their own options.

Page: 44

Question #11

Answer: A

Rationale: Patients must learn to differentiate among thoughts, feelings, and behavior.

Thoughts are related to our beliefs and to the stories that we tell ourselves. They are judgments, generalizations, and unfounded prognostications that we all make, and physicians must acknowledge patients' views before being able to challenge them.

Feelings are emotional responses to a situation that are based on thoughts and judgments. Feelings must be expressed and accepted. During this process, feelings change. Feelings also change when irrational thoughts and unrealistic expectations are altered.

Behavior consists of the actions we take, and it is the only thing in this life that we can control. Helping patients focus on their behavior and make positive adjustments to their lifestyles is probably the most important intervention that a physician can make to improve his or her patients' health.

Pages: 44, 45

Question #12

Answer: B

Rationale: When patients are overwhelmed by circumstances of their lives, they lose sight of the fact that they still have options. The physician's suggestion that there are always options and that the patient needs to explore them steers the patient in a positive direction. It is not the physician's task to generate these options; rather, it is the patient's. The physician communicates the expectation that the patient can and will discover these options and that he or she will return to report the results. This therapeutic intervention helps patients to be more open to possibilities, to look at their world—including themselves—in a new way, and to become aware of having options.

Pages: 44, 45

Question #13

Answer: B

Rationale: It is useful to encourage patients to reinterpret their situations. Every trying circumstance can be seen as an opportunity to learn a necessary lesson or to develop an essential skill. Physicians can point out that there are four healthy options for handling a bad situation:

1. *Leaving the situation:* This dictates exploring the best and worst possible outcomes that might result and planning for an appropriate time to make a move.
2. *Accepting the situation:* This requires recognizing that, if things could be different, they would be different.
3. *Changing the situation:* This requires an investigation of what is possible and what additional resources might be needed.
4. *Reframing the situation:* This means finding a way to interpret the situation as a positive experience or as a necessary learning experience.

Page: 45

Question #14

Answer: A

Rationale: Therapeutic talk is direct conversation that focuses patients on their strengths and choices. It makes patients feel better about themselves and more competent when it comes to dealing with the circumstances of their lives, and it also makes them feel connected in a positive relationship with the physician.

Page: 45

Question #15

Answer: E

Rationale: Groves[2] developed four stereotypes of hateful patients, which he labeled dependent clingers, manipulative help-rejecters, entitled demanders, and self-destructive deniers. These patients consistently trigger negative feelings in physicians, who cannot satisfy their endless demands and complaints. One approach to maintaining physician mental health while treating these patients is to recognize that these individuals are trying desperately to get their needs met in the only way that they see possible at the time. Because they

2. Groves JE: Taking care of the hateful patient. *N Engl J Med* 298:883, 1978.

experience little success, they become more frustrated and subsequently more difficult. It is important for the physician to acknowledge the suffering of these patients.

Page: 45

Question #16

Answer: A

Rationale: Except when there is an immediate threat to life, physicians must limit the time they spend with patients who arouse negative emotions to less than 15 minutes, regardless of the complexity of the problems or the number of complaints. If all problems cannot be addressed in one visit, the patient can be brought back the following week, which demonstrates the physician's interest and concern. With frequent brief sessions, these patients often feel less rejected. Also, they organize the details of their stories to fit into abbreviated time slots, after they are convinced that the physician will listen attentively and respond appropriately.

Page: 45

Question #17

Answer: B

Rationale: Barsky and colleagues[3] concluded that hypochondriacs believe "good health" means being relatively "symptom free," and they suggested that this accounts for these patients' numerous somatic complaints and resistance to reassurance. Hypochondriacs focus their attention on their physical symptoms and actually suffer from anxiety and depression while being unsuccessful in their efforts to find anyone to cure them. These patients will ultimately realize that the number and intensity of their somatic symptoms are correlated with their levels of stress and anxiety.

Page: 45

Question #18

Answer: B

Rationale: There are real differences between hypochondriacs, who are concerned about the state of their health ("the worried well"), and chronic complainers (Rittelmeyer[4]), who have multiple complaints, who demand to be seen frequently, who rarely get better, and who never appreciate the physician's efforts on their behalf. The best treatment is to acknowledge their suffering and to recognize the futility of trying to alleviate it. These patients seem to need their disease to function at all.

Page: 45

Question #19

Answer: A

Rationale: It is depressing to acknowledge that depression that is not diagnosed or treated by the primary care physician often results in long-lasting symptomatology, decreased quality of life, and suicide (Lecrubier[5]). Even mild to moderate depression affects people's lives negatively. Questioning the patient using the BATHE assessment results in the diagnosis, after which depression can be treated effectively using brief sessions, with or without medication.

Page: 45

Question #20

Answer: D

Rationale: Incorporating the psychosocial aspects of medicine into daily practice can be challenging but extremely gratifying, provided that the physician observes a number of basic rules for survival. Of the dozen rules that Stuart and Lieberman[1] prescribe, the most important ones are as follows: (1) do not take responsibility for things that you cannot control, (2) take care of yourself, or you cannot take care of anyone else, and (3) recognize that you have to start where the patient is, which means that it is crucial to do a psychosocial assessment along with a biomedical one.

Page: 45

3. Barsky AJ, Coeytaux RR, Sarnie MK, et al: Hypochondriacal patients' beliefs about good health. *Am J Psychol* 150:1085, 1993.

4. Rittelmeyer LF Jr: Coping with the chronic complainer. *Am Fam Physician* 31:211, 1985.

5. Lecrubier Y: The burden of depression and anxiety in general medicine. *J Clin Psychiatry* 62(Suppl 8):4-9, 2001.

Question #1

Answer: B

Rationale: Protocol compels mention that elder abuse first achieved notable recognition within the British medical literature under the title "Granny battering."[1]

Page: 47

Question #2

Answer: B

Rationale: Gender has not been found to be a reliable risk factor; numerous studies have indicated that males and females are equally likely to become victims of elder abuse.[2]

Page: 47

Question #3

Answer: B

Rationale: Although having more involvement with the partner's family than the male wants may be somewhat true, it is not a noted trigger for violence. The physician must recognize that a pregnancy often signals a crisis and a major threat for a bettering male; he is faced with no longer being central to his partner's life. Pathological jealousies are common; the male partner may question whether the child is even his.[3] Marital status is an additional marker.

Pages: 47, 48

Question #4

Answer: A

Rationale: Marriage is not a necessary condition nor is IPV exclusively a phenomenon of unhealthy heterosexual interaction. Violence rates have been shown to be higher among unmarried couples who are living together and among those couples who are dating.[4]

Page: 50

Question #5

Answer: A

Rationale: Younger white women appear more likely to use both formal and informal resources when seeking help.[5]

Page: 51

Question #6

Answer: B

Rationale: Pregnant women are more at risk for being victims of violence than they are for preeclampsia, gestational diabetes, or placenta previa.[6]

Page: 52

Question #7

Answer: B

Rationale: Barriers to communication include a patient's belief that doctors lack time and interest in discussing abuse, patient fears regarding legal ramifications and loss of confidentiality, their fears of retaliation from intimate partners, and the physician's own discomfort with regard to feeling capable of effectively addressing issues after they have been revealed.[7–10]

Page: 52

1. Burston GR: Granny-battering [letter]. *Br Med J* 3:592, 1975.
2. Kleinschmidt KC: Elder abuse: A review. Ann Emerg Med 30:463-472, 1997. 11 Koizumi LS, et al: The public health. In *1998 Health Care Almanac and Yearbook.* New York, Faulkner and Gray, 1998, p 263.
3. Meit SS, Meit HT: Domestic violence and primary care medicine: Building understanding—Improving assessment and treatment. *Prim Care Rep* 3:165-174, 1997.
4. Stringham P: Domestic violence. *Prim Care* 26:373, 1999.
5. West CM, Kantor GK, Jasinski JL: Sociodemographic predictors and cultural barriers to help-seeking behavior by Latina and Anglo American battered women. *Violence Vict* 13:361-375, 1998.
6. Petersen R, Saltzman LE, Goodwin M, Spitz A: *Key Scientific Issues for Research on Violence Occurring around the Time of Pregnancy.* Atlanta, Centers for Disease Control and Prevention, 1997.
7. Petersen R, Moracco KE, Goldstein KM, Clark KA: Moving beyond disclosure: Women's perspectives on barriers and motivators to seeking assistance for intimate partner violence. *Women Health* 40:63-76, 2004.
8. Rodriguez MA, Sheldon WR, Bauer HM, et al: The factors associated with disclosure of intimate partner abuse. *J Fam Pract* 50:338-344, 2001.
9. Rodriguez MA, Bauer HM, McLoughlin E, et al: Screening and intervention for intimate partner abuse: Practice and attitudes of primary care physicians. *JAMA* 282:468-474, 1999.
10. Sugg N, Thompson R, Thompson D, et al: Domestic violence and primary care. *Arch Fam Med* 8:301-306, 1999.

Question #8

Answer: B

Rationale: Research indicates that, in half of households in which a batterer beats a partner, children present in the home are also physically abused.[11] However, children of all ages are at risk for the adverse effects—both physical and psychological—of living in a home in which IPV is present.[12]

Page: 52

Question #9

Answer: A

Rationale: With respect to mental illness, the literature that has studied male perpetrators of partner violence includes descriptions of antisocial personality disorder and previous childhood victimizations.[13,14] However, it also includes the perhaps more frightening prospect that male batterers are not too different from nonviolent men.[15]

Page: 52

Question #10

Answer: C

Rationale: Being female, separated or divorced, and not having children are additional demographics that are associated with those who attempt suicide.[16]

Page: 52

Question #11

Answer: B

Rationale: The average age for husbands who murder their wives is 41 years, whereas the average age for wives who murder their husbands is 37 years.

Page: 52

Question #12

Answer: C

Rationale: Table 2 presents demographic and behavioral correlates of severe domestic violence and/or spousal homicide as reflected in the literature.[17–19] Of all of the risk factors, being a white female and being a black male are noted, but being a black female is not.

Page: 52

Question #13

Answer: B

Rationale: In family medicine, it is not unusual for a physician to treat both the victim of violence and the perpetrator. Fortunately, a published consensus statement offers clinical guidelines for managing IPV when both parties are patients of the same physician.[20] The expert panel felt that the patients should be dealt with independently, that the physician should not discuss the possibility of domestic violence with the offending partner unless specifically given permission to do so by the victim, and that joint counseling is generally not advisable and should only be attempted if the violence has ended.[20] When violence is ongoing, partners should be offered individual rather than couple's counseling.

Page: 54

Question #14

Answer: B

Rationale: In this era of evidence-based medicine, sufficient evidence has yet to demonstrate the efficacy

11. Saunders DG: Prediction of wife assault. In *Assessing Dangerousness: Violence by Sexual Offenders, Batterers, and Child Abusers.* Thousand Oaks, CA, Sage Publications, 1995.
12. Edleson JL: Children's witnessing of adult domestic violence. *J Interpers Violence* 14:839-870, 1999.
13. Hanson RK, Cadsky O, Harris A, Lalonde C: Correlates of battering among 997 men: Family history, adjustment, and attitudinal differences. *Violence Vict* 12:191-208, 1997.
14. Hamberger LK, Lohr JM, Bonge D, Tolin DF: A large sample empirical typology of male spouse abusers and its relationship to dimensions of abuse. *Violence Vict* 11:277-292, 1996.
15. Konchak PS: Domestic violence: A primer for the primary care physician. *J Am Osteopath Assoc* 98:S11-S14, 1998.
16. Fremouw WJ, de Perczel M, Ellis TE: *Suicide Risk: Assessment and Response Guidelines.* New York, Pergamon Press, 1990.

17. Lystad M, Domestic violence. In Kaplan SJ (ed): *Family Violence: A Clinical and Legal Guide.* Washington, DC, American Psychiatric Press, 1996.
18. Bachman R, Saltzman LE: National Crime Victimization Survey: Violence against Women: Estimates from the Redesigned Survey. Publication no. NCJ-154348. Washington, DC, US Department of Justice, 1995.
19. Campbell JC: Prediction of homicide of and by battered women. In *Assessing Dangerousness: Violence by Sexual Offenders, Batterers, and Child Abusers.* Thousand Oaks, CA, Sage Publications, 1995.
20. Ferris LE, Norton P, Dunn EV, Gort EH: Guidelines for managing domestic abuse when male and female partners are patients of the same physician. *JAMA* 278:851-957, 1997.

of physician screening, counseling, and referral in terms of improved clinical outcomes for those experiencing IPV.[21–23]

Page: 54

Question #15

Answer: B

Rationale: States have different standards for determining maltreatment. Some states require evidence of actual harm to a child, whereas other states require only evidence of potential harm.

Page: 55

Question #16

Answer: B

Rationale: Although reports of child maltreatment involving day care centers and foster care homes seem to attract media attention, only about 3% of confirmed abuse cases occurred in these or other institutional settings. This figure was constant over the 11 years prior to 1997.[24,25]

Page: 55

Question #17

Answer: B

Rationale: Rates of rape and sexual assault are highest among nonmarried women, women under the age of 35 years, women with low income, and women living in urban or suburban areas. An estimated 91% of victims are female, and 99% of attackers are male. Most rapes and sexual assaults involved a single attacker. Persons known to the victim committed 70% of rapes and sexual assaults.[26]

Page: 58

Question #18

Answer: A

Rationale: Most injured victims of rape or sexual assault do not receive medical care for their injuries.[27,28] Less than half of these victims report their attacks to a law-enforcement agency.

Page: 59

Question #19

Answer: B

Rationale: Sexual dysfunction occurs among 25% to 40% of victims of sexual assault.

Page: 59

Question #20

Answer: B

Rationale: Sexual intercourse without force may be considered rape when the victim is unable to give consent by virtue of mental illness, mental retardation, or intoxication.

Page: 59

Question #21

Answer: B

Rationale: Observed emotional reactions are variable, but they may be characterized as the "expressed style," with overt emotional expressions such as crying, sobbing, smiling, and restlessness, or as the "controlled style," with a calm, composed, or subdued affect. The two styles of emotional reaction occur with equal frequency among female victims, but the "controlled style" is more frequently seen among male victims.

Page: 59

21. Zink T, Putnam F: Intimate partner violence research in the health care setting: What are appropriate and feasible methodological standards? *J Interpers Violence* 20:365-372, 2005.
22. Rhodes KV, Levinson W: Interventions for intimate partner violence. *JAMA* 289:601-605, 2003.
23. Wathem CN, MacMillan HL: Interventions for violence against women. *JAMA* 289:589-600, 2003.
24. Finkelhor D, Williams L, Burns N: Nursery Crimes: Sexual abuse in day care. Newbury Park, CA, Sage Publications, 1998.
25. Wang CT: Current trends in child abuse reporting and fatalities: The results of the 1997 annual fifty state survey. Chicago, The Center on Child Abuse Prevention Research, 1998.
26. Castelano SM: Criminal Victimization, 2003. Publication no. 405255. Washington, DC, US Department of Justice, 2004.

27. Rennison CM: Rape and Sexual Assault: Reporting to Police and Medical Attention. Publication no. NCJ-194530. Washington, DC, U.S. Department of Justice, 2002.
28. Tjaden P, Thoennes N: Full report of the prevalence, incidence, and consequences of violence against women: Findings from the National Violence against Women Survey. Publication no. NCJ-183781. Washington, DC, U.S. Department of Justice, 2000.

7   Answers

Question #1

Answer: D

The aging of the global population will have a profound effect on the practice of medicine in the relatively near future. It is important that family physicians be aware of these changes and that they prepare to participate in the changes that will be necessary to care for this large wave of people that will require increasing medical attention.

Page: 68

Question #2

Answer: D

Rationale: Physicians who care for adult and elderly patients are responsible not only for diagnosis and treatment but for optimizing the patient's functional capabilities. Many medical conditions affect function. In addition to looking for poor health habits, poor nutrition, and polypharmacy, physicians need to assess an individual for psychosocial stress and depression, impaired cognition, impaired senses, immobility, impaired gait, and incontinence.

Page: 72

Question #3

Answer: D

Rationale: A geriatric health questionnaire should be one of the first items obtained when evaluating a geriatric patient. It will provide information about the patient's general health and about his or her ability to perform activities of daily living, and it will also provide a review of systems, which covers important geriatric syndromes. Information gleaned from this questionnaire can stimulate further investigations of important health and functional issues, and it can help prioritize concerns that need to be addressed immediately. Also to be included in the questionnaire are the following: (1) a comprehensive review of symptoms; (2) a fall assessment; (3) questions about the patients living environment; (4) a medication history; (5) a sexual history; (6) a vaccination history; and (7) a cognitive assessment.

Pages: 73–76

Question #4

Answer: A

Rationale: Although an assessment for depression is an important part of the evaluation for dementia, the Hamilton Depression Rating Scale is designed to screen for depression and not for cognitive function. The Folstein Mini-Mental Status Examination has become the most referenced screening test; it is widely used and easily administered, and it requires 10 to 15 minutes to administer and score. The Mini-Cog Test is a combination of a clock-drawing test and a three-word recall. It detects clinically significant cognitive impairment among multiethnic persons, and it is less biased by education and literacy than the Folstein Mini-Mental Status Examination. The Trail-Making Test may be a more appropriate screening tool for cognitive disorders when a clinician needs to provide a higher degree of difficulty (e.g., in a clinical situation in which the family's story is inconsistent with the findings of the Mini-Mental State Examination, such as a case in which a patient is becoming lost or confused when going to the grocery store but who scores a 28 out of 30 on the Mini-Mental State Examination).

Pages: 74, 77, 78

Question #5

Answer: B

Rationale: The Folstein Mini-Mental Status Examination is widely used as a screening test for cognitive impairment. A score of 20 or less, when adjusted for educational background, confirms dementia. Significant cognitive impairment may be present even with much higher scores, so the test cannot be used to rule out dementia. Naming the current president of the United States is not and never has been a part of this test.

Page: 74

Question #6

Answer: D

Rationale: Dementia is a common problem among the aged, and its frequency increases with age. Diagnosing Alzheimer's disease is extremely difficult, especially during its early stages. Most patients with dementia do not complain of memory loss.

Page: 77

Question #7

Answer: D

Rationale: Undertaking the elements of the history and physical examination should allow the physician to gather the information necessary to assess whether the patient meets the diagnostic criteria for dementia listed in the *Diagnostic and Statistical Manual of Mental Disorders, Fourth Edition,* which include the characteristics listed in A, B, and C. Dementia can occur as a result of chronic medical problems that lead to progressive impairment or as the result of a sudden insult to the central nervous system that leaves the patient with permanent residual cognitive impairment.

Page: 77

Question #8

Answer: B

Rationale: When one administers the Folstein Mini-Mental State Examination, the age and educational background of the patient must be known. Even in the absence of dementia, some errors are more common with advancing age or lower educational level.

Page: 78

Question #9

Answer: A

Rationale: There are multiple ways to score a clock drawing test. The key this test is assessing whether the clock is normal or abnormal. The clock drawing test is scored by assessing the severity of errors, and a perfect score is 1. A score of 6 would mean that no reasonable representation of a clock was drawn or that no attempt was made. Abnormal clocks are associated with a 3.7-times greater relative risk of Alzheimer's disease in the presence of dementia as compared with other dementing illnesses.

Page: 78

Question #10

Answer: B

Rationale: When assessing a patient for dementia, consideration also needs to be given to depression and delirium, because these two conditions are also prevalent in the elderly population and may have an impact on memory. Unlike dementia, which has an insidious onset, delirium has an acute onset, and depression usually has a recognized onset. Dementia is usually present for months to years before presentation, whereas delirium may occur in hours to days, and depression may occur weeks to months before presentation to the health care provider. The typical complainant in dementia cases is the family, whereas patients themselves report depression. Delirium has a variety of complainants, depending on the environment in which it is diagnosed.

Page: 78

Question #11

Answer: D

Rationale: After completing a history and physical and targeted neuropsychological testing, the family physician is faced with the task of ordering appropriate laboratory tests to evaluate the patient with dementia. There are no convincing data to support or refute ordering routine laboratory tests. The majority of consensus statements recommend ordering a complete blood cell count and determining thyroid function and B_{12} levels. Other routine laboratory tests that are mentioned include syphilis serology, electrolytes, calcium, glucose, blood urea nitrogen level, and liver function tests. Less often, other ordered tests include an electrocardiogram, a chest X-ray, and general anatomical neuroimaging, such as computed tomography scanning or magnetic resonance imaging of the brain. The presence of the apolipoprotein E epsilon 4 allele predicts an increased risk of developing Alzheimer's disease, but it is not diagnostic of the disorder and therefore would not be an appropriate test for the initial investigation.

Page: 78

Question #12

Answer: D

Rationale: Cholinesterase inhibitors are approved for the treatment of mild to moderate Alzheimer's disease. They can improve cognitive function in patients with Alzheimer's disease, vascular dementia, and dementia with Lewy bodies. Memantine, which is an *N*-methyl-D-aspartate receptor antagonist, appears to be effective for patients with moderate to severe Alzheimer's disease who have a Mini-Mental State Examination score of 3 to 14. Antibiotics—including doxycycline and rifampin—given for a 3-month period have been shown to reduce cognitive decline at 6 months among patients with mild to moderate Alzheimer's disease.

Page: 79

Question #13

Answer: B

Rationale: Although it may sound logical to screen geriatric patients for cognitive impairment, there is insufficient evidence to recommend screening for cognitive impairment in the absence of dementia. Memory complaints from the patient, the family, or other caretakers should be evaluated, and patients should be followed to assess progression. Cholinesterase inhibitors have been proven to improve function among patients with dementia; however, this improvement is modest, and the medications are expensive.

Page: 80

Question #14

Answer: D

Rationale: Falls are common. About one third of community-dwelling persons over the age of 65 years fall each year, and half of the people who have fallen each year will fall again in a given year. About half of falls in community-dwelling older persons occur in the home. The incidence of falls tends to increase with age and institutionalization. Each year, about 50% of persons over the age of 80 years and about 50% of nursing home residents will fall. Women fall more frequently than men, but men tend to have greater mortality as the result of falling. In 2002, unintentional injuries were the ninth leading cause of death in persons 65 years old and older, and falls were responsible for more than 60% of unintentional injuries among this age group. It is likely that injuries sustained from falls are an important cause of death among older individuals.

Pages: 80, 81

Question #15

Answer: A

Rationale: Physical restraint use in the nursing home and hospital settings does not reduce the risk of falling, and it is actually associated with an increased risk of injury. Since the 1980s, the use of physical restraints has been appropriately and dramatically reduced. Any

medication that sedates an individual—including benzodiazepines, antipsychotics, and antihistamines—may increase fall risk. Although only tricyclic antidepressants have been well documented to increase the risk of falls, selective serotonin reuptake inhibitors are probably associated with an increased fall risk as well. Other medications that have been associated with fall risk include narcotic analgesics and anticonvulsants. One guideline for preventing falls suggests that recurrent falls and single falls associated with an observed gait abnormality should be evaluated further, whereas single falls with a normal gait need not undergo further investigation. The examination of a person who has fallen should include a measurement of postural blood pressure and pulse. Up to 30% of older persons have orthostatic hypotension, and, although some may be asymptomatic, others will become lightheaded and dizzy when rising from a seated or recumbent position.

Page: 81

Question #16

Answer: D

Rationale: There are no simple cures for the faller; however, frequency of falls has been shown to be modifiable. The physician's goals are to identify the faller and to implement interventions to prevent future falls, especially injurious ones. Most single, untargeted interventions are unlikely to reduce the risk of falling, but some have been shown to help. Beneficial single interventions include the modification of environmental hazards in the home; the discontinuation of psychotropic drugs; and supervised exercise programs that improve gait, balance, and strength.

Page: 82

Question #17

Answer: B

Rationale: The presence of falls alone is not a strict contraindication to anticoagulation for atrial fibrillation. It has been estimated that a person on warfarin would need to fall 300 times per year for the risk of a fall-related bleed to outweigh the risk of stroke as a result of atrial fibrillation. The presence of cognitive impairment alters the fall evaluation, and current evidence suggests that multifactorial interventions are not likely to succeed for the cognitively impaired. Cardiac pacing for fallers with cardioinhibitory carotid sinus hypersensitivity reduces the risk of falling. If a patient is found to have orthostatic hypotension, antihypertensives and diuretics should be adjusted and consideration given to the use of other interventions, including wearing supportive stockings, instructing patients to rise carefully and ensure balance before ambulating, and liberalizing salt and fluid in the diet.

Page: 82

Question #18

Answer: D

Rationale: Perhaps the most useful test of integrated function is the "get up and go" test. This test may be scored, timed, or used as an overall assessment of the patient's gait, stability, balance, and strength. The patient is asked to stand from a seated position, walk about 10 feet (3 meters), turn around, walk back, and sit down again. Multiple aspects of this activity need to be observed so that a proper assessment or score may be given. The observer needs to note if the patient pushes off of the chair or rocks back and forth several times in an effort to arise, which would reflect leg strength being diminished. Gait abnormalities, such as poor step clearance and shuffling, need to be observed. A wide-based stance and slow, multiple-point turning may reveal poor balance.

Page: 82

Initial Evaluation of Falls

History
Circumstances of fall
Vision/hearing deficits
Medical conditions
Medications, especially sedatives, psychotropics, antihypertensives, narcotics, and anticonvulsants
Functional abilities

Physical Examination
Postural blood pressure
Heart rhythm
"Get up and go" test
Visual acuity
Targeted neurological examination
Targeted musculoskeletal examination
Hemodynamic response to carotid sinus massage, in appropriate patients

Diagnostic studies
None required routinely
If indicated in the appropriate patient: complete blood cell count, blood urea nitrogen level, creatinine level, electrolytes, glucose, thyroid function, vitamin B_{12}, Holter monitor

In Rakel RE, editor: *Textbook of family medicine*, ed 7, Philadelphia, WB Saunders, 2007.

Question #19

Answer: C

Rationale: Depression is a common disorder among the geriatric population. The diagnosis of depression requires skillful questioning of the patient. Frequently, the patient presenting with a complaint does not suspect the diagnosis of depression. The death of a spouse, which is rated among the most stressful of life events, can produce the symptoms of a major depressive disorder. Annually, 800,000 Americans lose their spouse. A third of widows meet the criteria for major depression 1 month after the death, and, of that third, half remain clinically depressed 1 year later. With uncomplicated bereavement, the most disturbing symptoms generally resolve within 2 months. Individuals who continue to meet the criteria for major depression after 2 months should receive antidepressants or other nonpharmacologic therapies. Although depression may be one of the first symptoms noted at the onset of a dementing illness, depression and dementia are often comorbid conditions rather than one disease mimicking the other.

Page: 83

Question #20

Answer: B

Rationale: The diagnosis of depression in patients with Alzheimer's disease is difficult in that the clinical manifestations of depression among these patients are even less typical than those seen among other older patients. Frank sadness is often less prominent than irritability, worry, fear, or anxiety. Functional decline may be manifested by the lack of ability to sustain activities of daily living. A common change in depressed patients with Alzheimer's disease is apathy, with a prominent loss of motivation. Guilt and suicidal thoughts among these patients are uncommon, and, although suicidal feelings are rare, they should be thoroughly evaluated. The Geriatric Depression Scale has been extensively studied and found to remain valid and reliable for individuals with Mini-Mental State Examination scores of 15 or more. Psychotic symptoms, such as delusions and hallucinations, are more likely to accompany depression in patients with Alzheimer's disease than in patients without dementia. This clinical picture can lead to mistaking the disturbance as psychosis rather than depression. If, in the clinical setting, there is doubt about the diagnosis of depression in the patient with cognitive impairment, an empiric treatment trial is usually warranted. However, the overall evidence offers weak support for the idea that antidepressants are an effective therapy for patients with depression and dementia.

Pages: 83, 84

Question #21

Answer: C

Rationale: Watchful waiting may be appropriate for patients who are reluctant to start depression-specific treatment, who have symptoms of recent onset that are not disabling, and who do not meet the criteria for major depression. Various antidepressants appear to be equally efficacious for treating major depressive illness among older adults. The selective serotonin reuptake inhibitors are considered first-line antidepressant therapy for late-life depression. Mirtazapine may be a useful alternative, especially for patients who would benefit from weight gain and improved sleep. Expert consensus findings recommend the combined use of psychotherapy and antidepressants for the treatment of late-life depression, specifically for episodes in which a clearly identified psychosocial stressor is present. Electroconvulsive therapy is a first-line treatment for patients who are at serious risk for suicide or life-threatening poor nutritional intake as a result of major depression. Amitriptyline offers no distinct advantage over other antidepressants, and it has many potential side effects that make it a second or third choice.

Page: 86

Question #22

Answer: C

Rationale: Hypothyroidism, diabetes, and glucocorticoid excess are frequent comorbidities of depression, but malignancy (especially pancreatic cancer) is the only true etiology for depression that was an option for this question. Physicians are taught to screen for underlying medical illnesses in a patient who presents with depression; however, the diagnostic yield is low for such evaluation when it is used in all cases. It is true that depression may be a presenting manifestation of a metabolic abnormality such as glucocorticoid excess or thyroid disease, but depression resulting from the biological effects of medical diseases or medications is less common than depression that simply coexists at higher rates among patients with these chronic physical illnesses. Vascular disease is another category of comorbid conditions that is associated with depression; depression is commonly seen among patients with coronary artery disease, stroke, and cerebral vascular disease. Depression and cancer of the pancreas often occur together, and symptoms of depression and anxiety may even precede knowledge of cancer diagnosis. Clinicians must have a strong suspicion for comorbid disease in the patient who presents with his or her first episode of depression late in life.

Page: 87

Question #23

Answer: D

Rationale: Late-life depression is associated with disproportionately high rates of completed suicide and high mortality rates independent of suicide. Rates of suicide increase markedly among Americans who are more than 75 years old, especially among white men. Rates are greater than five-fold higher as compared with the general population after the age of 85 years. Late-life suicide is characterized by less warning, higher lethality, and greater prevalence of depression and physical illness. The co-occurrence of alcohol-use disorders and depression increases suicide risk. A sobering fact for clinicians is that the majority of patients who attempt or complete a suicide have recently been seen by a health care provider.

Page: 87

Question #24

Answer: D

Rationale: Continence requires that the urinary system adequately perform its two main functions: storage and emptying. To achieve proper storage, the bladder must accommodate increasing amounts of urine under low pressure, the outlet must be closed at a relatively high pressure, fullness must be sensed, and no involuntary abnormal contractions should occur. Certain changes in the urinary system occur with aging, most of which result in increasing difficulty with maintaining continence. Bladder capacity tends to decline, whereas the post-void residual increases. Involuntary bladder contractions increase with age and are found more frequently among older incontinent persons. Among women, urethral resistance pressures decrease, whereas men have greater urethral resistance pressures as a result of enlargement of the prostrate gland and lengthening of the urethra. Although these age-related changes may contribute to incontinence, incontinence should not be considered part of normal aging.

Page: 88

Question #25

Answer: D

Rationale: Reversible causes of acute incontinence include urinary tract infection, vaginitis/urethritis, fecal impaction, volume overload, hyperglycemia, hypercalcemia, delirium, acutely restricted mobility, acute outlet obstruction, and medications (e.g., diuretics, anticholinergics, narcotics).

Page: 88

Question #26

Answer: D

Rationale: Stress incontinence is common among women, and it is unusual among men. Patients present with loss of urine when intra-abdominal pressure is increased, such as with laughing, coughing, sneezing, or lifting. Urge incontinence is so named because the patient experiences the sudden urge to void followed by urine loss. With overflow incontinence, patients may report continual urine loss, or they may have symptoms similar to those seen among patients with urge or stress incontinence. Functional incontinence occurs when a patient lacks the ability or the desire to reach the toilet when the need to urinate arises. Patients with functional incontinence often suffer from dementia or depression, and they have more frailty and comorbidities.

Page: 88

Question #27

Answer: B

Rationale: In addition to a urinalysis, the only other test that should be obtained at the initial evaluation of a patient with urine incontinence is the post-void residual (PVR). The urinalysis is used to screen for infection, glucosuria, and hematuria. To rule out overflow incontinence, PVR is measured by straight catheterization or bladder scanning after the patient attempts to completely empty his or her bladder. A PVR of less than 50 to 100 mL (depending on the reference) is normal, whereas a PVR of 200 mL or more signifies abnormal urine retention. The other tests listed may be appropriate based on the history or on the findings on the urinalysis or physical examination; however, they should not be considered routine.

Page: 89

Question #28

Answer: D

Rationale: The management of chronic urinary incontinence can be improved by encouraging patients to void frequently during the day and always before bedtime. For patients with nocturnal problems, fluids should be avoided 3 or 4 hours before bedtime. Caffeine and alcohol consumption should at least be curtailed and preferably avoided. In appropriate circumstances, diuretics may be reduced or eliminated. Patients should be educated about the use of protective undergarments, incontinence pads, and environmental modifications (e.g., bedside commodes, urinals). Additional specific treatment should then be implemented, depending on the cause or type of incontinence diagnosed during the evaluation. Finally, patients should be encouraged to pursue treatments until they are satisfied with the outcome and as functionally independent as possible.

Pages: 91, 92

Question #29

Answer: A

Rationale: For the statement given in option A to be correct, it should read as follows: Hormone replacement therapy (estrogen alone or estrogen plus progestin) in menopausal women is associated with an *increased* risk of all types of urinary incontinence and should *not* be used for the prevention or treatment of incontinence. The level of evidence for this statement is an A, and all of the other answers are true and carry a level of evidence of A as well.

Page: 93

Question #30

Answer: D

Rationale: The decision of whether or not to prescribe a drug must be made after the consideration of a number of factors, of which age is only one. The physician must also consider the patient's functional status, comorbidities, other medications, and personal preferences and values. Medications that are likely to benefit older patients should not be avoided to maintain some arbitrarily short drug list. Meanwhile, physicians must be extremely vigilant when prescribing, especially among the frail elderly, and they must continually review patients' medication lists with an eye for adverse effects, high-risk drugs, drug–drug interactions, and drug–disease interactions.

Page: 93

Question #31

Answer: D

Rationale: The mistreatment of older adults is a problem of unknown magnitude, with estimates ranging from 1% to 10% of the elderly population being affected annually. Perhaps the best estimate of elder abuse is available from National Center on Elder Abuse Study, which reported that nearly 550,000 adults over the age of 60 years were the victims of abuse in domestic settings in 1996. However, only about 20% of such cases were reported. One of the societal responses to the growing awareness of elder mistreatment is the creation of state mandatory reporting laws, which name health care providers as mandatory reporters. Although these statutes were instituted to increase awareness and decrease occurrence of elder mistreatment, there is no convincing evidence to support their effectiveness. The issue of elder mistreatment is especially significant for physicians, because they are in a unique position to detect abuse and neglect firsthand. It must be kept in mind that, like other forms of domestic violence, the situation tends to escalate if interventions are not initiated. In addition, the obligation to report elder abuse supersedes the privilege of confidential communications between physicians and patients.

Pages: 97, 98

Question #1

Answer: C

Rationale: Although discussing a terminal condition may be frightening to the patient, honest and frank discussions can relieve the patient's anxiety and promote open conversation. Hospital rounds made rapidly or statements such as "don't worry" can effectively close communication about the patient's concerns. Physicians can also be uncomfortable discussing a terminal condition, but coming to grips with these feelings can help the physician better address the patient's concerns and wishes.

Pages: 107, 108

Question #2

Answer: B

Rationale: Patients facing end-of-life care often experience an awakening or intensification of religious and spiritual issues; acknowledging this can improve communication with the patient. By listening respectfully, the patient will feel less isolated and alone during his or her final days.

Page: 111

Question #3

Answer: A

Rationale: Protraction of the dying process is a modern epidemic. Relieving the suffering rather than prolonging it should be the focus of the care of the terminally ill. Careful consideration of the quality of life should guide decisions before treatment options are exhausted.

Page: 112

Question #4

Answer: B

Rationale: The method of the administration of pain medication is often more important than the particular drug used. Ending the cycle of uncontrolled pain and preventing pain require the use of a narcotic medication on a regular schedule, around the clock. Additional booster doses of medication can be used for breakthrough pain, when necessary. Effective doses for booster medication are approximately half of the regular dose given at 4-hour intervals. As-needed use of larger doses of narcotics is likely to promote oversedation, and it is unlikely to break the cycle of uncontrolled pain.

Page: 113

Question #5

Answer: C

Rationale: Patients may benefit from nonpharmacologic techniques of pain management, including transcutaneous electrical nerve stimulation, exercise, heat, cold, acupuncture, relaxation, imagery, hypnosis, biofeedback, behavior therapy, psychotherapy, music therapy, and massage. Cold works especially well on neuropathic pain.

Page: 112

Question #6

Answer: B

Rationale: Meperidine has a short duration of action and a low oral potency, but it is also a toxic metabolite, which can cause seizures. Pentazocine has a high incidence of psychomimetic side effects, including hallucinations and confusion. Ibuprofen is an excellent co-analgesic that is useful for treating pain from bone lesions, but ibuprofen is not an opioid agent. Hydrocodone and oxycodone represent good initial choices. Additional alternatives include oral morphine and hydromorphone.

Page: 113

Question #7

Answer: B

Rationale: Dyspnea may have a variety of causes, all of which should be considered. When treatable etiologies have been addressed, the focus should be on symptom control. A careful titration of the booster dose of opioid is an effective way of treating the dyspnea, with little danger of respiratory depression. Oxygen is appropriate in select cases, but it is less convenient and more expensive, which may limit its use. Before prescribing antibiotics, the physician should consider whether their use will improve the quality of life or just prolong the process of dying.

Page: 118

Question #8

Answer: C

Rationale: Constipation is a very common problem that must be adequately treated to improve the patient's quality of life. Although regular stimulant laxatives may be needed, bulk agents are rarely successful, and they may make the patient's complaints worse as a result of increased gas production. Enemas and/or suppositories may be needed until an adequate regimen of laxatives is found.

Page: 118

Question #9

Answer: D

Rationale: Nausea and vomiting represent both common and challenging management issues for dying patients. Treatable causes of nausea and vomiting should be evaluated and corrected; overfeeding may be the problem when nasogastric or tube feeding is being used. Because there is no evidence that forced feeding prolongs life, discontinuing the tube feeding for a period of time is warranted. Combinations of antiemetics, which have different mechanisms of action, are also recommended. When simpler approaches of antiemetic agents fail, the subcutaneous infusion of these agents can be a very effective option.

Page: 118

Question #10

Answer: A

Rationale: The patient's dietary intake is often a focus of the patient's family during the treatment of cancer and terminal illness. The causes of the cancer cachexia are poorly understood, and there is no evidence that protein supplementation improves clinical outcomes. The evidence, based on a review of the clinical trials of parenteral nutrition among patients receiving

chemotherapy, suggests that the use of parenteral nutrition support was associated with net harm.

Page: 119

Question #11

Answer: D

Rationale: For maximum effectiveness, booster doses of pain medication should be quick acting. Slow-release morphine (MS Contin) and methadone are excellent choices for chronic pain management; however, their long duration of action make them less suited for booster dosage. Morphine solution (Roxanol) is an effective choice for booster analgesia; it can be given sublingually to patients who are too weak to swallow, and it can be used for a regular dosage every 4 hours as well as for a booster dosage. Pentazocine has a high incidence of psychomimetic side effects, including hallucinations and confusion, and it is no more effective than codeine; its use should be avoided.

Page: 119, 120

Question #12

Answer: C

Rationale: Persistent hiccupping in the terminally ill may arise from a variety of causes, including lesions affecting the phrenic nerve, gastric distention, and uremia. Baclofen, chlorpromazine, metoclopramide, and haloperidol have been used with success for managing this troublesome symptom.

Page: 118

Question #13

Answer: C

Rationale: Intramuscular injections are painful to the patient, and restarting intravenous infusions can be difficult to manage at home. At least 50 mL of medication per day can be delivered through a small butterfly needle placed into the subcutaneous space. Using a miniature pump, morphine, hydromorphone, metoclopramide, and haloperidol can all be given via a subcutaneous infusion. Fentanyl is available for use as a transdermal patch, which may be effective for a wide variety of patients. Because the patches depend on a subcutaneous fat reservoir to work, they are not the best choice for an emaciated patient.

Page: 113

Question #14

Answer: A

Rationale: The hospice concept is directed toward providing compassionate care for people facing a life-limiting illness or injury. The principle requirement for hospice admission is a life-limiting illness with a life expectancy of 6 months or less.

Page: 120

Question #15

Answer: D

Rationale: A living will is a type of advance directive that addresses the limitation of life-sustaining treatment in the face of life-threatening illness. Approximately 20% of Americans have living wills. Living wills are often ineffective because they are too vague, or they may attempt to cover too many scenarios. A health care surrogate serves as the health care proxy (medical power of attorney) to make medical decisions in the incapacitated patient's interest. A durable power of attorney designates a person to make health, financial, and legal decisions if the patient is unable to do so. It is best to have a patient both complete a living will and designate a health care surrogate.

Page: 123

Question #16

Answer: B

Rationale: Asking questions that convey empathy and honesty are most likely to allow the physician to understand the patient's needs and wishes. Encouraging an environment in which the patient is allowed to express his or her feelings and concerns is helpful.

Page: 108

Question #17

Answer: C

Rationale: Bad news is best delivered in person in a quiet, private location. Health Insurance Portability and Accountability Act (HIPAA) laws require identifying additional people present and their relationship to the patient. HIPAA violations can be avoided by simply asking, "Would you like for these people to be present while we discuss your personal health situation?"

Sitting at eye level and watching the patient's body language can alert the physician that the patient needs more time to react to the magnitude of the news. Family members who are present can provide a useful second set of ears.

Page: 111

Question #18

Answer: B

Rationale: Understanding oral morphine equivalents is a useful way to select a more potent agent when greater pain relief is needed. Table 4 lists several of the commonly used products for the treatment of chronic pain. Oxycodone is a potent agent that is roughly four times stronger than similar hydrocodone products (8-mg equivalent vs. 1- to 2-mg equivalent).

Page: 109

Question #19

Answer: D

Rationale: Commonly used 1-to-10 pain scale ratings are broken down as mild pain (1–3) moderate pain (4–7), and severe pain (8–10). For chronic moderate and severe pain, medication should be given around the clock to achieve a target level of relief level of less than 4. Complete absence of pain may be an unreasonable goal, and anxiety can exacerbate the perception of pain. Reassuring the patient that medication will be adjusted until the cycle of pain is broken is a good way to relieve this concern. The addition of an anxiolytic medication may be necessary when significant anxiety is also present.

Page: 112

Question #20

Answer: D

Rationale: Immediate-release opioids are more effective as a first step, and switching or adding slow-release products may be done after the pain cycle is controlled. When opioids cause side effects, switching to a comparable dose of a different opioid is useful. Other approaches include adding an adjuvant drug to the opioid. Anxiety is effectively addressed with benzodiazepines, but this class of drug will not control the pain cycle in the absence of an opioid.

Page: 112

Question #21

Answer: A

Rationale: Modern medical science has allowed for a greater lifespan. Instead of dying from acute infectious disease, many patients now deal with chronic disease. In the situation of terminal illness, medical care should focus on improving the quality rather than increasing the quantity of life.

Page: 110

Question #22

Answer: A

Rationale: Physicians can lose enthusiasm for the care of a patient after an illness is recognized as incurable. Studies have also demonstrated that nurses and other personnel spend less time with the terminally ill. Because abandonment is a major concern of this group of patients, physicians must be aware of the need to reduce the time that these patients spend alone each day.

Page: 112

Question #23

Answer: A

Rationale: Although the causes of the cachexia of cancer are not completely understood, a search for treatable etiologies is warranted. Oral candidiasis can certainly interfere with eating, and it is effectively treated after diagnosis.

Page: 119

Question #24

Answer: B

Rationale: The anticonvulsant gabapentin (Neurontin) given in a dose of 100–400 mg orally one to four times a day is a useful addition for the treatment of the burning, shooting pain caused by nerve damage. Amitriptyline, which is a tricyclic antidepressant, is also effective in a lower dosage (10–50 mg at bedtime) than the antidepressant dose. Newer agents like venlafaxine (Effexor) and duloxetine (Cymbalta) are also effective for neuropathic pain, and they have fewer side effects.

Page: 117

Question #25

Answer: B

Rationale: Assisted suicide involves the prescribing of large quantities of drugs for the purpose of empowering a patient to take his or her own life. Although many physicians are uncomfortable with this issue, this practice is legal in Oregon under certain circumstances.

Page: 123

Question #1

Answer: C

Rationale: Confusion about patient autonomy may place the physician in danger of becoming a "hired hand" of the patient, and it may convert the physician-patient relationship into a purely commercial arrangement. The physician and the patient can best work together through a cooperative effort. The physician-patient relationship may also suffer as a result of inappropriate intervention from outside parties.

Page: 127

Question #2

Answer: D

Rationale: Physicians have an obligation to practice within professional standards; however, at the same time, they may refrain from violation of their own moral and religious beliefs. The common goal in the physician-patient relationship is to maintain the health of the patient. The physician-patient relationship cannot exist exclusive of third-party influence, but the health of the patient must remain primary.

Page: 127

Question #3

Answer: E

Rationale: The purpose of the preplacement examination is not only to determine fitness and protect workers from illness and injury but also to protect employers and to collect baseline data for the future treatment of potential job-related illnesses and injuries. To complete such an evaluation, the employer must provide the physician with a specific job description to include physical and psychological requirements as well as potential exposures to toxins. The physician should then render an opinion about the prospective employee's ability to perform the job without posing a risk to himself or herself or to others.

Page: 127

Question #4

Answer: A

Rationale: Investigating nonmedical causes of absenteeism for employers or school administrators may damage the physician-patient relationship and foster patient mistrust. Physicians should encourage employers and school administrators to develop nonmedical strategies for policing casual absenteeism.

Page: 127

Question #5

Answer: C

Rationale: The Hippocratic Oath and the principles of medical ethics of the American Medical Association clearly define the principles of confidentiality, which remain widely accepted. Emphasis on the patient's right to privacy has always served as the cornerstone of those confidentiality principles. The recent change in emphasis has not been driven by the American Medical Association guidelines but by changes in health care delivery models, which have necessitated the increased sharing of information among members of the health care team.

Page: 128

Question #6

Answer: B

Rationale: Specific laws vary from jurisdiction to jurisdiction, but state laws commonly require the reporting of communicable diseases as well as child custody disputes, suspected child abuse, elder abuse, and gunshot wounds. Work releases, family inquiries, and third-party payer requests for information all require patient consent.

Page: 128

Question #7

Answer: B

Rationale: Information about pediatric patients is uniformly provided directly to the parents, and information about competent adult patients is provided directly to the patient. An adult patient who has been declared incompetent is generally not capable of medical decision-making; thus, patient information must be disclosed to a person serving as a durable power of attorney for health care. Considerable controversy exists, however, about the moral and legal approach to the confidentiality of information involving adolescent patients, particularly with respect to contraceptive issues, abortion, treatment for venereal diseases, substance abuse, and psychiatric problems.

Page: 128

Question #8

Answer: B

Rationale: The phrase *informed consent* was first documented in the court case *Salgo v. Leland Stanford, Jr. University Board of Trustees*, which was recorded in 1957. The fundamental principle of informed consent has come to be accepted in the relationships between patients and physicians.

Page: 129

Question #9

Answer: C

Rationale: Emergency exception and therapeutic privilege are both recognized exceptions to the principle of informed consent. Emergency exception is invoked when emergency treatment is necessary and consent cannot be obtained in a timely fashion. Therapeutic privilege is invoked when there is the perception that the conveyance of information will induce psychological harm to the patient.

Page: 129

Question #10

Answer: A

Rationale: It is standard practice in most institutions to obtain written documentation of informed consent in advance of invasive procedures; however, in reality, the principles of informed consent apply to all medical interventions, and they do not require a signed document. Signed consent forms are simply written evidence of informed consent that has already been obtained. Informed consent is believed to build trust through joint patient–physician decision-making that results in a clinical benefit.

Page: 129

Question #11

Answer: A

Rationale: The two informed consent proposals that have been adopted by America's courts are the professional practice standard and the reasonable person standard. The reasonable person standard maintains that consent is informed if the patient has been provided with the proper information that a reasonable person would require to make a decision about a particular health care option. The professional practice standard maintains that the consent is informed if the patient has been provided information that reasonable medical practitioners would ordinarily provide under similar circumstances.

Page: 129

Question #12

Answer: B

Rationale: The majority of courts have adopted the professional practice standard, because it is typically less demanding; however, many individuals believe that the reasonable person standard better corresponds with the goals of informed consent. Clinicians are best advised to use the reasonable person standard, which provides the clinical and moral benefits of informed consent while fulfilling the basic legal requirements.

Page: 129

Question #13

Answer: E

Rationale: The elements of informed consent under the reasonable person standard are clearly delineated in Table 9-1 from the text. Essential elements should include a description of the patient's condition and of the proposed treatment, with information about the benefits, risks, and costs of the treatment as well as alternative treatment options.

Page: 129

Question #14

Answer: A

Rationale: Although patient incompetence may certainly contribute to noncompliance, most cases of noncompliance are related to communication failure, lack of trust, and psychological factors. True value differences between the physician and the patient exist only in a minority of cases.

Page: 129

Question #15

Answer: B

Rationale: Physicians should not hesitate to discuss drug costs with their patients, and they should not hesitate to explore less expensive but satisfactory medications, even if they are not optimal choices. Decisions about unacceptable side effects should be based on the patient's values and tolerances. Barriers to compliance should be explored and addressed by the physician rather than simply accepting noncompliance as an inevitable consequence of health care.

Page: 130

Question #16

Answer: D

Rationale: Even after a primary care physician initiates a referral, he or she remains the patient's primary physician, and he or she remains responsible for the quality of the patient's care. The referral process is not complete until the consultant communicates findings, treatments, results, and recommendations to the primary care physician. The basic principles of informed consent apply to the referral process (as they do to other health-care decisions).

Page: 130

Question #17

Answer: B

Rationale: Although dedication to one's profession and commitment to perfection are desirable qualities, they are often coupled with unrealistic expectations, which may consequently lead to insecurity and guilt. Physicians who promote the recognition and expression of emotion in their patients as well as in themselves maintain humanistic qualities and allow the opportunity for self-healing and well-being. Improper expression, use, or interpretation of emotion can deprofessionalize the physician–patient relationship and lead to undesirable consequences.

Page: 131

Question #18

Answer: B

Rationale: Public support of assisted death has in fact increased over the past decade, according to public opinion polls. Most Americans favor the legalization of assisted death, and most terminally ill patients prefer palliative care. Physicians practicing in teaching hospitals were found to be particularly uncomfortable with death, less likely to disclose a terminal diagnosis, and more likely to provide curative treatment during the last months of life.

Page: 132

Question #19

Answer: C

Rationale: Physician-assisted suicide has been legal in the United States in the state of Oregon since October 27, 1997, when the Death With Dignity Act allowed physicians to prescribe lethal doses of controlled substances to patients who are terminally ill.

Pages: 132, 133

Question #20

Answer: B

Rationale: Recent published findings indicate that physicians continue to undertreat pain despite advances in pain management. It is also suggested that terminally ill patients are frequently overtreated against their will.

Page: 133

Question #21

Answer: E

Rationale: One of the unique qualities of the Terri Schiavo case was the unusually large number of intervening individuals, including family; religious organizations; both state and federal judicial systems; the state legislature, including the governor of Florida; and the federal legislature, including congressional physicians and the president of the United States.

Page: 133

Question #22

Answer: E

Rationale: The Karen Quinlan case in 1976, the Nancy Beth Cruzan case in 1990, and the Terri Schiavo case in 2005 all had an impact on right-to-die thinking and public opinion about right-to-die issues.

Page: 134

Question #23

Answer: C

Rationale: Surveys have repeatedly shown over the last 20 years that a majority of Americans would prefer to not be kept alive in a persistent vegetative state. Competent patients have the right to refuse cardiopulmonary resuscitation, mechanical respiration, chemotherapy, blood transfusion, renal dialysis, artificial nutrition, and hydration, even if the physician disagrees. Mentally incompetent patients have a right to refuse life-saving medical treatment based on their previously expressed desires.

Page: 129

Question #24

Answer: D

Rationale: Passage of the Patient Self-Determination Act after the Nancy Beth Cruzan case required clinics and hospitals to offer advance directives to all of their patients. U.S. citizens are not required to designate a durable power of attorney for health care unless they choose to do so. The intent of the legislation was to enable health care recipients and their families to make end-of-life decisions.

Page: 134

Question #25

Answer: C

Rationale: The authors recommend that physicians learn to distinguish between competence and perfectionism, dedication and workaholism, and compassion and sentimentalism. Doing so will help with their efforts to maintain personal health and well-being and to avoid the occupational hazards of the medical profession, including alcoholism, substance abuse, divorce, burnout, and suicide.

Page: 131

Question #1

Answer: B

Rationale: Multiple studies have failed to show a benefit of the periodic complete physical examination.[1] In addition, the Canadian Task Force on the Periodic Health Examination[2] and the USPSTF's Guide to Clinical Preventive Services[3] challenged the usefulness of the annual physical examination, both publishing guidelines that emphasized proven methods to screen for common causes of morbidity and mortality.

Page: 139

Question #2

Answer: D

Rationale: The financial cost to the patient and the use of the physician's time; the high false-positive rate, with potentially harmful follow-up evaluations; and the false sense of security provided to patients with normal findings have been reasons given for not performing the physical examination.[4]

Page: 139

Question #3

Answer: C

Rationale: The Denver Developmental Screening Test has a test-retest reliability of 97%. It assesses the categories of gross and fine motor movements and social and language development; sensory function is not evaluated. It is recommended by the AAP for all infants and children for screening purposes.

Page: 140

Question #4

Answer: A

Rationale: The AAFP and the AAP recommend height and weight measurements for all patients. The AAP recommends that infants have head-circumference measurements until they are 2 to 3 years old.

Page: 140

Question #5

Answer: C

Rationale: The AAP, the American Heart Association, and the American Medical Association (AMA) recommend the routine screening of asymptomatic children during well-child visits beginning at the age of 3 years. Before this time, measurements are limited by inherent inaccuracies. Elevated blood pressure in children is more commonly a result of secondary hypertension as compared with adults (28% vs. <5%, respectively),[5] and it may be reversible. However, the USPSTF and the AAFP cite insufficient evidence to recommend for or against routine screening.

Page: 140

Question #6

Answer: B

Rationale: The AAP and the USPSTF recommend screening for amblyopia, strabismus, and defects in visual acuity for all children who are less than 5 years old. However, the USPSTF finds insufficient evidence for or against screening for visual acuity in children who are more than 5 years old, whereas the AAP recommends continually screening for visual acuity every 1 to 2 years throughout childhood.

Page: 140

Question #7

Answer: B

Rationale: Universal newborn screening is not required by all states, and all states have not adopted this policy. The AAP, the American Speech-Language-Hearing Association, and the Bright Futures guidelines

1. Gordon PR, Senf J: Is the annual complete physical examination necessary? *Arch Intern Med* 159:909-910, 1999.
2. Canadian Task Force on the Periodic Health Examination (1979).
3. USPSTF's Guide to Clinical Preventive Services (1989).
4. Frame PS: The complete annual physical examination refuses to die [editorial; see comments]. *J Fam Pract* 40:543-545, 1995.

5. Feld LG, Springate JE: Hypertension in children. *Curr Probl Pediatr* 18:317373, 1988.

endorse universal screening before hospital discharge. The USPSTF has found good evidence that newborn hearing screening leads to the earlier identification of problems, but no sufficient evidence exists to support the idea that screening had an impact on future hearing abilities.

Pages: 140, 141

Question #8

Answer: A

Rationale: Although maple syrup urine disease may be included in the screening recommended by an individual state, it is not included in the recommendations of the AAP and the AAFP. Infants tested before they are 24 hours old should be retested when they are 2 weeks old. Ill and premature infants should be tested when they are approximately 7 days old.

Page: 141

Question #9

Answer: B

Rationale: The AAP, the CDC, and the USPSTF all recommend screening only those with a high risk of lead exposure for elevated blood lead levels (>10 g/dL). These high-risk individuals include children with significant exposure to homes built before 1950; those from areas where more than 12% of children screened have elevated blood lead levels; those living in areas of known lead industry or high lead water levels; those who have received lead-containing ethnic remedies; those who have close contacts with high lead levels; and those having close contact with individuals with hobbies or occupations that involve significant lead exposure.

Page: 141

Question #10

Answer: B

Rationale: The AAP and the AMA both recommend screening for elevated cholesterol beginning in children who are more than 2 years old who have a parent or grandparent with arteriosclerosis before the age of 55 years or who have a parent with a total serum cholesterol level of more than 240 mg/dL.

Pages: 141, 142

Question #11

Answer: A

Rationale: Universal PPD screening for all children is unnecessary, except for certain high-risk individuals.

Page: 142

Question #12

Answer: D

Rationale: Warning stickers such as the "Mr. Yuck" stickers have been found to draw children's attention and thus are not recommended. Childproof containers are helpful if the items cannot be stored away.

Page: 142

Question #13

Answer: A

Rationale: The AAFP strongly recommends counseling parents about the harmful effects of secondhand smoke. All of the choices listed except preterm labor are increased with exposure to secondhand smoke.

Page: 143

Question #14

Answer: B

Rationale: Accidental death is the leading cause of death during the school-aged and adolescent periods.[6]

Page: 146

Question #15

Answer: B

Rationale: The USPSTF and the AAFP strongly recommend screening all sexually active females—but not males—for chlamydia. Screening tests include DNA probes obtained by endocervical or urethral swabs. Significant declines in the prevalence of this disease have been noted over the past 10 years in areas in which screening has been instituted.

Pages: 144, 151

6. Kochanek KD, Smith BL, Anderson RN: Deaths: preliminary data for 1999. *Natl Vital Stat Rep* 49(3):1-48, 2001.

Question #16

Answer: C

Rationale: The USPSTF recommends all of the listed screenings except for HIV serology, which should only be offered to those at high risk. This category includes those adolescents being treated for other sexually transmitted diseases, those with a history of homosexual activity, past or present intravenous drug users, those who have had sex for money, and those who have had any partner with a known sexually transmitted disease. Chlamydia and gonorrhea testing is recommended by the USPSTF for female adolescents who are sexually active, who are 25 years old or younger, and who are considered high risk (i.e., having more than one sexual partner within 1 year). The USPSTF recommends that Pap smears should begin within 3 years after a woman becomes sexually active or at the age of 21 years. However, the AAFP, the AAP, the American College of Obstetricians and Gynecologists, and the AMA recommend Pap smears starting at time of sexual activity or at the age of 18 years.

Page: 145

Question #17

Answer: A

Rationale: Many of the problems facing adolescents are related to psychosocial and unintentional injury, and thus counseling becomes very important. The mnemonic *HEADS,* which addresses *h*ome, *e*ducation, *a*ctivities, *d*rugs and *d*epression, and *s*ex and *s*uicide is helpful to remember when interviewing teens.

Page: 146

Question #18

Answer: D

Rationale: Unintentional injuries and motor vehicle accidents are among the leading causes of death in the adolescent age group. Major areas of counseling for injury prevention include driving safety, bicycle safety, water safety, and firearm safety. The AAFP and the AAP recommend counseling this age group to wear helmets while biking and seat belts while riding in a car, to have appropriate supervision when swimming, and to avoid having guns in the home. Complete physicals, screening for anemia, and conducting hearing and vision screenings are not recommended for this age

group by the USPSTF. Lastly, adolescents should be interviewed, at least in part, without parents present.

Page: 146

Question #19

Answer: A

Rationale: The tetanus booster is now given to children who are between 11 and 12 years old. The pneumonia vaccine is given only to high-risk groups and to those over the age of 65 years. Varicella vaccine is given at the age of 12 months or 11 to 12 years if there is no history of varicella infection or serologic immunity. Inactivated polio vaccine is given before the age of 2 years.

Page: 147

Question #20

Answer: B

Rationale: The USPSTF makes no recommendation regarding the screening interval for hypertension. However, JNC V11 recommends screening every 2 years for patients with normal blood pressure (<120/80 mm Hg) and annually for those with blood pressures in the prehypertensive range (120–139/80–89 mm Hg).

Page: 148

Question #21

Answer: D

Rationale: The USPSTF recommends against screening for coronary artery disease among patients of average risk as a result of insufficient evidence to recommend either for or against screening. However, the American Heart Association and the American College of Cardiology recommend screening males who are more than 45 years old and females who are more than 55 years old with multiple risk factors who plan to start a vigorous exercise program or those employed in occupations in which their incapacitation could put others at risk (e.g., pilots).

Page: 149

Question #22

Answer: B

Rationale: The USPSTF and the AAFP recommend against screening asymptomatic patients for PVD, because no benefit has been demonstrated from the early treatment of asymptomatic PVD as compared with delaying treatment until patients develop symptoms.

Page: 149

Question #23

Answer: A

Rationale: The USPSTF recommends screening male smokers or past smokers between the ages of 65 and 75 years. Women have a low prevalence of abdominal aortic aneurysm, and the risk of repair outweighs the benefit of screening.

Page: 149

Question #24

Answer: C

Rationale: The USPSTF strongly recommends screening for cholesterol, hypertension, and chlamydia; in other words, there is good evidence for improved outcomes, and the benefit of screening significantly outweighs potential harms. Screening for PVD is not routinely recommended, but it is recommended for male smokers or past smokers between the ages of 65 and 75 years old. In these cases, there is at least fair evidence for improved outcomes, and the benefit outweighs potential harm. Screening for chlamydia is strongly recommended for all sexually active females who are 25 years old or younger.

Pages: 149, 150

Question #25

Answer: B

Rationale: Screening is recommended by the USPSTF for those adults with hypertension or hyperlipidemia. The American Diabetes Association recommends screening for diabetes and conducting an impaired fasting glucose test beginning at the age of 45 or even younger for those patients at high risk for diabetes or its complications.

Page: 150

Question #26

Answer: C

Rationale: The USPSTF, the AAFP, the American Geriatric Society, the American Academy of Orthopaedic Surgeons, and the American College of Radiology all recommend screening with dual-energy x-ray absorptiometry of the femoral neck beginning at age 65 routinely and at age 60 for women at increased risk, with the test being repeated every 2 years. A T-score value at the femoral neck of less than −2.5 correlates with a risk of hip fracture.

Page: 150

Question #27

Answer: A

Rationale: The USPSTF does not recommend screening for thyroid function, asymptomatic PVD, or coronary artery disease. However, cholesterol screening is strongly recommended, beginning at the age of 35 years for males and 45 years for females. The American Thyroid Association recommends screening all adults for subclinical thyroid dysfunction beginning at age 35 years.

Pages: 149, 150

Question #28

Answer: B

Rationale: CAGE is a screening tool that is used for the detection of problem drinking and alcoholism. However, it is not diagnostic for alcoholism. Asking the patient if they have tried to *c*ut down, if they have ever been *a*nnoyed when someone asked about their drinking, if they have ever felt *g*uilty for drinking, and if they have ever needed an *e*ye-opener to calm themselves in the morning has been shown to be highly sensitive for detecting alcohol abuse. Both the USPSTF and the AAFP recommend screening adults for alcohol misuse and to counsel patients who are identified as potentially having a problem.

Page: 151

Question #29

Answer: B

Rationale: The USPSTF and the AAFP recommend screening for obesity by calculating the body mass index (weight/meters square) and offering an intervention to help obese patients lose weight. Body mass index and mortality have shown a direct relationship.

Page: 149

Question #30

Answer: D

Rationale: The USPSTF recommends that mammography be performed on all women beginning at the age of 40 years. There is no evidence for or against performing mammography on women older than 70 years or for clinical breast examination or self breast examination. However, women with familial patterns that are suggestive of BRCA1 or BRCA2 mutations and that include the following should be offered genetic testing and counseling: three or more first- or second-degree relatives with breast cancer; two first-degree relatives with breast cancer if at least one of them was diagnosed before the age of 50 years; one first-degree relative with bilateral breast cancer; a first- or second-degree relative with both breast and ovarian cancers; or any male relative with breast cancer.

Page: 152

Question #31

Answer: A

Rationale: The USPSTF recommends against Pap smear screening for all women who have undergone hysterectomy for benign disease and for women more than 65 years old who have previously tested negative for dysplasia.

Page: 152

Question #32

Answer: D

Rationale: The sensitivity of a single fecal occult blood test is as low as 40%; therefore, multiple testing (usually three) on separate stool samples every 1 or 2 years is recommended. Sigmoidoscopy has a sensitivity of no more than 50%, which is similar to that of virtual colonoscopy. Colonoscopy has a sensitivity of almost 100%, and it is often the gold standard against which other colon cancer screening tests are compared.

Page: 152

Question #33

Answer: A

Rationale: Recent cost-effectiveness analysis demonstrates that all strategies are worthwhile and that none appear to be superior to the others with regard to cost per year of life saved. No direct evidence shows that colonoscopy, barium enema, or virtual colonoscopy decreases colorectal cancer mortality.

Page: 153

Question #34

Answer: A

Rationale: Studies have shown that the mortality of prostate cancer is linked to the grade of differentiation of the cancer rather than the stage of the cancer at the time of diagnosis. Therefore, screening is less useful.

Page: 153

Question #35

Answer: C

Rationale: Prostate cancer screening has not been shown to reduce mortality from prostate cancer. The USPSTF reports insufficient evidence to recommend either for or against prostate cancer screening with either the digital rectal examination or the prostate-specific antigen test.

Page: 153

Question #36

Answer: A

Rationale: Computed tomography scanning, chest x-ray, and sputum cytology studies for lung cancer may detect cancer during its asymptomatic stages, but no studies have demonstrated a decrease in mortality, so therefore there is no recommendation for or against routine screening. In addition, the high false-positive testing associated with screening women for ovarian cancer by pelvic exam, serum Ca-125 tumor marker, and pelvic ultrasound has lead the USPSTF to recommend against their use.

Page: 153

Question #37

Answer: A

Rationale: Counseling patients about smoking cessation is the only behavior that has been shown to have a decrease in mortality. Even so, the USPSTF does recommend that health-care providers counsel patients about alcohol misuse, obtaining regular physical activity, decreasing saturated fat and total caloric intake, and increasing the intake of fruits and vegetables.

Page: 154

Question #38

Answer: D

Rationale: A measles-mumps-rubella vaccine is recommended for adults born after 1957 and without prior adequate vaccination for measles.

Page: 155

11 Answers

Question #1

Answer: B

Rationale: Primary prevention is defined as interventions that reduce the risk of disease occurrence in otherwise healthy individuals. Counseling patients to avoid smoking and prescribing fluoride to children to prevent cavities are examples of primary prevention. Secondary prevention includes screening to identify risk factors for disease or the early detection of a disease among individuals who are asymptomatic and at risk for that disease. By contrast, tertiary prevention services are provided to individuals who clearly have a disease, and the goal is to prevent them from developing further complications.

Page: 159

Question #2

Answer: A

Rationale: The condition being screened for should be an important health problem. Screening for a rare disease is likely to produce many false-positive results and thus is unlikely to be cost effective.

Page: 160

Question #3

Answer: B

Rationale: Screening programs for breast cancer, cervical cancer, and colorectal cancer have all been shown to significantly reduce mortality. Screening for prostate cancer remains controversial as a result of a lack of a proven mortality reduction through treating screening-detected disease and as a result of the morbidity of diagnostic testing and treatment for prostate cancer.

Page: 168

Question #4

Answer: A

Rationale: Over one third of U.S. mortality is linked to four behaviors: tobacco use, alcohol consumption, poor diet, and physical inactivity. Achieving high rates of screening, improving immunization rates, and using chemoprophylaxis (e.g., aspirin use in patients with cardiovascular diseases) are important strategies for those populations. However, changing the health behaviors of Americans has the greatest potential impact of any current approach for decreasing morbidity and mortality and for improving the quality of life across diverse populations.

Page: 163

Question #5

Answer: B

Rationale: Sensitivity is defined as the proportion of people with the target disorder who have a positive test, and *specificity* the proportion of people without the target disorder who have a negative test. The *positive predictive value* is the proportion of people with a positive test who have the target disorder; the *negative predictive value* is the proportion of people with a negative test who are free of the target disorder.

Page: 163

Question #6

Answer: B

Rationale: Improving clinician knowledge and attitude has limited power to affect the quality, delivery, and effectiveness of prevention in the family physician's office. Further improvement requires changes in the office system.

Page: 163

Question #7

Answer: B

Rationale: All interventions—including preventive services—have harms, and, because screening occurs among asymptomatic patients, the standard of evidence must be very high to ensure that benefits truly outweigh harms. Benefits obtained through screening should be improvements in patient-oriented outcomes, such as mortality or quality of life, rather than in intermediate outcomes, such as laboratory values.

Page: 160

Question #8

Answer: A

Rationale: *Prevalence* is the proportion of a defined group of people who have a condition or disease at a given point in time. *Incidence* is the proportion of a group that, although initially disease-free, develops the disease over a given time period. *Morbidity* is the impact of the disease on health and functioning, and *mortality* is the degree to which a condition results in death.

Pages: 162–163

Question #9

Answer: A

Rationale: *Specificity* is the proportion of people without the target disorder who have a negative test. A test with high specificity may still have a small but substantial false-positive rate. When this is considered for a large population in which the target disease is rare, even if the test has a high specificity rate, most positive results will be falsely positive.

Page: 163

Question #10

Answer: B

Rationale: Although colonoscopy is considered the current gold standard for the detection of large colonic polyps, studies have shown that colonoscopy may miss some polyps that will be detected later. Colonoscopy is only about 90% sensitive for large polyps (>1 cm) and 75% sensitive for small polyps (<1 cm).

Page: 166

Question #11

Answer: E

Rationale: Acceptable screening strategies include fecal occult blood testing (FOBT) annually, FOBT testing annually plus flexible sigmoidoscopy every 3 to 5 years, double-contrast barium enema every 5 years, or colonoscopy every 10 years. FOBT has the lowest sensitivity but also the lowest cost of any screening strategy, whereas colonoscopy has the highest sensitivity but also the highest cost and direct risk to the patient.

Digital rectal exams are not a recommended screening method for colorectal cancer, because fewer than 10% of lesions will be within reach of an examiner's finger.

Page: 166

Question #12

Answer: D

Rationale: Colorectal cancer is the second leading cause of death from cancer, and it affects both men and women. The USPSTF strongly recommends screening for colorectal cancer among men and women who are more than 50 years old. Screening may be initiated earlier for those with risk factors.

Page: 166

Question #13

Answer: B

Rationale: The most important risk factor for cervical cancer is infection with human papillomavirus (HPV). HPV is considered a necessary but not sufficient condition for the development of cervical cancer. Cigarette smoking may alter the body's response to HPV and increase susceptibility to the disease, but it does not itself cause cervical cancer. Early onset of sexual intercourse and greater number of sexual partners are associated with cervical cancer, but they do not cause it; they are probably markers for an increased likelihood of acquiring HPV.

Pages: 166, 167

Question #14

Answer: C

Rationale: Cervical cancer is exceedingly rare among women who have had a hysterectomy for benign disease. The USPSTF recommends screening for cervical cancer among women who have been sexually active and who have a cervix. Most of the benefit of screening will be obtained by initiating screening within 3 years of the onset of sexual activity or at the age of 21 years, whichever comes first, and then screening at least every 3 years thereafter. The USPSTF recommends against routine Papanicolaou tests among low-risk women who are more than 65 years old and among women who have had a hysterectomy for benign disease.

Page: 167

Question #15

Answer: C

Rationale: Trials evaluating the efficacy of mammography have reported reductions in mortality of up to 32%. The accuracy of self breast examination is not known. Clinical breast examination has not been evaluated independent of mammography; screening with both clinical breast examination and mammography is comparable to using mammography alone. Breast ultrasound is a useful adjunct for the diagnostic evaluation of a patient with a palpable breast lump or a mammographic abnormality, but it has not been evaluated as a screening tool.

Page: 167

Question #16

Answer: B

Rationale: Potential screening methodologies for lung cancer have not been shown to affect lung cancer mortality, even among high-risk populations, and they have considerable harms as a result of the invasive procedures used to evaluate false positives. The USPSTF found insufficient evidence to recommend for or against screening asymptomatic individuals for lung cancer.

Page: 167

Question #17

Answer: D

Rationale: Screening for lung and ovarian cancer has not been shown to reduce mortality, and it would in fact carry substantial risks as a result of potential false-positive results and consequent unnecessary invasive diagnostic procedures. Screening for prostate cancer remains controversial, because, again, screening may carry substantial risk, and a mortality benefit has not been demonstrated. Screening programs for cervical cancer, on the other hand, have been highly successful at dramatically reducing mortality from the disease. The USPSTF strongly recommends screening sexually active women with a cervix for cervical cancer (A recommendation). The USPSTF recommends against screening for ovarian cancer (D recommendation), and there is currently insufficient evidence to recommend for or against screening for lung or prostate cancer (I recommendation).

Page: 167

Question #18

Answer: B

Rationale: Screening with prostate-specific antigen testing and digital rectal examination can detect prostate cancer during its early stages, but it is not clear whether this early detection actually improves health outcomes. Screening may result in several potential harms, including frequent false positives, biopsies, and anxiety. Treatment side effects may include erectile dysfunction, urinary incontinence, and bowel dysfunction. Treatment of all cases detected by screening is likely to result in many interventions for men who would never have experienced symptoms from their cancers. The USPSTF concluded that the evidence is insufficient to recommend for or against routine screening for prostate cancer using prostate-specific antigen testing or digital rectal examination.

Page: 168

Question #19

Answer: A

Rationale: Hypertension is the most common cardiovascular disease and the most common reason that patients visit family physicians. Approximately 35% of myocardial infarctions, 49% of heart failure, and 24% of premature deaths are the result of hypertension. Treating a patient for hypertension detected through screening appears to provide morbidity and mortality benefits. The USPSTF strongly recommends that clinicians screen all adults for high blood pressure (A recommendation).

Page: 168

Question #20

Answer: D

Rationale: Hypertension, hyperlipidemia, and tobacco use are all major cardiovascular risk factors. Treating screening-detected hypertension results in a reduction in mortality, and treating lipid abnormalities among persons at elevated cardiac risk reduces coronary events and mortality. Tobacco use contributes to other health problems, such as cancer, and it is the leading cause of preventable death in the United States. There is good evidence that even brief counseling interventions (lasting less than 3 minutes) increase tobacco abstinence rates, and several pharmacotherapies are also safe and effective for helping adults to quit smoking. The USPSTF strongly recommends that clinicians screen all adults for high blood pressure (A recommendation), and it strongly recommends screening men who are more than 35 years old and women who are more than 45 years old for lipid abnormalities (including high-density lipoprotein) and total cholesterol (A recommendation). The USPSTF recommends that clinicians screen all adults, including pregnant women, for tobacco use and that they provide tobacco-cessation interventions for those who use tobacco products. C-reactive protein levels may identify patients who are at risk for cardiovascular events, but its place in screening and its implications for patient management have not been determined.

Page: 168

Question #21

Answer: B

Rationale: The optimal duration and frequency of tobacco counseling interventions are not known, but there is good evidence that even brief counseling interventions (lasting less than 3 minutes) increase tobacco abstinence rates. Increasing the intensity of the counseling increases its efficacy.

Page: 170

Question #22

Answer: A

Rationale: Although electrocardiography and exercise stress testing can detect disease, the sensitivity and specificity of these tests limit their use among asymptomatic persons. Computed tomography scanning for coronary calcium may be useful for better defining risk in patients who are at intermediate risk based on traditional risk factors, but no mortality benefit of screening has been demonstrated. The USPSTF recommends against using electrocardiography, exercise testing, or computed tomography scanning to screen low-risk adults for coronary heart disease. Evidence is insufficient to recommend these techniques, even for adults who are at increased risk. Note that a lack of recommendation for screening does not alter these tests' usefulness as diagnostic tests for patients with clinical indicators of cardiovascular disease.

Page: 170

Question #23

Answer: B

Rationale: Screening programs reduce abdominal aortic aneurysm (AAA)–specific mortality among men. Although ultrasound can detect AAAs in women, women are unlikely to benefit from screening, because they tend to develop AAAs at an older age. Screening studies have not shown a benefit for women. The USPSTF recommends screening for AAA among men between the ages of 65 and 75 who have ever smoked; it makes no recommendation for or against screening men in this age group who never smoked, and it recommends against routine screening for women.

Page: 163

Question #24

Answer: D

Rationale: Effective screening strategies have been defined to detect tobacco use, alcoholism, and depression in primary care practice, and effective treatment strategies exist for screening-detected disease in each case. The USPSTF recommends that clinicians screen all adults, including pregnant women, for tobacco use and that they provide tobacco-cessation interventions for those who use tobacco products. The USPSTF recommends screening and behavioral counseling interventions to reduce alcohol misuse by adults, including pregnant women, in primary care settings. The USPSTF recommends screening adults for depression in clinical settings that have systems in place to ensure accurate diagnosis, effective treatment, and follow-up.

Pages: 170, 171

Question #25

Answer: B

Rationale: Age is the strongest predictor of chlamydia infection. Screening and treatment for chlamydia infection in a group of high-risk asymptomatic women significantly reduce the incidence of pelvic inflammatory disease and ectopic pregnancies, the prevalence of chlamydia in the population. However, although the treatment of men eradicates infection, there is no evidence that screening men reduces transmission, acute infection, or sequelae in women. The USPSTF recommends that clinicians routinely screen all sexually active women who are 25 years old and younger (including pregnant women) and all other asymptomatic women who are at increased risk for chlamydial infection.

Page: 171

Question #26

Answer: E

Rationale: Screening programs for chlamydia, gonorrhea, syphilis, and human immunodeficiency virus

(HIV) among targeted groups at high risk for these diseases are effective for reducing morbidity from those infections. The USPSTF makes the following recommendations: that clinicians routinely screen all sexually active women who are 25 years old and younger (including pregnant women) and all other asymptomatic women at increased risk for chlamydial infection; that clinicians screen all sexually active women who are at increased risk for gonorrheal infection; that clinicians screen persons at increased risk for syphilis infection; and that clinicians screen for HIV among all adolescents and adults who are at increased risk for HIV infection. The USPSTF recommends against screening asymptomatic adults who are not at increased risk for hepatitis infections for hepatitis B or C (D recommendation), and it finds insufficient evidence to recommend for or against screening individuals who are at high risk for hepatitis C (I recommendation).

Page: 173

Question #27

Answer: A

Rationale: The USPSTF recommends screening for type 2 diabetes only among adults with hypertension or hyperlipidemia, because the management of cardiovascular risk factors leads to reductions in major cardiovascular events.

Page: 173

Question #28

Answer: C

Rationale: The USPSTF recommends that women who are 65 years old and older be routinely screened for osteoporosis and that routine screening begin at the age of 60 years for women who are at increased risk for osteoporotic fractures. Risk factors for osteoporosis include older age (>70 years), low body mass index, not using estrogen replacement, white or Asian ancestry, positive family history, tobacco use, and low levels of weight-bearing physical activity.

Page: 174

Question #29

Answer: D

Rationale: Hormone-replacement therapy (HRT) increases bone density and reduces the risk of fractures. Contrary to prior thinking, there are now indications that HRT increases the incidence of coronary heart disease and

dementia. Other important harms of HRT include an increased risk of breast cancer, venous thromboembolism, and stroke. The USPSTF recommends against the routine use of HRT for the prevention of chronic diseases among postmenopausal women, because the evidence indicates that the harmful effects of combined estrogen and progestin or unopposed estrogen are likely to exceed the benefits of chronic disease prevention for most women.

Page: 175

Question #30

Answer: A

Rationale: Immunizations have resulted in the reduction or elimination of many important childhood diseases, and it represents the largest evidence base for preventive services to children. Aside from immunizations, the evidence base for other childhood services is generally much more limited. Some screening tests for genetic disorders are evidence based, whereas others may not be based on evidence but rather on concerns that certain high-risk populations will have conditions that may otherwise be missed. Counseling to prevent injuries and against the use of alcohol, tobacco, and drugs is considered an important component of preventive health care for adolescents. However, clear evidence of the benefits of screening and counseling for these conditions among adolescents is not clear.

Page: 176

Question #31

Answer: E

Rationale: Anticipatory guidance for children involves counseling caregivers to prepare for future normal child growth and development and to prepare caregivers for how these changes may need to be accommodated to promote development and to prevent injury or harm. Examples include providing counseling to caregivers about various safety issues, such as the use of infant and child car seats, bicycle helmets, water safety, poisoning prevention, and child-proofing the home; it also includes information about nutrition, appropriate dental care, and physical activity. Injury prevention is particularly important, because unintentional injury is the leading cause of death for both children and adolescents. Preventive care among adolescents also emphasizes anticipatory guidance and counseling: important topics to discuss include sexual activity; alcohol, tobacco, and drug use; healthy eating and physical activity; injury prevention; and mental health.

Pages: 176, 177

1. The condition being screened for should be an important health problem.
2. The natural history of the condition should be well understood.
3. There should be a detectable early stage.
4. Treatment at an early stage should be of more benefit than that at a later stage.
5. A suitable test should be devised to detect the early stage.
6. The test should be acceptable.
7. Intervals for repeating the test should be determined.
8. Adequate health service provision should be made for the extra clinical workload that will result from screening.
9. The risks—both physical and psychological—should be less than the benefits.
10. The costs should be balanced with the benefits.

From Wilson JMG, Jungner G: Principles and practice of screening for disease. Geneva: World Health Organisation, 1968. In Rakel RE, editor: *Textbook of family medicine,* ed 7, Philadelphia, WB Saunders, 2007.

12 Answers

Question #1

Answer: A

Rationale: According to Ewigman, the ultimate goal of EBM is to improve patient outcomes by considering the most current, valid, clinical research evidence when making patient care decisions. When combining the best evidence with clinical experience, the best patient outcome possible can be obtained.

Page: 186

Question #2

Answer: D

Rationale: A good RCT will be double blinded, which means that neither the participant nor the investigator knows whether the participant is in the treatment group or the control group. It will also include concealed allocation assignment. A good RCT also will make use of an intention-to-treat analysis. This means that patients lost to follow-up are included in the data of the group to which they were assigned. By including these patients in the final analysis in this way, the investigator eliminates potential bias from the study.

Page: 187

Question #3

Answer: C

Rationale: When looking at the hierarchy of EBM, expert opinion and clinical experience form the base of the pyramid, as they are the most prevalent but the least based on evidence. Next are the case-control and case-series studies, which compare two groups but allow for a large amount of bias. After that are observational studies, which by design have less bias. These are followed by RCTs, which are prospective in nature and designed to eliminate bias. At the top of the pyramid is meta-analysis, which combines in a systematic format multiple RCTs, thereby adding power to the study.

Page: 186

HIERARCHY OF EVIDENCE PYRAMID

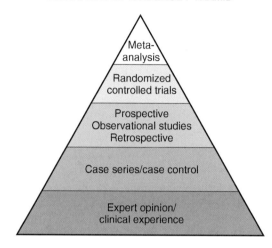

Question #4

Answer: B

Rationale: Table 2 of Ewigman's chapter lists the classic steps of EBM. It begins with formulating a clear, answerable, clinical question. Next, a systematic review of the medical literature is undertaken to find the most relevant article that might answer the question being posed. The third step involves critically appraising the article to make sure that it fits the patient population that is being inquired about and that the author's conclusions are appropriate. The final step involves the physician integrating his or her findings into the clinical decision-making involving the patient.

Page: 187

Question #5

Answer: A

Rationale: The apprentice model, deferral to authority, opinion based on experience, the pathophysiologic model, and consensus opinion are all forms of non-EBM approaches to patient care. The apprentice model involves a less-experienced physician (the apprentice) learning patterns of care from the more-experienced physician and emulating the teacher during subsequent care of patients. With this model, it is difficult for the apprentice to differentiate between helpful and harmful practices; therefore, the apprentice may make the wrong choice when making patient-care decisions. Deferral to authority happens when a physician seeks out and defers the decision-making to an expert when making a patient-care decision. Finally, although clinical experience is important, it is best used in conjunction with an EBM approach to clinical decision-making.

Page: 188

Question #6

Answer: B

Rationale: EBM is philosophically an empirical approach to clinical decision-making. It uses actual observations from real patient populations, and it makes use of careful and replicable methods. Its roots can be traced back to the Renaissance, when Vesalius made direct and accurate observations of human anatomy and functioning that disproved the anatomical theories of Galen. Empiricism holds that, when solid empirical evidence is found (even if it is in conflict with prevailing pathophysiological theory), it should be maintained as truth and not discarded. Finally, the scurvy experiment mentioned in option D is a good example of empiricism.

Page: 189

Question #7

Answer: D

Rationale: RCTs are below meta-analysis in the hierarchy of EBM.

Page: 190

Question #8

Answer: D

Rationale: InfoRetriever, DynaMed, and Cochrane Review are commonly used databases that systematically scan the literature and pre-appraise the findings, using a commonly accepted grading scale to help readers understand that strength of the conclusion that has been reached.

Page: 193

Question #9

Answer: C

Rationale: The term *POEM* implies outcomes that will be of clinical value to patients. This would include a

decrease in morbidity or mortality; a decrease in a clinical event rate, such as heart attack; or improved survival. A DOE, on the other hand, is an outcome that is measurable but that does not necessarily provide clinical relevance. Examples would include a decrease in systolic blood pressure of 5 mm Hg or an increase in the FEV_1. A medicine being shown to reduce the low-density lipoprotein level is an example of a DOE. Although these outcomes may portend clinical relevance to a patient, the values by themselves do not. Therefore, whenever possible, one should look for POEMs rather than DOEs.

Page: 194

Question #10

Answer: D

Rationale: The Clinical Inquiries network currently includes only 300 questions and answers.

Page: 194

Question #11

Answer: C

Rationale: The definition supplied is an example of a case-control study. A cohort study involves the identification of two groups of individuals, one of which received the exposure of interest and one of which did not. These groups are then evaluated over time for the outcome of interest. An RCT is a prospective study in which participants are randomly assigned to the treatment group or the control group and then evaluated over time for the outcome of interest. A retrospective case series looks at a group of individuals with a particular outcome and then retrospectively reviews the cases for similarities.

See Chapter 12

Question #12

Answer: B

Rationale: *Allocation concealment* involves a person enrolling a participant into a clinical trial and that person's being unaware if that participant will be in the intervention group or the control group.

Page: 187

Question #13

Answer: C

Rationale: The study described in this example is not a systematic review but simply a review by the author of the topic of atrial fibrillation. Option A is the definition of a systematic review, and B and D are examples of systematic reviews. A meta-analysis is a type of systematic review that includes statistical techniques to combine data from different studies. The Cochrane review, by definition, is a pre-appraised database that makes use of systematic and comprehensive review techniques.

Page: 187

Question #14

Answer: D

Rationale: Option D states the definition of *intention-to-treat analysis*. *Incidence* is the proportion of new cases of the target disorder in the population at risk during a specified time interval. The *summary statistic* is the number derived after combining studies in a meta-analysis.

Page: 190

Question #15

Answer: B

Rationale: The *confidence interval* is the range of values in which it can be certain that the truth lies. It is usually expressed as "the 95% confidence interval." This means that, if a particular study found the absolute risk reduction of death to be 10% with a 95% confidence interval of 5% to 15%, then readers of that study can be 95% confident that the true absolute risk reduction lies between 5% and 15%.

Page: 187

Question #16

Answer: A

Rationale: The *number needed to treat* may also be defined as "the inverse of the absolute risk reduction (1/absolute risk reduction)." The definition of the *negative predictive value* is the proportion of people with a negative test who are free of the target disorder. The *odds ratio* is the ratio of the odds of having the target disorder in

the experimental group relative to the odds in favor of having the target disorder in the control group.

Page: 188

Question #17

Answer: B

Rationale: *Selection bias* means that the population of the specialist does not resemble the general population as a whole; therefore, decisions about diagnosis and management cannot be generalized to the whole population. *Publication bias* occurs when studies with negative outcomes do not get published, and *allocation bias* occurs when the randomization is altered. An example might be a study of conservative versus operative management for small bowel obstruction in which all of the patients who present at night are placed in the conservative management group; although the same number of patients would be randomized to each group, the randomization was not truly random, and, therefore, a difference between the two groups may be related to the allocation rather than to the treatment alone.

Page: 191

Question #18

Answer: A

Rationale: An RCT that is double blinded and allocation concealed using intention-to-treat analysis is the best study when looking for an answer to a clinical question addressing treatment.

Page: 187

Question #19

Answer: B

Rationale: A cohort study is the gold standard for answering questions that pertain to diagnosis.

Page: 192

Question #20

Answer: D

Rationale: The distinguishing characteristics of EBM include the following:

1. Using explicit methods (describing the databases searched and the search strategies)

2. Performing systematic searches so that important evidence is not missed
3. Using standardized critical appraisal methods
4. Using a hierarchy of study design
5. Designating the level of evidence
6. Grading recommendations according to the strength of the accumulated evidence from research studies that support the recommendation

7. Providing verifiable findings that allow others to search and critically appraise the evidence and verify or refute the findings or recommendations.

Page: 186

Question #1

Answer: D

Rationale: Several barriers affecting family physicians work against the application of EBM in practice. The busy practices of many family physicians do not allow enough time for the adequate research of answers to clinical questions. Also, many family physicians have not been sufficiently trained with regard to performing the steps of practicing EBM, such as asking answerable clinical questions, determining the best information resources for finding answers to those questions, critically appraising these information resources, and incorporating this information when making clinical decisions. Often, individual patients have problems that have not been adequately addressed by studies. Finally, many practice settings lack the rapid access to the clinical information needed to practice EBM efficiently.

Page: 203

Question #2

Answer: D

Rationale: Several global factors affect the ability of family physicians to use EBM in practice. The amount of medical knowledge continues to grow at an exponential rate, making it difficult for family physicians to sort through evidence to find what is relevant and valid enough to apply to their patients. The breadth of family medicine contributes to this problem. The potential negative effects on the art of medicine includes the danger of not taking nonmedical factors into account when making medical decisions, practicing "cookbook" medicine, and not appreciating the importance of knowing a patient's preferences and personal circumstances when incorporating evidence into clinical decision making.

Page: 203

Question #3

Answer: D

Rationale: In an observational study, differences among groups of patients are observed without any attempt made to affect an outcome; rather, attempts are made to relate these differences to characteristics of the groups. In case reports or case series (a series of case reports), observations are noted in which patients exposed to the factor in question had a particular outcome. In a case-control study, a group of patients exposed to a particular factor is compared with a group of similar patient who have not been exposed, and observed outcomes in each group are tallied retrospectively. In a cohort study, patients exposed to a particular factor are identified and observed prospectively over a period of time to see if their rate of outcomes is different from a control group of similar patients not exposed. An RCT is distinct from these other types of studies, because patients are first randomized into groups and then either exposed or not exposed to a factor; they are then followed prospectively. In an RCT, patients are not simply observed; an intervention is made to attempt to effect an outcome.

Page: 203

Question #4

Answer: B

Rationale: A series of cases has already been reported that raises suspicion that drug A may be teratogenic. Investigators wish to do a study to see whether a more firm link exists between drug A and congenital heart defects. Because a case-control study is relatively inexpensive and rapid to perform, it would be the best design for a study to answer this question. If the case-control study shows an association between the exposure and the outcome, investigators may choose to do a higher-level study (e.g., a prospective cohort study) to confirm the findings.

Page: 203

Question #5

Answer: C

Rationale: An RCT is the best design for this study. Investigators would identify patients and randomly assign them to be treated with the drug-eluting stent or with usual care (treatment with the non–drug-eluting stent). The patients would then be evaluated over time to see whether the intervention results in fewer restenoses. Because this is a new device, it is likely that not enough evidence exists to perform a useful meta-analysis or a systematic review. An observational study such as a case-control study or a cohort study would not provide any more valid evidence than an RCT.

Page: 204

Question #6

Answer: E

Rationale: A systematic review provides the most valid evidence to determine what is currently known about the efficacy of treatment X for decreasing the intensity of musculoskeletal low back pain. An observational study (i.e., a case series, a case-control study, or a cohort study) would not be appropriate; the question lends itself well to an RCT. However, an RCT would not be the approach to take to determine what is currently known about this question.

Page: 204

Question #7

Answer: B

Rationale: In a case-control study, a group of patients who have been exposed to a particular factor is compared with a group of patients who have not been exposed, and observed outcomes are noted retrospectively. Case-control studies are relatively inexpensive, and they can be completed rapidly, because they involve only retrospective data review. The results of case-control studies are commonly affected by "recall bias"; this occurs if investigators cannot accurately determine whether control subjects were exposed to the same factor being studied as the case subjects.

Page: 203

Question #8

Answer: C

Rationale: In a cohort study, patients exposed to a particular factor are identified and observed prospectively over a period of time to see if their rate of outcomes differs from a control group of similar patients who were not exposed. Prospective cohort studies often require large numbers of participants to have enough statistical power to detect differences in the rate of outcomes between study groups. Because subjects must be identified ahead of time and because data must be collected and managed over a period of time, they are generally

more expensive and take longer to complete than case-control studies. Results are primarily reported as "relative risk," which is the likelihood that a person exposed to a factor will have the outcome being studied.

Pages: 203, 204

Question #9

Answer: C

Rationale: "Healthy-user bias," which occurs when subjects who are exposed to a factor also tend to make healthier lifestyle decisions that may affect the measured outcome, commonly influences the results of cohort studies. One example is weight-loss counseling. Patients who choose to have counseling for weight loss may tend to be more motivated to make lifestyle decisions that may also lead to weight loss apart from the counseling.

Page: 204

Question #10

Answer: D

Rationale: In structured reviews, authors retrieve data from studies on a particular topic, critically appraise them, combine their results, and summarize their findings. Meta-analysis is a method that is used to combine data from several studies using statistical techniques; doing this increases the power to determine the efficacy of interventions. The validity of meta-analysis also increases when studies are homogeneous (i.e., if they are similar in design, study similar populations of patients, and measure similar outcomes).

Page: 204

Question #11

Answer: A

Rationale: In an RCT, study participants are randomly allocated to two or more groups. Randomization helps minimize differences between treatment and control groups to control for any other factors that could confound the interpretation of the results should differences between the groups be found. Each group is assigned to receive either an intervention or no active treatment (placebo or usual care). The structure of RCTs helps eliminate many biases that affect observational studies, such as recall bias and healthy-user bias.

Page: 204

Question #12

Answer: A

Rationale: Relative risk is a summary measure of differences between the treatment and placebo groups. It is calculated as the ratio of the incidence rate for the treatment group divided by the incidence rate for the placebo group. The incidence rate for each group of study participants (treatment vs. placebo) is the rate at which the measured outcome occurs in each group during the study; it is calculated as the ratio of the number of outcomes in the group that occur over a specific period of time divided by the number of patients in the group. When relative risk is reported as the summary result of a study, the 95% confidence interval can be used to describe the statistical significance of the result; when the 95% confidence interval contains the value 1 within its range, this denotes a statistically significant difference in the measured outcome between the treatment and placebo groups.

Pages: 204, 205

Question #13

Answer: E

Rationale: Statistical significance can be measured in a number of ways. By convention, a P value of less than .05 denotes a statistically significant difference. Likewise, a 95% confidence interval for relative risk that does not include 1 within its range denotes a statistically significant difference. Although the NNT and the NNH can provide family physicians with useful information for determining whether a clinically significant difference may exist, they do not demonstrate whether the difference seen is statistically significant.

Page: 205

Question #14

Answer: B

Rationale: Although determining the statistical significance of a difference in study results is important, by itself, it does not tell us whether a clinically significant difference exists. For example, just because a study shows a statistically significant difference in one measured outcome does not mean that the outcome measured was appropriate (patient-oriented). The P value is the probability that the observed difference in the results between study groups was the result of chance alone; the higher this probability, the more difficult it is to prove that the observed difference is reproducible or that it

really exists. If the 95% confidence interval of a relative risk includes 1, it is not considered to be statistically significant.

Page: 205

Question #15

Answer: C

Rationale: Although relative risk is a good measure of differences in outcomes between study groups, it often overstates the difference between groups; this is why the relative risk is often used in media reports and advertising for medical treatments. However, a more clinically relevant measure would be the absolute risk difference, which is the difference in incidence rates between the intervention and control groups. The inverse of the absolute risk difference is the NNT, which is the number of patients who need to be treated with the study intervention over a period of time to affect one measured outcome. The NNT is the best measure of the clinical significance of a statistically significant observed difference in outcomes between study groups. Both the P value and the 95% confidence interval gauge statistical significance, but they do not take into account factors that determine the clinical significance of an observed difference.

Page: 205

Question #16

Answer: E

Rationale: All of the following are factors that determine whether the results of a study should lead to a change in clinical practice:

- Whether all relevant patient-oriented outcomes were considered
- Whether clinically important harms (risks) were measured
- Whether financial endpoints (costs and savings) were considered
- Whether appropriate competing alternative interventions were assessed
- Whether clinically significant differences were measured
- Whether the intervention is applicable to a physician's practice
- Whether the intervention is acceptable to both patients and physicians
- Whether the effectiveness of the intervention is likely to be seen in real-world practice, outside of the controlled conditions of the study

Pages: 205, 206

Question #17

Answer: D

Rationale: Physiologic outcomes include measures of biological function, such as electrolyte levels, body temperature, and blood pressure. Intermediate outcomes go one step beyond physiologic outcomes to measure disease-oriented outcomes that may (or may not) lead to clinically significant patient-oriented outcomes. One example is quantifying the amount of stenosis in a coronary artery. Although studies often report physiologic or intermediate outcomes, neither necessarily correlate with clinically significant outcomes. These patient-oriented outcomes measure morbidity, mortality, quality of life, and cost-effectiveness. Studies that measure these outcomes are called POEMs, and the results of such studies are potentially important enough to change clinical practice.

Page: 206

Question #18

Answer: B

Rationale: The level of follicle-stimulating hormone is an example of a physiologic outcome, but it does not necessarily correlate with any patient-oriented outcomes. However, mortality rate is an outcome that is important to patients. Other examples of patient-oriented outcomes include measures of morbidity, quality of life, and cost-effectiveness.

Page: 206

Question #19

Answer: B

Rationale: Power refers to the ability of a study to detect a difference between the treatment and the control groups. It depends on the number of patients in the study, the magnitude of the effect of the intervention, and the variability of the effect of the intervention from one subject to another. The number of patients excluded from the study is unrelated to the power of the study.

Page: 206

Question #20

Answer: D

Rationale: Systematic reviews (such as those written by the Cochrane Collaboration) use rigorous attempts in their search for and critical appraisal of evidence. They attempt to uncover all studies, published and unpublished, in English and other languages. After all of the studies are uncovered, they are critically appraised, and the most relevant and valid studies are incorporated into a summary. If appropriate, a systematic review may include a meta-analysis, which is a method of combining the results of the studies using statistical techniques. Unlike systematic reviews, qualitative reviews are summaries of information drawn from data synthesized according to the review author's overall judgment. It is difficult to assess the validity of qualitative reviews, because it requires assessing the validity of each reference, ensuring that the information from each reference was accurately incorporated into the review, and making certain that all relevant references were included in the review.

Page: 206

Question #21

Answer: E

Rationale: A local journal club can help clinicians sharpen their ability to read and evaluate studies. These clubs are often used to introduce clinicians to various study designs, biostatistical terms, and ways in which data are presented and interpreted. They also help clinicians stay updated with regard to new clinical information. The Family Practice Inquiries Network is a collaborative effort of family physicians to create a secondary source of information that is designed to answer common clinical questions quickly. Writing clinical reviews and assisting with the development of POEMs through the Family Practice Inquiries Network or other organizations are other ways in which clinicians can practice their critical appraisal skills. Clinicians can obtain additional training by attending an information mastery or EBM workshop.

Page: 206

Question #22

Answer: E

Rationale: Secondary sources of clinical information contain summaries of critically appraised clinical information obtained from individual studies such as RCTs (i.e., primary sources). Useful secondary sources of clinical information are created by experts through a systematic review of the medical literature, and they provide clinicians with practical guidance at the point of care. Evidence-based summaries report critically appraised clinical information and summarize the best evidence that exists to answer a clinical question.

Systematic reviews are a type of evidence-based summary; they use rigorous protocols to search, critically appraise, and summarize clinical evidence to answer a clinical question. Clinical guidelines summarize clinical information in the form of recommendations for clinicians to follow in practice. Evidence-based databases contain summaries of critically appraised clinical information in a searchable format.

Pages: 206, 207

Rationale for Questions 23–32:

It is useful to create two matrices that classify the study subjects by intervention and outcome.

One matrix looks at heart attacks:

	Heart attack	No heart attack	Total
Drug X	22	4378	4400
Placebo	42	4158	4200
Total	64	8536	8600

The other matrix looks at clinically significant abdominal pain:

	Abdominal pain	No abdominal pain	Total
Drug X	110	4290	4400
Placebo	30	4170	4200
Total	140	8460	8600

Remember that these outcomes are measured over a 2-year study period.

Question #23

Answer: A

Rationale: The incidence rate for heart attacks in the treatment group is determined by dividing the number of heart attacks in the treatment group by the number of patients in the treatment group. In this case, 22/4400 = 0.50%.

Page: 205

Question #24

Answer: C

Rationale: The incidence rate of heart attacks in the placebo group is determined by dividing the number of heart attacks in placebo group by the number of patients in placebo group. In this case, 42/4200 = 1.0%.

Page: 205

Question #25

Answer: B

Rationale: The incidence rate of clinically significant abdominal pain in the treatment group is determined by dividing the number of patients with clinically significant abdominal pain in the treatment group by the number of patients in the treatment group. In this case, 110/4400 = 2.5%.

Page: 205

Question #26

Answer: C

Rationale: The incidence rate of clinically significant abdominal pain in the placebo group is determined by dividing the number of patients with clinically significant abdominal pain in the placebo group by the number of patients in the placebo group. In this case, 30/4200 = 0.71%.

Page: 205

Question #27

Answer: E

Rationale: The relative risk of heart attacks in the treatment group is determined by dividing the incidence rate of heart attacks in the treatment group by the incidence rate of heart attacks in the placebo group. In this case, 0.5%/1.0% = 0.50.

Page: 205

Question #28

Answer: D

Rationale: The relative risk of clinically significant abdominal pain in the treatment group is determined by dividing the incidence rate of clinically significant abdominal pain in the treatment group by the incidence rate of clinically significant abdominal pain in the placebo group. In this case, 2.5%/0.71% = 3.5.

Page: 205

Question #29

Answer: A

Rationale: If a 95% confidence interval for relative risk excludes 1, it represents a statistically significant difference.

Page: 205

Question #30

Answer: B

Rationale: The absolute risk difference (or attributable risk) of heart attacks between the treatment group and the placebo group during the 2-year study is determined by subtracting the incidence rate of heart attacks in the treatment group from the incidence rate of heart attacks in the placebo group. In this case, $1.0\% - 0.5\% = 0.5\% = 0.005$.

Page: 204

Question #31

Answer: C

Rationale: The NNT for 1 year to prevent one heart attack is determined by dividing 1 by the absolute risk difference of heart attacks between the treatment and placebo groups. In this case, $1/0.005 = 200$.

Thus, 200 patients need to be treated with drug X for 2 years (remember that the study runs for 2 years) to prevent one heart attack. The NNT for 1 year is two times this number: 400. (Twice as many patients need to be treated in half the time to achieve the same result.)

Pages: 204, 205

Question #32

Answer: C

Rationale: The NNH for 1 year to cause one patient to have clinically significant abdominal pain is determined by dividing 1 by the absolute risk difference of abdominal pain between the treatment and placebo groups. This is also equal to dividing 1 by the incidence rate of abdominal pain in the treatment group minus the incidence rate of abdominal pain in the placebo group. In this case, $1/(2.5\% - 0.71\%) = 1/1.79\% = 1/0.0179 = 56$. (Note that the NNT and the NNH are rounded up to the nearest integer.)

So for every 56 patients taking drug X for 2 years, one patient will experience clinically significant abdominal pain. The NNH for 1 year is two times this number: 112. (Twice as many patients need to be treated in half the time to harm one patient.)

Page: 205

Question #1

Answer: B

Rationale: The family physician is faced with an ever-growing list of clinical questions. The computer and the various easily accessible electronic resources make answering the questions easier and more immediate. Computers have increased the power of practice management software, thereby allowing for efficient clinical/business information evaluation, and the use of e-mail has revolutionized patients' access to health care via the online exchange of health information with their physicians.
Page: 209

Question #2

Answer: D

Rationale: The opportunities to use the Internet as a medical resource are endless. There are many online interactive education resources that address clinical topics, offer improvement, and answer clinical questions. The powerful Internet search engines provide access to the literature to answer very specific questions.
Page: 209

Question #3

Answer: D

Rationale: The EHR has enhanced patient care and services by organizing information, increasing safety, and improving the process and efficiency of data collection. Ordering and reviewing laboratory tests, managing medications, and checking allergies for drug–drug interactions for multiple patients can be performed quickly and easily. This, along with the elimination of legibility issues, has made the EHR an enhancement for safer patient care.
Page: 210

Question #4

Answer: A

Rationale: The EHR allows for a variety of methods of health information capture. Dictation, voice recogni-

tion, keyboarding, and data point selection all have their advantages and disadvantages. A full assessment of how the health information will be used and a complete understanding of the pros and cons of each method will shed light on the primary method used in a specific office.
Page: 210

Question #5

Answer: C

Rationale: The past several years have seen the expansion of medical uses of the personal digital assistant and the rapid adoption of these handheld devices by physicians. The small size, instant access, and availability of many different types of software for medical information and everyday medical tasks have led to the widespread use of these devices in medicine.
Page: 210

Question #6

Answer: B

Rationale: With the EHR and the electronic billing system working together, it has become possible for billing information that is produced during the process of care to flow directly into the practice management software.
Page: 211

Question #7

Answer: C

Rationale: One of the greatest benefits of the EHR is the way that it supports office workflow. Remote access is critical for groups with multiple practice sites and for physicians who are on call from home or hospital.
Page: 211

Question #8

Answer: A

Rationale: The American Society for Testing and Materials, the International Massachusetts Medical

Society, the Health Information Management and Systems Society, the American Academy of Family Physicians, and the American Academy of Pediatrics have worked jointly to develop the continuity of care record. This record will speed up and improve the continuity of patient care, reduce medical errors, and increase the patient's role in managing his or her own health.

Page: 211

Question #9

Answer: D

Rationale: There is a great interest in monitoring and collecting data about the quality of care delivered to patients. Performance measures have been developed to monitor and improve office systems. The EHR should be designed to collect data about these elements of quality during the process of care.

Page: 211

Question #10

Answer: A

Rationale: Leadership and change management are important skills for physicians who are going through the transformation to the paperless office. Fronting a project team, good individualized training, and implementation strategies that minimize lost productivity are essential elements.

Page: 212

Chapter

15   Answers

Question #1

Answer: B

Rationale: As patient volume increases, clinicians are increasingly pressured to make clinical decisions on the fly, so the easiest knowledge base to fall back on is the most basic knowledge gained during early training.

Page: 215

Question #2

Answer: B

Rationale: Mindlines are a foundation that can be built on, but the knowledge that they provide can easily become stagnant and outdated. This knowledge should be continuously updated and refined.

Page: 215

Question #3

Answer: D

Rationale: Shared clinical decisions allow patients to be a part of their health, and they can empower patients to take control of their health. This is best achieved as a collaboration between the clinician and the patient. Clinicians are trusted to review the evidence using focused clinical questions and then discussing risks, benefits, and treatment options with patients. Using this evidence and incorporating patient preferences are the best ways to share clinical decision-making.

Page: 215

Question #4

Answer: B

Rationale: A study performed by Ely and colleagues[1] showed that answers were not sought by physicians for most questions that arise. However, when physicians do seek answers, they are usually successful in finding them.

Page: 216

1. Ely JW, Osheroff JA, Ebell MH, et al: Analysis of questions asked by family doctors regarding patient care. *BMJ* 319:358-361, 1999.

Question #5

Answer: B

Rationale: Background questions are the who, what, where, why, and how questions that are generally found in textbooks. At the next level, foreground questions focus on specific issues involving the patient, generally making use of current evidence and specific patient situations.

Page: 216

Question #6

Answer: C

Rationale: The best focused clinical question can be remembered using the acronym *PICO: p*roblem, *i*ntervention, *c*ontrol (or *c*omparison), and *o*utcome. The reference impact factor is an evidence term that compares how often references are cross-referenced; it is not part of the clinical question.

Page: 216

Question #7

Answer: B

Rationale: Reducing plasma glucose is a disease-oriented outcome. However, it cannot be directly linked to improved patient outcomes.

Page: 216

Question #8

Answer: B

Rationale: The evidence pyramid puts original research at the bottom, because it is the most plentiful. However, it is the least usable for a busy clinician.

Page: 216

Question #9

Answer: A

Rationale: Although all forms of evidence require some knowledge of statistical methods and study design, original research requires the most. To process and interpret the data, there must be an exhaustive evaluation of this material.

Page: 216

Question #10

Answer: B

Rationale: Systematic reviews and meta-analyses make up the second tier from the bottom of the evidence pyramid. They are studies that ask a single question and that review the volume of previously reported data to draw a single conclusion. These are better than original research, but they still require the reader to explore the methodology used to select and analyze the data.

Page: 213

Question #11

Answer: C

Rationale: As described, POEMs are strong, relevant evidence that uses a clinical question and a clinical outcome to determine the best evidence for treatment, diagnosis, and so on.

Page: 216

Question #12

Answer: B

Rationale: Although POEMs are the most useful research for answering clinical questions that can arise from patient visits, they are the least available. Many questions have not been addressed, and, therefore, the clinician would need to move down the pyramid of evidence to answer the question.

Page: 216

Question #13

Answer: C

Rationale: The National Library of Medicine maintains a database of more than 15 million articles—mostly original studies—called MEDLINE. There are many search engines, but PubMed is a free engine that helps search meta-analyses and systematic reviews using limits and clinical queries.

Page: 217

Question #14

Answer: D

Rationale: At the top of the evidence pyramid are clinical guidelines. These are updated every few years, and they reflect the consensus opinions of management based on solid evidence. These are often considered to be the standard of care. In addition, clinical guidelines require the least amount of additional interpretation by the clinician.

Page: 217

Question #15

Answer: B

Rationale: Shared decision-making as been called an ethical process; this means that physicians should inform patients about their options, data, and evidence, and they should factor patient values into their final decisions.

Pages: 217, 219

Question #16

Answer: B

Rationale: Many different studies and articles have shown that, when patients are included in the decision-making process, there is an increase in trust, in satisfaction, and, ultimately, in patient compliance. Whether a physician chooses to include the patient for avoidance of legal repercussion or for beneficence, the result is always better for the patient.

Page: 219

Question #17

Answer: E

Rationale: For decisions that have low risk and that have a single best course of action, sharing the decision is of little benefit. If there are multiple good alternatives that have equal benefit, the patient's preference should factor into the decision. If the decision involves significant risk, uncertain benefit, or morality, the patient should be encouraged to make the decision, with the physician acting as the informant.

Page: 220

Question #18

Answer: A

Rationale: Society places significant value on patients' relationships with their physicians. Therefore, physicians need to encourage patients to be a part of the decision and to then execute the plan. Physicians need to listen to their patients and help direct them through the health care system.

Page: 221

16 Answers

Question #1

Answer: B

Rationale: Although the terms *complementary, alternative, integrative,* and *holistic* medicine have been used interchangeably by both medical practitioners and the lay public, there are differences implied by all of these names. CAM is a group of diverse medical and health care systems, practices, and products that are not presently considered part of conventional medicine. Alternative medicine is practiced in place of conventional medicine; complementary medicine is practiced together with conventional medicine. The NCCAM classifies CAM into five categories or domains (Figure 16-1).

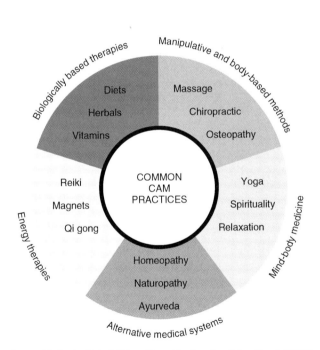

Figure 16-1 In Rakel RE, editor: *Textbook of family medicine,* ed 7, Philadelphia, WB Saunders, 2007.

According to the American Holistic Medical Association, the practice of holistic medicine integrates conventional and complementary therapies to promote optimal health and to prevent and treat disease by addressing contributing factors.

Page: 223

Question #2

Answer: C

Rationale: Women more than men, those with higher educational levels, those with higher income, and those who have been hospitalized during the past year are more likely to seek CAM therapies. In addition, Figure 16-2 shows the disease or condition for which patients are most likely to seek CAM. A national study by Astin and colleagues[1] found that, in addition to being more educated and reporting a poor health status, the majority of users of alternative medicine appear to be doing so not as a result of being dissatisfied with conventional medicine but rather largely because they find these health care alternatives to be more congruent with their own values, beliefs, and philosophical orientations toward health and life.

Page: 225

Question #3

Answer: D

Rationale: The first major study of CAM use in the United States was conducted in 1990 by Eisenburg and colleagues, and it was published as a landmark paper in the *New England Journal of Medicine* in 1993.[2] Eisenberg published a follow-up study in 1998 in the *Journal of the American Medical Association*[3] that was the result of a phone survey of English-speaking adults. Overall, 42% of Americans were estimated to be using at least one CAM therapy during the prior 12 months. Visits to CAM practitioners rose from 427 million to 629 million. Approximately 60% to 70% of CAM users in both the 1990 and the 1997 studies did not discuss their CAM use with their physicians. More recent data were published in May 2004; this included information about the use of prayer and megavitamin therapy, which had been excluded from the previous studies.

Pages: 226, 227

1. Astin JA: Why patients use alternative medicine: Results of a national study. *JAMA* 279:1548-1553, 1998.
2. Eisenberg DM, Davis RB, Ettner SL, et al: Trends in alternative medicine use in the United States, 1990-1997: Results of a follow-up national survey. *JAMA* 280:1569-1575, 1998.
3. Eisenberg DM, Kessler RC, Foster C, et al: Unconventional medicine in the United States: Prevalence, costs and patterns of use. *N Engl J Med* 328:246-252, 1993.

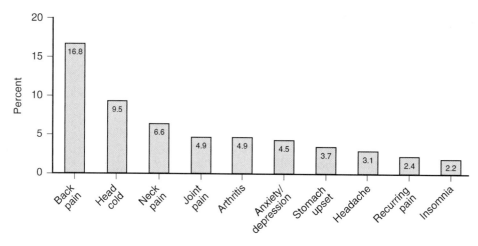

Figure 16-2 From Barnes PM, Towell-Griner E, McFann K, Nahin RL: Complementary and alternative medicine use among adults: United States, 2002. CDC Advance Data Report #343. 2004. In Rakel RE, editor: *Textbook of family medicine,* ed 7, Philadelphia, WB Saunders, 2007.

Question #4

Answer: C

Rationale: The White House Commission on CAM Policy, created in March 2002, was specifically formed to address the coordination of research to increase knowledge about CAM products, the education and training of health care practitioners of CAM, the provision of reliable and useful information about CAM practices and products to health care professionals, and the necessary guidance regarding appropriate access to and delivery of CAM. The 10 guiding principles are found in Box 4.

Page: 227

Question #5

Answer: B

Rationale: Acupuncture within traditional Chinese medicine is a component of the whole systems/nonallopathic medical system of care. It is based on the theory that health is determined by a balanced flow of energy (chi or qi), which is thought to be present in all living organisms. This energy circulates throughout the body along a series of energy pathways (meridians), each of which is linked to specific internal organs and organ systems. Within this system, there are more than 1000 acupoints that can be stimulated with the insertion of needles. Acupuncture has been used to treat a number of health problems. In 1997, the National Institutes of Health Consensus Development Panel concluded that there was clear evidence that acupuncture is efficacious

for adult postoperative and chemotherapy nausea and vomiting and for postoperative dental pain.

Page: 234

Question #6

Answer: C

Rationale: Yoga has its roots in India. There are many different styles practiced in the United States today. Most Yoga instructors are not medical professionals; however, the Yoga Alliance, formed in 1999, sets minimum training standards for yoga teachers. In addition, the International Association of Yoga Therapists is a worldwide organization for yoga teachers, therapists, and researchers. Both of these organizations provide sound resources for both professionals and the public. In 2005, an article stated that an integrated approach to yoga during pregnancy was safe and that it improved birth weight and decreased preterm labor and intrauterine growth restriction, with no complications.

Page: 234

Question #7

Answer: A

Rationale: Ayurveda was developed in India more than 5000 years ago, and it places equal emphasis on mind, body, and spirit. The practitioner identifies the individual's "constitution" or overall health profile by ascertaining the patient's metabolic body type through a series of personal history questions. The practice incorporates five elements and three types of energy, which are called *doshas*. The energies are *vata*, which is associated with movement; *pitta*, which governs metabolism; and *kapha*, which maintains structure. Foods, emotions, and behaviors are used to adjust dosha levels. *Panchakarma* is used to remove aggravated doshas and toxins. Methods include therapeutic vomiting, use of purgatives or laxatives, nasal administration of medications, blood purification, and therapeutic enemas. The CAM therapy that is based on the law of similars is homeopathy, which holds that medications can produce the same symptoms in healthy people that they can cure in those who are ill. Remedies are used in the smallest quantity possible.

Page: 233

Question #8

Answer: A

Rationale: The practice of homeopathy was founded by the German physician Samuel Hahnemann (1755–1843), and it has been practiced in Europe since that time. It is based on the theory that any substance that can produce symptoms of disease in a healthy person can cure those symptoms in a sick person. Therefore, the theory is that the more dilute the remedy, the more potent the effect. Remedies are used in the smallest quantity possible. The substances are naturally derived from plant, animal, metal, and mineral sources. Megavitamin therapy, although it is a CAM modality, is not a part of homeopathy. The evidence of the effectiveness for specific clinical conditions is scant; therefore, homeopathy offers options when conventional care has failed, is contraindicated, is not tolerated, or is not acceptable to patients.

Page: 233

Question #9

Answer B

Rationale: Chelation therapy involves the injection of a binding (chelating) agent such as the amino acid ethylenediaminetetraacetic acid. After they are injected, the binding agents travel through the bloodstream, attaching to toxic metals and wastes, which are subsequently excreted through the patient's urine. Used initially to treat lead poisoning, chelation therapy is used by a growing number of practitioners to treat and reverse the process of arteriosclerosis.

Page: 224

Question #10

Answer: D

Rationale: This answer reflects the ABC approach to patients seeking CAM therapies: *A*sk, don't tell; *B*e willing to listen and learn; *C*ommunicate and *C*ollaborate; *D*iagnose; and *E*xplain and explore options and preferences.

Page: 225

Question #11

Answer: A

Rationale: Although there can be overlap among them, NCCAM divides CAM practices into five domains. "Energy therapies" include Reiki, magnets, and qigong. Yoga is included in "mind-body medicine," along with spirituality and relaxation. Ayurveda is considered to be in the "alternative medical systems" group, along with naturopathy and homeopathy. Massage is include in "manipulation and body-based methods," along with chiropractic and osteopathy. The fifth domain is "biologically based therapies," which includes diets, herbal remedies, and vitamins.

Page: 231

Question #12

Answer: C

Rationale: The term *Reiki* means universal healing energy. During treatment, this healing energy is channeled through the hands of a practitioner into the client's body to restore a normal energy balance and health. It has been used to treat a wide variety of ailments and health problems, and it is often used in conjunction with other alternative and conventional medical treatments. The practice does not involve deep breathing, which is another CAM therapy. The visualization of peaceful images during relaxation is guided imagery.

Page: 234

Question #13

Answer: D

Rationale: Tai chi is an ancient form of Chinese self-defense and low-impact exercise used for health, relaxation, and self-exploration. It is considered a CAM therapy. Some of the proposed benefits include improved concentration, circulation, and posture; reduction of stress; and prevention of osteoporosis.

Page: 234

Question #14

Answer: B

Rationale: The body scan is one technique of mindful meditation in which the subject uses breathing to obtain a relaxed state while lying or sitting. The mind progressively focuses on different parts of the body, where it feels any and all of the sensations intentionally but nonjudgmentally before moving to another part of the body. During visualization/self-hypnosis, the subject uses visualization to recreate images that create a relaxed state, such as that of a place and time that were peaceful and comforting. It is best combined with breathing exercise.

Page: 231

Question #15

Answer: C

Rationale: Biofeedback was originated in the early 1960s by Neal Miller, an experimental psychologist. Its theory is that all autonomic responses can be brought under voluntary control. The process involves connecting electrodes to various parts of the body to monitor the autonomic response to various stimuli. The feedback may be visual or auditory. Controlled breathing is not a component of this CAM therapy.

Page: 232

Question #16

Answer: A

Rationale: A particular aspect of nutrition that has received increasing attention for its value in lessening inflammation is that of fish oil (omega-6 and omega-3 fatty acids). Inflammation has been shown to play a role in cardiovascular disease, asthma, arthritis, psoriasis, and inflammatory bowel disease. Omega-3 and omega-6 fatty acids are essential polyunsaturated fatty acids that cannot be made by the human body. The standard American diet has a ratio of omega-6 to omega-3 of greater than 20:1; the ideal range is less than 4:1.

Page: 233

Question #17

Answer: A

Rationale: All of these describe therapeutics of traditional Chinese medicine. Gua sha involves pressing the skin with a hard, round-edged instrument to create petechiae. Cupping involves the creation of a vacuum in a cup and applying the vacuum pressure to the skin. Moxibustion is the burning of moxa on or near meridian points, and acupuncture is the insertion of needles into various points along the qui meridians.

Page: 230

Question #18

Answer: D

Rationale: Acupuncture, ayurveda, biofeedback, chelation therapy, chiropractic care, energy healing therapy, massage, naturopathy, and Reiki are considered practitioner-based therapy.

Page: 226

Question #19

Answer: C

Rationale: Persons of all religions may practice transcendental meditation. To prevent distracting thoughts, the subject repeats a mantra, which can be a word or sound, over and over again while sitting in a comfortable position. If a distracting thought comes to mind, it is accepted and then let go, with the mind focusing again on the mantra. Yoga is a different mind–body CAM therapy that focuses on the use of postures and breathing exercises.

Page: 231

Question #20

Answer: C

Rationale: Many early clinical trials for CAM therapies have had serious flaws; however, rigorous clinical trials are possible. Clinical investigations have been made difficult as a result of the use of individualized, often complex treatments; a lack of standardization of herbal medicine; problems with accruing, randomizing, and retaining patients; and identifying placebo interventions.

Page: 228

Question #21

Answer: C

Rationale: Although the practice of naturopathy may include homeopathic treatment, the two CAM therapies hold different philosophies in their approach to healing. Naturopathy believes that the body is able to heal itself via the power of nature. Healing occurs through diet, exercise, avoidance of environmental toxins, elimination of body wastes, and positive thoughts and emotions. Key principles in naturopathy include taking a preventive approach and focusing on the maintenance of health rather than on the treatment of illness. When treating a disease with homeopathy, the philosophy is based on the law of similars, which holds that medicines can produce the same symptoms in healthy people that they cure in those who are ill. Remedies are used in the smallest quantity possible; they are often so dilute that not even a molecule of the original therapeutic substance remains in solution.

Page: 233

Question #22

Answer: A

Rationale: Transcendental meditation is not considered a movement therapy. Rather, it is a mind–body technique in which the subject repeats a mantra (word or sound) over and over again while sitting in a comfortable position. Movement therapies include tai chi, in which movement and breathing—often associated with specific flowing movement patterns—are used to affect the flow of energy or qi. Qigong is part of traditional Chinese medicine, and it is also used to cultivate qi. This practice included breathing exercises, meditation, and physical movement. It is used in martial arts and to generate energy to be used in healing. Feldenkrais, which was developed in the 1950s, involves gentle movements and

manipulation enlisted to retrain the body with new movement patterns. Yoga is also considered a movement therapy, and it focuses on postures and breathing exercise.

Page: 232

Question #23

Answer: C

Rationale: According to Barnes and colleagues in their article "CDC Advance Data Report #343, Complementary and Alternative Medicine Use Among Adults: United States, 2002,"[4] 16.8% of CAM therapy is for back pain. It is followed in descending order of treatment by head cold and neck pain (6.6%), arthritis (4.9%), anxiety/depression (4.5%), stomach upset, headache, and recurring pain and insomnia.

Page: 226

Question #24

Answer: B

Rationale: According to Barnes and colleagues in their article "CDC Advance Data Report #343, Complementary and Alternative Medicine Use Among Adults: United States, 2002,"[4] the most common CAM therapies used include, in descending order of use, prayer (self), prayer (others), natural products, deep breathing, prayer groups, meditation, chiropractic treatment, yoga, massage, and diet (Figure 16-3).

Page: 226

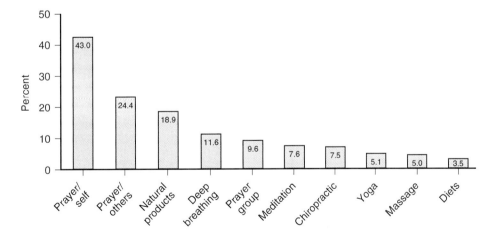

Figure 16-3 From Barnes PM, Towell-Griner E, McFann K, Nahin RL: Complementary and alternative medicine use among adults: United States, 2002. CDC Advance Data Report #343. 2004. In Rakel RE, editor: *Textbook of family medicine,* ed 7, Philadelphia, WB Saunders, 2007.

4. Barnes PM, Towell-Griner E, McFann K, Nahin RL: Complementary and Alternative Medicine Use Among Adults: United States, 2002. CDC Advance Data Report no. 343. 2004.

Question #25

Answer: B

Rationale: The NCCAM was established in 1998. Its predecessor, the Office of Alternative Medicine, was established in 1992. The American Holistic Medical Association was founded in 1978. In 2000, President Clinton appointed James S. Gordon, MD, to chair the first White House Commission on Complementary and Alternative Medicine Policy. The final report of this commission was submitted in 2002. In 2005, the Institute of Medicine released its report about CAM in the United States.

Page: 224

Question #26

Answer: C

Rationale: Prayer is communication with an absolute, imminent, or transcendent spiritual force, however it may be named. Such communication may take a variety of forms, and it may be theistic or nontheistic in nature; the practice transcends all religions and beliefs. Spirituality and prayer are considered a mind–body CAM therapy. In a 2002 study by Barnes and colleagues,[5] prayer ranked as the number one (self prayer) and number two (prayer/others) most common CAM therapies. Group prayer ranked number five.

Page: 226

Question #27

Answer: A

Rationale: A particular aspect of nutrition that has received increasing attention for its value in lessening inflammation is that of fish oil (omega-6 and omega-3 fatty acids). Inflammation has been shown to play a role in cardiovascular disease, asthma, arthritis, psoriasis, and inflammatory bowel disease. Omega-3 and omega-6 fatty acids are essential polyunsaturated fatty acids that cannot be made by the human body. To follow an anti-inflammatory diet, decrease red meats, poultry, and dairy intake; increase foods containing omega-3 fatty acids, including cold-water fish, flaxseed, walnuts, and green leafy vegetables; reduce foods containing omega-6 fatty acids, such as margarine and oils from corn, cottonseeds, grapeseeds, peanuts, safflowers, sesame seeds, soybeans, or sunflowers; and avoid foods with a long shelf life.

Page: 231

Question #28

Answer: A

Rationale: Hypnosis is a mind–body technique that may require referral; however, practitioners can learn the art of hypnosis without having medical or psychological degrees. Although the modality was previously known as "sleep healing," it is not sleep; rather, it is a relaxed state of focused awareness that eliminates critical judgment and distraction from daily thoughts. The procedure is used to access various levels of the mind to effect positive changes in a person's behavior and to treat numerous health conditions. It is an altered state of consciousness that is characterized by an increased responsiveness to suggestion, but no drugs are involved in the practice. A hypnosis session involves absorption, dissociation, and suggestibility.

Page: 231

Question #29

Answer: D

Rationale: The philosophy of traditional Chinese medicine is that qi and other substances flow through the body through various channels. Pain is a result of blocked qi. Yin and yang (passive and active characteristics) and the five elements (wood, fire, earth, metal, and water) have competing influences on various body parts. A specific diagnosis is not needed. Information is gathered through looking, asking, listening to the body's sounds, and palpation. Therapeutics include acupuncture, moxibustion, gua sha, cupping, tui na, plum blossom, and herbal therapies.

Page: 232

Question #30

Answer: B

Rationale: Therapeutic touch is an energy healing modality. It was developed in the 1970s, and there are currently more than 50,000 practitioners of this therapy. The hands are used to balance energy flows and chakra function in the body. The seven main chakras are energy vortices that project from the center of the body. Smaller chakras also exist in various locations. Therapeutic touch does not involve magnet therapy, which is a different energy therapy. Swedish and deep-tissue massage are massage therapies. Massage, chiropractic treatment, and osteopathy are considered manipulative and body-based methods according to the five domains of CAM therapies as grouped by the NCCAM.

Page: 231

---

5. Barnes and colleagues (2002).

Question #1

Answer: C

Rationale: Under the Dietary Supplements Health and Educations Act, herbs, vitamins, minerals, and other natural supplements are classified as dietary supplements. These products do not require prior marketing approval by the U.S. Food and Drug Administration (FDA). Indeed, the burden of proof has been placed on the FDA rather than the manufacturer if any suspicion develops about the safety of a supplement. The FDA may not question efficacy, whereas manufacturers are prohibited from making claims about specific disease therapy. Good manufacturing practices are the responsibility of the manufacturer.

Page: 243

Question #2

Answer: B

Rationale: Following the passage of the Dietary Supplements Health and Educations Act, the supplement market boomed with unprecedented promotion efforts by all available modes of communication. The use of supplements is widespread. According to the telephone survey of 8470 respondents referenced in the question, the prevalence of supplement use had increased from 14.2% in 1998 and 1999 to 18.8% in 2002.

Page: 243

Question #3

Answer: C

Rationale: The National Center for Complementary and Alternative Medicine was established in 1998 within the National Institutes of Health, and it funds research about supplements. Advising patients about supplement use is not without its challenges. The sheer numbers of available products and advertising claims can lead to confusion for both patients and health care professionals. Product safety and standardization are often variable, and research may be of poor quality or difficult to interpret.

Page: 244

Question #4

Answer: D

Rationale: A 2001 study revealed that only 70% of patients reported that they had even mentioned their use of supplements to their health care providers at all. Nearly half of those who regularly used supplements felt that their doctors were prejudiced against such use. Forty-four percent felt that their physicians had limited knowledge about such products. People who take supplements often value their independence with regard to making health care decisions, and many have spent a great deal of time researching various products online. Specifically asking about herbal and other supplement use when gathering a patient history is essential, given that patients may not always volunteer this information. It is also vital that clinicians have a working familiarity with supplement use. Physicians who are well informed about the commonly used herbs can educate and protect their patients from the potential hazards of dietary supplements.

Page: 244

Question #5

Answer: C

Rationale: Because it is not possible to patent individual supplement compounds, a manufacturer may sell a mixture of supplements as a "proprietary blend." When evaluating a combination product, it is important to consider each ingredient separately. Sometimes, products used in combination may have a synergistic or an antagonistic effect on each other. Therefore, a product involving a "proprietary blend" does not always mean that it is a high-quality product.

Page: 243

Question #6

Answer: B

Rationale: The quality of a product can be evaluated on the basis of its packaging information. It should be clear what ingredients the product contains. According to the Dietary Supplements Health and Educations Act, a supplement may not claim to cure, treat, or prevent disease, and it must state on its label that its claims "have not been evaluated by the FDA." Look for how the product's contents are standardized. Many botanicals will be standardized to a specific percentage content of one particular chemical. The manufacturer's name and address should be seen on the label. It may help to become familiar with a few manufacturers who produce reliable brands.

Page: 245

Question #7

Answer: D

Rationale: *Aristolochia* is commonly used as an aphrodisiac, an anticonvulsant, an immune stimulant, and a menstruation promoter. It contains aristolochic acid, which is nephrotoxic and carcinogenic; deaths have been linked to its use. The FDA considers it to be unsafe and adulterated.

Page: 246

Question #8

Answer: A

Rationale: Comfrey, chaparral, germander, and kava have been associated with liver damage. They are considered unsafe, and they should not be used at all. Milk thistle is used for liver disorders, including toxic liver damage caused by chemicals; it is usually well tolerated. Although ephedra does not cause liver damage, it has been linked to 155 deaths and to dozens of heart attacks and strokes. As a result, the sale of ephedra in the United States has been banned. Saw palmetto is considered safe when used orally and appropriately.

Page: 246

Question #9

Answer: B

Rationale: Yucca is commonly used to treat arthritis, hypertension, and hypercholesterolemia. Traditionally, it is used by American Indians as foods. In manufacturing, yucca extract is used as a foaming and flavoring agent in carbonated beverages. Yucca is likely safe when it is used in amounts that are commonly found in foods. Orally, it may cause stomach upset, bitter taste, nausea, and vomiting. Yohimbe is commonly used for erectile dysfunction. It can alter blood pressure, increase the risk of myocardial infarction, and cause respiratory depression; its use is generally not recommended. Pennyroyal oil is commonly used for intestinal disorders, respiratory aliments, and as

an abortifacient. The use of pennyroyal oil has been associated with renal and hepatic failure, nerve damage, and convulsion; hence, it is considered unsafe for general use. Skullcap is commonly used for insomnia, anxiety, and stroke; it has been linked to cases of liver damage and therefore is rated as likely hazardous.

Page: 254

Question #10

Answer: C

Rationale: Recent studies questioned the health benefits of vitamin E supplementation. A study by Zhang[1] showed that vitamin E may prevent Parkinson's disease if it is eaten in the diet, but it does not appear to have the same effect when it is taken as a supplement. A meta-analysis concluded that vitamin E at doses of more than 400 IU may increase all-cause mortality and should be avoided. Results from the Women's Health Study suggest that vitamin E supplementation does not seem to affect the incidence of cancer or major cardiovascular events among older women. A study by Lonn and colleagues[2] suggested a potential link between vitamin E consumption and the risk of developing heart failure among patients with vascular disease or diabetes.

Page: 245

Question #11

Answer: D

Rationale: St. John's wort has been shown to induce the cytochrome P450 isoenzymes and to decrease the blood levels of many drugs, such as indinavir, oral contraceptives, cyclosporine, digoxin, theophylline, and warfarin. Because one of the proposed mechanisms of action of St. John's wort is the inhibition of monoamine oxidase, it may cause serotonin syndrome if it is used with other antidepressants (including SSRIs) or other serotonergic drugs.

Pages: 247, 253

Question #12

Answer: B

Rationale: Stinging nettle has a high content of vitamin K; therefore, it may increase the potential for clot

1. Zhang SM, Hernan MA, Chen H, et al: Intakes of vitamins E and C, carotenoids, vitamin supplements, and PD risk. *Neurology* 59:1161-1169, 2002.
2. Lonne E, Bosch J, Yusuf S, et al: Effects of long-term vitamin E supplementation on cardiovascular events and cancer: A randomized controlled trial. *JAMA* 293:1338-1347, 2005.

formation. Alternatively, garlic, dong quai, and ginkgo leaves may increase the risk of bleeding by inhibiting platelet aggregation. Herbs that can increase hemorrhage risk should be stopped several weeks before surgery.
Page: 247

Question #13

Answer: B

Rationale: As a steroid hormone, DHEA may raise blood glucose. Alternatively, a few reports have suggested that ginseng, bitter melon, and fenugreek may lower blood glucose and that they can have a positive effect for diabetic patients.
Page: 247

Question #14

Answer: C

Rationale: Although American ginseng, ginger, licorice, and cayenne may raise blood pressure, black cohosh may lower it.
Page: 248

Questions #15 through #19

Answers: 15, B; 16, A; 17, D; 18, C; 19, E

Rationale: Herbal remedies are supplement preparations that are made from various parts of the plant, and they commonly contain numerous different chemical compounds. The potency and efficacy of a given remedy are influenced by a number of factors, including where an herb was grown, the particular species used in the formulation, which plant parts were used, the way in which the plant products were processed, and which compounds were used for chemical standardization. Some common herbal preparations are crude herb, juice, dry herb, infusion, decoction, tincture, and extract. Crude herb is used in the form in which it is harvested; ginger root is an example of this. Juice is obtained when an herb is crushed; concentrations of various compounds in the juice vary. Cranberry is commonly consumed as juice. Dry herb is a preparation in which the herb is air dried after picking, and it may then be powdered and packaged into capsules or pressed together to form tablets. Feverfew is an example of dry herb. Infusion is a water extract in which the herb parts are put in boiling water to make a tea. Chamomile is an example of an herb that is infused. A decoction is a water extract in which an herb and water are boiled

together; it is usually more concentrated than an infusion. Ginseng is usually consumed as a decoction. Tincture is a solvent extract in which the herb parts are put into an organic solvent (usually alcohol or glycerol). There are three kinds of extract: freeze-dried extract, fluid extract, and solid extract.
Page: 248

Question #20

Answer: C

Rationale: Herbs that have been used for menopause include black cohosh, dong quai, evening primrose, and soy. These herbs are called *phytoestrogens*. A recent review found black cohosh to be beneficial for treating hot flashes, but there is a lack of adequate long-term safety data. Soy may have modest effects on hot flashes, but most benefits disappear after 6 weeks. As for other herbs, clinical trials do not support their use during menopause.
Page: 250

Questions #21 through #26

Answers: 21, E; 22, C; 23, A; 24, B; 25, F; 26, D

Rationale: Echinacea is possibly effective when it is used for upper respiratory infections. It should be avoided for patients with systemic autoimmune disorders and for patients taking immunosuppressive drugs. Feverfew is commonly used to prevent migraines. However, it may cause withdrawal symptoms if it is stopped suddenly after long-term use. Ginkgo is often used for dementia and intermittent claudication, but it can increase bleeding when taken with aspirin and warfarin. Hawthorn is possibly effective when it is used for stage I or II heart failure; it enhances the effects of digoxin and reduces the toxicity. St. John's wort is likely effective for mild to moderate depression. At high doses, it can cause photosensitivity. Saw palmetto has been shown to be effective for treating benign prostatic hypertrophy; it may lower prostate-specific antigen levels.
Pages: 250–253

Question #27

Answer: D

Rationale: Panax ginseng is used to enhance the libido. It has been shown to have hypoglycemic activity, and it can also raise blood pressure and cause insomnia.
Page: 251

Question #28

Answer: C

Rationale: Valerian is commonly used for insomnia. It can cause morning drowsiness, and there is a possibility of withdrawal symptoms after long-term use.

Page: 253

Question #29

Answer: A

Rationale: Garlic can increase the risk of bleeding, and it should be discontinued at least 7 days before surgery. Because the effects of warfarin/antiplatelet agents can be increased by garlic, they should not be taken concomitantly with garlic. Garlic does not cause drowsiness. Some people use garlic to treat *H. pylori* infection, but there is not enough evidence to support such use.

Page: 251

Question #30

Answer: D

Rationale: Vitamin B_3 is niacin or niacinamide. Niacin is used to treat hyperlipidemia, and it can increase the risk of myopathy if it is given with statins.

Page: 249

Question #31

Answer: B

Rationale: Chromium is widely used by people with diabetes to lower blood glucose levels.

Page: 258

Question #32

Answer: D

Rationale: Creatine is used widely for athletic conditioning at high doses. It has been linked to dehydration and heat intolerance, and it may also cause muscle cramping and breakdown. It should be avoided among patients with renal and liver disease.

Page: 261

Question #33

Answer: B

Rationale: DHEA is an endogenous adrenal hormone. People use it for many reasons, including athletic performance, dementia, and sexual performance. It can raise androgen and estrogen levels, and it may possibly increase the risk of hormone-sensitive cancers.

Page: 261

Question #34

Answer: D

Rationale: Glucosamine is possibly effective for osteoarthritis. It is generally well tolerated, and palpitations resulting from its use are rare. It may alter the effects of drugs on glucose levels.

Page: 262

Question #35

Answer: C

Rationale: Melatonin is useful for delayed sleep phase syndrome and jet lag. It is generally safe, but it may cause sleepiness, headache, mood changes, drops in blood pressure drops, and hyperglycemia among patients with type 1 diabetes.

Page: 263

Question #36

Answer: A

Rationale: SAMe is likely useful for depression and osteoarthritis. It can precipitate manic episodes among bipolar patients, and it may augment the serotonergic effects of SSRIs and meperidine.

Page: 264

18 Answers

Question #1

Answers: A and C

Rationale: The establishment of rapport between the physician and the patient is highly conducive to instilling a sense of confidence in the patient. *Rapport* refers to the intangible element of a relationship that conveys warmth and trust. If rapport is established, the patient is much more likely to respond to recommended therapies and much more likely to forgive a less-than-perfect experience or poor clinical outcome.

Page: 269

Question #2

Answer: A

Rationale: Patient satisfaction is closely related to the quality of the physician–patient relationship. It is also related to the physician's ability to educate the patient regarding the disease process and to motivate the patient to partner in his or her own treatment or recovery.

Page: 269

Question #3

Answer: D

Rationale: A physician who fails to communicate well with his or her patient is much more likely to have a formal complaint made. It is also true that more complaints against a physician result from a perceived lack of caring than from office inefficiencies or from problems with treatment outcomes.

Pages: 269–270

Question #4

Answer: C

Rationale: Patients prefer to receive medical news from a physician whom they trust. This should be delivered carefully and in a setting in which the patient is absolutely confident that no one else can overhear the conversation. The patient can be given the choice of having a confidante present if he or she so chooses. The patient may prefer to have something to read, but this should not be used as an alternative to a face-to-face, unhurried meeting.

Pages: 269–270

Question #5

Answer: D

Rationale: It is important to convey a positive bedside manner for patients. However, the conveyance of this manner will be quite variable from physician to physician. One should develop a bedside manner that conveys trust and respect in the approach to the patient. Honesty and empathy incorporated into this approach will greatly help the development of this important component of the physician's role.

Page: 269

Question #6

Answer: C

Rationale: Each physician will need to develop his or her own style of dress. Circumstances of practice will vary widely, and the comfort level for the physician and the patient will also vary. However, in general, patients prefer that their physicians wear conventional clothes covered with a white coat. Studies have shown that patients consider house staff who wear white coats with conventional street clothes as more competent than those who wear scrub suits.

Page: 269

Question #7

Answer: B

Rationale: Studies have actually shown that a genuine smile is helpful for establishing a friendly atmosphere and developing a warm interpersonal relationship. A smile that is not genuine is considered to be "phony," and this is immediately detected by patients.

Page: 269

Question #8

Answer: E

Rationale: Knowing and pronouncing the patient's name is very important for both building rapport and for the safety of patients. Reviewing and commenting on the patient's record, including the last visit, establishes a sense of confidence on the part of the patient. Referring to the illness treated at another time, to family conditions, or to other events important to the patient will reassure the patient that the physician is genuinely interested in him or her and in the reason for and the outcome of his or her visit.

Page: 269

Question #9

Answer: B

Rationale: It is usually a lack of security that makes a physician appear aloof and unconcerned. This is combined with a lack of self-confidence, which causes the doctor to hide behind this protective stance. A physician with a positive self-image is much more likely to create a relaxed but professional image that does not impede the physician–patient relationship.

Page: 270

Question #10

Answer: D

Rationale: The establishment of mutual respect depends on the physician being able to convey a sense of quiet self-confidence. In addition, making positive comments about the patient or a colleague conveys respect for others. It can also be very helpful for establishing a respectful relationship if the physician is able to admit his or her own limitations; patients do understand and respect this in return.

Page: 270

Question #11

Answer: E

Rationale: A physician's emotions and how he or she manages them can have a powerful impact on the physician–patient relationship. Self-awareness is critical for helping to understand personal responses to patients. However, it is very rare for it to be beneficial for the physician to share his or her own emotions with the patient; the focus should be on the patient and the patient's emotions.

Page: 270

Question #12

Answer: A

Rationale: If a physician is feeling that he or she is seeing too many patients, the more likely he or she is to describe the patient's complaints as trivial, inappropriate, or bothersome. Patients who frequently seek help for nonspecific somatic and functional complaints may well be depressed.

Page: 270

Question #13

Answers: A and B

Rationale: Patient satisfaction with medical care is much more closely related to the desire for information and affective support than for further examination and testing. Furthermore, patients whose desire for information and attention to family and emotional problems have gone unmet have been found to be significantly less satisfied with their physicians. Patient satisfaction is closely tied to increased compliance with treatment regimens.

Page: 270

Question #14

Answer: C

Rationale: In a typical business, only 4% of customers actually voice their satisfaction; the other 96% say nothing, and 91% never return. It is strongly recommended that all physician practices conduct a patient satisfaction survey to identify any problems that might exist.

Page: 270

19 Answers

Question #1

Answer: E

Rationale: Developing a patient education plan has many benefits. Patients must have appropriate knowledge to make shared decisions and to participate more fully in their care. Patient education programs help deliver the knowledge and skills that patients need to plan and carry out a medical treatment. Numerous studies have shown the benefits of an active role for patients in their own care.[1,2] Two studies have shown enhanced treatment outcomes when patients are involved in making decisions about their health.[3,4]

Page: 285

Question #2

Answer: B

Rationale: Two studies have demonstrated better health outcomes when patients are involved in making decisions about their care.[3,4]

Pages: 285, 286

Question #3

Answer: A

Rationale: In the era of shorter visit lengths, many are concerned that providing patient-centered care may take longer. However, studies have shown that there are no differences in visit length for usual care as compared with patient-centered care.

Page: 286

Question #4

Answer: E

Rationale: Several studies have shown that patients are more likely to adhere to therapy when they have been properly informed with a patient education program.[5,6] Other benefits from a patient education program for physicians are improved patient satisfaction and good practice marketing.[7,8] Better education of patients can also reduce malpractice claims.[9,10]

Page: 286

Question #5

Answer: D

Rationale: The SOAPE format for progress notes includes a section for education in addition to the traditional SOAP components. Including education as a part of the format for documentation encourages patient education to occur during each encounter. This format also provides a convenient way to document any patient education that was offered during the visit.

Page: 286

Question #6

Answer: E

Rationale: Education is the key component of high-quality primary care. Education should be included in every interaction that occurs during the course of the care of patients. During the history-taking portion, knowledge, skills, and attitudes can be assessed. While

1. Toman C, Harrison MB, Logan J: Clinical practice guidelines: Necessary but not sufficient for evidence-based patient education and counseling. *Patient Educ Couns* 42:279-287, 2001.
2. Roter D: The medical visit context of treatment decision-making and the therapeutic relationship. *Health Expect* 3:17-25, 2000.
3. Epstein RM, Alper BS, Quill TE: Communicating evidence for participatory decision making. *JAMA* 291:2359-2366, 2004.
4. Stewart MA: Effective physician-patient communication and health outcomes: A review. *CMAJ* 152:1423-1433, 1995.
5. Rogers A, Kennedy A, Nelson E, Robinson A: Uncovering the limits of patientcenteredness: implementing a self-management trial for chronic illness. *Qual Health Res* 15:224-229, 2005.
6. Gray MJ, Elhai JD, Frueh BC: Enhancing patient satisfaction and increasing treatment compliance: Patient education as a fundamental component of PSD treatment. *Psychiatry Q* 75:321-332, 2004.
7. Aragon SJ: Commentary: A patient-centered theory of satisfaction. *Am J Med Qual* 18:225-228, 2003.
8. Ganz PA: What outcomes matter to patients: A physician-researcher point of view. *Med Care* 40(Suppl III):9-11, 2002.
9. Eastaugh SR: Reducing litigation costs through better patient communication. *Physician Exec* 30:36-38, 2004.
10. Wissow LS: Communication and malpractice claims—where are we now? *Patient Educ Couns* 52:3-5, 2004.

performing the physical examination, the physician can explain findings to the patient. When discussing the diagnosis, the physician can explain in easy-to-understand language and check for comprehension. When planning therapy, the physician can assess understanding and identify any barriers to the planned treatment. At every step of the office visit, there are opportunities to better educate the patients about their care and treatment plan.

Page: 286

Question #7

Answer: E

Rationale: Imagination is the only limitation to the many ways that physicians and practices can offer patient education and health promotion.

Page: 286

Question #8

Answer: E

Rationale: No physician is an island unto himself or herself. When planning a comprehensive patient education program, the physician should not overlook the available resources. Within the practice, there are many staff members who can be enlisted to assist with educational efforts. In communities, there are excellent local and national partners, such as the American Diabetes Association, the American Heart Association, the American Cancer Society, Weight Watchers, and Alcoholics Anonymous. There may also be courses offered by local libraries, YMCA chapters, or religious organizations. Knowing these resources within your community can facilitate patient education and care.

Page: 286

Question #9

Answer: A

Rationale: The principles of patient education include six key components: feedback, reinforcement, individualization, facilitation, relevance, and the use of multiple channels of communication. These principles have been incorporated into the U.S. Preventive Services Task Force for patient education and counseling.

Page: 286

Question #10

Answer: D

Rationale: When designing and planning patient education for a given patient, the concept of individualization requires that the physician consider all of the facets of the unique individual. The needs, desires, and characteristics of the patient should be the key determinants of how the educational material is delivered. This tailored approach enhances the effectiveness of the physician's message. In addition, this concept requires that specific goals and objectives be negotiated with each patient.

Page: 286

Question #11

Answer: D

Rationale: Facilitation is the assisting of patients with making lifestyle and treatment changes. This assistance can be in the form of materials, cues, or skill training. Each modality has its place in a comprehensive patient education program.

Page: 286

Question #12

Answer: C

Rationale: Prochaska studied the science of behavior change using the stages of change model to assess the percentages of people with behavioral problems. In this system, there are five stages of change: precontemplative, contemplative, preparation, action, and maintenance.

Page: 287

Question #13

Answer: A

Rationale: The *transtheoretical model* or the *stages of change model* is a practical way to classify different phases of behavioral change. As a patient considers a behavioral change, he or she moves through five distinct phases: precontemplative, contemplative, preparation, action, and maintenance. The precontemplative phase occurs before the patient has even begun to consider changing the behavior. After this, the patient begins to contemplate change; he or she then prepares for the change and finally takes action to change the behavior.

The final stage is the maintenance of the change. Practice is not a formal stage of change in this model.
Page: 287

Question #14

Answer: B

Rationale: This patient is considering beginning a behavioral change and therefore is in the contemplative stage of change.
Page: 287

Question #15

Answer: C

Rationale: After a patient has begun considering a change, the next step is preparation. During this phase, planning begins. Setting a quit date is a way to firmly plan action. At this time, the patient is preparing for action, which is the stage that follows preparation. The other strategies are more appropriate for patients in other stages. Trying to convince a smoker to quit is for those patients who are in the precontemplative phase. Keeping the door open for change is always useful, but it is really better geared toward the precontemplative patient as well. Nicotine replacement strategies are for the action phase.
Pages: 287, 288

Question #16

Answer: A

Rationale: This patient is in the precontemplative stage; she has yet to consider change.
Page: 287

Question #17

Answer: C

Rationale: This patient is in the precontemplative phase. The task for the physician is to move the patient to the contemplative stage. Research has shown that, if a person perceives significant benefit from a change, he or she is more likely to move from the precontemplative stage to the contemplative stage.
Page: 287

Question #18

Answer: C

Rationale: It is evidenced by the fact that she has set a date that she has been planning; therefore, she is in the preparation phase. She is ready to take action next.
Page: 287

Question #19

Answer: B

Rationale: Research has shown that the best strategy to help someone move to action is to address the perceived cons of the change. Each person is unique, and the physician must work to understand what is important to this patient. After the physician understands the patient's belief system, then he or she can address the patient's particular cons and help them move toward action.
Page: 287

Question #20

Answer: C

Rationale: Patients in the preparation phase are the most likely to succeed with behavioral change. Many patients are poorly motivated, and this can be very frustrating to physicians who are trying to achieve behavior change. As the physician becomes more skilled with regard to behavior modification, the more difficult groups (precontemplative and contemplative) can be tackled.
Page: 288

Question #21

Answer: B

Rationale: The first step in an educational process is to assess what the learner already knows. The physician can then plan to fill in the gaps in the patient's knowledge. A few simple questions can ascertain current knowledge. A physician can use any one of the following questions: "What have you been told the problem is?" "What does that mean to you?" "What questions do you have about the problem or its treatment?"
Page: 288

Question #22

Answer: E

Rationale: Poor literacy is very common in America, with more than 90 million adults being affected. The consequences of this problem are considerable for the health of these people. Lower literacy has an impact on just about every aspect of a person's healthcare; it not only affects written communication, but it may inhibit verbal communication as well.

Page: 288

Question #23

Answer: E

Rationale: Many factors lead to lower literacy levels. Intelligence, socioeconomic status, and learning disabilities all affect comprehension. Cultural differences between the physician and the patient can also lead to errors in communication.

Page: 288

Question #24

Answer: C

Rationale: Patients with literacy problems will often seek to conceal the fact that they have a problem. There is a strong social stigma attached to having difficulty reading or understanding information. As a result of the nature of this problem, physicians must be constantly vigilant to discover and assist patients with literacy difficulties.

Page: 288

Question #25

Answer: B

Rationale: Several studies have shown that patients with lower literacy levels can learn if their problem is identified and addressed. Sometimes additional time is needed to address the topic in an individualized way.

Page: 289

Question #26

Answer: E

Rationale: There are many strategies to use to assist with patient education for a patient with lower literacy. Using visual representations of topics may help the challenged patient understand more easily. Any written materials given to the patient should contain only the essential information, which should be organized in a logical sequence. Extra details should be omitted to limit potential confusion. When dealing with complex topics, it is often useful to break these down into simpler and more limited pieces. This also assists with conserving time during office visits.

Page: 289

Question #27

Answer: A

Rationale: Having the physician actually involved in part of the delivery of patient education enhances the credibility of the program. At a minimum, the physician should always be involved in developing the goals and objectives for the patient education plan for the office. The physical layout of the practice is also important. There should be bins for the display of brochures and other written materials. If group education sessions are going to be offered, then an appropriate room needs to be available.

Page: 289

Question #28

Answer: D

Rationale: Everyone should be involved. Formal studies have shown that the involvement of all of the office staff in patient education greatly enhances the overall impact of the program.

Page: 289

Question #29

Answer: D

Rationale: Patients live in intricate family systems; failure to recognize these interactions can limit the effectiveness of educational efforts. A smoking couple presents a challenge if only one wishes to quit. The person who cooks the meals has a greater impact on the composition of the diet than any member of the family with high cholesterol. Other family members can have behaviors that are harmful to a patient's disease, such as smoking around an asthmatic. When approaching patient education, it is important for physicians to consider the family system.

Page: 289

Question #30

Answer: E

Rationale: Creating an atmosphere of acceptance and avoiding a disparaging approach are prerequisites for effective communication. A judgmental environment limits disclosure and can hamper the discovery of important health behaviors that need to be addressed. Medical professionals use jargon without realizing it; this can be confusing and should be avoided. When teaching a patient, it is important to check frequently for understanding.

Pages: 289, 290

Question #31

Answer: D

Rationale: The use of written materials to support other methods of teaching patients is highly effective. When written materials are used alone, they have been shown to not be very effective. Unfortunately, this is often how these materials are used.

Page: 290

Question #32

Answer: E

Rationale: There are many sources of well-developed patient education material for purchase. Before using this material, the physician or a designee should review the information to ensure that the information is accurate and up to date. If there are published guidelines about the topic being addressed, the material should agree with these. There are educational materials that are provided by pharmaceutical companies, but they can be very biased; review of these materials is necessary to ensure that no partiality exists in these written materials.

Page: 290

Question #1

Answer: D

Rationale: The physician conveys interest and concern for the patient by giving the impression of having time for the patient and by conveying a sense of being unhurried. The physician must listen with the ears to what is being said, listen with the eyes for nonverbal behaviors, and listen with the fingers as examinations are completed.

Page: 293

Question #2

Answer: A

Rationale: It is the rapport, respect, and relationship that are enhanced by the physician taking the time to listen and understand the story of the patient's concerns.

Page: 293

Question #3

Answer: B

Rationale: Rapport is key to being a successful healer, especially in today's medical environment of technological sophistication and managed-care limitations. The physician must use the best listening skills to develop a positive rapport with his or her patients.

Pages: 293, 294

Question #4

Answer: C

Rationale: It is up to the physician to pay attention to the little internal message from the patient. Cluing in on how patients expresses themselves allows the physician to join with their sensory expansion. This allows the physician to have an understanding of the biopsychosocial aspects of the patients as they relate to the patients' lives and relationships.

Page: 294

Question #5

Answer: B

Rationale: Stone and colleagues[1] observed that physicians should encourage adherence rather than insist on compliance. "Compliance implies an involuntary act of submission to authority whereas adherence refers to a voluntary act of subscribing to a point of view."

Page: 295

Question #6

Answer: B

Rationale: Time is one of the greatest challenges for the busy physician. Few things disrupt effective communication like the perception by the patient that the physician does not have time to address his or her problem. Open-access scheduling helps predict urgent care needs and allows for the creation of adequate same-day appointment times.[2]

Pages: 295–296

Question #7

Answer: C

Rationale: Technology, complementary and alternative medicine, and various interruptions can impede the interview process. Keeping the patient informed, maintaining good eye contact, and being open to various approaches to health can foster the physician–patient relationship and keep the lines of communication open.

Page: 296

Question #8

Answer: B

Rationale: The emphasis on spiritual history-taking within medical schools increased from 13% to 66%

1. Stone SS, Bronkesh SJ, Gerbarg ZB, Wood SD: Improving patient compliance. Strategic Med January, 1998. Available at 7 www.hsmgroup.com/info/compli/compli.
2. Murray M, Tantau C: Same-day appointments: Exploding the access paradigm. Fam Pract Manage September 2000, available at http://www.aafp.org/fpm/20000900/45same.html.

between 1994 and 2004.[3] However, a report in 1991 indicated that only 10% of patients surveyed had ever been asked by their physician about their faith and the possible impact that their beliefs may have on their healthcare.[4]

Page: 297

Question #9

Answers: F, 3; I, 11; C, 1; A, 6

Rationale:

Faith: Do you consider yourself a spiritual person?

Importance: How important is your faith to you?

Community: Are you a part of a spiritual or religious community?

Address: How would you like me to address these issues in your health care?

Page: 297

Question #10

Answers: 3, Preparation; 5, Maintenance; 1, Pre-contemplation; 6, Termination; 2, Contemplation; 4, Action

Rationale:

Precontemplation: The person is not yet ready for any change.

Contemplation: The person is intending to change within the next 6 months.

Preparation: The person actually makes some behavioral lifestyle changes.

Maintenance: The person is consolidating gains and working to prevent relapse.

Termination: The person may reach the ultimate goal, and the problem or behavior is no longer a treat or temptation.

Pages: 297, 298

Question #11

Answer: D

Rationale: An analysis that compared CAGE screening to another alcohol screening reported that the CAGE tool had a sensitivity of 70% and a specificity of 90%.[5] However, this screening tool is less accurate for women and blacks.[6]

Page: 298

Question #12

Answers: C, E, A, H, B, G, D, F

Rationale: The act of interviewing and the various techniques used for each patient type are clinical skills that are learned, developed, and enhanced through clinical practice. This learning is an ongoing process that will change as the physician engages people from a variety of ages and circumstances and with a variety of health concerns. During every interview, however, listening is a key element for establishing and maintaining rapport, respect, and relationships with patients.

Page: 299

Question #13

Answer: B

Rationale: The LISTEN paradigm provides a structural mnemonic that moves the conversation logically and holistically throughout the interview. The key areas addressed are defined as follows: *l*istening, *i*nterpersonal, *s*omatic, *t*hinking, *e*motion, and *n*ormal.

Page: 297

---

3. Fortin AH, Barnett KG: Medical school curricula in spirituality and medicine. *JAMA* 291:2883, 2004.

4. Maugans TA, Wadland WC: Religion and family medicine: A survey of physicians and patients. *J Fam Pract* 39:349-352, 1991.

5. Vinson DC, Galliher JM, Reidinger C, Kappus A: Comfortably engaging: Which approach to alcohol screening should we use? *Ann Fam Med* 2:398-404, 2004.

6. Feldman MD, Christensen JF: *Behavioral Medicine in Primary Care: A Practical Guide*, 2nd ed. New York, Lange Medical Books/McGraw-Hill, 2003.

Question #1

Answer: A

Rationale: A serum creatinine level is recommended so that a creatinine clearance can be calculated. An estimate of renal function will assist the physician with making decisions about medications and dosages. Other tests that are useful include liver function testing, because many pain medications are metabolized by the liver. A complete metabolic panel would encompass both a serum creatinine and liver function tests. A complete blood cell count is not routinely recommended before starting pharmacotherapy for pain. However, if a patient is taking aspirin or NSAIDs chronically, it could be considered to look for anemia. A thyroid-stimulating hormone level is not routinely recommended, but it might be useful for the evaluation of an unexplained polyneuropathy. Urinalysis is not needed before starting pain medications, and an acetylneuraminic acid level is not useful and should not be obtained unless clinical suspicion for an autoimmune process is high.

Page: 305

Question #2

Answer: B

Rationale: Neuropathic pain is frequently diagnosed by history, so an understanding of the verbal descriptors used for this type of pain is important. Patients should be asked to describe the quality of their pain as well as the location, onset, intensity, and pattern. Other terms used may include "searing," "shooting," "raw," "numb," "shock-like," "pins and needles," and "tingling." Neuropathic pain responds well to anticonvulsants as pain medications. Musculoskeletal pain or somatic pain is more frequently localized to one area, and it is described as aching or throbbing.

Page: 307

Question #3

Answer: C

Rationale: Goals should be established to improve functional status and quality of life and to increase activities of daily living. It is helpful to address unrealistic expectations of achieving the complete relief of pain at the beginning of treatment. It is important to discuss potential side effects with the patient and the family, but it is unrealistic to find medications without side effects. Additionally, many opioids have side effects that are experienced initially but not over the long term. The achievement of euphoric states may be the goal of patients with addiction issues, but it is not the goal of pain management.

Page: 305

Question #4

Answer: D

Rationale: Common side effects of any opioid include pruritus and gastrointestinal side effects, such as nausea, vomiting, and constipation. However, these are not true allergies. The pruritus occurs from histamine release as a result of mu receptors on the mast cells. Premedication with diphenhydramine may help with the pruritus, and it can be given orally as well as intravenously. Patients should be told that these side effects often disappear with chronic opioid use. Patients commonly will tolerate a different opioid from the same class as one that caused pruritus and nausea, so the avoidance of similar drugs is not needed.

Page: 305

Question #5

Answer: C

Rationale: Continuous chronic pain is defined as pain that is present for the majority of a 24-hour period. Pain medications should be scheduled rather than used as needed for continuous chronic pain to maintain a therapeutic effect. Medications prescribed on an as-needed basis are useful for episodic or brief exacerbations of pain only.

It is ideal to use a time-contingent schedule for patients that uses the specific hours of the day and thus can be modified to their lifestyles. Terms such as *QID* or *four times a day* can be confusing and difficult for people to translate into their own life schedules.

Pages: 305, 306

Question #6

Answer: C

Rationale: Methadone has effects of blocking the reuptake of serotonin and norepinephrine; these are similar to the effects of antidepressants. This gives methadone a potential advantage for chronic pain syndromes and neuropathic pain. Other opioids with this effect include tramadol and meperidine.

Page: 307

Question #7

Answer: B

Rationale: *Maldynia* is a term used to describe chronic pain syndromes in which central sensitization and hypersensitivity lead to an abnormal pain response and the perception of pain. Maldynia is frequently associated with neuroendocrine changes and comorbidities. By contrast, the term *eudynia* is used to refer to acute pain that has only peripheral sensitization and an afferent nociceptive pathway that functions normally.

Page: 307

Question #8

Answer: D

Rationale: The woman described has chronic continuous pain, which will best respond to round-the-clock pain medications. Long-acting medications, such as methadone and sustained-release preparations of morphine and oxycodone, allow patients to achieve sustained therapeutic responses to the medications and thus less breakthrough pain.

Increasing her dose to two Vicodin at a time will not necessarily make the therapeutic effect last longer. Changing to a different short-acting opioid, such as oxycodone/APAP, is also unlikely to solve the issues of inadequate pain control as a result of their short length of therapeutic effect. Allowing her to take the medicine every 4 hours instead of every 6 hours may give her better pain control, but studies have shown that patients frequently take the medicine at the longest dosing interval suggested, even if they are in pain. A small amount of short-acting opioid to use for breakthrough pain along with long-acting opioids may be useful.

All of the opioid-acetaminophen combination products need to be used with caution regarding the maximum dose of acetaminophen (4 g/24 hr). The maximum daily dose of acetaminophen frequently is the limiting factor for dose escalation, and patients need to be educated about the use of additional acetaminophen (particularly that hidden in other over-the-counter products) and the risk of toxicity.

Page: 308

Question #9

Answer: B

Rationale: Meperidine (Demerol) is metabolized in the liver to a toxic metabolite, normeperidine, which can cause seizures. Meperidine is acceptable for short-term use, such as for procedure-related analgesia, but it should not be used chronically. It is not well tolerated in the elderly.

Page: 308

Question #10

Answer: E

Rationale: NSAIDs have significant risks, and cautious patient selection is important in their use. NSAIDs should be avoided for patients with renal dysfunction, with a creatinine clearance of 45 mL/min or less, with hypovolemia, or with congestive heart failure. Most patients with liver failure and ascites are chronically hypovolemic and at risk for renal dysfunction. Most patients with diabetes have some level of nephropathy or are at risk for renal dysfunction. People with diabetes are also at risk for hyporeninemic hypoaldosteronism, which can be induced by NSAIDs. Recently, concern about cardiovascular risks with NSAIDs has been raised.

Page: 310

Question #11

Answer: C

Rationale: Acetaminophen is relatively safe when it is used correctly. The maximum daily dose is 4000 mg/24 hr, but toxicity can occur at lower doses when it is used chronically or in combination with alcohol. Acetaminophen is frequently found in over-the-counter medications, so patients may be unaware of how much they are actually taking.

Pages: 311, 312

Question #12

Answer: A

Rationale: Antidepressants are useful adjuvant pain medications, even for patients who are not depressed. A variety of syndromes respond to antidepressants, and the mechanisms are not always well understood. Tricyclics have well-documented efficacy for the treatment of neuropathic pain. Serotonin and norepinephrine reuptake inhibitors such as venlafaxine and duloxetine have better evidence for pain reduction than SSRIs. People with chronic pain syndromes of all types may respond to antidepressants that work as adjuvant pain medications, and these drugs may also help them to cope with the experience of chronic pain.

Pages: 312–314

Question #13

Answer: B

Rationale: Pseudoaddiction refers to a situation in which inadequate pain control can cause a patient to be anxious and preoccupied with maintaining his or her medication supply. It can appear to be similar to "drug seeking" behavior, but it should not be misinterpreted. Pseudoaddictive behavior lessens when pain levels are improved, and the patient's functional status improves with better pain control. By contrast, addictive behavior is characterized by continued inappropriate behavior and worsening functional status as a result of psychological dependence on the drug. This patient may have developed tolerance to his medications, and this may be the reason for his inadequate pain control. However, tolerance does not include pseudoaddictive behavior.

Page: 307

Question #14

Answer: D

Rationale: Mental health disorders are significant comorbidities for people with chronic pain. Ineffective coping can occur until the patient learns to adapt his or her daily life demands to the presence of pain. The clinician should screen for any existing mental health disorders as part of a chronic pain workup. The mental illness may affect the patient's experience of pain, his or her ability to cope with pain, his or her social support systems, his or her communication about pain, and his or her ability to self-manage the pain. Both affective disorders and thought disorders will have an effect on a person's experience of chronic pain and his or her ability to communicate and to have to access health care. There are high rates of substance abuse among people with mental health issues, so communication and screening for substance abuse should be part of any management plan.

A family physician should treat the whole person, including the pain and mental health issues. An understanding of how these issues intersect can provide the patient with better overall care. Referral to mental health specialists can be a valuable part of a patient's care if care is well coordinated among the providers.

Page: 307

Question #15

Answers: D

Rationale: Skeletal muscle relaxants are centrally acting and have sedative properties. It is not fully known if their effect is the result of sedation or of an indirect effect on muscle relaxation. There is very little evidence to support their use for chronic pain, but there may be some benefit from short-term use. They have no direct effect on muscles or on the neuromuscular junction, and there is no evidence that they actually relax muscles or relieve tension. Caution should be used with carisoprodol (Soma), which is metabolized to a barbiturate-type substance that can cause dependence.

Page: 312

Question #16

Answer: C

Rationale: Caution should be used when prescribing medications for people who are elderly, particularly those with hepatic and renal dysfunction. Oxycodone is the correct answer in this case as a result of the relative contraindications of the other options. Propoxyphene has a toxic metabolite, as does meperidine. NSAIDs, such as indomethacin, could worsen the patient's renal dysfunction. Dosage adjustment is required for many opioids, NSAIDs, and adjuvant analgesics among elderly patients. Methadone is a good choice for a long-acting medication because it does not accumulate significantly in patients with renal impairment.

Pages: 309, 310

Question #17

Answer: B

Rationale: Constipation is a predictable and avoidable response to opioids; most patients taking opioids regularly develop constipation. Constipation is mediated by the opioid receptors (mu–2), which cause decreased gastrointestinal motility; it is caused by all opioids at all doses. Unlike other side effects of opioids, almost no tolerance develops to constipation. Most patients should be offered a prescription for stool softeners alone or in combination with a mild stimulant (e.g., Peri-Colace) to use as needed at the time of their first opioid prescription.

Page: 308

Question #18

Answer: B

Rationale: Nausea and vomiting occur as side effects of opioids that are thought to be mediated by opioid receptors at the chemoreceptor trigger zone. They are thought to occur in 30% to 60% of opioid-naïve patients. For most people, tolerance develops within 5 to 10 days. Prophylactic antiemetics are useful for patients until tolerance develops, and they can be used for people with a history of nausea and vomiting with previous opioid use. Suggested antiemetics include prochlorperazine, promethazine, and metoclopramide.

Page: 308

Question #19

Answer: D

Rationale: Formal written agreements or contracts between patients and physicians can improve communication in the setting of chronic pain treatment. Contracts can delineate provider concerns about the goals of chronic pain management and the appropriate use of pain medications. They can also emphasize patient concerns that their rights are respected and that their perceptions of pain are addressed. Contracts are not legally required in all states. They are useful in settings of difficult patient-physician relationships and suspected substance abuse, but they are ideally used in a positive, preventive role for all patients who are receiving chronic pain medications.

Page: 308

Question #20

Answer: A

Rationale: Mu1 receptors are primarily involved in analgesic effects, and mu2 receptors mediate gastrointestinal motility/constipation, respiratory depression, euphoria, and chemical dependency. The mu2 receptors—not the kappa receptors—are found in the gastrointestinal tract. Although mu1 receptors are primarily responsible for analgesia, kappa and delta receptors play a role in spinal analgesia and general analgesic effect, respectively.

Pages: 306, 308

Question #21

Answer: B

Rationale: Chronic pain should be viewed as a syndrome of neuronal plasticity and changes to the central and peripheral nervous systems. The way that a person responds to stimuli as well as the signaling and experience of pain changes over time. Hyperalgesia and allodynia are examples of this process. Chronic pain is defined as pain that lasts longer than 3 months. Both chronic and acute pain may respond to opioids.

Page: 307

Question #22

Answer: A

Rationale: The use of short-acting opioids for flares of breakthrough pain is recommended, and they should be prescribed along with long-acting opioids. Chronic intermittent pain may respond well to short-acting opioids, but the medications should be clearly dosed on a schedule for the patient's lifestyle or activities. As-needed dosing of short-acting opioids is not recommended, because this may lead to the overuse of the medications, to dependence on the euphoric effect of some medications, or to times of increased pain between doses. It is helpful to view chronic pain using a chronic illness model in which patients are scheduled for regular follow-up visits to ensure proper disease management and preventive health. A chronic illness model discourages patient appointments just for exacerbations of pain, acute crisis management, and refills of rescue medications.

Page: 306

Question #23

Answer: D

Rationale: If patches are always placed in the same anatomic location, that area of the body will begin to absorb the drug more rapidly, leading to toxicity. Areas with high levels of circulation, such as the suprascapular area, give the most even absorption of the drug over time. The transmucosal form of fentanyl is much more prone to abuse than the transdermal form, and its use should be limited to cancer pain managed by specialists in pain management or oncology. Seventy-five percent of a dose of transmucosal fentanyl is absorbed in the gastrointestinal tract.

Page: 309

Question #24

Answer: C

Rationale: The immediate-release form of oxycodone has a peak effect of 1 hour and a duration of 4 hours, similar to all of the short-acting opioids taken in oral form. The extended-release form (OxyContin) is formulated without acetaminophen, and it releases a bolus of 38% of the ingested doses within the first 2 hours. This unique characteristic allows for an initial increased analgesic effect that may be of benefit, but it may also make the drug more likely to be abused. The euphoric effect is mediated by mu2 receptors.

Page: 309

Question #25

Answer: D

Rationale: Propoxyphene is in the same chemical class as methadone; both are phenylheptanes. The cardiotoxic metabolite of propoxyphene is norpropoxyphene, which can lead to cardiac conduction abnormalities and pulmonary edema. Smoking tobacco induces the metabolism of propoxyphene, thereby reducing the efficacy of the drug. Propoxyphene does not provide good analgesia. It has effects that are similar to those of acetaminophen in head-to-head trials, but it can provide a significant euphoric effect.

Page: 309

Question #26

Answer: B

Rationale: All opioids are in pregnancy category C, with no controlled human studies showing adverse events for fetuses. Urinary retention is a problem with all opioids, and it is a particular consideration for males with benign prostatic hypertrophy. All opioids may precipitate seizures. Option B is incorrect in that the cytochrome P450 system undergoes decremental changes; this, coupled with changes in renal function, can lead to changes in drug levels.

Page: 308

Question #27

Answer: A

Rationale: The onset of action of tramadol is less than 1 hour, and it is dependent on the dose. Tramadol does not need to be taken on an empty stomach, because its bioavailability of 75% is unaffected by meals. It is not in the same schedule III category as hydrocodone/APAP (Vicodin), but it does require a prescription. Dosing should be adjusted for patients with a creatinine clearance of less than 30 mL/min.

Page: 310

Question #28

Answer: D

Rationale: Morphine is primarily excreted renally (85%). The immediate-release form has an onset of 30 to 60 minutes and a peak of 60 minutes if taken via the oral route. The extended-release form has a peak of 2 hours (120 minutes). Epidural analgesia lasts up to 24 hours. There are several extended-release forms, with durations ranging from 8 to 24 hours: MS Contin (8–12 hr), Kadian (12–24 hr), and Avinza (24 hr). The most commonly used form is MS Contin, and, although it was initially described as a 12-hour formulation, it is more frequently found to be effective for a duration of 8 hours.

Page: 309

Question #29

Answer: B

Rationale: Oxymorphone is currently available in the United States as an injectable medication, as a rectal medication, in an oral form as an immediate-release and an extended-release medication. It is metabolized in the liver and excreted by the kidneys. The peak effect parenterally is 15 to 90 minutes; rectally, it is 120 minutes. The duration of analgesia is 3 to 6 hours.

Page: 309

Question #30

Answer: A

Rationale: Hydromorphone is currently available in a short-acting form for both the oral and parenteral routes. It was marketed in a controlled-release form as Palladone, which was withdrawn from the U.S. market in July 2005 as a result of problems with alcohol changing the controlled-release mechanism and leading to "dose dumping." The onset of action parenterally is 15 minutes, and peak effect is achieved in 60 minutes. It is eliminated renally.

Page: 308

Question #31

Answer: B

Rationale: Etoricoxib is a COX-2 inhibitor that has not yet been approved by the U.S. Food and Drug Administration. Other COX-2 inhibitors include celecoxib (still on the market), rofecoxib (withdrawn voluntarily), and valdecoxib (withdrawn by the U.S. Food and Drug Administration). Diclofenac is a derivative of acetic acid, and it is nonselective. Meloxicam is also a nonselective NSAID. Abciximab is a IIb/IIIa inhibitor and not an analgesic or an NSAID. Several COX-2 inhibitors were withdrawn from the market as a result of concern about cardiovascular risks. Gastrointestinal bleeding is also a risk with these medications, and all NSAIDs should be used with caution among patients with renal insufficiency.

Pages: 310, 311

22   Answers

Question #1

Answer: E

Rationale: Community-acquired methicillin-resistant *S. aureus* is an emerging concern, as is increased resistance among such common organisms as *E. coli* and *S. pneumoniae.* Vector-borne illnesses such as West Nile fever and tick-associated infections are also emerging concerns. Bioterrorism is, of course, of increasing concern as well.
Page: 317

Question #2

Answer: E

Rationale: When seeing a patient with an infectious disease, a careful history must be taken and should include medications, travel history, and exposures to sick contacts, animals, and insects. A careful review of systems should be performed as well. Although, in general, it is preferable to obtain cultures before the start of antibiotic therapy, in life-threatening situations, empiric therapy may be started before diagnostic tests are performed. A surgery consult may be necessary for patients who need abscesses drained or foreign bodies removed. Physicians who are treating infectious diseases should be aware of the local antibiotic sensitivity patterns.
Page: 317

Question #3

Answer: C

Rationale: Infectious causes make up only 30% of causes of fevers of unknown origin. Of infectious causes, tuberculosis, endocarditis, and abdominal abscesses do make up a significant proportion of cases. The definition of fever of unknown origin no longer requires a week of hospitalization. Newborns with fever should be presumed to have a serious bacterial infection, regardless of their clinical appearance, and a response to antipyretic medication should not affect clinical decision-making.
Page: 317

Question #4

Answer: B

Rationale: Most cases of acute bronchitis are the result of viral agents, and they should not be treated with antibiotics. Atypical organisms are not common agents of acute bronchitis, and physicians should not routinely treat to cover these organisms. Empiric treatment with β-agonists should be avoided as well, because this has not been shown to improve symptoms. Patients with chronic cough should be screened for noninfectious causes, especially postnasal drip, asthma, and gastroesophageal reflux disease.
Page: 319

Question #5

Answer: C

Rationale: The majority of cases of acute exacerbations of chronic bronchitis are caused by viral agents, and they should be treated with supportive care. Antibiotics should be reserved for severe exacerbations. For patients requiring treatment with antibiotics, amoxicillin or doxycycline should be adequate. Sputum cultures have not been shown to be helpful, because they are just as likely to grow out a colonizer as a pathogen.
Page: 319

Question #6

Answer: A

Rationale: Patients with no comorbidities and no recent antibiotic use who do not require hospitalization should not be treated with a respiratory fluoroquinolone. Fluoroquinolones should be reserved for more complicated cases of pneumonia.
Page: 321

Question #7

Answer: E

Rationale: The Pneumonia Severity Index assigns points to patients presenting with pneumonia based on age, coexisting illnesses, physical examination findings, and laboratory and radiographic findings. Patients with advanced age, significant comorbidities, altered mental status, and abnormal arterial blood gasses are all at significantly increased risk, according to the scale.

Page: 321

Question #8

Answer: B

Rationale: Tuberculin skin tests should be read based on the measurement of the induration rather than the area of erythema. Tuberculosis skin tests with more than 15 mm of induration are positive in any group, whereas those with less than 5 mm of induration are negative in any group. A 5-mm area of induration is considered positive in patients who have been exposed to tuberculosis, who have changes that are suggestive of tuberculosis on x-ray, or who are immunosuppressed. A 10-mm area of induration is considered positive in recent immigrants from endemic areas, intravenous drug users, children less than 4 years old, children exposed to high-risk adults, and residents and employees of high-risk settings, including health care facilities, group homes, jails, and homeless shelters.

Page: 325

Question #9

Answer: A

Rationale: Latent tuberculosis infection is the term given to patients with a positive tuberculin skin test without evidence of active tuberculosis. The treatment of active tuberculosis is always with multiple agents with antituberculous activity. However, the treatment of choice for latent tuberculosis infection is isoniazid, 300 mg orally daily for a total duration of 9 months. Treatment with isoniazid should always include treatment with pyridoxine to prevent neuropathy. Patients with a newly positive tuberculin skin test need treatment to prevent active disease, regardless of whether they are asymptomatic and their chest x-ray is negative.

Page: 323

Question #10

Answer: E

Rationale: Antimicrobial prophylaxis is recommended for patients with a high-risk condition undergoing a procedure that may cause bacteremia. Patients with a high-risk condition include those with prosthetic heart valves (including bioprosthetic valves), patients with a history of endocarditis, patients with congenital cyanotic heart disease, and patients with surgically constructed shunts and conduits. Dental procedures considered at high risk for causing bacteremia include surgical procedures and any dental procedure that involves the gingival crevice (the space between the surface of the tooth and the gum), including routine teeth cleaning. Patients with a physiologic heart murmur are not at high risk for endocarditis.

Page: 326

Question #11

Answer: A

Rationale: SBP usually occurs in the setting of ascites, especially in the cirrhotic patient. Almost 70% of patients who develop SBP are Child-Pugh class B or C, and SBP is the most common infection among this group of patients. The presentation of SBP is variable, and patients may or may not have signs or symptoms of intra-abdominal infection and peritoneal signs. Therefore, SBP should be suspected in any patient with history of liver disease who suffers an acute decompensation. SBP is nearly always caused by a single organism, and the growth of more than one organism suggests secondary peritonitis. SBP is typically caused by enteric gram-negative rods; anaerobes are only rarely the causative agent.

Page: 327

Question #12

Answer: B

Rationale: The precipitating event in acute cholecystitis is the obstruction of bile drainage. Infection does not precipitate acute cholecystitis, but it may complicate 20% to 50% of cases. Patients with underlying comorbidities should be covered with antibiotics covering enteric gastrointestinal flora. Treatment with antibiotics is a temporizing measure; definitive treatment is with decompression or removal of the gallbladder. Diagnosis is usually by clinical presentation with ultrasound confirmation. Radionuclide cholescintigraphy (hepato-iminodiacetic acid scanning) may be used to confirm the diagnosis, if needed.

Page: 328

Question #13

Answer: C

Rationale: Patients with diverticulitis are typically older and have left lower quadrant pain, diarrhea (sometimes bloody), fever, and leukocytosis. Empiric antibiotics should cover gram-negative enteric and anaerobic organisms, and they may be given orally in uncomplicated cases. Conservative medical treatment is successful in 70% to 80% of hospitalized patients, and surgical treatment is usually not necessary. A colonoscopy is recommended after the episode of diverticulitis has resolved to rule out underlying colon cancer. Colonoscopy during an episode of acute diverticulitis is contraindicated as a result of the risk of colonic rupture.

Page: 329

Question #14

Answer: E

Rationale: Traveler's diarrhea is usually caused by enterotoxigenic *E. coli,* and it is usually self-limited. A short course of antibiotics may be needed if the diarrhea is bloody or associated with fever. If enterohemorrhagic *E. coli* (O157:H7) is suspected, antibiotics should be held. Patients needing antibiotics can be treated with Bactrim or a fluoroquinolone.

Page: 329

Question #15

Answer: E

Rationale: *C. difficile* is the cause of antibiotic-associated diarrhea in 50% to 75% of cases. The patient is typically one who has received antibiotics and who is now presenting with diarrhea, abdominal pain or cramping, and fever. Leukocytosis may be profound, even at levels that are consistent with a leukemoid reaction. The major offending antibiotics are clindamycin and the cephalosporins, although any antibiotic can be responsible.

Page: 331

Question #16

Answer: E

Rationale: Levels of pyuria as low as 2 to 5 white blood cells per high-power field in a centrifuged specimen are significant in a female with appropriate symptoms. Among pregnant women, asymptomatic bacteruria should be actively sought and aggressively treated, because 40% of pregnant women with bacteruria who are not treated later acquire pyelonephritis. Patients with long-term indwelling catheters should be treated with antibiotics only if they become symptomatic. Therapy in asymptomatic catheterized patients leads to increasingly resistant bacteria.

Page: 331

Question #17

Answer: D

Rationale: UTIs among young children suggest abnormalities of the urinary tract; therefore, every infant or young child with a first UTI and fever should undergo imaging of the urinary tract. Constipation, broad-spectrum antibiotics, incomplete bladder emptying, and infrequent voiding all predispose children to UTIs. Recurrent UTIs among men are most often the result of a chronic prostatic focus. Pregnant patients with UTIs should not be treated with fluoroquinolones because of the possible adverse affects on fetal cartilage development. In addition, Bactrim should be avoided during the first trimester because of possible teratogenic effects, and it should also be avoided near term as a result of its possible role in the development of kernicterus.

Page: 331

Question #18

Answer: E

Rationale: Sexually active patients presenting with genital ulcers may have genital herpes, syphilis, or chancroid. A diagnosis based only on the history and physical examination is often inaccurate, and not all genital ulcers are caused by sexually transmitted infections. Patients who present with genital ulcers should have serologic testing for syphilis and culture or antigen testing for herpes. If chancroid is prevalent in the area, a culture for *Haemophilus ducreyi* should also be performed. Chlamydia and gonorrhea affect the same anatomic sites, and clinically differentiating gonorrhea from chlamydia is inaccurate. In addition, coinfection may be present in up to 50% of patients. Laboratory confirmation is recommended for both chlamydia and gonorrhea infections.

Page: 333

Question #19

Answer: E

Rationale: Despite the necessary concern surrounding gonorrhea and chlamydia, the three most common causes of vaginal discharge are trichomoniasis, bacterial vaginosis, and candidiasis. Bacterial vaginosis may be treated with oral or intravaginal metronidazole or with clindamycin. Treatment of the sexual partners of patients presenting with acute vulvovaginal candidiasis is not usually necessary. However, for patients with recurrent candidiasis, the treatment of sexual partners may help achieve a cure. Patients with vulvovaginal candidiasis may be treated with oral or intravaginal imidazoles; both are equally effective.

Pages: 336–337

Question #20

Answer: E

Rationale: A brain computed tomography scan before lumbar puncture is necessary if the patient has papilledema, focal neurologic findings, or HIV or if a subarachnoid bleed is suspected. In addition, patients who are not alert on presentation should have such a scan performed before a lumbar puncture.

Page: 338

Question #21

Answer: E

Rationale: Edema-associated cellulitis is best treated by mobilizing edema fluid by elevating and immobilizing the affected limb. Immunocompetent patients should be treated for gram-positive cocci. Broader coverage is needed for diabetic patients, and it should include coverage for gram-positive aerobes, gram-negative aerobes, and gram-negative anaerobes.

Page: 340

Question #22

Answer: D

Rationale: Bactrim and clindamycin are both appropriate antibiotic treatments for recurrent furunculosis in patients with MRSA. However, a prolonged course of antibiotics has not been shown to be more effective than 10 to 14 days of treatment. The importance of good hygiene should be emphasized. Patients should wash their hands carefully after contact with the skin lesion, and lesions should be covered at all times. Separate towels and washcloths should be reserved for the patient. In addition, the patient's clothes and sheets should be changed daily and washed at a high temperature. In refractory cases, the elimination of nasal carriage using 2% mupirocin calcium ointment intranasally for 5 days should be considered.

Page: 341

Question #23

Answer: D

Rationale: Diabetic skin infections can be categorized into either non–limb threatening or limb threatening. Characteristics of non–limb threatening infections include superficial ulcers with minimal cellulitis (<2 cm from port entry) in patients with no limb ischemia and no systemic toxicity. *S. aureus* and facultative streptococci are the usual causes. Limb-threatening infections require broader antibiotic coverage, because polymicrobial infections with *S. aureus*, group B streptococci, enterococcus, facultative gram-negative bacilli, anaerobic gram-positive cocci, and bacteroides species are common.

Page: 342

Question #24

Answer: C

Rationale: Acute hematogenous osteomyelitis occurs primarily in children, with the metaphysis of the long bones being the most common location. Adults more typically have chronic osteomyelitis caused by trauma rather than hematogenous spread. Blood cultures in children are positive half of the time, and 90% of cases of osteomyelitis in children are caused by *S. aureus*.

Pages: 342–343

Question #25

Answer: C

Rationale: Rocky Mountain spotted fever, ehrlichiosis, and Lyme disease are all tick-borne diseases that may be treated with doxycycline. Although babesiosis is also a tick-borne disease, it is treated with clindamycin plus quinine or atovaquone plus azithromycin. Patients with Rocky Mountain spotted fever or ehrlichiosis are treated for 5 to 10 days, whereas patients with Lyme disease require more extensive treatment that lasts 3 to 4 weeks.

Page: 344

Question #26

Answer: E

Rationale: Human bites have a higher complication and infection rate than do animal bites. Bite wounds involving the hands should be evaluated by a hand surgeon because of the potential for severe infections involving tendons, bone, and joints. The treatment of bite wounds with Augmentin or with a penicillin plus a penicillinase-resistant penicillin or cephalosporin should be performed. A 7- to 14-day course is adequate for infections involving only the soft tissue. A minimum of 3 weeks of therapy is needed to treat infections involving joints or bones.

Page: 345

Question #27

Answer: B

Rationale: Patients with chickenpox are contagious for 48 hours before vesicle formation and until 4 to 5 days later, when all vesicles are crusted. Patients with vesicles at all stages of healing would still be contagious. In the normal host, chickenpox is a self-limited illness with a duration of less than a week.

Page: 346

Question #28

Answer: A

Rationale: Epstein-Barr virus is an infection of the B lymphocytes rather than the T lymphocytes. The classic presentation of infectious mononucleosis includes fever, sore throat, and lymphadenopathy. Fever is present in more than 90% of patients, and cervical lymphadenopathy (most commonly bilateral and posterior) is present in 80% to 90% of cases. Splenomegaly is present in about half of patients. Cytomegalovirus is clinically indistinguishable from Epstein-Barr virus, and it causes 20% of cases of infectious mononucleosis.

Page: 347

Question #29

Answer: A

Rationale: Infectious viral hepatitis is spread by either the fecal–oral route or the parenteral route. Hepatitis viruses A and E are spread by the fecal–oral route, whereas B, C, and D are spread by the parenteral route.

Page: 348

Question #30

Answer: E

Rationale: Hepatitis A is spread by the fecal–oral route. Multiple blood transfusions do not increase a person's risk of acquiring hepatitis A. Hepatitis A occurs with an increased incidence among lower socioeconomic groups, day care attendants, men who have sex with men, illicit drug users, and those who have traveled internationally to endemic areas.

Pages: 348, 349

Question #31

Answer: A

Rationale: The consumption of raw shellfish is a risk factor for hepatitis A and E but not for B, because B is spread by the parenteral route. Hepatitis B only causes about a third of the cases of acute icteric hepatitis in the United States. The hepatitis B vaccine is very effective, and it is available to any adult who is at risk for the virus and who is not immune. The universal vaccination of newborns and infants is now part of the standard vaccination series. Most children with acute hepatitis B do progress to a chronic infection, whereas most adults with acute hepatitis B clear the virus.

Page: 349

Question #32

Answer: E

Rationale: Hepatitis C, unlike hepatitis B, usually results in a chronic hepatitis. As with hepatitis B, the major long-term risks of chronic hepatitis C are progression to cirrhosis and the development of hepatocellular carcinoma. Before the widespread screening of blood, hepatitis C was a common cause of transfusion-associated hepatitis. Hepatitis C is predominately spread by parenteral transmission. Unlike hepatitis B, sexual transmission does not appear to play a major role in the spread of hepatitis C.

Pages: 349–350

23 Answers

Question #1

Answer: C

Rationale: The initially identified high-risk behaviors through which most people were infected with HIV included male–male sex, injection drug use, transfusion with infected blood products, and perinatal transmission.

Page: 354

Question #2

Answer: B

Rationale: In countries in the developing world, the HIV epidemic has always been most frequently transmitted through heterosexual sex.

Page: 355

Question #3

Answer: C

Rationale: Primary HIV infection, which has been described as a mononucleosis-like syndrome, has an incubation period from exposure to the development of an acute clinical illness of approximately 2 to 4 weeks. However, it can also be less than 1 week to more than 6 weeks.

Page: 356

Question #4

Answer: C

Rationale: At least half of infected people have symptomatic illness, but most elude diagnosis.

Page: 356

Question #5

Answer: D

Rationale: Some of the most common symptoms and signs include fever, lymphadenopathy, pharyngitis, and maculopapular rash. Less-frequent findings include myalgias or arthralgias, headache, and diarrhea.

Page: 356

Question #6

Answer: C

Rationale: A positive viral load with a negative or indeterminate antibody test is currently diagnostic of primary HIV infection.

Page: 357

Question #7

Answer: B

Rationale: For untreated patients, the average time from infection to a positive HIV antibody test is 2 months; almost all infected people have detectable antibody within 6 months of infection.

Page: 357

Question #8

Answer: D

Rationale: The commonly known HIV test is a test for antibodies to HIV, and it can be performed with a sample of blood, oral fluid, or urine.

Page: 357

Question #9

Answer: A

Rationale: A reactive enzyme immunoassay or ELISA test requires a confirmatory Western blot or immunofluorescence test. The combination of a repeatedly reactive enzyme immunoassay and a positive Western blot test gives a sensitivity of 99% and a specificity of generally more than 99.9%.

Page: 357

Question #10

Answer: D

Rationale: The physician should reconsider the likelihood of HIV infection when interpreting and explaining this result to the patient. In general, the HIV test should be repeated in 3 to 6 months.

Page: 357

Question #11

Answer: D

Rationale: The Centers for Disease Control and Prevention has guidelines for the management of health care workers who are exposed to blood or body fluids via percutaneous injury or contact with mucous membranes or nonintact skin.

Page: 358

Question #12

Answer: B

Rationale: Do not administer live vaccines to patients with advanced HIV or AIDS.

Page: 364

Question #13

Answer: A

Rationale: Chest x-ray is not necessary unless the history and physical examination warrant. A complete history and physical examination, and complete blood cell count and chemistry profile, and a determination of the CD4 and viral loads are all appropriate screening tools.

Page: 358

Question #14

Answer: A

Rationale: Because of the frequency with which HIV patients have hepatitis A antibodies or a history of hepatitis A or B, the patient should be checked for serum hepatitis A and B antibodies and hepatitis B surface antigen before immunization.

Page: 358

Question #15

Answer: A

Rationale: An asymptomatic patient with a CD4 count of greater than 350 and a viral load of less than 100,000 does not require therapy. However, follow-up evaluations should occur every 3 to 4 months.

Page: 359

Question #16

Answer: A

Rationale: As noted, patients with a CD4 count of less than $200/mm^3$ and people with symptomatic HIV infection (i.e., thrush or fevers for more than 2 weeks) should be encouraged to take antiretroviral drugs in combination.

Page: 359

Question #17

Answer: C

Rationale: The preferred initial treatment regimens include three to four drugs: two from the NRTI class and one or two from either the NNRTI group or the protease inhibitor group.

Page: 359

Question #18

Answer: D

Rationale: HIV classes of drugs are the NRTIs, the NNRTIs, the protease inhibitors, and the fusion inhibitors.

Page: 360

Question #19

Answer: A

Rationale: Gastrointestinal side effects, including nausea, diarrhea, and bloating, are common side effects that are associated with protease inhibitors.

Page: 361

Question #20

Answer: B

Rationale: If there are no major problems after the initiation of therapy, most providers will check the CD4 count and the viral load and perform other laboratory tests (depending on possible medication toxicities) every 3 months.

Page: 362

Question #21

Answer: B

Rationale: If the medication appears to be failing (as defined by an increase in viral load, a drop in CD4 count, or the development of an HIV-related illness), the provider must reconsider the effectiveness of the prescribed regimen. The major reason for failure is lack of adherence, and it may be difficult for the provider to obtain this history.

Page: 363

Question #22

Answer: C

Rationale: Elevated serum triglycerides were noted among HIV-infected patients before the use of antiretrovirals; however, more severe hypertriglyceridemia and severe hypercholesterolemia have been noted with the use of protease inhibitors and some of the NRTIs, sometimes to levels of triglycerides of more than 1000 mg/dL.

Pages: 361, 363

Question #23

Answer: D

Rationale: PCP prophylaxis is recommended for all patients with CD4 counts of less than 200.

Page: 364

Question #24

Answer: A

Rationale: Trimethoprim-sulfamethoxazole is the first-line recommendation. However, if the patient has a sulfa allergy, dapsone may be used.

Page: 364

Question #25

Answer: B

Rationale: Any HIV-infected person with a tuberculin skin test reaction of 5 mm or more or who is exposed to active tuberculosis (regardless of the size of his or her positive protein derivative test area) should receive chemoprophylaxis.

Page: 364

Question #26

Answer: A

Rationale: Data support the discontinuation of primary PCP prophylaxis (no prior episode) for patients with a sustained increase in CD4 lymphocyte count above 200 cells for at least 3 months.

Page: 364

Question #27

Answer: D

Rationale: *T. gondii* is an important cause of focal brain disease among patients with AIDS. Patients develop symptoms over days and present with headache, confusion, fever, seizures, or a stroke-like syndrome.

Page: 369

Question #28

Answer: B

Rationale: For patients with advanced HIV disease (usually those with CD4 counts of less than 50 cells/mm^3), the most frequent illnesses caused by cytomegalovirus are chorioretinitis and gastrointestinal disease.

Page: 369

Question #29

Answer: D

Rationale: For patients with only oral thrush, there are a variety of treatments, including nystatin oral suspension or clotrimazole (Mycelex) troches, but these must be used multiple times each day. Systemic therapy with fluconazole (Diflucan) is preferred; alternative, less-effective treatments include ketoconazole (Nizoral) and itraconazole (Sporanox).

Page: 370

Question #30

Answer: A

Rationale: Human papillomavirus is generally felt to be the most important etiologic factor for cervical cancer and anal neoplasia.

Page: 371

Question #31

Answer: C

Rationale: Pap smears are recommended twice during the first year after diagnosis and annually thereafter (if normal) for all HIV-positive women.

Page: 371

Question #32

Answer: A

Rationale: Because of the high frequency of coinfection, all HIV-infected patients should be screened for hepatitis C infection. Infection with HIV may result in a more rapid or more severe course of hepatitis C disease, including a more rapid progression to cirrhosis.

Pages: 358, 371

Question #33

Answer: B

Rationale: The greatest increases in HIV cases in the United States are occurring among women, especially women of low socioeconomic status and women of color.

Page: 372

Question #34

Answer: D

Rationale: Although the most commonly discussed issue in relation to HIV-infected women is the role of the vertical transmission of HIV infection from the infected woman to the newborn child, there are many other important pregnancy-related issues. Antiretroviral use during pregnancy reduces vertical transmission by at least two thirds.

Page: 372

Question #35

Answer: A

Rationale: Currently, the one antiretroviral about which there is most concern during pregnancy is efavirenz (Sustiva), which has been shown to cause birth defects in nonhuman primates.

Page: 372

Question #36

Answer: B

Rationale: HIV-infected women should be counseled to not breast-feed if other sources of infant nutrition are available because of the risk of HIV transmission.

Page: 372

24 Answers

Question #1

Answer: A

Rationale: Interventions that combine counseling plus education or group strategies plus pharmacologic treatment with nicotine replacement or specific antidepressant medications (bupropion and nortriptyline, but not selective serotonin reuptake inhibitors) can achieve sustained quit rates of 25% to 30%.

Page: 375

Question #2

Answer: D

Rationale: Table 2 defines a strategy for helping patients to quit smoking by a simple mnemonic of 5 As: Ask, Advise, Assess, Assist, and Arrange.

Page: 375

Question #3

Answer: A

Rationale: Localized egophony ("e-to-a" changes) also indicates the consolidation of that segment or lobe of the lung. This is not present in patients with pleural effusion, except in a small band just above the upper edge of the effusion.

Page: 376

Question #4

Answer: A

Rationale: Demonstrating an FEV_1/FVC ratio (or FEV_1/FEV_6) of less than 70% is the most accurate method of diagnosing airflow obstruction, although all of the options presented may be helpful as well.

Page: 377

Question #5

Answer: A

Rationale: Some asthma patients may have a normal FEV/FVC ratio, but they may also exhibit reversibility as defined in the question.

Page: 382

Question #6

Answer: D

Rationale: Other causes to consider include postnasal drip, foreign body, upper respiratory infection, and lung cancer, particularly in smokers.

Page: 380

Question #7

Answer: A

Rationale: It may be difficult to convince patients of this fact; many prefer the nebulizer because it is easy to use and often administered to hospitalized patients.

Page: 382

Question #8

Answer: C

Rationale: A Cochrane Database Systematic Review of 12 controlled trials found that long-acting β_2-agonists were more effective than leukotriene antagonists as add-on therapy to inhaled steroids. However, long-acting β_2-agonists should not be used as monotherapy; increased mortality rates have been noted.

Page: 383

Question #9

Answer: B

Rationale: Although dust mites are commonly mentioned as a controllable environmental trigger, a Cochrane Database Systematic Review of 49 controlled trials found no evidence that either physical or chemical methods aimed at reducing exposure to house dust mite allergens had any benefit.

Page: 385

Question #10

Answer: A

Rationale: All patients should be counseled about smoking cessation (Recommendation Level: A).
Page: 388

Question #11

Answer: D

Rationale: Note that combining inhaled corticosteroids with a long-acting β_2-agonist provided a modest additional benefit (a 30% reduction in exacerbations).
Page: 387

Question #12

Answer: D

Rationale: Other causes of acute respiratory distress syndrome include massive transfusions, acute pancreatitis, and drug overdose.
Page: 389

Question #13

Answer: B

Rationale: Bronchiectasis is both a chronic airway infection and a disease of chronic lung inflammation. Other causes include immunoglobulin deficiency, allergic bronchopulmonary aspergillosis, and cilia disorders.
Page: 389

Question #14

Answer: A

Rationale: Antibiotic use for acute bronchitis is controversial. Because the most frequent cause of bronchitis is viral, the condition has often been overtreated with antibiotics, which would be a preventable source of antibiotic resistance.
Page: 390

Question #15

Answer: A

Rationale: Legionella is another important cause of pneumonia. Patients with atypical pneumonias may present with atypical symptoms: headache, nausea, or vomiting. Pseudomonas pneumonia is usually a hospital-acquired pneumonia that is often seen among patients with bronchiectasis.
Page: 390

Question #16

Answer: A

Rationale: Other strong risk factors include human immunodeficiency virus infection and apical fibrosis.
Page: 393

Question #17

Answer: A

Rationale: This treatment of latent tuberculosis infection is a Level A evidence recommendation.
Page: 394

Question #18

Answer: B

Rationale: Histoplasmosis (*Histoplasma capsulatum*) is most common in the basins of the Ohio and Mississippi rivers. Blastomycosis (*Blastomyces dermatitidis*) is found in this same area of the United States, as well as in portions of Canada. Coccidiomycosis (*Coccidioides immitis*) is prevalent in desert areas of the southwestern United States, whereas paracoccidiomycosis (*Paracoccidioides brasiliensis*) is the most common endemic mycosis in Central and South America.
Page: 397

Question #19

Answer: B

Rationale: Arterial PaO_2 greater than 80 mm Hg on room air and a normal A-a gradient make the diagnosis of pulmonary embolus less likely, but they do not completely exclude the diagnosis. The patient described in the question was taking birth control pills and had an elevated D-dimer, thus making pulmonary embolus a likely diagnosis.
Page: 398

Question #20

Answer: D

Rationale: Other causes of pulmonary hypertension to consider include congestive heart failure, recurrent pulmonary emboli, and patent foramen ovale.

Page: 400

Question #21

Answer: C

Rationale: Wegener's granulomatosis is a vasculitis or inflammatory condition of the vascular bed that may present with either shortness of breath or hemoptysis or with progressive pulmonary fibrosis as a result of repeated small hemorrhages at the alveolar level. It is now categorized as a systemic antineutrophil-cytoplasmatic-antibody–associated, small-vessel vasculitis, and it usually combines pulmonary features with glomerulo-nephritis.

Page: 400

Question #22

Answer: D

Rationale: There are various pulmonary complications of sickle cell disease, but, among adults with sickle cell disease, pulmonary hypertension is a significant cause of morbidity, and it appears to be a significant predictor of mortality, even with relatively modest elevations of pulmonary artery pressure.

Page: 401

Question #23

Answer: A

Rationale: Although it is not the most common cancer, lung cancer is the leading cause of cancer deaths among both men and women in the United States. Lung cancer surpassed breast cancer as a cause of death among women in the 1990s, in part because of historical trends toward increased smoking among women and also because of improvements in the early detection and treatment of breast cancer, which have resulted in decreased breast cancer mortality.

Page: 401

Question #24

Answer: B

Rationale: Beta carotene may actually increase the chance of developing lung cancer.

Page: 402

Question #25

Answer: D

Rationale: Ninety percent of patients with sarcoidosis will develop evidence of hilar, paratracheal, or mediastinal adenopathy, but not all of these patients will have pulmonary symptoms. Travel to the Southwest would point to coccidiomycosis; constitutional symptoms would suggest any of the three options mentioned.

Page: 404

Question #26

Answer: B

Rationale: Neoplasia—whether congenital (tuberous sclerosis, neurofibromatosis) or malignant (lymphangitic carcinomatosis, bronchoalveolar carcinoma, pulmonary lymphoma)—may also lead to pulmonary fibrosis, as can certain drugs, such as bleomycin, nitrofurantoin, and amiodarone.

Page: 405

Question #27

Answer: D

Rationale: Pancreatitis is usually associated with an exudative effusion. Diagnostic thoracentesis for exudates will reveal a pleural to serum protein ratio of greater than 0.5, a pleural to serum lactate dehydrogenase ration of greater than 0.6 (or a measured pleural lactate dehydrogenase level of greater than 200 IU/dL), or a pleural protein level of greater than 3 gm/dL.

Page: 407

Question #28

Answer: C

Rationale: Patients with sleep apnea may present with symptoms of daytime drowsiness or sleepiness or a feeling of being inadequately rested. Family members often bring the problem to the attention of the patient or of the family physician after having observed loud snoring and interruptions in breathing during the patient's sleep. Sometimes a motor vehicle accident caused by somnolence while driving brings the condition to light. Depression can also develop. Polycythemia and edema are late findings.

Page: 407

Question #29

Answer: D

Rationale: Nasal continuous positive airway pressure is effective for obstructive sleep apnea patients who tolerate it. Various oral and dental devices are also available, with limited data available addressing effectiveness. Surgical procedures may attempt to reduce airway obstruction at the palate or at the tonsillopharyngeal or adenoidal levels. In extreme cases, tracheostomy may be curative.

Page: 407

Question #30

Answer: A

Rationale: Asthma is defined as an inflammatory, episodic, obstructive lung disease that is almost always reversible. Self-management focused on the control of environmental triggers, regular peak-flow monitoring, and "what-if" action plans can prevent or abort most flare-ups of asthma. Eliminating passive exposure to smokers is the most important intervention for eliminating environmental triggers.

Page: 384

25 Answers

Question #1

Answer: E

Rationale: Sore throat, high fever, the thumbprint sign on a lateral neck x-ray, and drooling are all classic signs and symptoms of epiglottitis. Because there is considerable overlap with the symptoms of croup, a lateral soft-tissue x-ray of the neck may help differentiate the cause. The thumbprint sign is usually diagnostic.

Page: 413

Question #2

Answer: A

Rationale: Tongue depressors have been known to precipitate an acute airway obstruction in an individual with epiglottitis. Any culture or other manipulation of the oropharynx should wait until the airway has been stabilized with intubation or tracheostomy.

Page: 413

Question #3

Answer: E

Rationale: The accumulation of purulent material dysphagia, fever, swelling, trismus, "hot potato" voice, and odynophagia are all characteristic of a peritonsillar abscess. These signs and symptoms may be accompanied by deviation of the uvula from the midline and fluctuance in the area surrounding the tonsil.

Page: 413

Question #4

Answer: A

Rationale: In a cooperative adult, the peritonsillar abscess may be drained in the office setting with appropriate anesthesia. Children are not usually cooperative enough to be a candidate for this procedure.

Page: 413

Question #5

Answer: C

Rationale: Button or disk-type batteries can cause significant tissue injury, and they may lead to esophageal perforation if they are not removed immediately.

Page: 414

Question #6

Answer: D

Rationale: Anytime a patient presents with new-onset wheezing without a previous history of reactive airway disease, aspiration of a foreign body must be excluded. A high level of suspicion must always be maintained, especially with children and adolescents. Often, there is a transient period between the time of aspiration and the beginning of wheezing. Direct laryngoscopy and bronchoscopy are the only definitive treatments; bronchodilator therapy alone is inadequate. A thorough history and a physical examination are mandatory to exclude foreign-body aspiration.

Page: 414

Question #7

Answer: B

Rationale: The Kiesselbach's plexus is a rich network of vessels in the anterior nasal septum, and it is the most frequent site of nose bleeds. These may be severe, but they are easier to control than posterior nosebleeds.

Page: 414

Question #8

Answer: C

Rationale: In all cases of patient management, the ABCs (airway, breathing, and circulation) must be evaluated first. Significant epistaxis may compromise the airway, and, therefore, rapid assessment of the airway must be made. Only after the airway has been stabilized

should the physician move forward with further evaluation of the nosebleed.
Page: 414

Question #9

Answer: D

Rationale: Nasal ala necrosis may occur if the pack is
expanded to the point of alar blanching; it also increases
the pain significantly. Make sure the tip of the packing
material or balloon is inserted far enough (straight back
and not superiorly) that, when inflated or expanded, the
ala is not blanched. The packing should not remain in
the nares for more than 5 days. Significant infection,
including toxic shock syndrome, may occur.
Page: 414

Question #10

Answer: B

Rationale: If a patient requires a posterior packing for
the control of bleeding, then an ear, nose, and throat consultation is warranted for pack removal or complications.
As compared with anterior packing, posterior packing
causes significant discomfort, often necessitating narcotic
pain control during and after the procedure.
Page: 415

Question #11

Answer: B

Rationale: Hypoxemia and carbon dioxide retention are
late signs of impending airway impingement. Any major
facial trauma can rapidly cause airway obstruction as well
as significant blood loss. Airway obstruction may present
as a muffled tone quality or as stridor. A thorough examination may also reveal subcutaneous emphysema.
Page: 417

Question #12

Answer: A

Rationale: When examining the TM, an otoscope with
a bright light and with the largest speculum that easily
fits in the canal should be used. The normal light reflex
is in the anterior-inferior portion of the TM.
Page: 417

Question #13

Answer: C

Rationale: When performing the Weber's test, the
vibrating fork is placed on the incisors or on the center
of the forehead.
Page: 418

Question #14

Answer: E

Rationale: Cranial nerves V, VII, IX, and X supply
innervation to the ear.
Page: 417

Question #15

Answer: D

Rationale: Although not pathognomonic of a laby-
rinthine disorder, true vertigo is a disorder of the inner
ear.
Page: 418

Question #16

Answer: B

Rationale: A patient presenting with classic Ménière's
disease will have all of the symptoms mentioned among
the answer options. However, the hearing loss is a low-
frequency sensorineural hearing loss rather than a
high-frequency loss.
Page: 423

Question #17

Answer: E

Rationale: Long-term treatments include a low-
sodium diet, thiazide diuretics, and a minimization of
caffeine and alcohol in the diet. More aggressive therapy
may include the placement of intratympanic gentamy-
cin. Surgical decompression or shunting procedures of
the endolymphatic sac are used as last-resort treatment
options.
Page: 423

Question #18

Answer: C

Rationale: Benign positional vertigo is more common among females. The Dix–Hallpike maneuver reproduces the vertigo in the patient and results in short-lived nystagmus. Treatment by repositioning (Epley maneuver) is safe and effective, but it may not lead to the long-term resolution of the vertigo.

Page: 423

Question #19

Answer: A

Rationale: Also known as herpes zoster oticus, Ramsay–Hunt syndrome is caused by herpetic involvement of the facial, vestibulocochlear, or trigeminal ganglia. Vestibular neuronitis is acute vertigo that is associated with vomiting and that originates in the vestibular nerve. It can be associated with a recent viral illness, but it can also occur spontaneously. Labyrinthitis can also cause sudden and severe vertigo. These patients also have hearing loss and tinnitus, and the hearing loss is sensorineural.

Page: 424

Question #20

Answer: A

Rationale: Magnetic resonance imaging is needed for any hearing loss that is unilateral (excluding external causes such as cerumen impaction). There are many other things that should be determined during the interview with the patient, including the laterality of the tinnitus, whether it is pulsatile, and whether it changes volume and pitch.

Page: 424

Question #21

Answer: C

Rationale: Itching—not pain—is the most common symptom of fungal ear infections.

Page: 425

Question #22

Answer: D

Rationale: Any hygroscopic object, such as a vegetable, a bean, or another food matter, may have the potential to swell. Batteries, when wetted, may leak electrolyte solution and cause necrosis of the ear canal.

Page: 427

Question #23

Answer: A

Rationale: The ear canal is self-cleaning. For most people, the use of a washcloth on the end of a finger is usually all that is needed. Cerumen impaction usually results from repeated attempts to clean the ear with cotton-tipped applicators; patients should be discouraged from this activity. Remember, your mother always told you to put nothing in your ear that is smaller than your elbow!

Page: 427

Question #24

Answer: B

Rationale: Cerumen impaction removal is a very common procedure that can be easily performed in the physician's office with relatively inexpensive equipment. However, impacted cerumen and a perforation of the tympanic membrane should be referred to an ear, nose, and throat specialist for appropriate treatment. The use of tepid or warm water is used to prevent nystagmus and associated vertigo. Irritation or bleeding may occur during curettage if the cerumen is hard and adherent to the canal.

Page: 427

Question #25

Answer: E

Rationale: The primary cause of otitis media is bacterial colonization of the middle ear by *S. pneumoniae* as a result of eustachian tube dysfunction. Child care outside of the home and exposure to cigarette smoke are significant contributors to otitis media.

Page: 428

Question #26

Answer: D

Rationale: The three criteria necessary to confirm the diagnosis of acute otitis media are acute onset, the presence of middle-ear effusion, and signs or symptoms of middle-ear inflammation. All of the symptoms described in the answer options are necessary to diagnose middle-ear effusion.

Page: 428

Question #27

Answer: D

Rationale: Amoxicillin at a dose of 80 to 90 mg/kg divided into two daily doses is the treatment of choice. If the patient has a nonanaphylactic allergic reaction to the penicillins, then cefdinir, cefpodoxime, or cefuroxime may be used. Patients with true anaphylaxis to the penicillins may take azithromycin or clarithromycin for treatment. Augmentin is reserved for treatment failures.

Page: 428

Question #28

Answer: B

Rationale: Magnetic resonance imaging is indicated only if there is suspicion of central nervous system involvement of the infection. Because of the high sensitivity of this type of imaging, there are a significant number of false positives. It is not uncommon for the magnetic resonance image to be read as evidence of chronic mastoiditis for a patient without otologic symptoms.

Page: 429

Question #29

Answer: B

Rationale: A cholesteatoma contains no cholesterol, but it contains squamous epithelium and keratin debris.

Page: 432

Question #30

Answer: A

Rationale: Otitis media with effusion is defined as persistent middle-ear fluid without pain, fever, or redness of the TM, and it usually resolves in 6 months. Tympanometry may be used to judge the presence of fluid in the middle ear, but this condition is best diagnosed with pneumatic otoscopy.

Page: 431

Question #31

Answer: B

Rationale: Three episodes of otitis media in 6 months with complete resolution or 4 episodes in 12 months warrants further evaluation. First-line antibiotic therapy is amoxicillin at 20/mg/kg for 3 to 6 months. Sulfasoxazole is indicated for those individuals who are allergic to penicillin.

Page: 431

Question #32

Answers: A, 2; B, 1; C, 4; D, 3

Rationale: Audiometry is essential for the evaluation of the hearing loss. Asymmetric hearing loss that is sensorineural may require an magnetic resonance imaging to rule out retrocochlear pathology.

Page: 433

Question #33

Answer: A

Rationale: Most types of hearing loss are not emergent. However, sudden sensorineural hearing loss is emergent, because early intervention may prevent permanent hearing loss. A complete history and physical examination are warranted. The most common urgent treatment is the use of high-dose corticosteroids.

Page: 434

Question #34

Answer: E

Rationale: A complete physical examination of the head and neck is warranted. Other studies include a tuning-fork examination, an audiogram, and magnetic resonance imaging of the head with gadolinium. This image should include fine cuts through the internal auditory canal, which can detect tumors as small as 2 mm.

Page: 435

Question #35

Answer: E

Rationale: If the hearing loss is sensorineural, it is not amenable to surgical correction, and a hearing aid is the only option for treatment. In rare cases, even a hearing aid may be of no benefit. With concussive or blast injury, a fistula of the labyrinth may form and cause severe vertigo. With bedrest, many fistulas will close spontaneously.

Page: 435

Question #36

Answer: C

Rationale: The most appropriate treatment for idiopathic Bell's palsy is an antiviral (e.g., Acyclovir) and oral steroids. It is thought that Bell's palsy is the reactivation of the herpes virus in the geniculate ganglion.

Page: 436

Question #37

Answer: D

Rationale: Most people have some mild form of nonsignificant septal deviation. Moderate to severe septal deviation may cause obstruction. Mucus production of the nose is about 1 quart a day, and only the inferior and medial turbinates can be seen during a routine examination. To visualize the superior turbinate, a flexible endoscope must be used.

Page: 437

Question #38

Answer: A

Rationale: Computerized tomography is the mainstay of the radiographic evaluation of the sinuses. Magnetic resonance imaging is too sensitive for the evaluation of inflammatory conditions, and it fails to show bony anatomy well.

Page: 438

Question #39

Answer: B

Rationale: Rebound congestion of the nasal mucosa is very common. Therefore, nasal decongestant sprays should be limited to 3 days of use.

Page: 442

Question #40

Answer: E

Rationale: In children, the presence of nasal polyps may represent cystic fibrosis; prompt testing should be initiated. Nasal polyps should appear grayish and translucent; infection may be present if they appear erythematous. Treatment includes topical steroids, allergy treatment, and the treatment of sinusitis.

Page: 446

Question #41

Answer: E

Rationale: History findings, a nasal crease, eosinophils, and boggy mucosa are all used to make the diagnosis of allergic rhinitis. Treatment includes allergen avoidance, both topical and oral antihistamines, decongestants, and topical steroids.

Page: 445

Question #42

Answer: B

Rationale: Although the diagnosis of sinusitis can be very difficult, the most common cause of acute rhinosinusitis is a viral. However, all of the other options are potential causes of sinusitis. Of course, antibiotics are not indicated for acute viral rhinosinusitis; the treatment of symptoms (decongestants and topical steroids) is the mainstay.

Page: 442

Question #43

Answer: E

Rationale: All the symptoms listed, in combination with clinical manifestations of sinusitis, require urgent evaluation. A high degree of suspicion is warranted in cases of complicated sinusitis, especially among small children. The proximity of the paranasal sinuses to the orbits of the eyes and the brain allows for the spread of infection to these locations.

Page: 442

Question #44

Answer: D

Rationale: Squamous papilloma is the most common benign lesion found inside of the nasal cavity. Other malignant tumors not listed among the answer options include squamous cell carcinoma and malignant melanoma.

Page: 445

Question #45

Answer: D

Rationale: The "asthma triad" is made up of asthma, polyps, and aspirin sensitivity. Penicillin allergy and chronic urticaria are unrelated. However, nasal polyps are often seen in atopic patients.

Page: 446

Question #46

Answer: E

Rationale: Recent studies have shown that cephalosporins appear to be superior to penicillin in terms of bacterial eradication and clinical cure. However, penicillin remains one of the most cost-effective options for treating individuals who have been diagnosed with group A β-hemolytic streptococcal pharyngitis.

Page: 447

Question #47

Answer: C

Rationale: Although each individual patient is different, six episodes within 1 year or three to four episodes in each of 2 years warrants further evaluation for possible tonsillectomy. However, the total number of missed work days or school days should be taken into account when considering tonsillectomy.

Page: 448

Question #48

Answer: E

Rationale: All the statements made in the answer options about obstructive sleep apnea are true. Individuals with this condition are at increased risk for hypertension, coronary artery disease, pulmonary hypertension, poor concentration, impotence, and motor vehicle accidents.

Page: 451

Question #49

Answer: B

Rationale: The most common midline neck mass is a thyroglossal duct cyst, whereas the most common congenital lateral neck mass is a branchial cleft cyst. Surgical excision is the treatment of choice for both types of masses.

Page: 456

Chapter

26 Answers

Question #1

Answer: C

Rationale: Allergic diseases are defined by their phenotype, and, for each allergic disease, there is an almost identical phenotypic expression that is unrelated to allergy.

Page: 463

Question #2

Answer: D

Rationale: Exposures to allergens are followed by complaints of paroxysmal sneezing, a watery nasal discharge with congestion, and nasal pruritus. Less-specific symptoms are postnasal drainage or fullness or aching in the frontal areas.

Page: 463

Question #3

Answer: D

Rationale: Season allergic rhinitis is often associated with allergic salute, allergic shiners, and sleep disruption as a result of nasal obstruction and mouth breathing. Otitis media may occur as a complication, but it is not commonly associated with seasonal allergic rhinitis.

Page: 463

Question #4

Answer: B

Rationale: Perennial allergic rhinitis commonly includes nasal congestion, itching, obstruction, and frequent sniffing. As a result, a loss of the senses of taste and smell, decreased hearing, and a popping of sensation of the ears may occur. Paroxysms of sneezing and rhinorrhea may result from changes in ambient temperature, head movement, odors from perfume, tobacco smoke, irritants, alcohol, and exposure to small quantities of antigen.

Page: 463

Question #5

Answer: B

Rationale: The nasal turbinates are usually swollen and edematous, and they may be mistaken for nasal polyps, which are pearl-gray gelatinous masses and unusual to find in patients with uncomplicated allergic rhinitis. In one third to one half of children with allergic rhinitis, eustachian tube obstruction may be present, with resultant serous otitis. Among patients with intact tympanic membranes, tympanometry to measure middle-ear pressures provides an indirect measure of eustachian tube function. Up to one third of patients may have a lower respiratory tract component, including exercise-induced asthma and mild persistent asthma.

Page: 464

Question #6

Answer: C

Rationale: A prime role for the patient and the family is the environmental control of house dust, which, although it is a heterogenous mixture of bacteria, fibrous matter of plant and animal origin, human epidermis, food remnants, fungi, insect debris, and animal dander, contains one major source of antigen: the dust mite. Mites are ubiquitous in households, and they are most prevalent in bedding, mattresses, carpeting, and upholstered furniture, particularly in areas in which warmth and humidity are high. High-efficiency particulate air filters are effective for the removal of dust and animal dander. The avoidance of use of fans is essential to allow for the settling of these lightweight particles.

Page: 464

Question #7

Answer: D

Rationale: For optimal results, the allergy drugs should be used before exposure to the known allergen. The second generation of drugs, with specific binding properties, allow little to no penetration into the central nervous system, thus markedly reducing their side effects (primarily sedation). Fexofenadine (Allegra), which is an analog of terfenadine, is safe and effective, and it is available in 30-mg (twice a day), 60-mg (twice a day) and 180-mg (once a day) tablets. Through its effects on T cells, fexofenadine may diminish airway inflammation. Cetirizine (Zyrtec), which is a metabolite of hydroxyzine, is also available in once-daily dosing as 5-mg/mL syrup or a 10-mg tablet. Cetirizine's chemical properties, however, allow for greater central nervous system penetration, and sedation is its chief side effect (16% vs. 4% for fexofenadine and loratadine).

Page: 465

Question #8

Answer: C

Rationale: Topical intranasal glucocorticoids—beclomethasone, fluticasone, mometasone, triamcinolone, flunisolide, and budesonide—are extremely effective. Their effectiveness is directly related to proper and daily use, which can pose problems with patient compliance. Using saline as a moisturizer can help negate these side effects. Approximately 1 to 3 weeks may be required for some patients to achieve maximal benefit. The use of intramuscular long-acting steroids should be avoided as the primary treatment of seasonal allergies because of pituitary-adrenal axis suppression and decreased efficacy with repeated use.

Page: 465

Question #9

Answer: A

Rationale: When skin tests identify sensitivity to an unavoidable inhalant allergen, immunotherapy may be indicated for the treatment of allergic rhinitis. Its efficacy has been shown to be 80% for pollen symptom control and 60% for molds and house dust symptom control. It is more effective for seasonal allergic rhinitis than for perennial allergic rhinitis. Immunotherapy is an effective treatment for allergic rhinitis; it is well tolerated and works well for children. The use of immunotherapy for the treatment of allergic rhinitis may prevent the development of asthma among children.

Page: 466

Question #10

Answer: B

Rationale: Perennial allergic rhinitis may be associated with nasal polyps, but usually only when the condition

is complicated by sinus infection. In adults, the presence of polyps may be associated with a sensitivity to aspirin manifested by the aggravation of rhinitis, asthma, and even shock. Nasal polyps often develop in the absence of or only coincidentally with allergy. The size of nasal polyps may be reduced by brief treatment with systemic glucocorticoids and the daily use of topical glucocorticoids for longer periods.

Page: 466

Question #11

Answer: C

Rationale: Chronic allergic rhinitis predisposes individuals to sinus disease, although sinus disease can develop in the absence of allergy. Acute sinusitis is characterized by persistent rhinorrhea, postnasal drip, purulent drip or discharge after an upper respiratory infection, dull throbbing pain over the affected sinus, and fever. Among both children and adults, the ethmoid and maxillary sinuses are the most frequently infected. With complicating allergic rhinitis, sinus disease may be associated with a sore throat, middle-ear disease, and, characteristically, a persistent cough, especially at night. Periorbital edema, facial pallor, and circles under the eyes may be striking.

Page: 466

Question #12

Answer: A

Rationale: Some patients with perennial rhinitis are not atopic by history or skin testing.

Page: 466

Question #13

Answer: A

Rationale: Chronic nasal obstruction is the predominant symptom, and the condition may be associated with sinus disease and nasal polyps.

Page: 466

Question #14

Answer: A

Rationale: Although there is no evidence of allergy by skin testing, numerous eosinophils are present, and the diagnosis is readily made by examining the nasal secretions for eosinophils and eosinophilic cationic protein. The condition is also called nonallergic rhinitis with eosinophilia.

Page: 466

Question #15

Answer: B

Rationale: Topical glucocorticoid therapy is much more effective than antihistamines or decongestants for the treatment of eosinophilic nonallergic rhinitis.

Page: 466

Question #16

Answer: C

Rationale: Conjunctivitis is the usual ocular reaction to airborne allergens. Vernal conjunctivitis is so called because of its occurrence during spring and summer. Vernal conjunctivitis commonly occurs in patients who are between the ages of 5 and 20 years. It often spontaneously resolves in 10 years. Azelastine (Optivar), epinastine (Elestat), ketotifen (Zaditor), and olopatadine (Patanol) are dual-acting drugs; they prevent mast-cell releases and exert antihistamine activity as well. Ketorolac (Acular) is a nonsteroidal anti-inflammatory medication.

Page: 467

Question #17

Answer: A

Rationale: The definition of asthma has undergone many changes over the years, but three elements are key to the diagnosis: reversible airway obstruction, airway inflammation, and increased airway responsiveness to a variety of stimuli.

Page: 467

Question #18

Answer: B

Rationale: Asthma is a chronic inflammatory disorder of the airways in which many different cells play a role. Among individuals with this condition, this inflammation causes breathlessness, chest tightness, recurrent epi-

sodes of wheezing, and cough, particularly at night. These symptoms are usually associated with variable airflow limitation that is partly reversible with treatment or that sometimes resolves spontaneously. This inflammation causes an associated increase in airway responsiveness to a variety of stimuli. Pulmonary function testing is the gold standard of testing for the diagnosis and management of asthma, and it is the second stage in the diagnosis. Spirometry includes measurements of FEV_1, which is the amount of forced expiratory volume of air in 1 second, and the forced vital capacity, which is the amount of air one can expel during forced expiration. FEV_1 is the most important value for the assessment of airflow obstruction.

Page: 467

Question #19

Answer: B

Rationale: The diagnosis of asthma should occur in three stages. First, suggestive symptoms referable to the chest with precipitating factors should raise the possibility of asthma. Second, further testing should be performed to confirm the diagnosis. Third, the patient should have symptomatic improvement with the appropriate asthma therapy. When all of the stages have been performed and meet the criteria, then the diagnosis of asthma can be made. Positive findings on the PA and lateral views are helpful, but they are not diagnostic.

Page: 467

Question #20

Answer: B

Rationale: The administration of a bronchodilator such as albuterol is indicated when spirometry is being performed. The improvement of FEV_1 by 12% or 200 mL after the use of a bronchodilator suggests significant reversibility of the airway obstruction. The home use of peak flow meters is helpful for the self-management of asthma but not for the diagnosis. The patient should establish a baseline peak flow in the absence of asthma symptoms. Three zones on the meter are then set: green, yellow, and red. The green zone is 80% to 100% of the personal best, and it helps reassure the patient to continue his or her current regimen. Asthma often begins during childhood, and it is frequently found in association with atopic dermatitis. The classification of asthma has four categories that are based on both subjective symptoms of frequency and severity and on objective measurements of pulmonary function. These categories are mild intermittent asthma, mild persistent asthma, moderate persistent asthma, and severe persistent asthma.

Page: 468

Question #21

Answer: B

Rationale: All patients with mild persistent asthma should be considered to receive daily treatment with inhaled corticosteroids, although there is some new controversy about this. Leukotriene modifiers such as cromolyn and nedocromil may be considered as alternative—not preferred—controller medications for those with persistent asthma. Inhaled corticosteroids are now the preferred controller medication based on their greater efficacy. The most important question to monitor symptom control is the use of short-acting β_2-agonists, which should be used less than two times per week.

Page: 469

Question #22

Answer: A

Rationale: Moderate persistent asthma is defined as a patient's having daily symptoms of asthma, a daily need for bronchodilator medications, the development of

asthmatic attacks that interfere with activity, nocturnal awakenings more than once per week, and a peak expiratory flow rate that is 60% to 80% of normal.

Page: 469

Question #23

Answer: A

Rationale: Severe persistent asthma is defined when patients are usually awakened from sleep four to seven nights per week; when they have frequent asthma exacerbations, even from minor exposures to viruses, allergens, exercise, or air pollutants; when they have an FEV_1 of less than 60% of predicted; and when they are unable to achieve normal lung function despite appropriate treatment.

Page: 469

Question #24

Answer: A

Rationale: Exercise-induced bronchospasm is a bronchospastic event that usually occurs during or minutes after vigorous activity. The peak of the bronchospasm occurs within 5 to 10 minutes after stopping the activity, and it usually resolves within 30 minutes.

Page: 471

Question #1

Answer: A

Rationale: Once thought to be a problem mainly confined to the tropics and developing countries, parasitic infections are now being seen in developed countries. This reemergence is primarily the result of increases in world travel, immigration, and immunodeficiency (either from human immunodeficiency virus or iatrogenesis).
Page: 477

Question #2

Answer: D

Rationale: Giardiasis is the most common protozoan cause of human enteric disease, although it causes less than 5% of all cases of "traveler's diarrhea." Other less-common causes include amebiasis and ascariasis. *E. vermicularis* and *T. gondii* are not usually associated with diarrhea.
Page: 477

Question #3

Answer: B

Rationale: Giardiasis caused by the protozoan *G. lamblia* is usually transmitted by water or food, and it is frequently spread throughout daycare centers. Infants, young children, travelers, and those who are immuno-compromised are at highest risk for disease. The *G. lamblia* cysts are resistant to the low-level chlorination of water supplies and/or swimming pools, which accounts for an occasional outbreak of disease in the community. On the other hand, the cysts are rendered inert by boiling.
Page: 477

Question #4

Answer: B

Rationale: Giardiasis can produce a wide spectrum of illness, from an asymptomatic carrier state to acute diarrhea with abdominal pain, flatulence, and lassitude to chronic diarrhea with malabsorption, steatorrhea, and weight loss. Acute nausea, vomiting, and fever are rarely seen with giardiasis.
Page: 477

Question #5

Answer: C

Rationale: The interval between infection with giardiasis and the development of symptoms ranges from 3 to 20 days, with an average of 7 days. As such, travelers who will develop symptoms usually do so during or right after their trips. Most symptomatic patients will have a spontaneous resolution of their illness and will not require treatment. However, up to 25% may have symptoms that persist for 7 weeks or more. Reasonable first-line agents to treat giardiasis include tinidazole (Tindamax) and metronidazole (Flagyl), although the latter is not approved by the U.S. Food and Drug Administration for this condition.
Page: 479

Question #6

Answer: A

Rationale: Ascariasis is the most common parasitic infection worldwide, with up to 20% of the world's population infected.
Page: 479

Question #7

Answer: D

Rationale: Although pneumonitis can occur, it is usually a self-limited illness; rarely will the appendix or biliary system become obstructed. Although some authorities believe that ascariasis can impair cognitive development, this impairment has not yet been proved by reliable research. Intestinal obstruction is the most common cause of serious morbidity and mortality among people infected with ascariasis. Obstruction usually occurs when more than 60 worms are present; most commonly, it occurs in the terminal ileum.

Complete obstruction can lead to intussusception, infarction of the bowel, and perforation.

Page: 479

Question #8

Answer: B

Rationale: Single-dose oral therapy with albendazole (Albenza) 400 mg or mebendazole (Vermox) 500 mg is the best treatment for ascariasis. Alternatively, pyrantel pamoate (Antiminth) 11 mg/kg as a single oral dose or mebendazole 100 mg twice daily for 3 days may be used. There is no need for the intravenous treatment of ascariasis.

Page: 479

Question #9

Answer: B

Rationale: After schistosomiasis and malaria, amebiasis is the third most common cause of death from parasitic infection.

Page: 480

Question #10

Answer: B

Rationale: The trophozoites of *E. histolytica* invade the mucosa of the colon, resulting in the destruction of tissue, with deeper extension into the submucosa. Lateral extension of this damage produces the classic "flask-shaped" ulcer.

Page: 480

Question #11

Answer: B

Rationale: The most common extraintestinal manifestation of amebiasis is hepatic involvement with abscess formation. In about 80% of cases, this will present as a febrile illness with right upper quadrant abdominal pain, leukocytosis, and abdominal tenderness on examination. For some unknown reason, men have a 10-fold greater risk of extraintestinal amebiasis as compared with women.

Page: 480

Question #12

Answer: C

Rationale: Amebiasis can be treated with either metronidazole (Flagyl) or Tinidazole (Tindamax) in the doses and frequencies noted in the question. Most authorities also recommend a course of therapy with an intraluminal drug such as iodoquinol (Yodoxin) or paromomycin (Humatin) to reduce the rate of relapse. The correct length of treatment with iodoquinol is 20 days rather than 5 days; the other doses noted are correct. It is also recommended that follow-up stool examinations be performed to confirm that patients are no longer infectious.

Page: 480

Question #13

Answer: C

Rationale: Enterobiasis is the most common helminth infection in the developed world, with an estimated prevalence range of 10% among the general population and of nearly 100% among selected groups.

Page: 481

Question #14

Answer: A

Rationale: Enterobiasis is more common among those who live in crowded conditions, such as children in daycare, institutionalized persons, and families. Poverty or lower socioeconomic status is not an increased risk unless it is associated with poor hygiene.

Page: 481

Question #15

Answer: C

Rationale: The adult *E. vermicularis* lives in the cecum and the adjacent intestines. Gravid females migrate to the anus and deposit their eggs on the perianal skin, causing intense itching (pruritus ani). The diagnosis of enterobiasis is by visually demonstrating worms or eggs on perianal skin, which is most effectively done by placing a piece of cellophane tape on the skin and then examining it under the microscope.

Page: 481

Question #16

Answer: B

Rationale: All family members and close household contacts, regardless of whether they are symptomatic, should be treated at the same time as the index case to reduce the risk of reinfection or retransmission. Thorough cleaning of bedding and clothing also helps to reduce the risk of transmission. Mebendazole (Vermox), albendazole (Albenza), and pyrantel pamoate (Antiminth) are all effective for the treatment of enterobiasis.

Page: 481

Question #17

Answer: A

Rationale: Humans can be exposed to the larvae of the nematode worms of the family Anisakidae through the ingestion of raw or poorly prepared fish. Commonly affected fish include herring, mackerel, salmon, cod, pollock, halibut, and sardines.

Page: 481

Question #18

Answer: A

Rationale: Anisakid larvae will be killed by cooking at 60°C for 10 minutes or more or by freezing at −20°C for 24 hours but not by salting, smoking, or marinating.

Page: 482

Question #19

Answer: C

Rationale: Symptoms of anisakiasis vary, and they can range from mild abdominal pain to severe abdominal pain that mimics a surgical abdomen. In cases of allergic anisakiasis, angioedema and anaphylaxis may occur. Upper gastrointestinal endoscopy is usually necessary to confirm the diagnosis of gastric anisakiasis. Treatment is rarely needed, because this condition is self-limited.

Page: 482

Question #20

Answer: B

Rationale: Babesiosis is usually transmitted from an animal reservoir (e.g., white-footed deer mice, other rodents) to man by an *Ixodes* tick bite. Less than 50% of patients diagnosed with babesiosis remember having a tick bite.

Page: 482

Question #21

Answer: B

Rationale: Babesiosis is endemic to New England along the Northeastern Seaboard. Cases have also been found along the upper Atlantic coast, in the northern Midwest, and along the Pacific coast. Most cases occur during the summer and fall. Infection occurs as a result of an *Ixodes* tick bite, a transfusion, or transplacental/perinatal transmission. Infection is usually subclinical. When symptomatic, it most often presents as a nonspecific, gradually appearing, flu-like syndrome; rarely will it produce severe disease.

Page: 482

Question #22

Answer: C

Rationale: Babesiosis is usually asymptomatic. If symptomatic, it usually presents as a self-limited flu-like illness. Occasionally, disease can be severe, and it may include acute respiratory distress syndrome, severe anemia, and renal failure. Individuals at increased risk for severe disease include the elderly, those who have had a splenectomy, and those who are immunodeficient.

Page: 482

Question #23

Answer: D

Rationale: Antibiotic therapy is reserved for those patients who are moderately or seriously ill with babesiosis, because patients with mild cases usually recover without treatment. The preferred treatment is a combination of clindamycin and quinine. Atovaquone plus azithromycin is an alternative treatment. Exchange transfusions are for those who have hemolysis and high levels of parasitemia.

Page: 482

Question #24

Answer: E

Rationale: The transmission of *T. gondii* occurs either through eating the tissue cysts (i.e., raw or undercooked infected meat) or having contact with the oocysts (i.e., vegetables or water, contaminated cat feces, poor hand washing after cleaning cat litter).

Page: 483

Question #25

Answer: D

Rationale: Toxoplasma infections are asymptomatic in 90% of immunocompetent patients. For those who develop symptoms, the most common presentation is self-limited focal tender adenopathy in the head and neck region. The fetus is susceptible to toxoplasmosis, and infection during pregnancy can be quite devastating. If infection occurs during the first trimester, it will likely end in fetal or neonatal death. For those infections that occur during the second or third trimester, more than 80% of the newborns will go on to eventually develop chorioretinitis, learning disabilities, or mental retardation. In these children, immunoglobulin G remains elevated for life. A positive immunoglobulin G test does not distinguish acute from past infection. A four-fold rise in immunoglobulin G titer or seroconversion is supportive of acute infection, but a confirmatory immunoglobulin M level is required.

Page: 483

Question #26

Answer: A

Rationale: Because the majority of toxoplasma infections in immunocompetent and nonpregnant patients are asymptomatic, no therapy is required.

Page: 484

Question #27

Answer: C

Rationale: Because congenital toxoplasmosis is devastating, women who are contemplating pregnancy or

who have just become pregnant should be counseled about ways to avoid getting infected. However, toxoplasmosis is not transmitted by swimming in public pools.

Page: 484

Question #28

Answer: A

Rationale: Treatment for cercarial dermatitis (swimmer's itch) is symptomatic. Antihistamines and topical or oral corticosteroids are effective; antibiotics are rarely required.

Page: 485

Question #29

Answer: C

Rationale: Scabies is transmitted primarily by direct contact. Children in daycare and primary school are at particular risk, and they are the principal route of entry into a family. Institutionalized individuals—whether they are elderly, mentally ill, disabled, or imprisoned—are at increased risk for infection. Unlike pediculosis, poor hygiene does not seem to be a significant risk factor for scabies.

Page: 486

Question #30

Answer: D

Rationale: This description is a classic presentation of a patient with scabies. The intense pruritus that is worse at night is the result of a delayed hypersensitivity reaction (type IV) to the feces and to other secretions from the larvae and mites. Erythematous papules and nodules can usually be found in the web spaces of the fingers or toes, the flexor aspect of the wrist, the extensor aspect of the elbow, the axilla, the inframammary area, the belt line, the areola, the groin, and the intertriginous areas.

Page: 486

Question #31

Answer: D

Rationale: Permethrin 5% (Elimite) is the drug of choice for the treatment of scabies, with an excellent efficacy and safety profile. Cure rates are generally in the 90% to 100% range. Gamma benzene hexachloride 1% (lindane, Kwell) is effective, but it is associated with more side effects, some of which can be quite serious. Ivermectin is not approved by the U.S. Food and Drug Administration for the treatment of scabies. However, it has been shown to be effective for cases in which multiple other treatments have failed.

Page: 487

Question #32

Answer: C

Rationale: Symptoms from a scabies infection may persist for several weeks, despite successful treatment, because the hypersensitivity reaction does not stop until the skin bearing the mites and their feces is shed. All clothing, bedding, cloth toys, and dolls that the patient has used during the prior 4 days should be washed with hot water and dried in a hot dryer for 10 minutes; an alternative is to store these items in a closed plastic container for at least a week. Reinfection may occur if all physical contacts and family members are not treated, even if they are asymptomatic. After treatment, children do not have to wait for symptoms to resolve to return to day care or school.

Page: 487

Question #33

Answer: D

Rationale: Body lice, unlike pubic and head lice, serve as vectors, carrying epidemic typhus, trench fever, and louse-borne relapsing fever. The mode of transmission of lice depends on the type; head lice are transmitted through direct head-to-head contact and, less frequently, through shared combs, brushes, and hats. Body lice are spread through contact with infested clothing, bedding, towels, or cloth-covered seats. Pubic lice are transmitted via physical and sexual contact.

Page: 487

28 Answers

Question #1

Answer: C

Rationale: Immigrants returning home to visit friends and family in developing countries may be at high risk for travel-related illnesses. Because they may have been away from their home country for years, they may have lost immunity to endemic diseases. While visiting, they drink the local water and are exposed to mosquitoes, and oftentimes they do not have access to travel medical services. In 2002, immigrants visiting friends and relatives accounted for 45% of the civilian cases of malaria in the United States. Members of the military and the Peace Corps are immunized and provided with information about local health hazards, and they receive ongoing care while overseas. Medical missionaries often live in difficult conditions, but they hopefully have the knowledge to protect themselves.

Page: 491

Question #2

Answer: A

Rationale: Traveler's diarrhea is by far the most common illness among travelers, and it is estimated to affect 30% to 80% of them. Up to 11% of returning travelers will report fever.

Page: 491

Question #3

Answer: B

Rationale: Cardiovascular events are the most common cause of death among travelers, followed by motor vehicle accidents and drowning. Infectious diseases account for only 1% to 4% of deaths. Although natural disasters and airline crashes are newsworthy, they account for relatively few deaths on average. Common causes of death at home are also the common causes of death while traveling.

Page: 491

Question #4

Answer: D

Rationale: Unless the traveler has symptoms to suggest an infectious illness, screening is not usually performed during the pretravel examination. The exception would be pretravel purified protein derivative screening for health care workers going to endemic areas. Travelers returning home with significant fever should undergo an infectious disease workup. In addition, travelers with chronic diseases that would put them at risk may have screening performed when they return.

Page: 491

Question #5

Answer: B

Rationale: Six weeks before travel allows enough time to immunize, to stabilize any current medical problems, and to work up any new problems that are uncovered. Six months may be too long, because significant problems could develop or worsen before departure.

Page: 491

Question #6

Answer: C

Rationale: The Centers for Disease Control and Prevention Web site is an excellent source for current travel information and advisories. Textbooks may not provide the most current information about specific countries, and travel agents and tourism bureaus work to attract travelers to destinations rather than provide health information.

Page: 491

Question #7

Answer: D

Rationale: Although travel at any time during pregnancy may entail some risk, travel after 36 weeks' gestation should be discouraged. If travel cannot be postponed, a country-specific list of high-quality care can be found at www.iamat.org.

Page: 492

Question #8

Answer: B

Rationale: Exposure to elevation above 8000 feet may result in altitude illness in some travelers. Those travelers coming from a coastal sea level will be less acclimatized than those beginning their trip at a higher elevation, such as Denver, Colo (5000 feet). The higher the elevation change, the greater the incidence of altitude illness. Physical fitness does not protect an individual from altitude illness.

Page: 492

Question #9

Answer: A

Rationale: Acetazolamide is the only drug approved by the U.S. Food and Drug Administration for the prevention of acute mountain sickness. Dexamethasone is also effective, but it is less commonly used because of its side-effect profile. Dehydration as a result of diuretics or alcohol can worsen altitude illness. Multivitamins with iron are of no proven value.

Page: 492

Question #10

Answer: D

Rationale: Descent to a lower altitude is the mainstay of treatment. Supplemental oxygen, especially if given by positive pressure, is also helpful. Dexamethasone is used for high-altitude cerebral edema. Morphine is not currently used, and sedatives may worsen the condition.

Page: 492

Question #11

Answer: C

Rationale: Chloroquine is the drug of choice for areas in which the malaria parasite is sensitive to chloroquine. It is contraindicated among patients with retinopathy. Mefloquine is indicated only in areas of CRPF. If there

is chloroquine resistance and the patient is allergic to mefloquine, other antimalarials must be used. Primaquine can cause fatal hemolysis in G6PD-deficient patients; it is only indicated in areas with CRPF.

Page: 493

Question #12

Answer: A

Rationale: Chloramphenicol is not used to treat malaria. Doxycycline is indicated in areas with CRPF and for chloroquine-allergic patients. Malarone and Mefloquine are also first-line drugs in areas with CRPF.

Page: 493

Question #13

Answer: B

Rationale: Malarone and doxycycline are both started 1 day before travel, and they are taken daily. Malarone is continued for 1 week after return. All other preventive medications are continued for 4 weeks. Both chloroquine and mefloquine are taken weekly, starting 1 week before travel and continuing for 4 weeks after return.

Page: 493

Question #14

Answer: D

Rationale: A G6PD level in the normal range must be documented before the patient is given primaquine. It is also contraindicated during pregnancy.

Page: 493

Question #15

Answer: D

Rationale: Use of Fansidar has been greatly limited as a result of increasing drug resistance among CRPF. Mefloquine and Malarone may be used, provided that they were not previously being used for prophylaxis. Significant mefloquine-associated neuropsychiatric symptoms have been seen when higher treatment dosages are used.

Page: 493

Question #16

Answer: B

Rationale: Permethrin is both an insecticide and a repellent. When sprayed onto clothing or bed netting, it will repel insects for 4 weeks or more. When rinsed into clothing, it will repel insects for up to 1 year or 30 washings.

Page: 493

Question #17

Answer: A

Rationale: For an adult who has completed his or her childhood immunization series, the Centers for Disease Control and Prevention currently recommends a single lifetime booster dose of inactivated polio vaccine for travel to polio-endemic areas in West Africa and South Asia.

Page: 494

Question #18

Answer: A

Rationale: The yellow fever vaccine is a live virus vaccine, and it should not be given to pregnant women. If travel to an endemic area is unavoidable, then the risks and benefits must be considered and the vaccine given or a waiver given. If travel to a high-risk area is absolutely necessary, the benefits outweigh the risks to both mother and fetus.

Page: 494

Question #19

Answer: C

Rationale: Hepatitis A infection is the leading cause of vaccine-preventable illness among travelers. Hepatitis A vaccine is given in two doses, 6 to 12 months apart. The first dose is up to 90% effective after 2 weeks. If traveling to a high-risk area will occur within 2 weeks of the initial dosage, a dose of immunoglobulin should be given. Because it is an inactivated vaccine, the Hepatitis A vaccine is safe for use during pregnancy.

Page: 494

Question #20

Answer: D

Rationale: On a worldwide basis, enterotoxigenic *E. coli* is the most common cause of traveler's diarrhea in developing and tropical countries. It can produce both heat-stable and heat-labile enterotoxins, which stimulate the secretion of fluid throughout the small bowel. In general, bacteria are responsible for the majority of cases of traveler's diarrhea. Viruses, parasites, and toxins are less common.

Page: 494

Question #21

Answer: C

Rationale: Antibiotic prophylaxis is no longer recommended by the Centers for Disease Control and Prevention. Antibiotics may be given when symptoms develop. Ice and uncooked vegetables are high-risk foods in developing and tropical countries; carbonated beverages without ice are generally safe. If cans or bottles are submerged in ice water, dry off the outside of the container. No known human pathogens can be found in beer.

Page: 494

Question #22

Answer: A

Rationale: A fluoroquinolone antibiotic (ciprofloxin, levofloxin, or ofloxin) for 3 days is the drug of choice for adults with persistent or distressing diarrhea. Systemic fluoroquinolones have not been proven safe for patients who are less than 18 years old. Doxycycline is contraindicated during pregnancy. Azithromycin may be used for children and pregnant women. Metronidazole is not active against many of the common bacterial pathogens of this condition.

Page: 494

Question #23

Answer: B

Rationale: The World Health Organization recommends screening any traveler who suffers from a chronic disease that would place him or her at an increased risk of infection or complication. This includes cardiovascular disease, diabetes, and chronic respiratory disease. Screening is also recommended for travelers who have spent more than 3 months in a developing country. Panels of screening tests for asymptomatic short-term travelers are of unproven value. Any traveler who thinks that he or she may have been exposed to a serious infectious disease while traveling should be screened.

Page: 495

Question #24

Answer: C

Rationale: Overseas health care workers should be screened for tuberculosis with a purified protein derivative before travel, annually, and on return. Hepatitis C, human immunodeficiency virus, and sexually transmitted diseases should be screened for on the basis of individual exposure history.

Page: 495

Question #25

Answer: B

Rationale: Fever in a returning traveler is a medical emergency. If the traveler has been in an area in which malaria is endemic, then malaria should be considered in the differential diagnosis. Intestinal parasites and ciguatera poisoning usually do not present with fever, and cutaneous leishmaniasis rarely presents with fever. However, visceral leishmaniasis (Kala-azar) will have fever as an early symptom.

Page: 495

Question #26

Answer: A

Rationale: Conjunctival suffusion is a dilation of the conjunctival vessels without inflammation; it is not conjunctivitis, and it is frequently found in patients with leptospirosis. It usually appears on the third or fourth day of illness, and it may be mild and often overlooked. Although it may rarely be seen with viral hemorrhagic fevers, some experts consider its presence to be pathognomonic for leptospirosis. Conjunctival suffusion is not seen with Dengue fever, Yellow fever, or malaria.

Page: 495

Question #27

Answer: D

Rationale: Strongyloides are roundworms that inhabit the intestinal tract. They may be acquired by ingestion or skin contact with contaminated soil. Their life cycle may include passage through the lung, which can cause cough. It is not uncommon for stool examinations to be negative for Strongyloides on multiple specimens. If Strongyloides is suspected, then a serologic test should obtained. Giardia, *C. difficile,* and *H. pylori* do not cause cough or eosinophilia.

Page: 496

Question #28

Answer: A

Rationale: Leishmaniasis is caused by a protozoan parasite, leishmania. Its vector is the sandfly. In the cutaneous form, it can cause a non- or slow-healing ulcer on the face, arms, or legs. Diagnosis can be made by smears from lesions, cultures, or biopsy. The classic skin lesion of early Lyme disease is erythema migrans, which is a round or oval well-demarcated erythematous lesion at the site of the tick bite. Classic scabies lesions are excoriated 2-mm papules seen on the finger webs, the flexor aspects of the wrist, the breast, the genitals, the buttocks, and the feet; they are rarely on the face or scalp, except among the very young or the very old. Cutaneous larva migrans is caused by the penetration of the barefoot traveler's feet by hookworm larvae, causing a distinctive serpiginous rash.

Page: 496

Question #29

Answer: B

Rationale: Chagas disease is caused by *Trypanosoma cruzi,* and it is not sensitive to doxycycline. Malaria, leptospirosis, and cholera can all be prevented or treated with doxycycline, which makes doxycycline a very useful medication for travelers in a variety of situations.

Page: 493

Question #30

Answer: C

Rationale: The measles vaccine is a live virus vaccine; thus, it is not to be used during pregnancy. Hepatitis A is an inactivated virus vaccine and is safe during pregnancy. Meningococcal vaccine is a killed bacteria vaccine, and tetanus and diphtheria is a toxoid vaccine; both are considered safe for the pregnant patient.

Page: 495

29   Answers

Question #1

Answer: D

Rationale: The United States consistently ranks poorly with regard to measures such as maternal and infant mortality. In 1994, the World Health Organization ranked the United States as 25th for infant mortality rates, behind the other listed countries in the question. In 2002, the National Center for Health Statistics reported an increase in infant deaths in the United States as a result of premature births, birth defects, and maternal complications of pregnancy. The poor rankings reflect, in part, the disparities in health access and delivery for citizens.

Page: 497

Question #2

Answer: D

Rationale: Folic acid supplementation has been shown to reduce the occurrence and recurrence of neural tube defects. For low-risk women, folic acid supplementation of 0.4 mg/day is recommended, because nutritional sources alone are insufficient. Folic acid supplementation of 4 mg/day is recommended for all women at high risk of neural tube defects, including a previous pregnancy that involved such a defect.

Page: 498

Question #3

Answer: B

Rationale: Biochemical testing measures certain biochemicals in maternal blood that can be predictive of fetal abnormalities. Maternal serum alpha-fetoprotein is an effective screening test for neural tube defects, and it should be offered to all pregnant women. The addition of beta subunit of human chorionic gonadotropin and estriols (the triple screen) has improved sensitivity for the detection of chromosomal abnormalities. Maternal blood samples can be obtained at 15 to 20 weeks' gestation, but they are most sensitive at 16 to 18 weeks' gestation. A quadruple screen is identical to the triple screen but with the addition of inhibin A to increase the sensitivity of the detection of Down syndrome.

Page: 501

Question #4

Answer: A

Rationale: Inaccurate menstrual age assignment and maternal obesity are the most common reasons for inconsistent fundal measurements. Larger-than-expected fundal heights may be the result of obesity, uterine fibroids, multiple gestation, polyhydramnios, and a large-for-gestational-age fetus. Smaller-than-expected fundal heights can be the result of oligohydramnios, fetal growth restriction, and fetal demise. Inaccurate menstrual age assignment can result in either larger-than-expected or smaller-than-expected fundal heights.

Page: 502

Question #5

Answer: D

Rationale: Screening for group B streptococcus colonization significantly reduces early-onset infection with this disease among neonates. Original strategies issued in 1996 were based on risk; however, compelling evidence for a strong protective effect of this screening-based strategy led to a new recommendation in 2002 for universal screening at 35 to 37 weeks' gestation.

Page: 502

Question #6

Answer: D

Rationale: There are few absolutes in the field of human teratology. However, Category X drugs are contraindicated for women who are or who may become pregnant. The abbreviated definitions of the other risk categories are as follows:

- Category A: Controlled studies in women fail to demonstrate a risk to the fetus.
- Category B: Either animal-reproduction studies have not demonstrated a fetal risk but there are no controlled studies in pregnant women, or animal-reproduction studies have shown an adverse effect.
- Category C: Either studies in animals have revealed adverse effects on the fetus, or there are no controlled studies in women. Drugs should be

given only if the potential benefit justifies the potential risk to the fetus.

- Category D: There is positive evidence of human fetal risk, but the benefits of use for pregnant women may be acceptable.

Page: 504

Question #7

Answer: A

Rationale: The safety of a trial of labor in women with a history of one low transverse uterine incision has been documented. Rupture of these incisions is only 0.5%. After careful patient selection, approximately 7 out of 10 women will have a successful vaginal birth after Cesarean delivery. Women with a classical uterine incision or any other variation that penetrates into the upper uterine segment have as much as a 12% risk of rupture. Oxytocin use is not contraindicated in this setting, although it should be used cautiously. There is not sufficient information to determine whether a trial of labor is completely safe for vaginal birth after Cesarean delivery candidates with suspected macrosomia and a gestational age beyond 40 weeks. However, based on the findings of several retrospective studies, this may be a reasonable birthing method option.

Page: 504

Question #8

Answer: D

Rationale: Maternal HIV is not teratogenic or associated with increased fetal loss, except during end-stage disease. The most serious consequence of HIV infection in pregnancy is transmission to the fetus; this results in an infected newborn, and this condition may ultimately prove to be lethal. Cataracts and chorioretinitis are associated with congenital rubella syndrome. Congenital hearing loss is a feature of cytomegalovirus infection. Syphilis may result in an increase in miscarriages, hydrops fetalis, stillborn, and preterm deliveries.

Page: 506

Question #9

Answer: D

Rationale: Alpha-methyldopa (Aldomet), a central-acting alpha adrenergic agent, is the drug of choice for the treatment of chronic hypertension during pregnancy. Other medications that can be used are nifedi-

pine, hydralazine, and labetalol. Angiotensin-converting enzyme inhibitors and diuretics are contraindicated during pregnancy.

Page: 509

Question #10

Answer: B

Rationale: The treatment of gestational diabetes reduces serious perinatal morbidity, and it may also improve the woman's health-related quality of life. Therefore, screening is recommended for all pregnant women. The initial screening test is performed in a non-fasting state using a mixture that contains 50 g of glucose. A plasma glucose level is drawn 1 hour after ingestion. If the result is greater than or equal to 140 mg/dL, a 3-hour glucose challenge test is needed. The patient should fast the night before and receive 100 g of glucose. Venous blood glucose is drawn after fasting and at 1, 2, and 3 hours after the glucose challenge. Two abnormal values make the diagnosis of gestational diabetes.

Page: 509

Question #11

Answer: A

Rationale: Approximately 3% to 5% of pregnant women will have asymptomatic bacteriuria. This can also be found in up to 10% of pregnant women with the sickle-cell trait. Although this percentage may seem low, 30% will progress to pyelonephritis. Periodic cultures for screening should be performed among pregnant women with the sickle-cell trait, with urine dipsticks suggestive of bacterial growth, and with a history of recurrent urinary tract infections.

Page: 510

Question #12

Answer: B

Rationale: Serum human chorionic gonadotropin levels drawn 48 hours apart can be helpful for the diagnosis of ectopic pregnancy. In general, human chorionic gonadotropin values will double during that time. A plateauing of human chorionic gonadotropin is consistent with an ectopic pregnancy or an abnormal uterine pregnancy. Ultrasonography can be used to help differentiate the two, although as much as 20% to 30% of ectopic gestations have no detectable abnormalities. A serum progesterone level of less than 15 µg/mL is suggestive of an abnormal pregnancy and warrants further investigation. A serum progesterone level of more than 25 μg/mL is probably a normal pregnancy. Alpha-fetoprotein is used as a screen for neural tube defects but not for the evaluation of ectopic pregnancy.

Page: 510

Question #13

Answer: C

Rationale: If preterm delivery is a possibility, antibiotic prophylaxis should be given. In addition, betamethasone is recommended for patients between 24 and 34 weeks' gestation in an effort to accelerate fetal lung maturity. Common tocolytics used to reduce or stop contractions include terbutaline, ritodrine, and magnesium sulfate. Plasma magnesium levels must be monitored, because magnesium toxicity can occur. Although calcium gluconate is the usual treatment for magnesium toxicity, it has no role in the initial treatment of preterm labor.

Page: 512

Question #14

Answer: C

Rationale: Intrauterine growth restriction can be described as *symmetric* or *asymmetric.* If inadequate delivery of oxygen and nutrients is early, persistent, or profound, all organs and tissues may be affected, and symmetric intrauterine growth restriction results. Asymmetric intrauterine growth restriction results when inadequate oxygen and nutrients are present and the fetus shunts blood flow to important organs, such as the brain, while hypoperfusing other areas, such as muscle and viscera. Although acute infections and conditions should be treated with appropriate fluids and antibiotics and genetic testing may reveal an underlying condition, the only treatment modality thought to be of benefit is bedrest in a lateral recumbent position. This position maximizes venous return to the heart, improving cardiac output and uteroplacental perfusion.

Page: 513

Question #15

Answer: C

Rationale: *HELLP* is an acronym for *h*emolysis, *el*evated *l*iver enzymes, and *l*ow *p*latelets. This may be a complication of seemingly stable patients with pree-

clampsia. These patients frequently present with right upper quadrant pain and epigastric pain. A peripheral blood smear will show a microangiopathic hemolytic anemia, platelet counts will be low, and liver enzymes will be increased. This is a life-threatening emergency that requires prompt delivery. Lumbar puncture has no role in this disorder.

Page: 514

Question #16

Answer: A

Rationale: Abruptio placenta is a clinical diagnosis, because ultrasonography has a high false-negative rate. Painful vaginal bleeding during the third trimester is the hallmark. First-trimester bleeding is associated with spontaneous miscarriage. Other common presenting features include abdominal pain, back pain, uterine tenderness, and fetal distress. There is a noted causal relationship with cocaine usage.

Page: 514

Question #17

Answer: B

Rationale: The incidence of placenta previa is about 1 in every 200 to 250 pregnancies. The placenta may take up 25% to 50% of the uterine surface area during the second trimester. Approximately 5% of routine ultrasounds performed during the second trimester will detect a complete previa, and approximately 90% will resolve by term as a result of placenta migration and the growth of the lower uterine segment. Painless vaginal bleeding is characteristic of placenta previa, whereas painful vaginal bleeding is consistent with abruptio placenta.

Page: 515

Question #18

Answer: A

Rationale: There are three forms of abnormal placental attachment in which the trophoblasts invade beyond the normal location and into the uterine muscle. A minimally invasive placenta (accreta) can be removed manually or by curettage. Deeper invasions into the myometrium (increta) or through the myometrium (percreta) often require hysterectomy. A low-lying placenta is implantation in the lower uterine segment.

Page: 515

Question #19

Answer: D

Rationale: Women with a twin gestation have an increased risk of placenta previa, kidney infection, and hypertension. They are also more likely to experience premature labor, gestational diabetes, and early miscarriage.

Page: 516

Question #20

Answer: A

Rationale: The three most common methods used to evaluate fetal well-being in utero are the nonstress test, the contraction stress test, and the biophysical profile. Vibroacoustic stimulation is also used to provoke accelerations in the fetal heart rate. Although all of these tests evaluate fetal heart rate and maternal contractions, only the biophysical profile includes the ultrasound assessment of amniotic fluid volume, fetal breathing, movement, and tone.

Page: 516

Question #21

Answer: C

Rationale: The first hour after delivery has the highest risk of uterine atony and excessive vaginal bleeding. If fundal massage does not stop bleeding, then intravenous oxytocin as well as intramuscular oxytocin, methylergonovine (Methergine), or prostaglandin F_2-alpha (Hemabate) may be used. However, methylergonovine should not be used to treat hypertensive women.

Page: 530

Question #22

Answer: B

Rationale: Misoprostol (Cytotec), a synthetic E_1 prostaglandin, is approved by the U.S. Food and Drug Administration for the prevention of gastric ulcers, but it is used off-label for cervical ripening and the induction of labor. It is a strong uterotonic agent that may be associated with a higher incidence of uterine rupture. As such, it is best not used in women with previous uterine surgery, including Cesarean section. Both low- and high-dose oxytocin regimens are used for the induction of labor.

Page: 520

Question #23

Answer: C

Rationale: The management of the prolonged latent phase of labor is primarily conservative, and it often includes rest and observation. Unless there is a need to deliver the fetus quickly, the prolonged latent phase by itself is not an indication for Cesarean section. Amniotomy should be avoided, because it increases the risk for chorioamnionitis. Maternal rest can be induced by an appropriate dose of morphine. Oxytocin induction may be useful, especially if uterine inertia is an underlying etiology.

Page: 520

Question #24

Answer: B

Rationale: The first stage of labor consists of both the latent phase and the active phase of cervical dilatation up to complete dilatation. The second stage is the period between complete dilatation and the delivery of the infant. The third stage begins after the delivery of the infant and includes the interval to the delivery of the placenta. The first hour after the delivery of the placenta is considered to be the fourth stage of labor.

Page: 521

Question #25

Answer: C

Rationale: Shoulder dystocia is a life-threatening event that needs to be recognized early and managed quickly. Shoulder dystocia is defined as the impaction of the anterior shoulder of the fetus against the pubic symphysis. Multiple complications can occur. Erb's palsy is the most common brachial plexus injury, and it involves the fifth and sixth cervical roots. Klumpke's palsy involves the eighth cervical and first thoracic roots. Although a number of conditions are associated with the development of shoulder dystocia, their predictive value is low, and approximately half of all shoulder dystocias occur in normal-weight fetuses.

Page: 521

Question #26

Answer: C

Rationale: The McRoberts maneuver is used for the initial management of shoulder dystocia. This involves the flexion of the maternal thighs onto the abdomen, which increases the inlet diameter. Suprapubic pressure can often dislodge the anterior shoulder from behind the maternal pubic symphysis. Fundal pressure should not be exerted, because it can exacerbate the situation. As a measure of last resort, cephalic replacement of the fetus followed by Cesarean delivery can be tried.

Page: 521

Question #27

Answer: D

Rationale: EFM has become the standard practice for the management of both high- and low-risk pregnancies. However, although it can be predictive of good outcomes, it is not accurate or predictive of bad outcomes. In fact, in a 1996 report, the U.S. Preventative Services Task Force could not recommend its routine use for the management of low-risk deliveries. Recognizing the limits of this technology, the American College of Obstetricians and Gynecologists concur that EFM appears to have no inherent benefit over properly performed auscultation for low-risk pregnancies.

Pages: 521–522

Question #28

Answer: A

Rationale: Fetal tachycardia is defined as a baseline fetal heart rate of greater than 160 bpm. Common causes of fetal tachycardia include anxiety, fever, and hypoxia. However, fetal tachycardia of more than 200 bpm is usually the result of a fetal tachyarrhythmia or, rarely, a congenital anomaly.

Page: 524

Question #29

Answer: A

Rationale: Early decelerations are caused by a vagal response to fetal head compression. They have a smooth uniform shape that is a mirror image of the contraction. They are reassuring and associated with a good outcome. Variable decelerations are almost always the result of umbilical cord compression. They have variable shapes, recoveries, and relationships with contractions.

Page: 524

Question #30

Answer: D

Rationale: During the postpartum period or the puerperium, the mother undergoes many changes that are normal and that should not be confused with pathological conditions. Among the normal changes are a drop in the pulse rate, a slight elevation in temperature, and the development of a leukocytosis of up to 20,000/μL. Any bleeding that results in hemodynamic instability is considered postpartum hemorrhage, which is a potentially life-threatening complication.

Page: 529

Question #1

Answer: A

Rationale: Neonatal GBS infection is fulminant, life threatening, and unpredictable. Routine screening for GBS during the prenatal period and the use of antepartum antibiotics for all women who have tested positive for GBS have been shown to significantly reduce early-onset GBS infection. The highest risk for neonatal GBS infection after delivery is early during the first 48 hours of life, and, thus, recommendations include a minimum of 48 hours of observation, regardless of antepartum antibiotic use. If antibiotic prophylaxis is given for more than 4 hours before delivery, neonates of more than 35 weeks' gestation do not require evaluation other than observation. However, neonates of less than 35 weeks' gestation are recommended to be evaluated with a complete blood cell count and a blood culture.

Page: 536

Question #2

Answer: B

Rationale: The risk reduction for neural tube defects afforded by preconceptual folic acid supplementation is well documented at doses of 400 μg per day. If a pregnant woman already has a child with a neural tube defect, the recommended dose increases to 4000 μg per day. The risks of known genetic diseases as well as the benefits of avoiding known environmental hazards (including abuse of substances and medications) should be explained before conception.

Page: 535

Question #3

Answer: A

Rationale: Tracheal suctioning for meconium-stained amniotic fluid has benefited depressed newborns but not vigorous infants with heart rates of more than 100 beats per minute, spontaneous respirations, and spontaneous movement or extremity flexion.

Page: 537

Question #4

Answer: A

Rationale: Newborn infants go through significant changes during the first few hours of life, and, thus, they should be examined during the first 12 to 18 hours of life. Maternal and prenatal historical information helps determine an infant's risk factors for various conditions to be evaluated during a physical examination. Examining infants in uncomfortable environments often contributes to an upset, uncooperative infant who is difficult to completely examine.

Page: 539

Question #5

Answer: C

Rationale: Macular hemangiomas (also called "stork bites") are extremely common among newborns. Newborn respiratory rates tend to vary significantly within a 1-minute period ("periodic breathing"), and, thus, respiratory rates should be measured only after 60 seconds of monitoring. All limbs should move symmetrically, and, if this does not occur, further evaluation is required. Fine crackles (or "wet lungs") in a newborn can be normal, especially after a Cesarean section, because the interstitial fluid from intrauterine life is being cleared.

Page: 539

Question #6

Answer: A

Rationale: Infants can lose up to 10 percent of their birth weight in the first few days of life. These infants should return to or exceed their birth weight by 2 weeks of age.[1]

Page: 539

1. Thureen PJ, Deacon J, Hernandez JA, Hall DM: *Assessment and care of the well newborn*, 2nd ed, Philadelphia, WB Saunders, 2005.

Question #7

Answer: D

Rationale: Immediately after delivery, all infants require proper airway positioning and suctioning to open their airways. Drying, which stimulates the infant to breath, is also required. Occasionally, an infant may require positive-pressure ventilation to overcome apnea or persistent cyanosis. Epinephrine is only indicated when basic ABCs have been adequately attempted and bradycardia persists. (See Figure 30-1.)

Page: 538

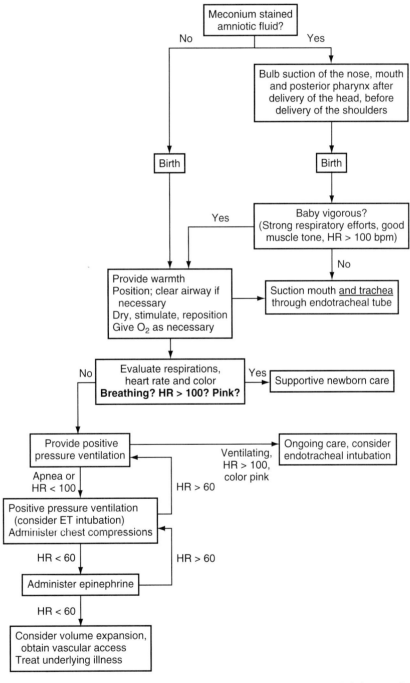

Figure 30-1 Adapted from American Academy of Pediatrics, American Heart Association; Kattwinkel JMF, editor: *Textbook of neonatal resuscitation,* ed 4, American Academy of Pediatrics and American Heart Association, 2000. In Rakel RE, editor: *Textbook of family medicine,* ed 7, Philadelphia, 2007, WB Saunders. Adapted from: American Academy of Pediatrics, American Heart Association. John Kattwinkel MF, editor. *Textbook of neonatal resuscitation,* ed 5, American Academy of Pediatrics and American Heart Association; 2006. In Rakel RE (ed). *Textbook of family medicine,* ed 7, Philadelphia, WB Saunders, 2007.

Question #8

Answer: B

Rationale: Apgar scoring assesses heart rate, respirations, muscle tone, reflex irritability to tactile stimulation, and color. Neonatal resuscitation decisions do not require all of this information; rather, only breathing, color, and heart rate need to be considered. An Apgar score should not be a determining factor for whether further resuscitation is required, and obtaining the Apgar score should not interrupt resuscitation.

Page: 537

Sign	Score		
	0	1	2
Heart rate	Absent	<100 bpm	≥100 bpm
Respirations	Absent	Irregular and slow	Strong breaths, crying
Muscle tone	Limp	Some flexion	Good flexion, active motion
Reflex irritability to tactile stimulation	No response	Grimace	Coughing, sneezing, crying
Color	Blue or pale	Blue extremities, pink body	Completely pink

Adapted from American Academy of Pediatrics, American Heart Association; Kattwinkel JMF, editor: *Textbook of neonatal resuscitation,* ed 4, American Academy of Pediatrics and American Heart Association, 2000. In Rakel RE, editor: *Textbook of family medicine,* ed 7, Philadelphia, WB Saunders, 2007.

Question #9

Answer: B

Rationale: Neonatal asphyxia diagnosis requires more than an abnormal Apgar score. Although 5-minute Apgar scores may be more predictive of outcome than 1-minute Apgar scores and a 5-minute Apgar score of less than 7 is correlated with a significantly increased risk of neonatal death, neonatal death is still a very uncommon event.

Page: 537

Question #10

Answer: C

Rationale: Periodic breathing is a common benign finding in the neonate. However, infants with pulmonary problems can present simply with grunting that lasts beyond the first hour of life. Bradycardia may be asso-

ciated with sepsis, asphyxia, heart block, and other conditions. Hypothermia is more common than hyperthermia in the septic neonate. Jaundice—especially that found during the first 24 hours of life—could represent hemolysis or other bilirubin-clearance issues, which could lead to kernicterus without adequate investigation.

Page: 539

Question #11

Answer: B

Rationale: Although the U.S. Preventive Services Task Force has found insufficient evidence to recommend for or against universal screening, 35 states have mandatory universal newborn hearing screening, which may be performed using one of three acceptable screening tests: automated auditory brainstem response, transient evoked otoacoustic emissions, or distortion product otoacoustic emissions. Any failed screening test requires pediatric audiologic evaluation.

Page: 542

Question #12

Answer: A

Rationale: GBS is a leading cause of neonatal morbidity and mortality in the United States. Symptoms of GBS sepsis include respiratory symptoms of tachypnea, grunting, or retractions or nonspecific symptoms of poor feeding, intolerance to feeds, lethargy, or an inability to maintain body temperature. GBS sepsis risks factors are identifiable before a newborn's delivery, and sepsis can be reduced with intrapartum antibiotic prophylaxis. Prompt evaluation and treatment are required when GBS sepsis is suspected.

Page: 545

Question #13

Answer: E

Rationale: Disorders that affect a newborn's ability to oxygenate or that impact his or her metabolic status will result in tachypnea. Pulmonary disorders such as surfactant deficiency (respiratory distress syndrome), persisting fetal lung fluid (transient tachypnea of the newborn), and congenital pneumonia cause impaired delivery of oxygen to alveoli. Congenital heart disease can result in an abnormal mixture of oxygenated and deoxygenated blood in the newborn's circulation. Circulatory compromise from neonatal sepsis often causes tachypnea. Simple neonatal hyperbilirubinemia in itself is not associated with tachypnea.

Page: 546

Question #14

Answer: A

Rationale: Respiratory distress syndrome is most commonly found among preterm infants, but can also occur among infants who have been carried to term, especially those of diabetic mothers. Respiratory distress syndrome usually presents with respiratory distress and a gradual worsening cyanosis as the disease worsens. Preterm infants who present with symptoms of respiratory distress syndrome are also high risk for GBS sepsis and thus should be treated for both, pending further evaluation. Risk for preterm-related respiratory distress syndrome can be reduced with the use of steroids for mothers who are experiencing preterm labor.

Pages: 545, 546

Question #15

Answer: B

Rationale: Meconium aspiration syndrome may lead to congenital pneumonia, and, thus, antibiotic treatment is often required pending recovery. During the stabilization of either condition, intubation may be necessary to adequately oxygenate and ventilate severely affected infants. A complication of meconium aspiration syndrome may be subsequent persistent pulmonary hypertension.

Page: 546

Question #16

Answer: D

Rationale: The most common cause of tachypnea in the term newborn is transient tachypnea of the newborn, which is probably caused by the delayed clearing of fetal lung fluid. Transient tachypnea of the newborn presents with tachypnea at birth that may persist.

Pages: 546, 547

Question #17

Answer: C

Rationale: Newborns with highly suspected congenital heart disease should be promptly transferred to a facility with a pediatric echocardiography department and a neonatal intensive care. Infants with congenital heart lesions may not have audible murmurs, but the oxygen challenge test may help distinguish heart disease from pulmonary disease. Infants without congenital heart disease who are placed on 100% oxygen should have an increase in pO_2 to more than 150 mm Hg.

Page: 546

Question #18

Answer: B

Rationale: The blood glucose level that defines hypoglycemia is controversial, but plasma levels of less than 36 mg/dL warrant close monitoring. Hypoglycemia is often observed in term infants with hypoglycemia risk factors as liver glycogen stores rapidly decline within the first few hours after birth. These glucose levels decline until 1 to 3 hours of life, at which time they tend to rise.

Page: 547

Question #19

Answer: D

Rationale: Infants who are at risk for hypoglycemia include those born from diabetic mothers, those who are small for gestational age, those with perinatal hypoxia, those with hypothermia, and those with sepsis. Routine blood glucose monitoring of large-for-gestational-age infants without other risk factors is not necessary.

Page: 547

Question #20

Answer: C

Rationale: Hypoglycemia is uncommon among infants who are healthy, asymptomatic, and without other risk factors, such as being small for gestational age, having hypothermia, having sepsis, or having diabetic mothers. Without symptoms and other risk factors, healthy premature and large-for-gestational-age infants do not specifically require glucose monitoring.

Page: 547

Question #21

Answer: C

Rationale: Intravenous glucose doses are determined by serum glucose levels. Asymptomatic and alert infants can be treated with either breastfeeding or bottle feeding. Hypoglycemia after treatment may reoccur, and, thus, follow-up glucose testing is recommended.

Page: 547

Question #22

Answer: B

Rationale: Infants born to diabetic mothers have higher rates of morbidity and mortality than the general newborn population. They may become macrosomic, which increases their risk for various birth traumas. Gestational diabetes with vascular complications can cause poor intrauterine growth, which results in the birth of an infant who is small for gestational age. Polycythemia and hyperviscosity are more common among these infants as a result of increased erythropoieses and the shift of blood from the placenta to the fetus during chronic hypoxia.

Page: 547

Question #23

Answer: E

Rationale: Umbilical hernias are common, but they are not any more common among infants of diabetic mothers. Respiratory distress syndrome occurs five to six times more often in infants born after 38 weeks' gestation to diabetic mothers than to infants of the same age born to nondiabetic mothers. Cardiac and central nervous system malformations are four to eight times more common among infants of mothers with poorly controlled diabetes. Newborns from diabetic gestations have an increased risk for hyperbilirubinemia.

Page: 547

Question #24

Answer: B

Rationale: Neonatal jaundice is the most common condition requiring medical attention for the term newborn and requiring readmission during the first week of life. Impaired bilirubin clearance from an infant's body often leads to rising bilirubin levels, which, if they reach high enough levels for long enough, can cause permanent neurologic disability from kernicterus. The American Academic of Pediatrics recommends assessing hyperbilirubinemia severity with serum or transcutaneous bilirubin levels and not by physical examination alone.

Pages: 547, 548

Question #25

Answer: C

Rationale: The American Academy of Pediatrics has published guidelines for hyperbilirubinemia in healthy, term neonates, which importantly include determining severe hyperbilirubinemia risk before hospital discharge based on various risk factors and bilirubin levels plotted on a nomogram according to the infant's age in hours.

Pages: 547, 548

Question #26

Answer: D

Rationale: Asymmetric Moro reflex or movement of the arms can be associated with osseous or neurologic injuries of the newborn's neck, shoulder, or arm, such as clavicle fractures, brachial plexus injuries, and cervical spinal injuries. Cephalohematomata are another example of birth-related trauma, but they are not directly related to impaired arm function.

Page: 549

Question #27

Answer: C

Rationale: The American Academy of Pediatrics has recommended initial newborn follow-up within 48 to 72 hours of discharge; this usually reflects 4 to 5 days of life rather than a week. Breastfeeding mothers should be offered help with establishing breastfeeding, observation to correct breastfeeding problems, and reassurance that supplementation is only necessary when medically indicated.

Page: 549

Question #28

Answer: C

Rationale: Infants who are put to sleep in a position other than on the back and who have a soft sleeping surface with extra bedding (e.g., quilts, comforters) have an increased risk for sudden infant death syndrome. Infants who are co-bedding with parents—especially smoking parents—are at an increased risk of infant death. Pacifier use in infants is not associated with increased risk of death.

Page: 550

Question #29

Answer: B

Rationale: Baths with standing water are not necessary for an infant, because postural reflexes are not developed enough to prevent a newborn from submersion. Parents should be instructed to avoid shaking an infant in frustration and to place an infant in an adequately secured, rear-facing car seat in the middle portion of the rear seat. Signs and symptoms of infection in a newborn (e.g., fever, respiratory distress, poor feeding, difficulty sleeping or awakening) should be reviewed, and immediate return to the hospital should be advised.

Page: 550

Question #30

Answer: B

Rationale: Although some medical benefits of circumcision have been suggested by some studies, neonatal circumcision is still considered primarily an elective procedure with no absolute medical indication. Parents should be given full information about the risks and benefits before committing to this procedure; the most common risk is bleeding, but infection is also a possibility. The procedure does cause pain, which can be reduced with a dorsal penile or ring block. The care of the uncircumcised penis is no different during the first 3 to 5 years of life.

Page: 550

Question #1

Answer: B

Rationale: Growth is the result of increasing cell size and number in various tissues, which leads to an increase in physical size.

Page: 555

Question #2

Answer: D

Rationale: Nutritional, family, emotional, sociocultural, community, and physical factors play a role in shaping a child's psychological and physiological development.

Page: 555

Question #3

Answer: C

Rationale: Head circumference reflects the growth of the cranium, and it should be determined and recorded for the first 2 years of life.

Page: 555

Question #4

Answer: B

Rationale: Macrocephaly is most frequently caused by hydrocephalus. Other reasons for this condition include familial causes; intracranial bleeding, masses, or thickening of the skull; and association with fragile X syndrome or other conditions.

Page: 555

Question #5

Answer: C

Rationale: Premature infants should have their chronologic age adjusted according to their degree of prematurity up to the age of 2 years, because most catch-up growth is complete by this time.

Page: 555

Question #6

Answer: B

Rationale: Linear growth in infants has been shown to occur in incremental bursts rather than continuously.

Page: 555

Question #7

Answer: A

Rationale: Children with genetic short stature have normal length and weight at birth, but their growth percentiles decline within the first 2 to 3 years of life as they reach their genetic potential.

Page: 555

Question #8

Answer: D

Rationale: If a child's growth falls outside of the range of normal, it is useful to obtain a bone-age radiograph, usually of the left hand and wrist, and to compare with age-specific standards.

Page: 567

Question #9

Answer: E

Rationale: If an organic cause of short stature has been excluded, children with delayed bone age are likely to have constitutional growth delay. Children and adolescents of short stature whose bone age is delayed as compared with their chronologic age have more growth potential than do children with a skeletal age that is appropriate for their chronologic age.

Page: 567

Question #10

Answer: D

Rationale: The onset of puberty generally occurs at the age of 9 years among American girls, with the peak height velocity occurring at the age of 11.5 years (range, 9.7–13.5 years for early to late maturers). American boys have onset of puberty at the age of 11 years and peak height velocity at the age of 13.5 years (range, 11.7–15.3 years.)

Page: 568

Question #11

Answer: A

Rationale: Girls who demonstrate signs of puberty before they are 7 to 8 years old and boys who show signs before the age of 9 years should be evaluated for precocious puberty. Conversely, girls who do not show signs of puberty by the time they are 13 years old and boys without such signs at the age of 14 years should be evaluated for pubertal delay.

Page: 568

Question #12

Answer: C

Rationale: Although the peak height velocity has been passed, girls may grow an average of 6 cm more after menarche.

Page: 568

Question #13

Answer: B

Rationale: Infant formulas contain almost 50% more protein than human milk.

Page: 569

Question #14

Answer: D

Rationale: Whole cow's milk is not suitable for infants, because the higher intake of sodium, potassium, and protein increases renal solute loaf. In addition, the lower concentrations of iron, zinc, essential fatty acids, and

vitamin E may result in deficiencies.[1] Significant intestinal blood loss may occur among infants who are less than 12 months old and who are receiving whole cow's milk.

Page: 569

Question #15

Answer: C

Rationale: Honey is associated with infant botulism, and it should not be given to infants who are younger than 1 year old.

Page: 570

Question #16

Answer: A

Rationale: Children who eat only vegetables but no dairy products, meat, or eggs require supplemental vitamin B_{12}, and they are at risk for vitamin D deficiency, especially if they lack adequate sunlight exposure.

Page: 570

Question #17

Answer: B

Rationale: Universal screening for hypercholesterolemia among children is not currently recommended. A serum lipid profile should be obtained for children who have a family history of premature (55 years old or younger) coronary heart disease or peripheral vascular or cerebrovascular disease in parents or grandparents.

Page: 570

Question #18

Answer: B

Rationale: Temperament is a set of consistent, inborn characteristics that influence how individuals interact with and learn from their environment. The individual's temperament characteristics are innate to his or her personality. Three basic temperament profiles based on nine separate infant characteristics are outlined in Table 31-8 of Rakel's *Textbook of Family Medicine.*

Pages: 571–572

1. American Academy of Pediatrics (AAP): *Pediatric Nutrition Handbook,* 5th ed. Elk Grove Village, Ill, American Academy of Pediatrics, 2004.

Question #19

Answer: B

Rationale: Delays in one developmental domain may impair development in another domain. For example, an 18-month-old youngster with motor impairments as a result of spina bifida lacks the freedom to explore his or her environment and thus to learn how two pieces of furniture are oriented in space.

Page: 572

Question #20

Answer: A

Rationale: Research shows that clinical impression alone is quite poor for the detection of developmental delay. This has led to recommendations from the American Academy of Pediatrics, the American Academy of Neurology, and the Child Neurology Society for the routine use of standardized developmental screening tools at periodic intervals.

Page: 573

Question #21

Answer: D

Rationale: A majority of children will walk by the age of 14.5 months. Certain red flags should prompt referral for further evaluation.

Page: 576

Age	Sign
12 months	No babbling
12 months	No pointing
12 months	No gestures
16 months	No single words
24 months	No two-word phrases
Any age	Loss of language or social skills

From Filipek PA, Accardo PJ, Ashwal S, et al: Practice parameter: screening and diagnosis of autism: report of the Quality Standards Subcommittee of the American Academy of Neurology and the Child Neurology Society, *Neurology* 55:468–479, 2000. In Rakel RE, editor: *Textbook of family medicine*, ed 7, Philadelphia, WB Saunders, 2007.

Question #22

Answer: C

Rationale: It is important to keep in mind that most young children with autism present to their physicians with the chief complaint of language delay. Global developmental delay is defined as a significant delay in two or more areas of development (i.e., gross/fine motor, speech/language, cognition, social/personal, activities of daily living).

Pages: 575–576

Question #23

Answer: D

Rationale: The Individuals with Disabilities Act mandates a free and appropriate education for all children, regardless of handicapping condition. Therefore, if a child is suspected to have a learning disability, the school is obligated to evaluate and provide necessary services free of charge. The Multi-Factored Evaluation must be performed within 60 days of suspension of the learning disability. If the child is eligible for special education services, these services may occur in the regular classroom or in a separate one, although the law requires that services be provided in the least restrictive environment.

Page: 576

Question #24

Answer: B

Rationale: Minor febrile illnesses are not contraindications to vaccine administration. General contraindications to immunizations are moderate or severe illnesses with or without fever, a previous anaphylactic reaction to the specific vaccine, and a severe hypersensitivity reaction to vaccine constituents, such as gelatin, or to antibiotics, such as neomycin, streptomycin, or polymyxin B.

Page: 577

Question #25

Answer: A

Rationale: Theoretical concerns exist that immune responses may be impaired if two live virus vaccines are given within 28 days of each other. Live virus vaccines must be given either simultaneously or at least 4 weeks apart.

Page: 577

Question #26

Answer: D

Rationale: Doses of any vaccine should not be divided or reduced, because this can result in an inadequate response.

Page: 577

Question #27

Answer: B

Rationale: From 1980 to 1996, there were approximately eight cases per year of vaccine-associated paralytic poliomyelitis as a result of oral poliovirus vaccine in the United States. Consequently, inactivated poliovirus vaccine is recommended for all routine childhood polio vaccinations in the United States, and the oral vaccine is no longer distributed.

Page: 577

Question #28

Answer: A

Rationale: The use of Hib conjugate vaccines has lowered the U.S. incidence of invasive Hib disease among children younger than 5 years old by 99%.

Page: 577

Question #29

Answer: B

Rationale: Two vaccines that contain reduced concentrations of diphtheria toxoid and pertussis antigens in combination with tetanus toxoid are now licensed for adolescents between the ages of 10 and 18 years (BOOSTRIX) and for persons between the ages of 11 and 64 years (ADACEL). The vaccines are recommended for adolescents who are 11 or 12 years old in place of the tetanus and diphtheria booster or for ages 13 to 18 years old who have not yet received a tetanus and diphtheria booster to decrease the reservoir of *Bordetella pertussis* in this population.

Page: 579

Question #30

Answer: C

Rationale: An infant born to a mother who is positive for hepatitis B surface antigen should receive an initial dose of 5 μg of Recombivax HB or of 10 μg of Engerix-B and 0.5 mL of hepatitis B immunoglobulin intramuscularly at separate sites within 12 hours of birth. Repeat vaccine doses should be given at the ages of 1 month and 6 months.

Page: 582

Question #31

Answer: D

Rationale: Infants should be immunized at 2, 4, 6, and 12 to 15 months of age. Children between 7 and 11 months old require two doses 6 to 8 weeks apart followed by a third dose at 12 to 15 months of age. Children 12 to 23 months old require two doses 6 to 8 weeks apart. Only one dose is required for children between the ages of 24 and 59 months. The vaccine is recommended for all children up through the age of 23 months. Children 24 to 59 months old at high risk for invasive pneumococcal disease should receive two doses of vaccine 6 to 8 weeks apart if they have not been previously immunized.

Page: 582

Question #32

Answer: A

Rationale: The meningococcal vaccines contain serogroups A, C, Y, and W-135. Serogroups C, Y, and W-135 cause 75% of all cases of meningococcal disease in persons who are more than 11 years old in the United States. Neither vaccine is protective against serogroup B, which accounts for most of the remaining cases

Page: 582

32   Answers

Question #1

Answer: B

Rationale: Half of all deaths that occur during childhood are attributable to accidents. The type of accidents that result in fatalities are most commonly motor vehicle accidents, followed by drownings, fires and burns, and aspirations and asphyxiation.

Page: 598

Question #2

Answer: C

Rationale: Oral and transdermal contraceptives are the contraceptive method of choice for the sexually active adolescent female. They can be safely recommended for most patients, with only the usual absolute contraindications restricting their use. The diaphragm has the lowest likelihood of continued use in adolescent females. Condoms pose no significant medical risk to adolescents, and they also provide protection against sexually transmitted diseases. Depo-Provera does not offer the additional health benefits of combined hormonal oral contraceptives. Many clinicians recommend Depo-Provera as a second-line agent.

Page: 606

Question #3

Answers: (1), A; (2), B; (3), B; (4), A

Rationale: Universal screening for iron-deficiency anemia is recommended for children whose diet puts them at risk or who live in communities in which a significant level of iron-deficiency anemia exists. The Centers for Disease Control and Prevention recommends routine lead testing of children at about 9 to 12 months of age and again at about 24 months of age. The U.S. Preventive Services Task Force does not recommend routine urinalysis because of the high false-positive rates for hematuria and proteinuria. Cholesterol screening during childhood remains controversial. According to the National Cholesterol Education Program, children more than 2 years old with a family history of early heart disease (<55 years) or with a parent with a total cholesterol level of more than 240 should receive cholesterol screening.

Pages: 590, 591

Question #4

Answer: D

Rationale: Gastroenteritis is a common problem in children. About 80% of the pathogens that cause it are viral. The rotavirus has been implicated as a major cause of gastroenteritis in children.

Page: 596

Question #5

Answer: C

Rationale: Failure to thrive is an uncommon diagnosis for children who are more than 2 years old. Failure to grow or to gain weight can be a consequence of many physical and psychological problems. There is no universal definition of failure to thrive, but various authors have suggested that the definition include children whose weight falls below the third or fifth percentiles for age or children whose growth declines and crosses two major growth percentiles during a short period of time. In most cases, individual, familial, or ethnic variations are responsible for deviations from accepted growth standards.

Page: 586

Questions #6 through #8

Answers: 6, C; 7, B; 8, A

Rationale: Croup is characterized by hoarseness, cough, and inspiratory stridor. Bronchiolitis is characterized by expiratory wheezing with or without tachypnea, air trapping, and substernal retractions. Pneumonia has evidence of pulmonary consolidation or rales.

Page: 595

Question #9

Answer: D

Rationale: Osgood–Schlatter disease is a painful swelling of the tibial tubercle at the insertion of the infrapatellar tendon. It is a common problem in males around Tanner stage 2 or 3. X-rays are not essential for the diagnosis, and they are only used in atypical cases. Treatment recommendations include ice, mild anti-inflammatories, and the restriction of running and jumping activities.

Page: 607

Question #10

Answer: A

Rationale: Inhaled corticosteroids are the first-line controller therapy for all children more than 12 months old with chronic asthma. For acute asthma episodes, initial treatment includes an inhalation therapy with β-agonists and steroids. The addition of ipratropium bromide to albuterol reduces the risk of hospitalization.

Page: 594

Question #11

Answer: C

Rationale: Among males, the first sign of puberty is testicular enlargement, which typically begins between 9½ and 13½ years of age. The growth spurt in males occurs later in puberty, usually around Tanner stage 4.

Page: 601

Question #12

Answer: D

Rationale: Febrile children 3 to 36 months old without a focus for the fever need laboratory testing to guide decision-making. A urine culture is recommended for boys who are less than 6 months old and for girls who are less than 2 years old. Children with a white blood cell count of more than 20,000 or labored breathing need to have a chest x-ray to look for pneumonia. Empiric treatment with antibiotics is recommended after a blood culture is done for children with white blood cell counts of more than 15,000.

Pages: 595–596

Question #13

Answer: B

Rationale: Cervicitis among adolescent females is diagnosed by finding mucopurulent cervical discharge and cervical friability. Cultures are positive for chlamydia or gonorrhea in more than 50% of cases. Herpes simplex is less commonly found.

Pages: 604, 605

Questions #14 through #16

Answers: 14, B; 15, A; 16, C

Rationale: Campylobacter is the most common bacterial cause of childhood diarrhea. Prolonged episodes should be treated with erythromycin. Shigella may be associated with bloody diarrhea. Oral ampicillin or trimethoprim–sulfamethoxazole will shorten the duration of symptoms. Salmonella usually causes relatively mild symptoms, with no treatment indicated for normal children. Giardia is a protozoan that may cause diarrhea and that should be treated with Metronidazole in symptomatic children.

Page: 596

Question #17

Answers: (1), A; (2), A; (3), A; (4), A

Rationale: Corporal punishment is ineffective as a primary means of discipline, and it is potentially detrimental to childhood development and health. Children should be encouraged to get about 30 minutes of exercise daily. Physicians should review with parents the appropriate car safety seat for the child. It is imperative that parents provide direct supervision and that they monitor children's television viewing and access to the Internet.

Pages: 591, 592

Question #18

Answer: A

Rationale: Streptococcal pharyngitis presents with symptoms of high fever, beefy red tonsils with exudates, swollen tender anterior cervical lymph nodes, and the absence of cough. Hand, foot, and mouth disease presents with papulovesicular lesions on the buccal mucosa, the palms of the hands, and the soles of the feet. Herpangina presents with small vesicles or ulcers on the tonsillar pillars or the soft palate. Infectious mononucleosis causes petechial lesions of the soft palate in addition to sore throat and cervical adenopathy.

Page: 593

Question #19

Answer: A

Rationale: Croup is an acute respiratory illness that is characterized by barking cough, hoarseness, and inspiratory stridor. The most common causes of croup are viral, primarily parainfluenza virus types I and II and influenza virus.

Page: 595

Question #20

Answer: C

Rationale: Although upper respiratory infections predispose children to middle-ear infections, having a recent upper respiratory infection is not a requirement for the diagnosis of acute otitis media.

Page: 596

Question #21

Answer: B

Rationale: Primary dentition is usually complete by the age of 2 years. Permanent teeth begin erupting when a child is around 6 to 7 years old, and the process is complete by the age of 12 to 13 years. Routine dental appointments should begin at the age of 2 or 3 years; it is recommended by pediatric dentists that these visits occur twice yearly.

Page: 589

Question #22

Answer: D

Rationale: The child has followed the usual recommended schedule of immunizations. Preschool children require the final diphtheria, tetanus, and pertussis (DTaP) and polio boosters to complete the childhood schedule. These are given between 4 and 6 years of age. A second measles, mumps, and rubella (MMR) vac-

cine is also required before the start of kindergarten or first grade.

Page: 593

Question #23

Answers: (1), A; (2), B; (3), B; 4, (A)

Rationale: Nationally obtained data substantiate growing rates of substance use among both younger and older adolescents. The use of alcohol or cigarettes is predictive of experimentation with marijuana and other drugs. The critical time for experimentation appears to be 7th and 8th grades. Adolescents who regularly use illegal substances should be referred to a professional who is trained in adolescent substance abuse.

Page: 606

Questions #24 through #26

Answers: 26, A; 27, B; 28, D

Rationale: Antibiotics for acute otitis media should be prescribed for severely ill children with a certain diagnosis of acute otitis media. Observation is an option for less severely ill children or for when the diagnosis is less certain. If antibiotics are used, amoxicillin is the first-line choice. High-dose amoxicillin–clavulanate (Augmentin) is an appropriate choice for severely ill patients for whom coverage against β-lactamase–positive species is desired. Azithromycin (Zithromax) is an option for penicillin-allergic patients. Single-dose, parenteral ceftriaxone (Rocephin) is effective for patients who cannot tolerate oral therapy.

Page: 596

Questions #27 through #30

Answers: 29, B; 30, A; 31, B; 32, C

Rationale: The early adolescent is preoccupied with self and pubertal changes, relationships with same-sex peers, and increased need for privacy. During middle adolescence, the peak of parental conflicts occurs; conformity with peer values and risk-taking behaviors are also seen. Late adolescence is characterized by the reacceptance of parental values, the capacity to form intimate relationships, and the formation of practical, realistic vocational goals.

Pages: 602, 603; Table 32-15

33 Answers

Question #1

Answer: C

Rationale: Problems with sleep initiation and nighttime awakening are most common during infancy. Parasomnias and obstructive sleep apnea syndrome are most common among children who are 3 to 8 years old. Sleep deprivation, delayed sleep-phase syndrome, and narcolepsy are common problems among the adolescent age group.

Page: 612

Question #2

Answer: A

Rationale: Night terrors happen early in the night and last for only a few minutes. The child will sit up and scream or cry, but he or she is not awake and will go quickly back to sleep if not awakened by the parents; there will be no recollection of the event by the child the next morning. Night terrors occur most often among children who are between the ages of 2 and 6 years, and they are more likely to occur during times of stress.

Page: 612

Question #3

Answer: D

Rationale: Children do not have the associated drop in oxygen levels because of frequent, brief awakenings to reestablish their airway.

Page: 613

Question #4

Answer: B

Rationale: Asperger's syndrome involves autistic behaviors and impaired social interactions but no language delay.

Page: 614

Question #5

Answer: A

Rationale: A comprehensive meta-analysis discounted the assertion that vaccines containing thimerosal contributed to the development of autism.[1]

Page: 614

Question #6

Answer: C

Rationale: Screening tests for autism lack sensitivity, so any parental concern about language delays should be taken seriously. Screening for hearing loss should also be performed, because this can present as a speech delay. The Denver Developmental Screening Tool lacks sensitivity and specificity for autism.

Page: 614

Question #7

Answer: A

Rationale: Although only a portion of anxiety problems will cause serious impairment, these children will often present to their primary care physician's office. Many anxiety disorders have their onset during childhood, and they will remain unchanged into adulthood unless they are treated.

Page: 614

Question #8

Answer: D

Rationale: Encopresis is the repeated passage of stool in inappropriate places after the age of 4 years. It is usually involuntary, and it accompanies constipation. The encopresis is often overflow incontinence around the impaction of stool. It is caused by a combination of physiologic and psychological factors, and it can be caused by organic disease. It is accompanied by enuresis 40% of the time, and it occurs more often among boys than girls.

Page: 615

1. Parker SK, Schwartz B, Todd J, Pickering LK: Thimerosal-containing vaccines and autistic spectrum disorder: A critical review of published original data. *Pediatrics* 114:793-804, 2004.

Question #9

Answer: C

Rationale: Medical management includes enemas, laxatives, and stool softeners to allow soft, painless stools to pass at least once daily. As the stooling becomes more regular, the laxatives are decreased, and fiber supplementation is started. The child should not be punished for soiling clothes, because this is involuntary. Regular toileting times and close parental supervision are also important.

Page: 615

Question #10

Answer: A

Rationale: Enuresis is the second most common chronic ailment in childhood, affecting 15% to 20% of 5-year-old children, 5% to 10% of 10-year-old children, and 1% to 2% of 18-year-old adolescents. It can be primary or secondary. If a child who was continent suddenly becomes incontinent, an evaluation to determine the cause should be performed. The incidence of enuresis goes up significantly with a history in either parent, and it increases to 75% if both parents were affected.

Page: 615

Question #11

Answer: A

Rationale: Anything not discovered by an examination and a urine test is considered complicated and warrants further workup. A workup should also be performed if enuresis occurs only during the day or if it is secondary.

Page: 616

Question #12

Answer: A

Rationale: Enuresis alarms are an effective and safe treatment, and they work by waking the child before voiding is finished so that the process can be completed in the toilet. Medications including Desmopressin and Imipramine can be effective, but both can have serious side effects. Fluid restriction and scheduled voiding can help decrease incontinent episodes. If constipation is present, treating it can spontaneously resolve enuresis.

Page: 616

Question #13

Answer: D

Rationale: ADHD is the most commonly diagnosed behavioral disorder of childhood, with a prevalence of 4% to 12% per the DSM-IV-TR. It will account for 10% of behavior problems seen in a general pediatric practice, with boys presenting more than girls. The diagnosis should be considered for any child presenting with inattention, hyperactivity, impulsivity, academic underachievement, or behavior problems.

Page: 617

Question #14

Answer: B

Rationale: ADHD is a chronic disorder that persists from childhood through adolescence and into adulthood. Symptoms decrease by half every 5 years between the ages of 10 and 25 years, with hyperactivity disappearing first. Inattention seems to persist.

Page: 617

Question #15

Answer: A

Rationale: It is always imperative to get information from as many sources as possible, including home, school, and any other available areas. It is important to make the diagnosis using the criteria established in the DSM-IV-TR, although only 30% of physicians currently use this.

Pages: 617–618

Question #16

Answer: A

Rationale: The first-line treatment for ADHD is stimulant medication. Psychosocial treatments alone have not been shown to be more effective or to even provide additional benefit unless there are comorbid diagnoses.

Page: 618

Question #17

Answer: B

Rationale: If the first stimulant medication is not effective, it is appropriate to sequentially try each available stimulant medication before moving on to another class of medications.

Page: 618

Question #18

Answer: C

Rationale: Strattera is the third-line treatment after at least a trial of two stimulant medications. It can take up to 4 weeks to reach full effect. It is not scheduled, and it has no abuse potential. It has a side-effect profile that is similar to the stimulant medications.

Page: 619

Question #19

Answer: A

Rationale: Poor parenting behaviors (e.g., inconsistent discipline, impulsivity, immaturity) are predisposing characteristics to a child having ODD. These behaviors lead to a child's impulsivity, inconsistency, and acting out.

Page: 620

Question #20

Answer: D

Rationale: This is the DSM-IV-TR description of ODD.

Page: 620

Question #21

Answer: A

Rationale: Children with conduct disorder are more likely to die by homicide, suicide, violent accident, or drug overdose. The natural history includes developing ADHD at an early age, which will be followed by ODD and then by conduct disorder. Alcohol and substance abuse develop during adolescence.

Page: 620

Question #22

Answer: A

Rationale: Children with conduct disorder will often increase negative behaviors when punished as opposed

to normal children, who will decrease negative behaviors when punished. Family interventions and social-skills training are important management tools.

Page: 621

Question #23

Answer: A

Rationale: These are the DSM-IV-TR criteria for conduct disorder.

Page: 621

Question #24

Answer: D

Rationale: Between 40% and 70% of depressed children and adolescents will have at least one comorbid diagnosis, and 20% to 50% will have two or more.

Page: 622

Question #25

Answer: A

Rationale: At least one of the following should be present nearly every day for at least 2 weeks for the diagnosis of depression to be made in either children or adults: (1) a persistent sad and depressed mood; or (2) markedly diminished interest or pleasure in daily activities. Children may report frequent irritability rather than depressed mood.

Page: 622

Question #26

Answer: A

Rationale: Selective serotonin reuptake inhibitors are the first-line medication treatment for depression among children and adolescents. The side-effect profile is the same as it is for adults, with gastrointestinal symptoms and sleep problems being the most common. No causal link between selective serotonin reuptake inhibitor use and suicide has been found. Tricyclics have not been found to be effective treatment for depression among children and adolescents.

Page: 623

Question #27

Answer: A

Rationale: Thirty percent of high-school seniors report behaviors that correspond with patterns of problem drinking. Five percent report daily marijuana use. Among teenagers, the lifetime prevalence of alcohol abuse or dependence is 5% to 32%, whereas the prevalence of drug abuse is 3% to 10%.

Page: 623

Question #28

Answer: A

Rationale: Kits can be purchased online to invalidate drug tests. Not all substances are checked for with routine tests. The half-life varies widely, so it is important to know how long certain drugs and metabolites remain in the body. There is always a possibility for error, so personal and family histories and reports are important for placing test results in context.

Page: 624

Question #29

Answer: D

Rationale: Failure to thrive can be caused by gastrointestinal, endocrinological, and neurological conditions.

If the failure to thrive does not seem to fall into one of these categories, a psychosocial component must be looked for, including caregiver issues related to knowledge deficits or to neglect and abuse.

Page: 624

Question #30

Answer: A

Rationale: The incidence of diagnosis of eating disorders is increasing as a result of improved recognition and reporting as well as a true increase in incidence. Ninety-five percent of these patients are female, with athletes and diabetics being at increased risk.

Page: 624

Question #31

Answer: B

Rationale: Bulimia is more common than anorexia, with a prevalence of 1% to 3%. However, the mortality rate of anorexia is 6% to 20%, which is much higher than that of anorexia.

Page: 624

Question #1

Answer: A

Rationale: Ginkgo biloba has platelet-inhibiting properties, and it has been reported in at least one study to have resulted in bilateral spontaneous subdural hematomas.

Page: 628

Question #2

Answer: C

Rationale: Infection after needlestick exposure from a needle used on a patient who has tested positive for hepatitis B virus surface antigen ranges from 6% to 30%; this is much higher than the risk of human immunodeficiency virus infection following a similar needlestick exposure.

Page: 628

Question #3

Answer: A

Rationale: Level I procedures include minor surgery performed under topical or local anesthesia and not involving a drug-induced alteration of consciousness. Level II involves procedures requiring moderate sedation anesthesia with postoperative monitoring, and level III involves procedures requiring deep sedation/analgesia. Most office-based procedures fall into the level I category.

Page: 628

Question #4

Answer: A

Rationale: When applied to abraded skin, most topical agents result in peak blood levels similar to those that result from local infiltration.

Page: 629

Question #5

Answer: E

Rationale: The major concern with the use of EMLA cream is methemoglobinemia. The risk of methemoglobinemia is increased among infants who are less than 3 months old and among those patients taking certain medications (e.g., acetaminophen, nitrates, sulfonamides, antimalarials), those with anemia, those with cardiopulmonary disease, and those with glucose–6-phosphate dehydrogenase deficiency.

Page: 629

Question #6

Answer: C

Rationale: The maximal dose of lidocaine for cutaneous infiltration in adults and children should not exceed 5 mg/kg. If a procedure requires a dose exceeding this limit, then a field block should be considered.

Page: 630

Question #7

Answer: C

Rationale: After infiltrative local anesthesia, allergic reactions occur in 1% to 2% of patients, and they can be prevented with prior knowledge of a patient's history of allergic reactions. Vasovagal reactions occur in 2% to 3% of patients.

Page: 631

Question #8

Answer: D

Rationale: Oral doses of Valium should not exceed 10 mg before an office procedure. If respiratory distress occurs, it can be reversed promptly and temporarily by using the medication flumazenil, 0.02 mg/kg intramuscularly in children and 0.1 to 0.2 mg in adults.

Page: 632

Question #9

Answer: A

Rationale: The inflammatory phase of wound healing begins immediately after vessel injury occurs as a result of skin disruption. The aggregation of platelets and the activation of the clotting cascade with cytokines are followed by leukocyte infiltration to clean up wound byproducts. These neutrophils are part of wound healing, but they may occasionally be mistaken for purulence.

Page: 632

Question #10

Answer: B

Rationale: Keloids, unlike hypertrophic scars, are examples of excessive wound healing that extends beyond the original scar margin and that develops months to years after the original skin disruption.

Page: 633

Question #11

Answer: E

Rationale: Many factors—including diabetes, anemia, jaundice, uremia, human immunodeficiency virus, cancer, immunocompromise, peripheral vascular disease, age, and smoking—increase a person's risk for wounds that won't heal.

Page: 633

Question #12

Answer: B

Rationale: Basic principles of wound repair include the following: (1) avoiding skin tension on the wound; (2) minimizing trauma to tissue; and (3) accurately approximating wound edges. To adhere to the above principles, excisions should be parallel to the skin tension lines of Langer, and only clean wounds should be undermined to avoid infection. In addition, layered closure should be used for wounds with skin tension to avoid infection, and the excision of a lesion should employ an ellipse with a length-to-width ratio of 3:1 to 4:1.

Page: 634

Question #13

Answer: A

Rationale: The closure of wounds on the face should be single layered, preferably using 6–0 nylon, and the sutures should be removed in 3 to 5 days to avoid sinus tracts.

Page: 634

Question #14

Answer: A

Rationale: The wound closure of superficial lacerations by tissue adhesives is quicker and less painful as compared with conventional suturing (strength of evidence = A).

Page: 635

Question #15

Answer: A

Rationale: A wound that has separated after suture removal should be left open to heal by secondary intention. Wound infections usually occur by day 4 or 5 after repair. Increasing, severe pain within 12 hours after surgery rarely signifies a clostridial or necrotizing infection, and wounds left to heal by secondary intention can be revised in the future.

Page: 636

Question #16

Answer: C

Rationale: Punch biopsies of less than 5 mm do not need suturing. Bleeding can be controlled with direct pressure or with a topical hemostatic agent such as silver nitrate or mensal solution.

Page: 636

Question #17

Answer: B

Rationale: The evaluation of a wound using the ABCDE criteria is considered positive if one or more of the criteria are met (strength of recommendation =

A). This is felt to be a useful clinical predictor of malignant melanoma.

Page: 637

Question #18

Answer: D

Rationale: Animal bites to the distal extremities should be left open to heal by secondary intention to reduce the risk of infection. Dog bites to the scalp, face, and trunk can be debrided, irrigated, and primarily closed.

Page: 639

Question #19

Answer: C

Rationale: Absolute contraindications to cryosurgery include patients with a known history of Raynaud's disease and patients with malignant melanoma in whom the preservation of tissue for pathologic examination is a must.

Page: 639

Question #20

Answer: D

Rationale: Local intradermal infiltration with lidocaine is at times unrewarding in an abscess, because the local pH of the infected tissue causes the deactivation of the anesthetic.

Page: 641

Question #21

Answer: B

Rationale: A subungual hematoma is bleeding that occurs between the nailbed and the fingernail. It is caused by a crush injury, and it is best treated by nailbed decompression. The optimal treatment for onychomycosis is with continuous treatment with oral antifungal (Lamisil) for a minimum of 4 weeks. Acute paronychia is a bacterial infection with local abscess formation, and it is best treated with the incision and drainage of the abscess. Antibiotics are only helpful if there is a secondary cellulitis. Chronic paronychia is an inflammatory condition of the nails—not an infection—that is found among people with repeated exposure to moisture.

The mainstay of treatment of this condition is the avoidance of moisture; there is little or no role for systemic antibiotics or antifungals.

Page: 641

Question #22

Answer: B

Rationale: Anoscopy detects a higher percentage of lesions in the anorectal region than flexible sigmoidoscopy does, and it is the procedure of choice for the evaluation of rectal disease. Internal hemorrhoids are above the pectinate line; they have no sensory innervation, and they are usually painless. External hemorrhoids are located below the pectinate line; they are covered by anoderm, and they are extremely sensitive.

Page: 642

Question #23

Answer: B

Rationale: Hemorrhoids are very common in the United States, with a prevalence of up to 4.4% of the adult population. Predisposing factors include chronic constipation, prostate enlargement, chronic cough, pregnancy, and familial (hereditary) factors. Alcoholics appear to be predisposed to hemorrhoids as a result of portal hypertension that may be a contributing factor to venous engorgement.

Page: 643

Question #24

Answer: B

Rationale: Although rubber-band ligation was more effective and required fewer treatments for the symptomatic recurrence of grade I, II (those that do not respond to medical therapy), and III hemorrhoids than did infrared coagulation and sclerotherapy, it produced more complications (strength of recommendation = A).

Page: 643

Question #25

Answer: D

Rationale: The rubber rings cause tissue necrosis, leaving an ulcerated area. Pain is natural after the procedure, but, if the pain is not tolerated, the rings should be removed as soon as possible, because tissue swelling makes it more difficult later on. Symptomatic relief is accomplished with sitz baths.

Page: 643

Question #26

Answer: D

Rationale: Acute thrombosed external hemorrhoids present with acute anal pain and with or without minimal bleeding. Thrombosed external hemorrhoids should be excised rather than incised because of the high probability of a recurrent thrombosis if the hemorrhoid is incised only; this can result in worsening pain.

Page: 644

Question #27

Answer: C

Rationale: Anorectal abscesses arise in the anal crypts from the blockade of anal ducts. There are four types: perianal, ischiorectal, intersphincteric, and supralevator. Perianal (or perirectal) abscesses are the most common, making up to 40% to 45% of all rectal abscesses. Definitive management is by incision and drainage in a timely manner. Perirectal abscesses can be drained in the office; deeper abscesses should be referred for prompt surgical debridement.

Page: 644

Question #28

Answer: A

Rationale: Colposcopy is performed to investigate abnormal Pap smears or lesions found during a routine pelvic examination. Although there are no absolute contraindications to colposcopy, pregnancy, active infection, and acute cervicitis are absolute contraindications to endocervical curettage.

Page: 645

Question #29

Answer: D

Rationale: Endometrial biopsy is useful for the evaluation of unexplained uterine bleeding and infertility, and it is reported to have a diagnostic accuracy equal to or superior to dilation and curettage with regard to endometrial cancer (highly sensitive). However, it is not very specific for detecting interluminal pathology, and it should be used in conjunction with transvaginal ultrasound or hysteroscopy in these circumstances.

Page: 646

Question #30

Answer: A

Rationale: Knee joint aspiration injection can be used diagnostically and therapeutically for a variety of conditions, including large effusions, posttraumatic hemarthroses, and unexplained monarthritis. Intra-articular steroid injections of the knee are recommended for inflammatory exacerbations of osteoarthritis (strength of recommendation = A). Steroid injections should not be given more frequently than four times in a 12-month period. A recent meta-analysis revealed superior outcomes with Synvisc instillation as compared with placebo after 6 months for patients with osteoarthritis that have not responded to standard pharmacologic and nonpharmacologic therapies.

Page: 647

Question #31

Answer: B

Rationale: Neonatal circumcision is one of the most common procedures performed in the United States. Despite its popularity, little is known about its long-term risks and benefits. The dorsal penile nerve block is more effective than EMLA cream for pain control during the procedure (strength of recommendation = A). Contraindications to circumcision include hypospadias, ambiguous genitalia, balanitis, or phimosis. Circumcisions should be delayed 24 hours to ensure that the infant is medically stable.

Page: 648

Chapter

35   Answers

Question #1

Answers: (1), A; (2), B; (3), A; (4), A; (5), B

Rationale: There are four basic principles of perioperative care: (1) preoperative risk is ultimately related to the condition of the patient, the proposed surgery, and the type of anesthesia needed; (2) interventions to lower preoperative risk should be made regardless of surgery, excluding prophylaxis of venous thromboembolism; (3) always consider preoperatively what can be done before surgery to lessen or prevent complications postoperatively; and (4) excellent communication among the family physician, the surgeon, and the anesthesiologist is essential for the best perioperative outcomes.

Page: 653

Question #2

Answer: E

Rationale: A good history requires a thorough medication history, because many patients do not think of oral contraceptive pills, aspirin, nonsteroidal anti-inflammatory drugs, herbal preparations, and over-the-counter agents as medications. Edema of the lower extremities could be from heart failure, poor nutrition, liver or kidney disease, or hypothyroidism. No single test is routinely indicated for patients having surgery. Coagulation studies are unnecessary without a history of easy bruising, a coagulation disorder, a family history of bleeding problems, or the use of antiplatelet or anticoagulation medications. A complete blood cell count—although a common preoperative test—is not required for minor surgery. It is reasonable to obtain a serum creatinine level for geriatric patients (especially those 75 years old and older) to assess for renal disorders.

Pages: 653–654

Question #3

Answer: C

Rationale: Pathologic Q-waves represent an intermediate risk for perioperative cardiac mortality. Men and women who are more than 45 years old with two or more atherosclerotic risk factors and patients with angina or diabetes should undergo a 12-lead EKG. Stress imaging is appropriate for those who are having major vascular surgery. Any patient with an unexplained heart murmur requires an EKG and an echocardiogram.

Page: 654

Question #4

Answer: B

Rationale: The perioperative executive summary by the American College of Cardiology and the American Heart Association Perioperative Executive Summary defined the clinical predictors of increased perioperative cardiovascular risk as major, intermediate, and minor.[1] Major clinical predictors that have an increased perioperative cardiovascular risk include unstable coronary syndromes, decompensated heart failure, significant arrhythmias, and severe valvular disease. Intermediate clinical predictors include minor angina pectoris, previous myocardial infarction by history or pathologic Q waves, compensated heart failure, diabetes mellitus, and renal insufficiency. Minor clinical predictors include advanced age, abnormal EKG, a rhythm other than sinus, low functional capacity, a history of stroke, and uncontrolled systemic hypertension.

Page: 654

Question #5

Answer: A

Rationale: Minor clinical predictors that have an increased perioperative cardiovascular risk include advanced age, abnormal EKG (left ventricular hypertrophy, left bundle-branch block, and/or ST-T abnormality), a rhythm other than sinus (e.g., atrial fibrillation), a low functional capacity, a history of stroke, and uncontrolled systemic hypertension. Intermediate clinical predictors that have an increased perioperative cardiovascular risk include mild angina pectoris (Canadian Class I or II), previous myocardial infarction by history or pathologic Q waves, compensated or prior heart failure, diabetes mellitus (particularly if it is insulin dependent), and renal insufficiency. Major clinical predictors that have an

---

1. Eagle KA, Berger PB, Calkins H, et al: ACC/AHA guideline for perioperative cardiovascular evaluation for noncardiac surgery: Executive summary: A report of the American College of Cardiology/American Heart Association Task Force on Practice Guidelines (Committee to Update the 1996 Guidelines on Perioperative Cardiovascular Evaluation for Noncardiac Surgery). *Circulation* 105:1257-1267, 2002.

increased perioperative cardiovascular risk include unstable coronary syndromes, decompensated heart failure, significant arrhythmias, and severe valvular disease.

Page: 654

Question #6

Answer: B

Rationale: Determining a patient's underlying cardiac function is the centerpiece of preoperative risk assessment. Patients with poor functional capacity are at high risk for perioperative cardiac morbidity and mortality. Poor functional status is an indication for noninvasive cardiac testing before all surgeries, except among those patients who are scheduled for low-risk surgeries. Hypertrophic and dilated cardiomyopathy increases the risk of perioperative heart failure. Testing patients with prior heart failure or dyspnea of unknown origin should be considered.

Pages: 654, 656

Question #7

Answers: (1), B; (2), A; (3), A; (4), B; (5), A

Rationale: If valvular heart disease is suspected during the preoperative history and physical, the workup and treatment are the same for both perioperative and nonoperative patients. Rarely is a patient so compromised that his or her lung function precludes surgery altogether. Symptom severity is important, because almost all patients with a baseline of stable mild to moderate disease can proceed directly to surgery after a thorough history and physical. Carbon dioxide retention can be exacerbated by respiratory depressants used during the postoperative period. Surgery and anesthesia can often lead to an acute worsening of the restrictive defect as a result of altered neuromuscular function, pain, or immobility.

Pages: 656–657

Question #8

Answer: D

Rationale: Surgery with symptomatic vertebrobasilar stenosis has the greatest perioperative ischemic stroke risk rate: 6%. Other surgeries have lower perioperative ischemic stroke risk rates, including general surgery (0.2%), general surgery with or without carotid bruit (0.5%), general surgery after a prior stroke (2.9%), and general surgery with carotid stenosis and bruit or prior symptoms (3.6%).

Page: 659

Question #9

Answer: A

Rationale: It is essential to make preoperative adjustments to common medications. Antiplatelet medications, such as aspirin, clopidogrel, and ticlopidine, require stopping 7 days before surgery, whereas others, including nonsteroidal anti-inflammatory drugs, COX-2 inhibitors, and cilostazol, require 3 days. Oral antidiabetic medications (e.g., metformin), angiotensin-converting enzyme inhibitors, and angiotensin-II receptor blockers require the last dose on the day before the surgery. Anticonvulsants, insulin, and many cardiac medications (e.g., digoxin, β-blockers, nitrates) can be taken on the morning of surgery.

Page: 659

Question #10

Answer: B

Rationale: There are a number of indications for perioperative β-blockers, including high-risk surgery, patients with chronic β-blocker use, known coronary artery disease, history of transient ischemic attack or cerebral vascular accident, and chronic renal insufficiency. Having two or more cardiac risk factors requiring perioperative β-blocker use include an age of more than 65 years, hypertension, non-insulin-dependent diabetes, a cholesterol level of more than 239, and current smoking or having quit within the last 6 months. Contraindications to β-blockers include a resting heart rate of less than 60 beats per minute, second-degree heart block, hypotension, and allergy to β-blockers. There are relative contraindications to perioperative β-blocker use, including asthma, chronic obstructive pulmonary disease, and heart failure.

Page: 660

Question #11

Answer: A

Rationale: Pulmonary function tests monitor the effectiveness of preoperative medical treatment for patients with severe pulmonary compromise who are undergoing surgery. Among type 2 diabetics who are controlled with oral agents preoperatively, the stress response plus hepatic, renal, and respiratory abnormalities that can occur among postoperative patients may preclude oral agents and necessitate the use of insulin. Autonomic dysfunction is present in up to 40% of type 1 diabetics and up to 17% of type 2 diabetics, and it can result in gastroparesis and, thus, regurgitation, aspiration, orthostatic hypotension, and diabetic diarrhea. Patients with hypothyroidism should continue receiving thyroid hormone during the perioperative period.

Pages: 657–658

Question #12

Answer: C

Rationale: Glucose levels of more than 180 mg/dL may involve glycosuria, osmotic diuresis, and dehydration. Poor glycemic control is associated with a higher risk of infection and poor wound healing as a result of inhibited white blood cell chemotaxis and functions and impaired collagen formation. Tight glycemic control among both diabetic and nondiabetic subjects improves survival. The subcutaneous administration of insulin can be unpredictable perioperatively, and infusions allow for the rapid fine-tuning of glucose levels. Continuous insulin drips are superior to intermittent insulin for glycemic control in type 1 diabetics and type 2 diabetics who use insulin.

Pages: 657–658

Question #13

Answer: D

Rationale: The anesthetic technique can make a difference with regard to stress response. Increases in circulating glucose, cortisol, and norepinephrine are blocked in non-diabetic patients by epidural anesthesia below T3-S5 for pelvic surgery. Advantages of regional anesthetic techniques include having an awake patient who can report hypoglycemic symptoms and who can describe the quality of pain control.

Page: 658

Question #14

Answer: B

Rationale: Hypothyroid patients can be very sensitive to sedative medications. The administration of thyroid hormone to the severely hypothyroid surgical patient without steroid replacement may precipitate an adrenal crisis. In the patient with hyperthyroidism, the level of thyrotoxicosis must be measured preoperatively, because there is a direct correlation between the severity of the disease and the intraoperative risk. When possible, patients with hyperthyroidism should be made euthyroid

(e.g., with elective surgery). β-Blockers can provide adrenergic antagonism for hyperthyroid patients that are not euthyroid, and they block the peripheral conversion of T4 to T3.

Page: 658

Question #15

Answer: D

Rationale: It is essential to make sure that patients with cardiac conditions are stable before they undergo any operation, because the additional stress may exacerbate the underlying disorder. The patient with challenging heart failure can be precipitated by total body water overload, decreased intravascular volume, diminished stroke volume, and rare pericardial effusion. This is especially true for patients with concomitant metabolic disorders, such as the severely hypothyroid patient.

Reference: Chapter 35

Question #16

Answer: B

Rationale: Having a pulmonary embolism is a significant postoperative complication. The first step when considering a pulmonary embolism is a good history, physical examination, and initial testing, which may involve the determination of arterial blood gases, an EKG, and a chest X-ray. The Wells Clinical Prediction Rules for Pulmonary Embolism assigns points for certain clinical features that can guide the clinician with regard to seeking additional testing, especially if the total risk interpretation score is significantly elevated.

The presence of hemoptysis or malignancy is assigned 1 point, and 1.5 points are assigned to each of the following three clinical conditions: (1) a heart rate of more than 100 beats per minute; (2) immobilization or surgery within the past 4 weeks; and (3) previous deep venous thrombosis or pulmonary embolism. The clinical conditions that give the most points are clinical symptoms of deep venous thrombosis and other diagnoses that are less likely than pulmonary embolism, which are assigned 3 points each. The more total points, the higher the patient's risk for pulmonary embolism. Having more than 6 points puts a patient at a high risk of a pulmonary embolism (78.4%), whereas 2 to 6 points constitutes moderate risk (27.8%), and less than 2 points is a low risk (3.4%).

Reference: Chapter 35

Question #17

Answer: C

Rationale: Patients with wound infections are 60% more likely to be admitted to an intensive care unit and five times more likely to be readmitted to the hospital, and they have twice the mortality rate as compared with patients without a wound infection. The National Surgical Infection Prevention Project recommends the following: (1) that the infusion of the first antimicrobial dose should begin within 1 hour of surgical incision; and (2) that prophylactic antimicrobial agents should be discontinued within 24 hours of the end of surgery. Two additional simple interventions can reduce the incidence of wound infections: (1) the routine use of 80% inspired supplemental oxygen during surgery and for the first 2 hours after surgery; and (2) the avoidance of perioperative hypothermia.

Pages: 661–662

Question #18

Answers: (1), B; (2), B; (3), B; (4), A; (5), B

Rationale: Primary adrenal insufficiency (AI) is the result of conditions that damage the adrenal glands themselves. Secondary AI is the result of disorders of the hypothalamus or of the pituitary gland that result in the suppression of the secretion of adrenocorticotropic hormone. This is most commonly caused by the use of chronic steroids. Suppression blunts the adrenal gland's response to stress, which results in adrenal crisis. The effect of an adrenal crisis on blood pressure and fluid status is potentially life threatening. Perioperative doses of corticosteroids are given to prevent an adrenal crisis among patients with known or suspected primary or secondary AI. The dosing of corticosteroids is much higher among patients with adrenal crisis than it is among those with adrenal insufficiency. The dosing of steroids depends on the clinical situation, because major surgery and general anesthesia cause a greater stress than minor surgery or local anesthesia.

Page: 658

Question #19

Answer: A

Rationale: The risk factor that is most consistently associated with perioperative ischemic stroke is a history of having had a stroke. Other risk factors include peptic ulcer disease, chronic obstructive pulmonary disease, and postoperative cardiac arrhythmia. Patients with well-controlled blood pressure—especially those with cerebrovascular insufficiency or prior stroke—can lower the risk of neurological injury during surgery as compared with patients with poorly controlled blood pressure.

Page: 659

Question #20

Answer: D

Rationale: There is no current evidence to support one method of postoperative pain relief as being clearly better under all circumstances. The goal for all patients is to maximize their activity level while minimizing and avoiding side effects. Intravenous narcotics have been proved over time, and they are considered the standard with which all other pain-control regimens are compared. Postoperative epidural analgesia has been consistently shown to provide superior pain relief as compared with intravenous narcotics. Intravenous narcotics can be supplemented with nonsteroidal anti-inflammatory drugs for mild to moderate postoperative pain.

Page: 659

Question #21

Answer: C

Rationale: The prevention of postoperative bleeding starts with the consideration of preoperative events. A preoperative review of medications, including over-the-counter medications and herbal remedies, may require stopping the medications that affect clotting early during the preoperative period. Other historical factors to consider include a history of excessive bleeding with previous surgeries, recent changes in bruisability, and a family history of coagulopathy. Medical illnesses that increase the risk for operative and postoperative bleeding include liver, renal, and collagen vascular diseases. When evaluating excessive bright-red bleeding postoperatively, the patient should have a prothrombin time, partial thromboplastin time, and platelet count measured to help establish whether bleeding is the result of a coagulopathy or of a surgical problem. When values are normal, unless the underlying disease suggests a more complex coagulopathy, the exploration of the wound of a bleeder may be necessary. If the values are abnormal, correction with a specific replacement therapy is indicated.

Page: 664

Question #22

Answers: (1), B; (2), A; (3), B; (4), A; (5), A

Rationale: When considering the diagnosis of a pulmonary embolism, begin with a careful history and a physical examination. Initial diagnostic studies to determine if there is a pulmonary embolism could possibly include the determination of arterial blood gas levels, an EKG, and a chest X-ray. Further pulmonary imaging is warranted if, after these initial steps, findings still leave a possible diagnosis of pulmonary embolism. There is no consensus as to the best clinical prediction rule for pulmonary embolism, but a landmark study demonstrated that a physician's clinical judgment was nearly as good as the clinical prediction rule used.[2] Patients with signs and symptoms of pulmonary embolism who are found to have a deep venous thrombosis but who have negative imaging studies—including a computed tomography pulmonary angiogram or a nondiagnostic (low or intermediate probability) ventilation-perfusion scan—should be treated for a pulmonary embolism.

Page: 666

Question #23

Answer: D

Rationale: The management of a pulmonary embolism requires hospitalization with close monitoring, supportive care, and anticoagulation. Unfractionated heparin is usually given, although low-molecular-weight heparin is an acceptable alternative. Thrombolysis is reserved for massive pulmonary with hemodynamic compromise. Long-term anticoagulation is accomplished with warfarin to achieve an International normalized ratio of 2.0 to 3.0 for at least 3 months if the pulmonary embolism was the patient's first and if it was solely attributable to surgery.

Pages: 666–667

Question #24

Answers: (1), A; (2), B; (3), B; (4), A; (5), A

Rationale: In the vast majority of cases, patients can take their oral medications the morning of surgery, because most medications do not interfere with anesthesia, and they are well tolerated during surgery. Unless a medication is completely unnecessary or contraindicated,

it should be continued through the morning of surgery. This is especially true for antihypertensive, anticonvulsive, and psychiatric medications, with the exception of certain medications, such as angiotensin-converting enzyme inhibitors or angiotensin-II receptor blockers. Serum levels should be checked preoperatively, if available. Certain medications, such as β-blockers, are especially important to continue uninterrupted through the perioperative period. The discontinuation of β-blockers can increase the incidence of perioperative myocardial infarctions and death. Medications with long half-lives, such as antiarrhythmic formulations, should be continued right up until surgery, and they can usually be held for a few days postoperatively until the patient is eating.

Page: 659

Question #25

Answer: E

Rationale: Postoperative epidural analgesia has been consistently shown to provide superior pain relief as compared with intravenous narcotics. Other benefits include earlier extubation, earlier ambulation, decreased cardiac arrhythmias, decreased pulmonary complications, decreased ileus, and shorter hospitals stays.

Page: 663

Question #26

Answer: C

Rationale: The most common infectious causes of postoperative fevers are pneumonia, urinary tract infection, wound infection, and intravascular-catheter–associated infection. Medications are the most common cause of noninfectious postoperative fever. Malignant hyperthermia is a rare, dominantly inherited, genetic disorder that is caused by anesthetics, most commonly succinylcholine and halothane. Neuroleptic malignant syndrome can cause high fever and rigidity among patients who are receiving antipsychotics, especially haloperidol. Other causes of fever include surgical wound inflammation (e.g., seroma, hematoma).

Page: 664

Question #27

Answer: A

Rationale: Postoperative fever, which is defined as a temperature of more than 38°C (100°F), is common during the first few days after a major surgery. The

---

2. The PIOPED Investigators: Value of the ventilation/perfusion scan in acute pulmonary embolism. Results of the Prospective Investigation of Pulmonary Embolism Diagnosis (PIOPED). *JAMA* 263:2753-2759, 1990.

timing of onset and the type of surgery are essential for focusing the differential diagnosis of a postoperative fever. Fevers are infectious or noninfectious, and they can be categorized into immediate, acute, subacute, or delayed. Most early fevers are caused by the inflammatory response to surgery. Delayed fevers (i.e., those having an onset of more than a month after surgery) are typically caused by infectious etiologies, such as viral infections from blood products and parasitic infections. Fever should be treated to decrease physiologic stress and to help make the patient more comfortable, which are stronger arguments than concerns about masking a fever.

Page: 664

Question #28

Answers: (1), A; (2), B; (3), B; (4), A; (5), A

Rationale: Malnutrition is associated with an increase in surgical morbidity and mortality. This is especially true for cardiac patients, who are at risk of a higher mortality rate with a low serum albumin level (<3.2 g/dL), a low total cell count (<3000 per μL), and a low body mass index (<24). Postoperatively, oral nutrition is best, when possible, but it requires an awake patient with an intact gag reflex and swallowing mechanism and with a functioning digestive tract. For patients who cannot have oral feedings after surgery, enteral feedings (usually by a nasogastric tube) or parenteral feedings should be considered. Consider parenteral feedings if enteral nutrition is impossible and the anticipated length of the patient taking nothing by mouth is less than 5 days. In summary, meeting the nutritional needs of the surgical patient has its challenges, including the perioperative illness, the injury of the surgery itself, the surgical stress response, and the postoperative condition, which can involve starvation as a result of nothing-by-mouth status.

Page: 663

Question #1

Answer: B

Rationale: The U.S. Preventive Services Task Force gives an A-level recommendation to the following: all patients more than 18 years old being screened for high blood pressure; all adults being screened for tobacco use and offered cessation interventions; women over age 21 (or earlier for those who have been sexually active) being screened for cervical cancer; all women 25 years old and younger being screened for chlamydia; and all adults and adolescents at increased risk for syphilis, chlamydia, and HIV being screened for these. Women over the age of 45 years should be screened for lipid disorders, and abnormal lipid levels should be treated among those with increased risk of heart disease. There is no recommendation for screening for thyroid disease in asymptomatic women.

Page: 669

Question #2

Answer: C

Rationale: Women are considered low risk for cervical cancer if they have had two or fewer sexual partners, if they did not have intercourse before the age of 20 years, if they do not smoke, if they have not had any sexually transmitted diseases, and if they have never had an abnormal Pap smear. After three consecutive normal pap smears or after the age of 30 years, these women can be screened at 2- to 3-year intervals. Women who have had exposure to diethylstilbestrol in utero or who are HIV-positive or otherwise immunocompromised should be screened annually. There are no recommendations to use liquid-based cytology for specific populations.

Page: 670

Question #3

Answer: D

Rationale: Specimens are collected in the same manner for both conventional Pap smears and liquid-based cytology. The spatula is used to sample the entire transformation zone by sweeping it around the entire os.

The endocervical brush is inserted into the endometrial canal and rotated. Both samples can be sent on the same slide or in the same container if liquid-based screening is done. The spatula and brush are rinsed (swished) in the liquid media for liquid-based testing. Reflex HPV testing can be done on liquid-based specimens showing ASCUS.

Page: 670

Question #4

Answers: B

Rationale: Colposcopy is used to evaluate abnormal Pap smears by visualizing the genital tract—particularly the cervix—under magnification. Acetic acid (vinegar) is picked up by abnormal cells and turns them white. The glandular cells of the columnar epithelium have a grape-like appearance as seen during colposcopy. A colposcopy is considered adequate when the entire transformation zone (i.e., the junction of the columnar epithelium of the cervical canal with the squamous epithelium of the cervix) is seen and when the full extent of any lesions is seen. Abnormal areas should be biopsied and the specimens sent to pathology.

Page: 671

Question #5

Answer: A

Rationale: Patients with ASCUS Pap smears may be managed by repeat cytology, high-risk HPV typing, or colposcopy. If the repeat Pap shows ASCUS or a higher-grade abnormality or if the HPV high-risk type is positive, colposcopy is indicated.

Page: 671

Question #6

Answer: B

Rationale: Patients with glandular-cell abnormalities require an endometrial biopsy and colposcopy for complete evaluation. HPV testing is indicated for ASCUS Pap smears but not for those showing atypical glandular cells of undetermined significance.

Page: 671

Question #7

Answer: B

Rationale: Colposcopy rather than HPV testing is indicated for women with Pap smears showing atypical squamous cells—one cannot exclude high-grade squamous intraepithelial lesion, atypical glandular cells of undetermined significance, or low-grade squamous intraepithelial lesion. Reflex HPV testing can be done on liquid cytology specimens, and this is a more sensitive triage tool for ASCUS Pap smears than repeat cytology. Condyloma caused by HPV can be treated with cryotherapy, trichloroacetic acid, podophyllin, laser cautery, or imiquimod; however, these are not appropriate treatments for HPV-positive precancerous Pap smears.

Page: 671

Question #8

Answer: C

Rationale: Normal menstrual cycles that are controlled by hormones produced by the hypothalamus, the pituitary gland, and the ovaries are 28 days in length (± 5 to 7 days), with bleeding lasting 3 to 7 days. *Menorrhagia* is bleeding that is excessive in amount and duration that occurs at regular intervals. *Metrorrhagia* is bleeding that occurs at irregular intervals. *Menometrorrhagia* is frequent, irregular, excessive bleeding. *Oligomenorrhea* is infrequent, irregular bleeding that occurs at intervals of more than 45 days.

Page: 672

Question #9

Answer: D

Rationale: Pregnancy-related causes of abnormal uterine bleeding include ectopic pregnancy; threatened, incomplete, complete, or missed abortion; and gestational trophoblastic disease. Bleeding may also occur in otherwise normal pregnancies. Contraceptive methods may be the source of abnormal bleeding. Breakthrough bleeding associated with oral contraceptive pills usually resolves after 3 months of use; however, if it is persistent, it can be managed by changing the dosage or type of pill. Bleeding associated with progestin-only contraceptive methods may be managed by reassurance, estrogen supplementation, or nonsteroidal anti-inflammatory drugs. Blood dyscrasias, although they are infrequent causes of abnormal bleeding, may be seen among adolescent patients. Other causes of bleeding include polyps, fibroids, ovarian neoplasms, and thyroid, renal, or liver disease.

Page: 672

Question #10

Answer: A

Rationale: Risk factors for endometrial hyperplasia include obesity, diabetes, hypertension, age of more than 35 years, and anovulation.

Page: 672

Question #11

Answer: D

Rationale: Anovulation leads to the overgrowth of the endometrium, which can lead to amenorrhea or to irregular, prolonged, and/or excessive bleeding. The chronic estrogen stimulation places patients at risk for endometrial hyperplasia and endometrial cancer. The treatment of choice is medical therapy with oral contraceptives; cyclic progestins are also effective. Ovulation induction is indicated for women who would like to become pregnant.

Page: 673

Question #12

Answer: A

Rationale: Primary amenorrhea is diagnosed when an adolescent has not had a menstrual period by the age of 16 years. Evaluation includes ascertaining the presence and stage of secondary sexual characteristics; evaluating the reproductive tract for an imperforate hymen of the absence of the uterus or vagina; and, in some cases, referral to a geneticist or a reproductive endocrinologist.

Page: 673

Question #13

Answer: D

Rationale: The first step in the workup of a woman with secondary amenorrhea is a history and a physical, followed by a pregnancy test. If the pregnancy test is negative, a progesterone challenge (10 days of 10 mg medroxyprogesterone acetate) is done. The normal response of an estrogen-primed endometrium is a withdrawal bleed

2 to 7 days after the completion of this medication. Possible etiologies for the amenorrhea in this case include polycystic ovarian syndrome and other causes of anovulation.

Page: 673

Question #14

Answer: C

Rationale: Physiologic vaginal discharge is comprised of secretions from the vagina and cervix, shedding epithelial cells, and bacterial products. It can vary in amount and consistency with stress and the menstrual cycle. The pH is usually 3.8 to 4.5, and the discharge pools in the posterior fornix rather than adhering to the vaginal walls. There is a predominance of long, rod-shaped bacteria (lactobacilli); there are few white blood cells, and there is an absence of clue cells.

Page: 674

Question #15

Answer: D

Rationale: Bacterial vaginosis is the most common cause of abnormal vaginal discharge in the adult heterosexual woman, accounting for 10% to 37% of symptomatic cases. It may be even more common among lesbian patients.

Page: 675

Question #16

Answer: B

Rationale: Bacterial vaginosis is thought to begin with a decrease in lactobacilli leading to an increase in vaginal pH, which allows for the overgrowth of anaerobic bacteria such as *Gardnerella vaginalis, Mycoplasma hominis, Bacteroides* species, and *Mobiluncus* species. This type of infection has been associated with pelvic inflammatory disease, premature rupture of membranes, preterm delivery, postpartum endometritis, posthysterectomy cuff cellulitis, and postabortion infection. It is diagnosed by the examination of the discharge, which includes microscopic examination of a wet preparation looking for clue cells, a vaginal pH of more than 4.5, a fishy odor noted with the application of 10% potassium hydroxide to the discharge, and a speculum examination showing discharge that is adherent to the vaginal walls.

Page: 675

Question #17

Answer: C

Rationale: Treatment of bacterial vaginosis is indicated for symptomatic discharge and only for those asymptomatic women with high-risk pregnancies or who are undergoing vaginal surgery. Metronidazole or clindamycin orally or topically is most commonly used to treat bacterial vaginosis. Triple sulfa cream, erythromycin, tetracycline, and povidone-iodine douches have not been successful for the treatment of bacterial vaginosis. Even with effective treatment, it recurs in 20% to 30% of patients within 3 months.

Page: 675

Question #18

Answer: C

Rationale: Candidal infections caused by *Candida albicans, Candida glabrata,* or *Candida tropicalis* are characterized by a pruritic and often curd-like vaginal discharge. Topical, over-the-counter, or prescription preparations of oral fluconazole are used for treatment. Oral antifungals are contraindicated during pregnancy. Women who are immunosuppressed, who have been on antibiotics recently, or who are diabetic or pregnant are at increased risk. Although culture can be used for symptomatic women with negative microscopic examinations or for those who fail usual treatment, it is not indicated for asymptomatic women, as up to 20% of women may be colonized.

Page: 675

Question #19

Answer: A

Rationale: Trichomonas is usually transmitted by sexual contact. The classically described "strawberry" cervix is seen in only about 5% of cases. Diagnosis is made by identifying the organism on saline microscopy. Treatment is with oral metronidazole, because topical therapy does not adequately treat organisms harbored in the perivaginal glands and in the urethra. The treatment of sexual partners is important, because most cases of treatment failure are the result of contact with an untreated partner. A relative resistance to metronidazole has been reported; this usually responds to a higher dose of this medication.

Page: 676

Question #20

Answer: D

Rationale: Atrophic vaginitis is typically a problem of postmenopausal women, but it can occur in any situation in which there is a relative estrogen deficiency, such as during lactation, postpartum, or during therapy with medications such as tamoxifen or danazol. Estrogen decrease leads to the thinning of the vaginal tissue, causing pallor, dryness, and decreased rugae. Clinically, this is manifested by itching, vaginal soreness, spotting, dyspareunia, and urinary retention. The thinner vaginal tissue produces less glycogen, which leads to decreased lactic acid production by the lactobacilli, and the pH rises. Atrophic vaginitis is treated with topical or oral estrogens, with the lowest possible dose used to control symptoms.

Page: 677

Question #21

Answer: A

Rationale: When evaluating the woman with pelvic pain and a positive pregnancy test, it is important to rule out ectopic pregnancy. If the patient is stable, a combination of quantitative human chorionic gonadotropin measurement and ultrasound can help determine the location of the pregnancy. An intrauterine gestational sac should be visible on transvaginal ultrasound when the human chorionic gonadotropin level is 2000 or higher. A human chorionic gonadotropin level that doubles over 48 hours is reassuring for a normal pregnancy, as is a progesterone level of 25 or more. A history of tubal trauma, pelvic inflammatory disease, bilateral tubal ligation, or previous ectopic pregnancy increases the risk for ectopic pregnancy.

Page: 678

Question #22

Answer: A

Rationale: A woman who has had an ectopic pregnancy has a 25% chance of recurrence with a subsequent pregnancy. These women should have an ultrasound to verify an intrauterine pregnancy when a subsequent pregnancy is confirmed.

Page: 678

Question #23

Answer: C

Rationale: Pelvic inflammatory disease is usually considered a sexually transmitted disease; however, ordinary vaginal organisms may be involved. Antibiotic regimens covering *Neisseria gonorrhea*, *Chlamydia trachomatis*, and anaerobes are recommended. Outpatient treatment is the norm. Indications for inpatient treatment include severe nausea and vomiting, pregnancy, high fever, and failure to respond to or comply with outpatient treatment; it may also occur when observation is needed to rule out a surgical cause of symptoms.

Page: 679

Question #24

Answer: D

Rationale: Endometriosis is the most common cause of chronic pelvic pain identified by laparoscopy. Findings may include "powder burn" implants on pelvic structures; cystic, brown, fluid-filled lesions; and adhesions caused by inflammation.

Page: 679

Question #25

Answer: C

Rationale: The diagnosis of endometriosis is suspected on the basis of the history and the physical examination. Although nodularity of the uterosacral ligaments, pain in the posterior cul-de-sac, or a fixed retroverted uterus is suggestive of endometriosis, physical examination is usually normal. Laparoscopy is the gold standard for diagnosis. Treatment with nonsteroidal anti-inflammatory drugs or hormones such as oral contraceptives, Depo-Provera, or danazol may decrease pelvic pain, but they do not improve fertility. Surgical treatments improve fertility rates, and they may be effective for reducing pain among those for whom medical treatment fails. However, over time, about half of these patients will have recurrent pain.

Page: 680

Question #26

Answer: D

Rationale: Adenomyosis, which is sometimes referred to as *internal endometriosis*, is characterized by endometrial tissue growing within the muscle of the uterus. Patients present with chronic pelvic pain, and the physical examination may reveal a tender, enlarged uterus. When the diagnosis is suspected, magnetic resonance imaging should be performed. Definitive treatment is a hysterectomy.

Page: 680

Question #27

Answer: C

Rationale: Chronic pelvic pain is pelvic pain that has been present for 6 months or more. It can come from a variety of gynecologic causes, or it may be a presentation of irritable bowel syndrome, interstitial cystitis, or musculoskeletal disorders, such as pelvic muscle spasm. Non-gynecologic causes, such as irritable bowel syndrome, may worsen with menstruation. *Mittelschmerz,* which is painful ovulation, occurs mid-cycle, between periods. When no physical reason for the pain is found, it is important to address psychosocial issues. Chronic pain can result from exposure to sexual violence or from sexual abuse as a child. Sometimes a source of pain is not identified; in those cases, the focus is on symptom relief.

Page: 680

Question #28

Answer: A

Rationale: Fibroids or leiomyomas are benign tumors that arise from the connective tissue of the uterus, and they are a common cause of pelvic mass. They may be asymptomatic, or they may be associated with heavy bleeding and with pelvic pain or pressure on surrounding structures, such as the bladder or bowel. Medical treatment with progesterone, danazol, or gonadotropin-releasing hormone agonists aims to reduce the effect of estrogen on the tumor. Ovarian cysts are common among women of reproductive age.

Page: 681

Question #29

Answer: A

Rationale: Most adnexal masses in nonpregnant women of reproductive age are benign ovarian cysts. Small, simple (fluid-only) cysts in premenopausal women are unlikely to be malignant, and they can be monitored clinically over several months; 70% will resolve spontaneously. Cysts that are larger than 5 cm

are more prone to rupture, and, like complex cysts, they are more likely to harbor malignancy. Monophasic oral contraceptive pills have been used for several cycles to aid in the resolution of ovarian cysts.

Page: 682

Question #30

Answer: C

Rationale: Ovarian cancer, which is the fifth leading cause of death in women, is difficult to detect early. Symptoms, if present, are vague, and they include bloating, pelvic heaviness, and urinary frequency. There is no good screening test for ovarian cancer. CA-125 levels are sensitive but not specific, and they may be elevated in the presence of other conditions, such as endometriosis. Risk is increased among women with a family history of breast or ovarian cancer, a personal history of breast cancer, and delayed childbearing. The use of oral contraceptive pills for 5 years has been shown to decrease risk. Five-year survival rate for all stages of this type of cancer is 35%.

Page: 682

Question #31

Answer: A

Rationale: Vulvar lesions should usually be biopsied, because appearance alone does not distinguish benign from premalignant or malignant lesions. In particular, white areas that may indicate vulvar dysplasia or lichen sclerosis and condyloma that appear irregular in consistency and color or that do not respond to traditional treatment should be biopsied. Treatment for an asymptomatic Bartholin's gland cyst is not necessary. A large bothersome cyst or a Bartholin's gland abscess should be incised and drained. A Word catheter or gauze packing can be used to allow drainage to continue. Condylomatous lesions may be treated with trichloroacetic acid, podophyllin, cryotherapy, imiquimod, or laser therapy. Lichen sclerosis is treated with topical steroids after biopsy has confirmed the diagnosis and ruled out dysplasia or cancer.

Page: 682

Question #32

Answer: C

Rationale: Impaired ovulation is one of the most common causes of female infertility. A woman who is having regular periods at normal intervals is probably ovulating, especially if she is having premenstrual symptoms. Indications that ovulation has occurred include a serum progesterone level of 15 drawn 7 days after presumed ovulation, an endometrial biopsy showing histologic evidence of ovulation, and a positive home ovulation detection test (i.e., the detection of urinary luteinizing hormone).

Page: 682

Question #33

Answer: B

Rationale: Female infertility is often caused by impaired ovulation or tubal blockage. After ovulation has been confirmed or, simultaneously, if the evaluation for infertility is urgent, semen analysis should be performed to identify any abnormalities in sperm volume, count, concentration, motility, or morphology. Because an hysterosalpingogram is an invasive test, it is performed after semen analysis. Hysterosalpingogram using oil- or water-based contrast can show tubal patency. There is evidence that the use of oil-based contrast leads to higher pregnancy outcomes than the use of water-based contrast. Infertility is usually defined as the failure to conceive after 1 year of unprotected intercourse. However, earlier evaluation may be appropriate for couples over the age of 30 or for those with significant infertility risks. In about 20% of couples trying to get pregnant, both the man and the woman have some form of infertility.

Page: 682

Question #34

Answer: B

Rationale: Classic symptoms of menopause (i.e., hot flashes, vaginal dryness, sleep disturbances) can be relieved with hormone therapy. Because hormone therapy was found to be associated with increased cases of coronary heart disease, breast cancer, pulmonary embolism, and stroke, it is recommended to use the lowest possible dose for the shortest duration of time, and it is not recommended for the prevention of chronic diseases, including heart disease. Selective estrogen receptor modulators (e.g., raloxifene, tamoxifen) can help prevent bone loss in women who are at risk for osteoporosis, and they can be used to treat women with established osteoporosis. These drugs should not be used for women with a history of venous thromboembolic events.

Page: 684

Question #35

Answer: C

Rationale: The most common cause of urinary incontinence among women is stress incontinence, which is the loss of urine after a Valsalva-type (bearing down) action, such as coughing, laughing, or sneezing. It is caused by hypermobility of the urethra or weakness of the sphincter. Urge incontinence is the involuntary loss of urine that is associated with a strong urge to void. Common causes are involuntary contractions of the bladder and detrusor instability. Treatment is with anticholinergic medication.

Page: 685

37 Answers

Question #1

Answer: D

Rationale: Half of the pregnancies each year in the United States are unintended, and a little more than half of the women in whom they occur were using contraception at the time. These unintended pregnancies account for most of the 1.3 million abortions in the United States each year. In addition to decreasing unintended pregnancy and abortion, effective birth control can provide the primary prevention of STIs and of some medical conditions. The role of the physician is to be knowledgeable about all options for contraception, to present the information to the patient, and to let her make the best decision for her individual situation.

Page: 689

Question #2

Answer: A

Rationale: The absolute number of past pregnancies does not limit the contraceptive options, although the desire for the timing of future pregnancies can influence the selection of a short-term versus longer-term option. The number of sexual partners, compliance with contraception methods, methods of STI prevention, and personal beliefs are all important factors to consider with regard to the choice of contraception. In addition, the partner's willingness to participate in prevention, comorbid medical conditions, and the financial ability to pay for contraception must be considered.

Page: 689

Question #3

Answer: E

Rationale: There are multiple formulations of combination oral contraceptives available today. All have equal efficacy, although varying amounts of estrogen may help symptoms or side effects. The current range of ethinyl estradiol in commercially available pills is 20 to 50 μg. Higher doses of estrogen have been used in the past, but they are no longer available.

Pages: 690, 692

Question #4

Answer: E

Rationale: COCs provide more benefits than contraception alone. In addition to the benefits listed in the question, COCs reduce the risk of endometrial and ovarian cancer; they regulate irregular menstrual cycles; they suppress symptomatic endometriosis, and they improve acne. COCs do not decrease STI transmission, although they can decrease the risk of symptomatic pelvic inflammatory disease.

Pages: 690, 691

Question #5

Answer: C

Rationale: Most recent research does not show an increase in breast cancer among COC users. The risk of deep venous thrombosis is higher during pregnancy (4× to 6× increase) than it is with the use of COCs (3× increase.) COC use has not been associated with an increased risk of cervical cancer. Arterial events associated with COC use, such as myocardial infarction or cerebrovascular accident, are limited to women 35 years old or older with additional risk factors. COC use can accelerate gallbladder disease progression among women who are already susceptible; however, COC use does not cause gallbladder disease.

Page: 691

Question #6

Answer: B

Rationale: BTB is a common and typically transient side effect of COC use. If BTB persists for more than three cycles, then the pill formulation should be changed. Lower-dose estrogen pills and prolonged COC regimens have a higher risk of BTB. Smokers are more likely to experience BTB, most likely from increased hepatic metabolism of the COC.

Page: 691

Question #7

Answer: D

Rationale: Breast tenderness, nausea, and headaches are common side effects of COC use. Switching to a lower-dose estrogen pill may help decrease or eliminate these side effects. Headaches can also happen during the placebo week, in which case they are associated with estrogen withdrawal. Those patients may benefit from continuous COC dosing or low-dose estrogen supplementation during the placebo week. Amenorrhea is a physiologically normal consequence of COC use that is the result of a lack of buildup of the endometrial lining. Pill formulations do not need to be changed because of amenorrhea, unless the patient desires cyclic bleeding. Heart palpitations are not one of the common side effects of COC.

Page: 691

Question #8

Answer: B

Rationale: Progestin-only pills (POPs) are appropriate for women in whom estrogen is not tolerated or in whom it is contraindicated. Because estrogen can reduce breast milk production, POPs are preferred over COCs for lactating women. Nausea is an estrogen-related side effect, so the use of POPs would be helpful for patients with that side effect when taking COCs. POPs have not been shown to increase the risk of cardiovascular complications, so they would be a good option for women with high blood pressure as well as for women 35 years old or older who smoke. Because POPs are less effective than COCs and more likely to cause BTB, they are less suitable for adolescents.

Page: 693

Question #9

Answer: D

Rationale: The transdermal contraceptive patch (Ortho Evra) is a combination estrogen and progestin hormonal contraceptive. The main advantage of the patch is compliance, because patients only need to remember to change patches once per week. Fewer contraceptive failures have been reported with the patch than with COCs, most likely for this reason. Patch users tend to experience more in the way of breast tenderness side effects than COC users. Despite recent media reports, there is insufficient evidence to determine if the mortality rate and the incidence of nonfatal venous thromboembolisms is higher among patch users than COC users. The absolute risk is still very low, especially as compared with the mortality and nonfatal venous thromboembolism risk from pregnancy. There is some concern that the patch may be less effective for women who weigh more than 198 lb.

Page: 693

Question #10

Answer: A

Rationale: The vaginal contraceptive ring (NuvaRing) is a combination estrogen and progestin hormonal contraceptive. Hormones are released continuously and absorbed systemically through the vaginal mucosa. Because of lower peak serum hormone levels and less hormonal fluctuation, the ring causes less nausea and BTB. The ring is made out of ethylene vinyl acetate, so it is safe for those with latex allergy. The ring is placed intravaginally for 3 weeks and then removed for 1 week. It does not need to be over the cervix, because it does not act as a barrier contraceptive. The ring can be left out for short periods of time, but it should be replaced within 3 hours to maintain its efficacy. Vaginitis, headache, and leukorrhea are the most commonly reported side effects.

Pages: 693, 694

Question #11

Answer: D

Rationale: DMPA is a long-acting progesterone-only contraceptive that is injected intramuscularly (and recently approved for subcutaneous dosing) every 12 weeks. DMPA does inhibit ovulation very effectively, and it also decreases the pain from endometriosis. There is a long return to fertility of 6 to 12 months after the discontinuation of DMPA. The U.S. Food and Drug Administration did add a black-box warning to DMPA in 2004, stating that it may result in loss of bone density; therefore, the manufacturer recommends limiting use to 2 years unless other birth-control methods are inadequate.

Page: 694

Question #12

Answer: B

Rationale: The etonogestrel implant, Implanon, is a single-rod, progestin-only, subcutaneous form of hormonal contraception. It provides highly effective contraception for 3 years. Special training is required for the insertion and removal of the device, but this system is associated with fewer difficulties than the prior six-rod device, Norplant. After removal, the return to fertility is rapid. Irregular bleeding and amenorrhea can occur with Implanon, but, over time, bleeding becomes more regular.

Page: 695

Question #13

Answer: A

Rationale: A significant benefit of the levonorgestrel-secreting IUD is endometrial suppression, which causes a 90% decrease in the average amount of menstrual blood loss among users. This is helpful for the prevention of anemia from heavy menses. This IUD provides 5 years of effective contraception. IUD users are twice as likely to develop pelvic inflammatory disease as women who do not use contraceptives. The primary mechanisms of action of this IUD are thickening of cervical mucus, inhibition of sperm survival, endometrial suppression, and induction of a local endometrial foreign-body effect. The systemic absorption of levonorgestrel is low, which causes ovulation suppression only among some women.

Page: 695

Question #14

Answer: B

Rationale: Condoms made from latex and polyurethane offer protection from many bacterial and viral STIs. Natural membrane condoms do not offer significant STI protection. The Reality condom is made of polyurethane, and it is therefore is safe for latex-allergic individuals. Male condom use can be associated with decreased penile sensitivity.

Page: 696

Question #15

Answer: D

Rationale: Case-control and cross-sectional studies support that the use of a diaphragm is associated with protection from cervical gonorrhea, chlamydia, trichomoniasis, and pelvic inflammatory disease. There is no evidence to support protection from HIV, and so the diaphragm should not be used by women to prevent HIV transmission.

Page: 696

Question #16

Answer: D

Rationale: Studies of nonoxynol-9 and its effect on STI and HIV transmission have had conflicting results. A recent meta-analysis concludes that spermicides with nonoxynol-9 protect against gonorrhea and chlamydia infection, but evidence of its effect on HIV transmission is inconclusive. Therefore, the World Health Organization and the Centers for Disease Control and Prevention have recommended against the use of spermicides with nonoxynol-9 alone for the purposes of STI prevention. Nonoxynol-9–containing spermicides are available in multiple delivery systems, including gels, films, suppositories, foams, and creams. With typical use, pregnancy failure rates are 20% to 25% at 1 year. A dose of spermicide remains effective for approximately 1 hour after insertion. The spermicide sponge can be left in place for up to 30 hours after intercourse; however, prolonged contraceptive sponge placement can increase the risk of toxic shock syndrome.

Page: 697

Question #17

Answer: E

Rationale: The copper-T IUD provides effective contraception for 10 years (as compared with 5 years with the levonorgestrel IUD). Both IUDs cause a significant decrease in the absolute number of ectopic pregnancies. However, in the rare event that a pregnancy does occur with an IUD in place, there is a higher likelihood that the pregnancy will be ectopic. Both IUDs are associated with a short return to fertility after removal. Neither IUD will disrupt an established pregnancy; thus, they are not abortifacients. The copper-T IUD does cause increased menstrual bleeding, cramping, and risk of anemia as compared with the levonorgestrel-secreting IUD, which decreases all of those phenomena.

Page: 698

Question #18

Answer: A

Rationale: Although breast sensitivity is cyclic in many women, it is not used as a fertility-awareness–based method. The other methods listed are all used, and their goal is to identify potentially fertile days of the cycle and to use either abstinence or barrier contraception on those days to prevent pregnancy. Counting days of the cycle, detecting a change in basal-body temperature signaling ovulation, monitoring the consistency of cervical mucus, or a combination of all of these methods may be used as fertility-awareness–based contraception.

Page: 698

Question #19

Answer: B

Rationale: The lactation amenorrhea method is more than 98% effective as contraception, provided that the infant is exclusively or nearly exclusively breastfeeding, that the woman is less than 6 months postpartum, and that the woman has not experienced her first menses postpartum. No additional formula or solids should be introduced during this period.

Page: 699

Question #20

Answer: C

Rationale: Ultrasound-guided tubal ligation is not an approach that is currently used for tubal ligation. Laparoscopy, laparotomy, and mini-laparotomy can all be used to close the fallopian tubes with clips, rings, or electrocoagulation. A new technique involves placement of a coil device (Essure) into the proximal portion of the fallopian tubes through a hysteroscope. A fibrotic tissue-growth reaction is stimulated, effectively causing occlusion of the tubes.

Page: 700

Question #21

Answer: B

Rationale: There are three main regimens of EC available in the United States: a combination estrogen and progestin (Yuzpe) method, a progestin-only regimen (Plan B), and the insertion of a copper-T IUD. Currently available combination and progestin-only oral contraceptives are commonly used for EC, in addition to the commercially available Plan B.

Page: 701

Question #22

Answer: A

Rationale: The progestin-only regimen of EC has recently been shown to be highly effective as a single dose of 1.5 mg of levonorgestrel for up to 120 hours after intercourse. The combination estrogen and progestin regimen should be given within 72 hours of intercourse. The copper-T IUD can be inserted up to 5 days after intercourse and still be highly effective.

Page: 701

Question #23

Answer: C

Rationale: The Yuzpe regimen consists of two doses of 100 μg of ethinyl estradiol and 50 μg of levonorgestrel given 12 hours apart. The high estrogen dose causes significant nausea (42%) and vomiting (16%) among women using this regimen, so antiemetics are often prescribed with this form of EC. EC is extremely safe and 75% or more effective for the prevention of unintended pregnancy when used properly. It is important to counsel the patient about routine contraception methods after prescribing EC. Providing patients with advance prescriptions for EC does not increase promiscuity or the risk of STIs.

Page: 701

Question #24

Answer: E

Rationale: Those patients who choose abstinence as a form of contraception should be reassured that this is common, normal, and acceptable. The term *abstinence* means different things to different people, and it is not strictly defined. Abstinence can be primary or secondary. Patients who choose abstinence often need support as a result of peer or partner pressure.

Page: 702

Question #25

Answer: E

Rationale: If no method of contraception is being used, the percentage of pregnancies that occur during the first year is a significant 85%. With the multiple current available options, family doctors can help counsel patients to find the best regimen to prevent unintended pregnancies and STIs.

Pages: 689, 690

Question #26

Answer: A

Rationale: Ortho Evra is a combination estrogen and progesterone contraceptive patch that provides similar benefits and risks to those of COCs. One of the absolute contraindications for COCs is smoking over the age of 35 years, because this is associated with an increase in venous thromboembolism and other serious side effects. All of the other options listed in the question can be used for these patients without increased risk.

Pages: 690, 691

Question #27

Answer: B

Rationale: Polyurethane condoms are actually more likely to slip or break during intercourse. They are also thinner than latex condoms, thus improving penile sensation. Latex and polyurethane condoms offer similar protection from STI transmission. Polyurethane condoms are less likely to degrade when exposed to oil-based products.

Page: 696

Question #28

Answer: D

Rationale: Lea's Shield is a cervical cap that is made of silicone rubber. It is only available in one size, and it is intended to fit all and to make fitting easier. Efficacy is improved among patients who are nulliparous and among those who use a spermicide with the device.

Page: 697

Question #29

Answer: C

Rationale: "No-scalpel" vasectomy is a technique that is faster, is less invasive, requires fewer instruments, and is most often performed in the office setting. Complications are rare, but they include bleeding, hematomas, and infection. Vasectomy is slightly more effective than female sterilization, although both are considered permanent. In addition to young age and unstable marriage, risk factors for regret after sterilization include recent pregnancy, low socioeconomic status, and Hispanic origin. There is no evidence to support an association between vasectomy and prostate cancer.

Page: 700

Question #30

Answer: E

Rationale: COCs require daily compliance, which would make them a noncompliant patient. The other methods listed require much less frequent patient intervention for effective contraception. The Ortho Evra patch only has to be changed weekly. The NuvaRing is placed for 3 weeks at a time and then removed for 1 week to induce a menstrual cycle. The DMPA shot is only given once every 12 weeks, and the IUD can be effective for 5 to 10 years, depending on the type.

Page: 691

Question #1

Answer: B

Rationale: The electromotive forces generated by the heart during systole are recorded as follows: (1) P wave caused by depolarization of the atria; (2) QRS wave of depolarization of the ventricles; and (3) T wave as a result of repolarization of the ventricles (Figure 38-2). The U wave is an afterwave of repolarization. It may always occur, but, in general, it has a very small magnitude, and it can only be detected in those precordial leads in which the electrodes are close to the myocardial mass. Certain electrolyte disturbances (e.g., hypokalemia) produce a large U wave in practically all leads.

Page: 705

Question #2

Answer: B

Rationale: The electrical field is three dimensional, but its projection in a frontal plane can be assessed by analyzing the standard limb leads (I, II, III, aVR, aVL, and aVF), and its projection in a horizontal plane can be assessed by analyzing the precordial or chest leads (V_1 through V_6).

Page: 705

Question #3

Answer: C

Rationale: The direction of QRS is normally between 0 and +90 degrees, although some textbooks indicate

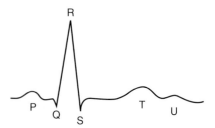

Figure 38-2 In Rakel RE, editor: *Textbook of family medicine*, ed 7, Philadelphia, WB Saunders, 2007.

that the normal range is from −20 to +110 degrees. It is clear from this figure that, normally, the axis of QRS is projected in the positive part of leads I and aVF, whereas a right atrial defect will cause a negative QRS in I and a left atrial defect will cause a negative QRS in aVF. In the rare cases of extreme right atrial defect, QRS will be negative in both lead I and aVF. Thus, a much simplified pattern analysis of the QRS axis can be done by assessing leads I and aVF. Extreme right atrial defect occurs if the axis falls between 180 and −90 degrees. The mean QRS axis projects itself in all of the leads. There is right atrial defect because of the relative preponderance of right ventricular forces during the neonatal period.

Page: 707

Question #4

Answer: B

Rationale: There is a horizontal axis or slight left atrial defect because of the preponderance of left ventricular forces in the majority of persons beyond the sixth decade of life.

Page: 708

Question #5

Answer: D

Rationale: V_1 is placed in the fourth intercostal space at the right sternal border. The electrical center of the heart is actually displaced to the left and to the front of the center of the transverse plane; this precludes accurate measurements of the amplitude and direction of QRS axis. The close proximity of the electrodes to the heart causes the amplitudes on V_3, V_4, and V_5 to be approximately 150% larger than the true amplitudes that would be recorded if the electrical center of the heart coincided with the center of the transverse plane. Thus, high voltages of QRS, T, and ST in these leads may not necessarily indicate the presence of pathology. There is a gradual increase in voltage of the R wave as it progresses from V_1 to V_5. Absence of the anteriorly displaced initial forces depolarization is called poor R progression. These criteria could indicate an old anterior wall myocardial infarction, but the presence of a P-pulmonale and the clinical history would help establish the diagnosis of chronic obstructive pulmonary disease.

Page: 709

Question #6

Answer: D

Rationale: The P axis has almost the same direction as that of QRS, but the range of normal is from +20 to +70 degrees. The magnitude is less than 0.25 mV. In a pattern analysis, P is considered normal if it is positive in lead II. If P is negative in aVF, it suggests a marked left atrial enlargement or a nodal rhythm. If P is very small, isoelectric, or negative in lead I, it is likely the result of right atrial enlargement. Practically all V leads show a positive P (Figure 38-3).

Page: 708

Question #7

Answer: A

Rationale: The atrial repolarization is seldom detected, because it takes place at the time of recording of the QRS complex, which is of greater magnitude and therefore cancels out the atrial repolarization forces.

Page: 706

Question #8

Answer: E

Rationale: The condition referred to as ventricular strain occurs when the T is negative in the lead of highest QRS positivity or, alternatively, when it is positive in the lead of highest QRS negativity. Practically all V leads show a positive T, with the exception of V_1, which may be isoelectric or negative (see Figure 38-3). Negative T waves in V_1 through V_3 indicate strain in the right (anterior) ventricle or in the anterior (anteroseptal) wall of the left ventricle (Figure 38-4, *A*). Negative T waves in V_4 through

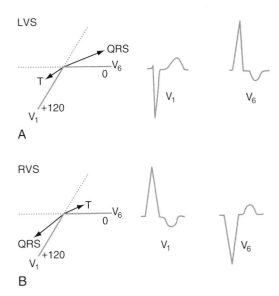

Figure 38-4 A and B. In Rakel RE, editor: *Textbook of family medicine,* ed 7, Philadelphia, WB Saunders, 2007.

V_6 indicate strain in the left (posterior) ventricle. This pattern is referred to as "flipped Ts," because normally the T waves are positive in these leads (see Figure 38-4, *B*).

Page: 710

Question #9

Answer: A

Rationale: High magnitude, according to the index of Sokolow and Lyon, is demonstrated by the following equation: $S_1 + R_5 > 3.5$ mV. This empirical index states that, when the total of the negative portion of QRS in V_1 (S_1) added to the positive portion of QRS (R) in V_5 exceeds 35 mm (equivalent to 3.5 mV), the diagnosis of left ventricular hypertrophy should be considered.

Page: 713

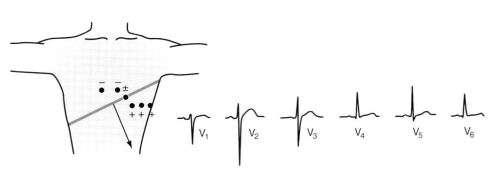

Figure 38-3 In Rakel RE, editor: *Textbook of family medicine,* ed 7, Philadelphia, WB Saunders, 2007.

Question #10

Answer: E

Rationale: Whenever the angle between the QRS and T axis exceeds 60 degrees counterclockwise or 45 degrees clockwise, the diagnosis of electrical strain is warranted. A T axis of strain points away from the ventricle where the strain occurs. Usual causes of strain are hypertrophy, bundle branch block, ischemia, digitalis, catecholamine-epinephrine effect, metabolic disturbances, and cerebral hemorrhage.

Pages: 713–714

Question #11

Answer: B

Rationale:
Frontal Plane

- Left-axis deviation
- Magnitude of QRS within normal limits in the lead of the mean axis (except when there is also left ventricular hypertrophy)
- Left ventricular strain very often (as a result of a change in the sequence of repolarization)
- QRS duration: >0.12 sec
- Slurring of QRS in several leads

Horizontal Plane

- Posterior axis (transitional lead at V_3 or V_4)
- Magnitude within normal limits (except when there is also left ventricular hypertrophy)
- Left ventricular strain very often (i.e., flipped T waves in V_4, V_5, and V_6)
- QRS duration: >0.12 sec
- Slurring of QRS in several leads

Page: 715

Question #12

Answer: C

Rationale:
Frontal Plane

- Left axis deviation of at least −30 degrees (not as a result of other causes)
- Low or normal magnitude of QRS
- Initial forces of depolarization away from the main axis (with Q wave in aVL and occasionally in I)
- No slurring or only a small notch in one or two leads
- QRS duration: <0.12 sec

Conduction disturbances may occur as a result of a lesion in one or several locations of the bundle of His. A clinical history usually reveals the existence of coronary artery disease in most cases of hemiblock.

Left Posterior Hemiblock or Left Posterior Fascicular Block

This type of hemiblock occurs much less frequently than left anterior hemiblock.

Page: 717

Question #13

Answer: D

Rationale: As a result of the increased size of the right atrium, most electromagnetic fields originate in that atrium and proceed in a slightly more rightward direction than normal (Figure 38-5). Because most cases of right atrial enlargement are the result of chronic obstructive pulmonary disease, pulmonic valve disease, or pulmonary artery disease, the term *P-pulmonale* may be used interchangeably with *right atrial enlargement.*

Frontal Plane

- Direction of the axis of P is vertical, almost vertical, or deviated to the right (small P in I and negative P in aVL).
- Magnitude: >0.25 mV (peaked P wave in II)
- Duration of P: ≤0.08 sec

Horizontal Plane

- P axis may be anterior (with a prominent upright P in V_1).

Page: 719

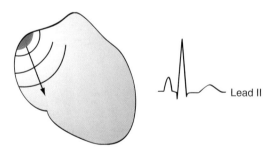

Figure 38-5 In Rakel RE, editor: *Textbook of family medicine,* ed 7, Philadelphia, WB Saunders, 2007.

Question #14

Answer: E

Rationale: The increased size of the left atrium causes a shift of late atrial electromagnetic fields to the left, but the normal forces of depolarization of the right atrium occur earlier and in the normal direction; this explains the existence of two P waves. The first is the result of depolarization of the right atrium, and the second is the result of depolarization of the left atrium. The P wave in several of the standard limb leads shows a double-hump pattern (Figure 38-6). Because most cases of left atrial enlargement are the result mitral valve disease, the term *P-mitrale* may be used interchangeably with left atrial enlargement. Among patients with diffuse myocardial damage of the left atrium (e.g., those with atherosclerotic cardiovascular disease), the depolarization progresses slowly, first to the right atrium and then to the left. As a result, the P wave is broad and small, and it has a double hump resembling a P-mitrale. Because the problem here is not hypertrophy but rather delayed depolarization through a damaged myocardium, the preferred term is *left atrial abnormality.*

Frontal Plane

- Usually there are two small axes of P, the first in the normal direction of about +60 degrees and the second (and often smaller) 30 to 60 degrees to the left of the first. This causes a double-humped P wave in lead II.
- Highest amplitude of either one of the two P waves is 2.5 mm (0.25 mV). In cases of left atrial abnormality, the magnitude is very small.
- Duration of P: usually >0.08 sec

Horizontal Plane

- The two axes of P (one anterior and quite small, the other posterior and larger) usually produce a biphasic P wave in V_1.

Page: 720

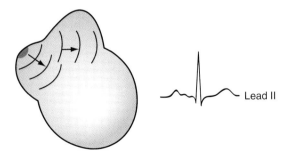

Figure 38-6 In Rakel RE, editor: *Textbook of family medicine,* ed 7, Philadelphia, WB Saunders, 2007.

Question #15

Answer: A

Rationale: As a result of the effect of chronic obstructive pulmonary on electrical impedance, the changes described in the question and attributable to the cor pulmonale syndrome may be masked by a distorted transmission of electromagnetic fields from the heart to the precordial electrodes. As a result, the following changes are noticeable.

ECG Changes Attributable to the Effect of Chronic Obstructive Pulmonary Disease on Cardiac Dynamics

Frontal Plane

- Right atrial enlargement (or P-pulmonale)
- Vertical axis or right axis deviation (sometimes, the axis of QRS is <+90 degrees)
- Right ventricular strain
- Overall decrease in the magnitude of the QRS in the frontal plane
- Undifferentiated axis or left axis deviation that mimics a left anterior hemiblock

The presence of P-pulmonale and the clinical history help to establish the diagnosis of chronic obstructive pulmonary disease.

Horizontal Plane

- Decrease in the amplitude of QRS
- Absence of the anteriorly displaced initial forces of depolarization (poor R progression)

Page: 721

Question #16

Answer: A

Rationale: Criteria for the Diagnosis of the Stage of Myocardial Infarction

Acute Stage (about 1 week)

- A prominent ST displacement (up or down)
- Deep and wide Q waves may be present in leads that do not normally have Q waves.

Subacute Stage (1–8 weeks)

- A prominent negative T is present in the leads with a positive QRS (strain pattern).
- Deep and wide Q waves may be present.

Old Myocardial Infarction (>8 weeks)

- Deep and wide Q waves
- Slurring in S waves

Page: 723

Questions #17 through #20

Answers: 17, D; 18, C; 19, B; 20, A

Rationale:

- Anterior or anteroseptal: caused by an occlusion of the left anterior descending artery or one of each of the lateral branches
- Anterolateral or anterobasal or superior: caused by an occlusion of the circumflex artery
- Apical: caused by an occlusion of the terminal portion of the left anterior descending artery
- Posterior: caused by an occlusion of the posterior segment of the right coronary artery (or one of its branches); may affect the sinoatrial and atrioventricular nodes and cause dysrhythmia
- Inferior or diaphragmatic: caused by an occlusion of the dominant right or left coronary artery; if it results from an occlusion of the right coronary artery, may affect the sinoatrial and atrioventricular nodes and cause dysrhythmia

Page: 723

Question #21

Answer: B

Rationale: This syndrome consists of brief periods of anginal chest pain at rest as a result of spasm of the epicardial coronary arteries. It produces a transient ST elevation, which is a manifestation of an injury current in the subepicardial region.

The ST changes and pain usually are not detected during exercise, unless a coronary spasm occurs. Most of the recorded ST changes are of brief duration and obtained with a Holter monitor.

Criteria for Diagnosis

- Displacement of ST of variable magnitude (usually small, but sometimes large)
- Axis of ST almost in the same direction of the QRS vector in the frontal plane (ST elevated in leads in which QRS is positive)
- Axis of ST anterior in the horizontal plane (ST elevated in anterior leads)
- Usually observed in young or middle-aged women
- No clinical manifestations of pericarditis; brief duration of pain that occurs at rest

Page: 727

Question #22

Answer: B

Rationale: Digitalis usually speeds up the repolarization process (short QT time), but the effect is slightly different in the subepicardial and subendocardial areas. The difference accounts for the ST displacement.

Criteria for Diagnosis

- Small ST depression, usually ≤2 mm (0.2 mV), with downsloping and coving in leads with a positive QRS

During exercise, patients with coronary artery disease may develop acute insufficiency of coronary blood flow (ischemia); this is reflected in a significant ST displacement. The mechanism for this displacement may be a difference in the sequence of repolarization between the subendocardial area and the subepicardial area. The ST displacement must be at least 0.08 sec long and either horizontal or downsloping.

The presence of an ST ischemic pattern on an ECG obtained at rest suggests the existence of subendocardial ischemia. Left ventricular hypertrophy or left bundle branch block may cause an ST displacement that is not caused by ischemia.

As a result of the inflammation of the pericardial sac, there is a small current of injury in the subepicardial area, which is oriented toward the front. This current causes an ST displacement with an axis that points downward and forward (i.e., toward the anterior wall of the ventricles).

Criteria for Diagnosis

- Displacement of ST: ≤2 mm (0.2 mV)
- Axis of ST almost in the same direction of the QRS axis in the frontal plane (ST elevated in leads in which QRS is positive)
- Axis of ST anterior in the horizontal plane (ST elevated in anterior V leads)

Page: 727

Question #23

Answer: E

Rationale: As a result of the inflammation of the pericardial sac, there is a small current of injury in the subepicardial area, which is oriented toward the front. This current causes an ST displacement with an axis that points downward and forward (i.e., toward the anterior wall of the ventricles).

In some healthy persons, there may be a difference in the sequence of repolarization between the subepicardial and subendocardial areas. As a result, there is an ST displacement that apparently does not have any clinical significance. It may be confused with pericarditis, but there are no signs or symptoms of it.

Page: 728

Questions #24 through #27

Answers: 24, C; 25, D; 26, B; 27, A

Rationale: See the tracings from the text.

Anterior or Anteroseptal

- ST positive in the first or anterior V leads (acute)
- T negative in the first V leads (subacute)
- QS pattern in V_1 and V_2 (i.e., poor R progression [old])

Anterolateral or Superior

- ST negative in the inferior lead aVF (acute)
- T positive in III and possibly in aVL (subacute)
- Q in the lateral leads I and aVL (old)

Apical

- ST positive in I (acute)
- T negative in I (subacute)
- Q in I (old)

Posterior

- ST negative in the first or anterior V leads (acute)
- T positive in the first V leads (subacute)
- R prominent in the first or anterior V leads (old)

Inferior or Diaphragmatic

- ST positive in the inferior leads, II, III, and aVF (acute)
- T negative in II, III, and aVF (subacute)
- Q in II, III, and aVF (old)

Pages: 724, 725, 726

Question #28

Answer: E

Rationale: In cases of a postmyocardial infarction ventricular aneurysm of the anterior or anteroseptal wall, there is an ST displacement that is produced by a difference in the speed of repolarization at the subendocardial and subepicardial areas of the anterior wall. It is not the result of an injury potential.

Criteria for Diagnosis

- Very small or nonexistent ST displacement in the frontal plane
- Axis of ST anterior and prominent ≥2 mm (0.2 mV) in the horizontal plane (ST is elevated in anterior leads)
- Evidence of dead zone effect in anterior wall (very poor R progression or QS pattern in V_1 through V_4 leads)
- History of anterior wall myocardial infarction

Pages: 727, 728

Question #29

Answer: A

Rationale: Causes of prolonged PR interval include the following: (1) first-degree atrioventricular block as result of coronary artery disease, rheumatic fever, or diphtheria (infrequent in the United States); (2) digitalis; and (3) increased vagal tone. Causes of short PR interval include the following: (1) Wolff-Parkinson-White syndrome; (2) other pre-excitation syndromes, especially Lown-Ganong-Levine syndrome; (3) wandering pacemaker; (4) nodal rhythm; and (5) premature atrial beats or contractions.

Page: 731

Question #30

Answer: E

Rationale: The QT interval (electrical systole time) is directly proportional to the duration of the cardiac cycle and inversely proportional to the heart rate. The QT time is shorter than predicted in patients with hyperkalemia and hypercalcemia and in those who are in the early stages of digitalization. It is longer than predicted in patients with hypokalemia and hypocalcemia and in those who are under the influence of quinidine or some psychotropic drugs (especially tricyclic antidepressants and thioridazine).

Another way to determine the normal duration of QT is as follows:

$$QT_c = QT/\sqrt{R\text{-}R}$$

For adults, a QT_c value of more than 0.44 sec is considered abnormal.

There are two rare congenital syndromes of prolonged QT that may occur in families and that may cause episodes of syncope with a special pattern of ventricular tachycardia (torsade des pointes) and sometimes death. The congenital Jervell-Lange-Nielsen syndrome is associated with deafness, whereas while the Romano-Ward syndrome is not.

Page: 732

Question #31

Answer: B

Rationale: The original description of Lown-Ganong-Levine syndrome indicated the occurrence of episodes of supraventricular tachycardia. Subsequently, the diagnosis of this syndrome has been made on the basis of the above criteria, regardless of supraventricular tachycardia. The World Health Organization recommends the term *short PR interval syndrome* rather than *Lown-Ganong-Levine syndrome.*

Criteria for Diagnosis

- Short PR
- Normal P
- No delta (Δ) wave
- Normal QRS
- Normal QT

Page: 734

39 Answers

Question #1

Answer: C

Rationale: The development and progression of atherosclerosis is driven by a variety of risk factors, including dyslipidemia, hypertension, impairments in glycemic control, age, family history, cigarette smoking, obesity, and systemic inflammation.

Page: 735

Question #2

Answer: C

Rationale: Endothelial dysfunction and atherosclerosis development are dynamic processes that encompass a diverse array of biochemical and histological changes. When endothelium is stressed by increased inflammatory or oxidative insult, hyperlipidemia, and hypertension, its functional characteristics change. Dysfunctional endothelium has less vasodilatory capacity; it is more thrombogenic, and it upregulates the expression of a variety of cell adhesion molecules, such as vascular cell adhesion molecule-1 and intercellular adhesion molecule-1.

Page: 735

Question #3

Answer: B

Rationale: In the majority of cases, culprit lesions giving rise to AMI are not flow limiting.

Page: 736

Question #4

Answer: E

Rationale: HDL extracts excess intracellular cholesterol from macrophages and delivers it back to the liver for elimination as bile salts through the gastrointestinal tract in a process referred to as *reverse cholesterol transport*. HDL has also been shown to reduce endothelial cell adhesion molecule expression, to augment endothelial nitric oxide and prostacyclin production, to reduce oxidized LDL, to decrease platelet aggregation, and to

inhibit endothelial cell apoptosis, among other beneficial effects.

Page: 736

Question #5

Answer: D

Rationale: In the Adult Treatment Panel III, the National Cholesterol Education Program also implemented the following conceptual changes: (1) an optimal LDL-C is defined as being less than 100 mg/dL for all patients, independent of race or gender; and (2) an HDL of less than 40 mg/dL is now defined as a categorical risk factor for CAD. LDL-C reduction is the primary goal of therapy for patients with dyslipidemia.

Page: 738

Question #6

Answer: A

Rationale: Based on such trials as the Heart Protection Study,[1] the Treating to New Targets study,[2] and the Pravastatin or Atorvastatin Evaluation and Infection Therapy-Thrombolysis in Myocardial Infarction trial,[3] when it comes to LDL-C reduction and reducing risk for CAD-related morbidity and mortality, "the lower the better."[4] In a recent white paper, the National Cholesterol Education Program recommended that physicians consider treating LDL-C to less than 70 mg/dL and non–HDL-C to less than 100 mg/dL for very-high-risk patients (e.g., a patient with recent ACS or a diabetic with multiple poorly controlled risk factors).

Page: 738

1. Heart Protection Study Collaborative Group: MRC/BHF Heart Protection Study of cholesterol lowering with simvastatin in 20,536 high-risk individuals: A randomised placebo-controlled trial. *Lancet* 360:7–22, 2002.
2. LaRosa JC, Grundy SM, Waters DD, et al: Intensive lipid lowering with atorvastatin in patients with stable coronary disease. *N Engl J Med* 352:1425–1435, 2005.
3. Cannon CP, Braunwald E, McCabe CH, et al, for the Pravastatin or Atorvastatin Evaluation and Infection Therapy—Thrombolysis in Myocardial Infarction 22 Investigators: Comparison of intensive and moderate lipid lowering with statins after acute coronary syndromes. *N Engl J Med* 350:1495–1504, 2004.
4. Toth PP: Low-density lipoprotein reduction in high-risk patients: How low do you go? *Curr Atheroscler Rep* 6:348–352, 2004.

Question #7

Answer D

Rationale: In a large number of prospective, placebo-controlled, clinical trials, the statins have been shown to significantly reduce rates of myocardial infarction, stroke, and coronary and all-cause mortality in the primary and secondary prevention settings. Statins reduce the frequency of stable and unstable angina and decrease atheromatous plaque progression. In addition, on the basis of intravascular ultrasonographic measurements and magnetic resonance imaging, they even stimulate some degree of plaque resorption.

Page: 738

Question #8

Answer: E

Rationale: There is no documented evidence that the statins increase the risk of liver failure. The most important adverse events associated with statin therapy are rhabdomyolysis, myoglobinuria, and renal failure. Mild elevations in serum transaminase levels early during the course of therapy are relatively common, and they usually resolve spontaneously.

Page: 738

Question #9

Answer: F

Rationale: Like the statins, fibrates are associated with a low incidence of myopathy and mild elevations in serum transaminases. Fibrate therapy can increase the risk for cholelithiasis, and it can raise prothrombin times by displacing warfarin from albumin-binding sites.

Page: 740

Question #10

Answer: B

Rationale: Fish-oil capsules enriched with omega-3 (eicosapentaenoic acid) and omega-6 (docosahexaenoic acid) fatty acids can reduce serum triglyceride and very-low-density lipoprotein levels and raise HDL-C in a dose-dependent manner.

Page: 739

Question #11

Answer: D

Rationale: The incidence of hypertension increases as a function of age, and patients who are normotensive at age 55 have a 90% risk of developing hypertension at some point during their lives. For every 20/10 mm Hg increase in blood pressure above 115/75 mm Hg, risk for CVD increases two-fold. Contrary to a widely held misconception in medicine, among patients older than 50 years, the treatment of systolic blood pressure reduces the risk for CVD and renal disease significantly more than the treatment of diastolic blood pressure. Despite the recognized dangers of hypertension and the large number of medications available to treat it, only one third of patients with this disorder are treated to target levels in the United States.

Page: 741

Question #12

Answer: A

Rationale: In response to recent epidemiologic and clinical trial data, "The Seventh Report of the Joint National Committee on Prevention, Detection, Evaluation, and Treatment of High Blood Pressure" made a series of new recommendations for addressing the hypertension epidemic, which now includes more than 50 million patients in the United States alone. Patients with systolic blood pressure of 120 to 139 mm Hg and diastolic blood pressure of 80 to 89 mm Hg are defined as "prehypertensive," and aggressive lifestyle modification is warranted to prevent progression to hypertension. Thiazide diuretics such as hydrochlorothiazide or chlorthalidone, used either alone or in combination with other antihypertensive medications, should be used to treat most patients with hypertension. If the baseline blood pressure reading is more than 20/10 mm Hg above the target level, then initial therapy should consist of two antihypertensive agents (one of which should be a thiazide diuretic, unless there is a contraindication) started simultaneously.

Page: 741

Question #13

Answer: A

Rationale: For patients requiring inhibition of the renin-angiotensin-aldosterone axis (i.e., those with CHF, CAD, postmyocardial infarction, nephropathy, and left ventricular hypertrophy), an elevation in serum creatinine

	Diuretic	BB	Angiotensin-Converting Enzyme Inhibitors	Angiotensin II Receptor Blockers	Calcium-Channel Blockers	AA
Heart failure	✓	✓	✓	✓		✓
Postmyocardial infarction		✓	✓			✓
Coronary artery disease risk	✓	✓	✓		✓	
Diabetes mellitus	✓	✓	✓	✓	✓	
Renal disease			✓	✓		
Recurrent stroke prevention	✓		✓			

In Rakel RE, editor: *Textbook of family medicine,* ed 7, Philadelphia, WB Saunders, 2007.

of up to 35% is tolerable, and it is not an indication for discontinuing an ACEI or an ARB. Men with hypertension and benign prostatic hypertrophy or low serum HDL can be treated with an α-blocking agent.

Page: 742

Question #14

Answer: B

Rationale:

Risk Factor	Defining Level
Abdominal obesity	
Men	Waist >40 inches
Women	Waist >35 inches
Triglycerides	≥150 mg/dL
HDL-C	
Men	<40 mg/dL
Women	<50 mg/dL
Blood pressure	≥130/≥85 mm Hg
Fasting glucose	≥100 mg/dL

In Rakel RE, editor: *Textbook of family medicine,* ed 7, Philadelphia, WB Saunders, 2007.

Page: 745

Question #15

Answer: A

Rationale: Visceral adipose tissue is metabolically highly active. As the mass of visceral adipose tissue increases, adiponectin production decreases, which is associated with increased insulin resistance in adipose tissue, skeletal muscle, and the hepatic parenchyma. Serum levels of free fatty acids rise; this results in both increased triglyceride deposition within the liver (nonalcoholic steatohepatitis or fatty liver) and increased very-low-density lipoprotein secretion, resulting in hypertriglyceridemia.

Page: 746

Question #16

Answer: A

Rationale: Metabolic syndrome should be treated with aggressive lifestyle modification, including weight loss, exercise, smoking cessation, and dietary modification. As shown in the Diabetes Prevention Project, lifestyle modification can reduce risk of the development of diabetes mellitus by 58%.

Page: 747

Question #17

Answer: C

Rationale: Diabetes significantly magnifies the risk for myocardial infarction, sudden death, stroke, CHF, adult-onset blindness, loss of the lower extremities, and end-stage renal disease. Nearly 80% of diabetics will die of cardiovascular disease. Unfortunately, because of increasing obesity and metabolic syndrome among adolescents and young adults, type 2 diabetes is becoming relatively common among those who are less than 21 years old. Diabetics also tend to have hypercoagulability. This hypercoagulability and disordered fibrinolysis increase the likelihood that, if a diabetic experiences acute plaque rupture, it will result in a greater and perhaps a complete vascular luminal obstruction, with acute ischemia and infarction.

Page: 749

Question #18

Answer: C

Rationale: The United Kingdom Prospective Diabetes Study 35 demonstrated that, for every 1% drop in hemoglobin A1c, diabetics experience a 21% reduction in any diabetes-related endpoint, a 14% drop in myocardial infarction, a 12% reduction in stroke, and a 37% reduction in the risk of microvascular disease. In that study, it was shown that metformin therapy reduced the risk for acute cardiovascular events by 38%. Hypertension commonly accompanies diabetes. Diabetic patients require, on average, three or more antihypertensive medications to meet blood-pressure targets. Based on data from the National Health and Nutrition Examination Survey III, 65% to 80% of diabetic men and women—whether white, Hispanic, or black—have either hypertension or a blood pressure level of more than 130/80 mm Hg. Among diabetic hypertensive patients with and without nephropathy, the percentage that reaches blood-pressure goals are 11% and less than 10%, respectively. The Hypertension Optimal Treatment trial evaluated the effect of blood-pressure reduction on cardiovascular event rates among 1501 diabetic patients. Importantly, this trial found no confirmation of the "J-curve" hypothesis (i.e., that the incidence of cardiovascular events increases as diastolic blood pressure decreases as a result of a reduction in coronary perfusion pressure during diastole).

Page: 750

Question #19

Answer: A

Rationale: Among diabetic patients with nephropathy, ACEI and ARBs should be used as first-line therapy, and the drugs should be titrated as tolerated to reduce blood pressure and urinary albumin and protein excretion as much as possible. Among diabetic patients with albuminuria, both ACEIs[5] and ARBs[6] have been shown to reduce the magnitude of albumin excretion and to decrease rates of progression to nephropathy.

Page: 750

Question #20

Answer: B

Rationale: In the Physicians' Health Study, men in the highest quartile of CRP levels had a three-fold higher risk for myocardial infarction over 8 years of evaluation as compared with men in the lowest quartile. Among

women enrolled in the Women's Health Study, an elevated CRP level portends a risk for cardiovascular disease, and it emerged as a better predictor of risk than serum LDL-C. Elevated CRP levels are also associated with increased risk for stroke, metabolic syndrome, and new-onset diabetes mellitus. Patients at low (10-year risk of <5%) and high (CAD, CAD risk equivalent, or 10-year risk of >20%) risk should not be screened for CRP. In the primary prevention setting, the target population consists of patients at moderate risk (10-year risk of 5%–20%). CRP levels of less than 1.0 mg/L, 1.0 to 3.0 mg/L, and more than 3.0 mg/L portend low, intermediate, and high risk for cardiovascular disease.

Page: 751

Question #21

Answer: B

Rationale: Although it is widely assumed that homocysteine is an established risk factor for atherosclerotic disease, there is little prospective clinical trial or epidemiologic evidence to support this. It has been known for decades that patients with homocystinuria have an increased risk for CAD, stroke, peripheral arterial disease, and thromboembolic events. Two clinical trials evaluating folate, B_6, and B_{12} supplementation among patients with CAD and undergoing percutaneous transluminal coronary angioplasty demonstrate the contradictory nature of some of the data in this field. In one study, triple vitamin therapy resulted in reduced rates of atheromatous plaque progression, in-stent restenosis, and the need for subsequent revascularization of the target lesion.[7] In a subsequent study, triple vitamin therapy showed increased rates of plaque progression as well as increased in-stent restenosis and the need for target-lesion revascularization.[8] The American Heart Association and the American College of Cardiology currently discourage widespread screening for hyperhomocysteinemia.

Page: 751

Question #22

Answer: E

Rationale: On an annualized basis, cigarette smoking in the United States incurs more than $159 billion in lost productivity and direct health care costs. Approximately 25.2% of American men and 20.7% of American

5. Heart Outcomes Prevention Evaluation (HOPE) Study Investigators: Effects of ramipril on cardiovascular and microvascular outcomes in people with diabetes mellitus: Results of the HOPE study and MICRO-HOPE Substudy. *Lancet* 355:253–259, 2000.
6. Parving H-H, Lehnert H, Brochner-Mortensen J, et al, for the Irbesartan in Patients with Type 2 Diabetes and Microalbuminuria Study Group: The effect of irbesartan on the development of diabetic nephropathy in patients with type 2 diabetes. *N Engl J Med* 345:870–878, 2001.

7. Schnyder G, Roffi M, Pin R, et al: Decreased rate of coronary restenosis after lowering of plasma homocysteine levels. *N Engl J Med* 345:1593–1600, 2001.
8. Lange H, Suryapranata H, De Luca G, et al: Folate therapy and in-stent restenosis after coronary stenting. *N Engl J Med* 350:2673–2681, 2004.

women are smokers. Smoking is the single most preventable cause of mortality in the United States. Smoking cessation results in a 36% reduction in the risk for myocardial infarction and mortality.[9] Smoking cessation is facilitated by patient education about the dangers of smoking and pharmacologic intervention with nicotine-replacement products and bupropion. Bupropion (Zyban, 150–300 mg orally per day) reduces the intensity of withdrawal symptoms among patients who are trying to quit smoking by inhibiting the neuronal reuptake of norepinephrine, serotonin, and dopamine.

Page: 751

Question #23

Answer: E

Rationale: Coronary supply is determined by oxygen transport capacity and delivery and by conditions that regulate the coronary circulatory system, such as endothelial cell substances (e.g., nitric oxide, endothelin), the autonomic nervous system, metabolic activity, neural control, and perfusion pressure. Most coronary flow occurs during systole, whereas only 25% of flow occurs during diastole.[10–12] As observed among patients with longstanding diabetes, myocardial ischemia can be silent, with no angina reported.

Page: 752

Question #24

Answer: D

Rationale: The electrocardiogram quite often does not show ischemic changes in patients with stable angina who are at rest and who have no symptoms. However, the resting electrocardiogram might show nonspecific ST and T abnormalities in a patient with known severe CAD. False positives are common among patients with left ventricular hypertrophy, digoxin intake, electrolyte imbalances, or electrical conduction anomalies such as bundle branch blocks or pre-excitation syndromes.

Page: 753

Question #25

Answer: B

Rationale: The mean sensitivity of this test is 68%, and the specificity is 77%.[13] Some studies indicate that, when selection bias is removed, the sensitivity can be as low as 40% to 50%, but the specificity may be as high as 85% to 90%.[13–15]

The test specificity is reduced when baseline electrocardiograms are abnormal, with left ventricular hypertrophy, preexcitation syndrome, or a bundle branch block or if the patient is receiving digoxin[16,17] or if he or she has electrolyte abnormalities.[13,18] Also, if a patient cannot reach the target heart rate, the diagnostic accuracy of the test is diminished. If a patient experiences chest pain and 1-mm ST-segment depression during exercise, the test can be 90% predictive of the presence of CAD. A 2-mm ST-segment depression accompanied by chest pain is almost pathognomonic of the presence of obstructive CAD. It should be noted that the presence of anti-ischemic agents (i.e., nitrates, β-blockers and calcium-channel blockers) can reduce the sensitivity of the test; thus, if the intent from the test is to diagnose the presence of obstructive disease, long-acting drugs should be withheld for 2 to 3 days before the procedure, and short-acting drugs should be withheld for 24 hours.[13]

Page: 753

Question #26

Answer: C

Rationale: The absolute contraindications to stress testing are decompensated CHF, symptomatic severe aortic valve stenosis, ongoing chest pain at rest, a recent myocardial infarction (within the past week), severe

9. van Berkel TFM, Boersma H, Roos-Heeselink JW, et al: Impact of smoking cessation and smoking interventions in patients with coronary heart disease. *Eur Heart J* 20:1773–1782, 1999.

10. Verma S, Wang CH, Li SH, et al: A self-fulfilling prophecy: C-reactive protein attenuates nitric oxide production and inhibits angiogenesis. *Circulation* 106:913–919, 2002.

11. Yada T, Richmond KN, Van Bibber R, et al: Role of adenosine in local metabolic coronary vasodilation. *Am J Physiol* 276:H1425–H1433, 1999.

12. Feigl EO: Neural control of coronary blood flow. *J Vasc Res* 35:85–92, 1998.

13. Gibbons RJ, Antman EM, Alpert JS, et al: ACC/AHA 2002 Guideline Update for Exercise Testing. A Report of the American College of Cardiology/American Heart Association Task Force on Practice Guidelines (Committee to Update the 1997 Exercise Testing Guidelines). *Circulation* 106:1883–1892, 2002.

14. Detrano R, Gianrossi R, Froelicher V: The diagnostic accuracy of the exercise electrocardiogram: A meta-analysis of 22 years of research. *Prog Cardiovasc Dis* 32:173–206, 1989.

15. Gianrossi R, Detrano R, Mulvihill D, et al: Exercise induced ST depression in the diagnosis of coronary artery disease: A meta analysis. *Circulation* 80:87–98, 1989.

16. Sundqvist K, Atterhög JH, Jogestrand T: Effect of digoxin on the electrocardiogram at rest and during exercise in healthy subjects. *Am J Cardiol* 57:661–665, 1986.

17. Sketch MH, Mooss AN, Butler ML, et al: Digoxin induced positive exercise tests: Their clinical and prognostic significance. *Am J Cardiol* 48:655–659, 1981.

18. Froelicher VF, Fearon WF, Ferguson CM et al: Lessons learned from studies of the standard exercise ECG test. *Chest* 116:1442–1451, 1999.

hypertension, and intractable arrhythmias. When patients have conditions that reduce the specificity of a stress test, an imaging stress test (nuclear or echocardiographic) can be an alternative, more accurate means by which to evaluate for CAD.

Page: 753

Question #27

Answer: C

Rationale: Myocardial perfusion imaging can be also performed with the induction of pharmacologic stress. Adenosine and dobutamine are the most commonly used pharmacologic agents. Adenosine is a vasodilator, and it stresses the heart by a "steal phenomenon." Adenosine and dipyridamole dilate normal coronaries, shunting blood from abnormal regions of the myocardium and creating a discrepancy in perfusion between normal and abnormal regions. Dobutamine increases heart rate and contractility, and it therefore increases myocardial oxygen demand. Adenosine causes flushing, shortness of breath, nausea, chest pain and a "strange" feeling in most patients; however, this does not reflect the presence of CAD.

Page: 753

Question #28

Answer: E

Rationale: Nitrate therapy reduces myocardial oxygen demand by increasing venous capacitance and, therefore, reducing venous return and ventricular wall stress. In addition, nitrates increase coronary blood supply by dilating the coronary arteries.[19,20] Administering nitrates to patients with stable angina increases their symptom-free walking distance and reduces the frequency and severity of their anginal episodes. Nitrates are not known to significantly reduce risk for myocardial infarction or to prolong survival. β-Blockers reduce myocardial oxygen demand primarily by reducing heart rate and contractility, and they are essential for patients with stable angina and a history of prior myocardial infarction or reduced left ventricular function. In these conditions, β-blockers can prolong survival, and they should be administered

to those patients unless they are absolutely contraindicated.[21] Generally, short-acting calcium blockers need to be avoided, because they could potentially increase adverse events. For high-risk patients, aspirin (81 mg) reduces vascular events by approximately 35%, and it is a prime therapy for patients with stable angina.[22] Aspirin is very effective for the reduction of myocardial infarction among healthy subjects and also for the reduction of elevated serum CRP levels.[23]

Page: 754

Question #29

Answer: A

Rationale: Coronary artery bypass surgery is reserved for patients with the following: (1) left main artery disease or severe three-vessel coronary artery disease, particularly diabetic patients or those with reduced left ventricular function; and (2) unsuitable anatomy for coronary angioplasty or those with disease in multiple bypass grafts, especially if the graft to the left anterior descending coronary artery is involved and can be considered for bypass surgery.

Page: 755

Question #30

Answer: A

Rationale: Several crucial facts need to be considered by the practicing family physician when treating an ACS. First, a large percentage of angiographically "normal" coronaries have significant plaque burden according to intravascular ultrasound or magnetic resonance imaging, particularly in patients over the age of 40 years. Second, more than 60% of myocardial infarctions are induced by culprit lesions that initially obstruct less than 50% of the arterial lumen. These lesions are generally not detected by stress testing. Third, when an ACS occurs, multiple vulnerable plaques generally coexist at the same time throughout the vascular tree. In an inadequately managed patient, any one of these lesions could suddenly rupture and precipitate an ACS.

Page: 755

19. Parker JD, Parker JO: Nitrate therapy for stable angina pectoris. *N Engl J Med* 38:520–531, 1998.
20. Parker JO, Amies MH, Hawkinson RW, et al: Intermittent transdermal nitroglycerin therapy in angina pectoris. Clinically effective without tolerance or rebound. Minitran Efficacy Study Group. *Circulation* 91:1368–1374, 1995.
21. Gottlieb SS, McCarter RJ, Vogel RA: Effect of β-blockade on mortality among high-risk and low-risk patients after myocardial infarction. *N Engl J Med* 339:489–497, 1998.
22. Antiplatelet Trialists' Collaboration: Collaborative overview of randomized trials of antiplatelet therapy: I. Prevention of death, myocardial infarction, and stroke by prolonged antiplatelet therapy in various categories of patients. *BMJ* 308:81–106, 1994.
23. Ridker PM, Cushman M, Stampfer MJ, et al: Inflammation, aspirin, and the risk of cardiovascular disease in apparently healthy men. *N Engl J Med* 336:973–979, 1997.

Acute Pharmacologic Therapy of the Unstable Angina/Non-ST Elevation Myocardial Infarction Supported by Level of Evidence A, American College of Cardiology/American Heart Association Guidelines

---

1. Aspirin (or clopidogrel in patients who cannot take aspirin) should be administered as soon as possible after the onset of symptoms and continued indefinitely.
2. Clopidogrel should be added to aspirin for the hospitalized patient and continued for at least 1 month, whether the patient will be undergoing percutaneous intervention or treated conservatively. Continuing clopidogrel and aspirin for up to 9 months is based on Level B evidence.
3. Antithrombin therapy with unfractionated heparin or low-molecular-weight heparin (preferred over unfractionated heparin, unless bypass surgery is planned within 24 hours) should be started with clopidogrel and aspirin.
4. Glycoprotein IIb/IIIa inhibitors should be added to aspirin, clopidogrel, and antithrombin for patients with planned revascularization or for those with no planned revascularization but with undergoing ischemia or abnormal cardiac biomarkers. However, abciximab should be avoided for patients with no planned revascularization.
5. Fibrinolytics are contraindicated for patients with unstable angina or non–ST-segment elevation myocardial infarction.

From Braunwald E, Antman EM, Beasley JW, et al: ACC/AHA 2002 guideline update for the management of patients with unstable angina and non-ST-segment elevation myocardial infarction: a report of the American College of Cardiology/American Heart Association Task Force on Practice Guidelines (Committee on the Management of Patients With Unstable Angina), *J Am Coll Cardiol* 40:366–374, 2002. In Rakel RE, editor: *Textbook of family medicine*, ed 7, Philadelphia, WB Saunders, 2007.

Question #31

Answer: B

Rationale: A more sensitive and specific marker than myoglobin is creatine kinase and its cardiac isoform, creatine kinase, myocardial bound. This marker is 90% accurate for the diagnosis of myocardial infarction at 6 hours from symptom onset. Creatine kinase reaches its peak within about 24 hours of symptom onset, and it returns to normal or near normal by 72 hours.

Page: 756

Question #32

Answer: D

Rationale: See the box at the top of the page.

Page: 756

Question #33

Answer: D

Rationale: Plaque rupture is the predominant mechanism of ST elevation myocardial infarction, with subsequent platelet and fibrin deposition. It is estimated that there are half a million ST elevation myocardial infarctions in the United States every year. Current guidelines indicate that a patient with symptoms and signs of ST elevation myocardial infarction should receive either thrombolytics within 30 minutes or angioplasty within 90 minutes of arrival to the emergency room[24]. Currently, angioplasty is considered the first choice of therapy, because it leads to overall superior results[25], primarily reducing the rate of nonfatal myocardial infarction and resulting in fewer intracranial bleeds as compared with thrombolysis.

Page: 756

Question #34

Answer: C

Rationale: Irrespective of the injury precipitating CHF, neurohormonal mechanisms are activated, and they promote the remodeling process. These include the renin-angiotensin-aldosterone system and the sympathetic nervous system. A rise in endothelin-1 production, which is a product of dysfunctional endothelium, also occurs and contributes to vasoconstriction. In addition, inflammatory markers and cytokines are increased, thereby further exacerbating endothelial dysfunction.[26,27]

---

24. Antman EM, Anbe DT, Armstrong PW et al: ACC/AHA guidelines for the management of patients with ST-elevation myocardial infarction—executive summary. A report of the American College of Cardiology/American Heart Association Task Force on Practice Guidelines (Writing Committee to revise the 1999 guidelines for the management of patients with acute myocardial infarction). *J Am Coll Cardiol* 44:671–719, 2004.
25. Magid DJ, Calonge BN, Rumsfeld JS, et al, for the National Registry of Myocardial Infarction 2 and 3 Investigators: Relation between hospital primary angioplasty volume and mortality for patients with acute MI treated with primary angioplasty vs thrombolytic therapy. *JAMA* 284:3131–3138, 2000.
26. Francis GS: Neurohumoral activation and progression of heart failure: Hypothetical and clinical considerations. *J Cardiovasc Pharmacol* 32: S16–S21, 1998.
27. Blum A, Miller H: Pathophysiological role of cytokines in congestive heart failure. *Annu Rev Med* 52:15–27, 2001.

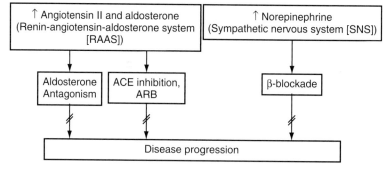

Figure 39-1 In Rakel RE, editor: *Textbook of family medicine,* ed 7, Philadelphia, WB Saunders, 2007.

Pharmacologic interventions that block neurohormonal activation can reduce mortality and morbidity in patients with CHF.

A rise in angiotensin II promotes programmed cell death (apoptosis), hypertrophy, and fibrosis. Angiotensin II also causes an increase in aldosterone secretion (Figure 39-1). This in turn augments the harmful effects of angiotensin II on the myocardium, and it promotes adverse remodeling. A rise in the circulating levels of catecholamines in response to the activation of the sympathetic nervous system can lead to the suppression of adrenergic receptors,[28] and it has direct toxic effects on the myocardium.[29] Catecholamines mediate toxicity as a result of the β-adrenoceptor-mediated cyclic adenosine monophosphate-dependent calcium overload of cardiac myocytes (Figure 39-2).[30]

Page: 759

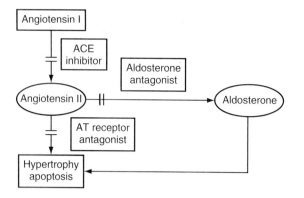

Figure 39-2 In Rakel RE, editor: *Textbook of family medicine,* ed 7, Philadelphia, WB Saunders, 2007.

28. Bristow MR: Changes in myocardial and vascular receptors in heart failure. *J Am Coll Cardiol* 22:61A–71A, 1993.

29. Mann DL, Kent RL, Parsons B, Cooper G 4th: Adrenergic effects on the biology of the adult mammalian cardiocyte. *Circulation* 85:790–804, 1992.

30. Mann DL: Basic mechanisms of disease progression in the failing heart: The role of excessive adrenergic drive. *Prog Cardiovasc Dis* 41:1–8, 1998.

Question #35

Answer: E

Rationale: Patients with CHF should have their cardiovascular risk factors aggressively modified. Hypertension is strongly linked to the development of CHF, and it should be very aggressively treated.[31] The target blood pressure should be less than 130/85 mm Hg, except among diabetics, in whom the target is lowered to less than 125/85 mm Hg. Control of dyslipidemia and diabetes is also very important for the management of patients with CHF. [32]Screening for sleep apnea and thyroid disease and aggressively treating these conditions needs to be done. The avoidance of alcohol, illicit drug use, and smoking is strongly advised. Losing weight and establishing a routine exercise program are also important preventative measures for the CHF patient to take.

Pages: 759, 780

Question #36

Answer: B

Rationale: There are no data to support that diuretics or digoxin alter a patient's long-term survival. ACEIs reduce mortality by an absolute 4% and a relative 15% to 20% among patients with left ventricular systolic dysfunction (i.e., an ejection fraction of <40%).[32] β-Blockers have been shown to reduce mortality by approximately 35% when added to ACEIs in mild to moderate CHF (MERIT-HF with metoprolol succinate, U.S. Carvedilol trials with carvedilol and CIBIS-II trial

31. Vasan RS, Levy D: The role of hypertension in the pathogenesis of heart failure. A clinical mechanistic overview. *Arch Intern Med* 156 (16):1789–1796, 1996.

32. The Randomized Aldactone Evaluation Study, Pitt (1999).

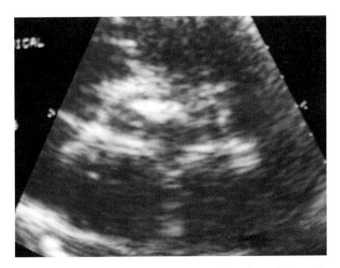

Figure 39-3 In Rakel RE, editor: *Textbook of family medicine,* ed 7, Philadelphia, WB Saunders, 2007.

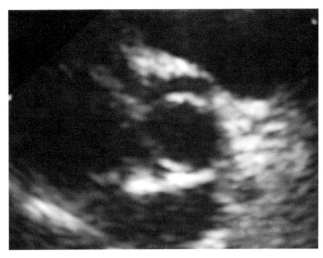

Figure 39-4 In Rakel RE, editor: *Textbook of family medicine,* ed 7, Philadelphia, WB Saunders, 2007.

with bisoprolol)[33–35] or in very advanced CHF (Copernicus trial with carvedilol).[36] β-Blockers also reduce hospitalizations by 33% to 38%,[33,34,37] and they work in synergy with ACEIs to reduce cardiac remodeling, to reduce cavity size, and to improve ejection fraction.[38] Patients with advanced CHF and ejection fractions of less than 35% may receive spironolactone 25 mg daily or placebo in addition to standard therapy. After a mean follow-up period of 24 months, spironolactone reduced mortality by 30% as a result of the reduction of the progression of CHF and sudden cardiac death.

Page: 762

Question #37

Answer: C

Rationale: Aortic valvular stenosis is the most common valvular abnormality in the United States. It

can be congential, rheumatic, or calcific/degenerative. Calcific aortic valve stenosis (Figure 39-3) is most prevalent among patients who are more than 70 years old, whereas congenital, mostly bicuspid valve disease (Figure 39-4) is more common among younger patients. As disease progresses, left ventricular mass increases, and diastolic dysfunction becomes evident, with an increase in left ventricular filling pressure. Myocardial oxygen demand typically increases, and, even in the absence of CAD, patients may experience angina.

Page: 764

Question #38

Answer: B

Rationale: Patients with severe aortic valve stenosis describe progressive dyspnea, chest pain, and syncope with exertion, and symptoms of CHF, including orthopnea, paroxysmal nocturnal dyspnea, and edema. Syncope at rest is typically induced by arrhythmia.

Page: 764

Question #39

Answer: C

Rationale: Surgery is typically not advisable for patients with asymptomatic severe valvular stenosis. Patients with dyspnea and with an indication of progressive left ventricular dysfunction need to be considered

33. Packer M, Bristow MR, Cohn JN, et al: The effect of carvedilol on morbidity and mortality in patients with chronic heart failure. US Carvedilol Heart Failure Study Group. *N Engl J Med* 334:1349–1355, 1996.
34. MERIT-HF Study Group: Effect of metoprolol CR/XL in chronic heart failure: Metoprolol CR/XL Randomised Intervention Trial in Congestive Heart Failure (MERIT-HF). *Lancet* 253:2001–2007, 1999.
35. CIBIS-II Investigators: The Cardiac Insufficiency Bisoprolol Study II (CIBISII): A randomised trial. *Lancet* 353:9–13, 1999.
36. Packer M, Coats AJ, Fowler MB, et al; Carvedilol Prospective Randomized Cumulative Survival Study Group: Effect of carvedilol on survival in severe chronic heart failure. *N Engl J Med* 344:1651–1658, 2001.
37. Fowler MB, Vera-Llonch M, Oster G, et al: Influence of carvedilol on hospitalizations in heart failure: Incidence, resource utilization and costs. U.S. Carvedilol Heart Failure Study Group. *J Am Coll Cardiol* 37:1692–1699, 2001.
38. Remme WJ, Riegger G, Hildebrandt P et al: The benefits of early combination treatment of carvedilol and an ACE-inhibitor in mild heart failure and left ventricular systolic dysfunction. The carvedilol and ACE-inhibitor remodeling mild heart failure evaluation trial (CARMEN). *Cardiovasc Drugs Ther* 18:57–66, 2004.

for valve replacement. Most patients with asymptomatic and severe aortic valve stenosis will, however, develop symptoms within 5 years of follow-up. Aortic valvuloplasty carries a poor outcome, and it is reserved as a palliative therapy for inoperable patients. Aortic valve surgery with or without coronary artery bypass grafting is the treatment of choice.[39,40] Aortic valve replacement can be performed with a mechanical valve or a tissue valve, depending on the clinical situation. For instance, patients who have a contraindication to anticoagulation with warfarin should receive a bioprosthetic valve. These valves typically do not require anticoagulation with warfarin, and patients are generally put only on an aspirin subsequent to the procedure. Patients in their 60s or 70s with no contraindication to Coumadin are best served with mechanical valves, because these last longer and hopefully will obviate the need for another valve surgery in the future.

Page: 765

Question #40

Answer: C

Rationale: Mitral stenosis is defined as the reduced ability of the blood to move from the left atrium to the left ventricle during diastole. It is mostly caused by dysfunction in the mitral valve, which lacks the ability to open its leaflets during diastole. Mitral valve stenosis (see below) is predominantly caused by rheumatic carditis, and it is more prevalent among females.[41] The main symptom of mitral valve stenosis is slowly progressive dyspnea and fatigue. In patients with advanced mitral valve stenosis, left atrial pressure and a redistribution of blood to the chest occur. Patients may complain of orthopnea and paroxysmal nocturnal dyspnea. Pulmonary hypertension can become severe, and right-sided ventricular failure can then lead to dependent edema, hepatomegaly, and right-upper-quadrant pain. (See Figure 39-5.)

Page: 766

39. Schwarz F, Baumann P, Manthey J, et al: The effect of aortic valve replacement on survival. *Circulation* 66:1105–1110, 1982.
40. Lund O: Preoperative risk evaluation and stratification of long-term survival after valve replacement for aortic stenosis: reasons for earlier operative intervention. *Circulation* 82:124–139, 1990.
41. Bonow RO, Carabello B, de Leon AC Jr, et al: Guidelines for the management of patients with valvular heart disease: Executive summary. A report of the American College of Cardiology/American Heart Association Task Force on Practice Guidelines (Committee on Management of Patients with Valvular Heart Disease). *Circulation* 98:1949–1984, 1998.

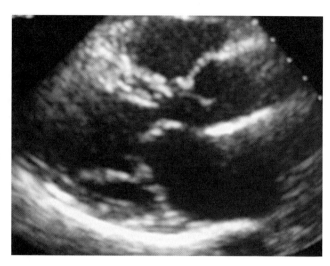

Figure 39-5   In Rakel RE, editor: *Textbook of family medicine*, ed 7, Philadelphia, WB Saunders, 2007.

Question #41

Answer: D

Rationale: All patients with rheumatic mitral valve disease require bacterial endocarditis prophylaxis before dental, genitourinary, or gastrointestinal procedures. Increasing diastolic filling time is important for the treatment of moderate to severe mitral valve stenosis; therefore, drugs such as β-blockers or verapamil may be used. Patients with atrial fibrillation need to be aggressively treated with rate control and anticoagulation with warfarin to reduce embolic strokes.

Page: 766

Question #42

Answer: D

Rationale: On examination, patients with mitral regurgitation will display a systolic murmur that is most often holosystolic, high-pitched, and present at the apex, with radiation to the axilla, the left scapula, the mid back, or the left sternal border, depending on the direction of the regurgitant jet. The chest x-ray may show an enlarged cardiac silhouette, a calcified mitral valve, or increased pulmonary vascular congestion. Patients might provide a history of rheumatic fever, endocarditis, coronary artery disease, or CHF. A lower threshold for surgical intervention is generally agreed upon as compared with AR. Intervention should occur among symptomatic patients (NYHC II-IV) or asymptomatic patients with a left ventricular end-systolic dimension approaching 4.5 cm or a left ventricular ejection fraction of 60% or less.

Page: 769

Question #43

Answer: A

Rationale: Although it has previously been thought that strokes occur more frequently among patients with mitral valve prolapse, recent data do not support this conclusion.[42] Asymptomatic patients with mitral valve prolapse generally do not require treatment, unless they have severe associated mitral regurgitation.[43] A high-pitched, mid-systolic click is often heard that occurs shortly after the first heart sound, and it can be associated with a systolic murmur.

Page: 768

Question #44

Answer: A

Rationale: Atherosclerotic peripheral vascular disease (PVD) is an underdiagnosed, undertreated, age-dependent disease that has a profound impact on patient quality of life, and it is an independent predictor of mortality.[44–47] On average, the mortality rate of claudicant patients is 2.5 times higher than that of non-claudicant patients.

Page: 769

Question #45

Answer: B

Rationale: Intermittent claudication is only a symptom of peripheral vascular disease (PVD), and it can be misleading for measuring the prevalence of PVD. For example, a patient with advanced PVD may not have significant IC as a result of functional decline and inactivity, whereas someone who is very active may have significant IC, even if he or she has only mild disease. More than 50% of patients with PVD are asymptomatic, and they may only be identified by noninva-

sive testing, such as the ABI. The fate of the amputee is poor, particularly among the elderly. The level of amputation also dictates the overall prognosis: although two to three times as many below-the-knee amputees achieve full mobility as compared with above-the-knee amputees, the initial rehabilitation may take up to 9 months.

Page: 769

Question #46

Answer: F

Rationale: The prevalence of PVD increases with age. The incidence of IC in five large population–based studies is four times higher and the prevalence is eight times higher comparing the 35- to 39-year-old age group to the 70- to 74-year-old age group.[48] Smoking is a very strong independent cause of atherosclerotic PVD. The severity of PVD increases with the number of cigarettes smoked.[49,50] Diabetes/glucose intolerance is one of the most powerful independent modifiable risk factors that contributes to the development of PVD, IC, and CLI.[51–53] As in CAD, low-density lipoprotein cholesterol (LDL-C) and triglyceride levels are directly related, whereas high-density lipoprotein cholesterol (HDL-C) levels are indirectly related to the progression of PVD, and the observed risk seems to demonstrate a linear relationship.[52,54] Hypertension is a major risk factor for PVD and carries a 2.5-fold age-adjusted risk for men and a 3.9-fold age-adjusted risk for women.[51,55]

Page: 769

Question #47

Answer: B

42. Gilon D, Buonanno FS, Joffe MM, et al: Lack of evidence of an association between mitral-valve prolapse and stroke in young patients. *N Engl J Med* 341:8–13, 1999.
43. Devereux RB, Kramer-Fox R, Kligfield P: Mitral valve prolapse: Causes, clinical manifestations, and management. *Ann Intern Med* 111:305–317, 1989.
44. Criqui MH, Langer RD, Fronek A, et al: Mortality over a period of 10 years in patients with peripheral arterial disease. *N Engl J Med* 326:381–386, 1992.
45. Vogt MT, Cauley JA, Newman AB, et al: Decreased ankle/arm blood pressure index and mortality in elderly women. *JAMA* 270:465–469, 1993.
46. Vogt MT, McKenna M, Anderson SJ, et al: The relationship between anklearm index and mortality in older men and women. *J Am Geriatr Soc* 41:523–530, 1993.
47. Nikolsky E, Mehran R, Dangas GD, et al: Prognostic significance of cerebrovascular and peripheral arterial disease in patients having percutaneous coronary intervention. *Am J Cardiol* 93:1536–1539, 2004.
48. Dormandy JA, Rutherford DB: Management of peripheral arterial disease (PAD). TASC Working Group. TransAtlantic Inter-Society Consensus (TASC). *J Vasc Surg* 31(1 Pt 2):S1–S296, 2000.
49. Powell JT, Edwards RJ, Worrell PC, et al: Risk factors associated with the development of peripheral arterial disease in smokers: a case-control study. *Atherosclerosis* 129(1):41–48, 1997.
50. Cronenwett JL, Warner KG, Zelenock GB, et al: Intermittent claudication. Current results of nonoperative management. *Arch Surg* 119(4):430–436, 1984.
51. Murabito JM, D'Agostino RB, Silbershatz H, Wilson WF: Intermittent claudication. A risk profile from The Framingham Heart Study, *Circulation* 96(1):44–49, 1997.
52. Fowkes FG, Housley E, Riemersma RA, et al: Smoking, lipids, glucose intolerance, and blood pressure as risk factors for peripheral atherosclerosis compared with ischemic heart disease in the Edinburgh Artery Study, *Am J Epidemiol* 135(4):331–340, 1992.
53. Kannel WB, McGee DL: Diabetes and cardiovascular disease. The Framingham study. *JAMA* 241(19):2035–2038, 1979.
54. Murabito JM, Evans JC, Nieto K, et al: Prevalence and clinical correlates of peripheral arterial disease in the Framingham Offspring Study. *Am Heart J* 143(6):961–965, 2002.
55. Kannel WB, McGee DL: Epidemiology of sudden death: insights from the Framingham Study. *Cardiovasc Clin* 15(3):93–105, 1985.

Rationale: Approximately 40% of patients with atherosclerotic vascular disease manifest symptoms in more than one vascular bed. The all-cause mortality rate among patients with PVD is approximately equal between men and women, and it is elevated even among asymptomatic patients. The lower the ABI, the greater the risk for cardiovascular events. Patients with critical limb ischemia, who typically have the lowest ABIs, have an annual mortality rate of 25%.

Page: 769

Question #48

Answer: B

Rationale: A classical description of nocturnal pain from critical limb ischemia is a moderate to severe aching paresthesia/dysesthesia while lying horizontally that is alleviated by dangling the leg over the side of the bed. Observations should note any asymmetry between the limbs, joint deformities, varicose veins, skin discoloration, absence of hair, swelling, ulcerations, tissue loss, and gangrene. A cadaveric pallor upon elevating the limb to more than 45 degrees above the horizontal plane for 1 to 2 minutes followed by slow venous filling with rubor after returning to a dependent position (Buerger's sign) is also a sign of advanced critical limb ischemia.

Page: 770

Question #49

Answer: A

Rationale: Not uncommonly, patients with mild PVD may have an ABI that is actually normal at rest. However, it may be significantly decreased with exercise.

Page: 769

Question #50

Answer: C

Rationale: Even a mildly depressed resting ABI implies there is a considerable burden of disease. Therefore, ABIs that are performed at rest only and not with exercise will have a relatively high false-negative rate, and many patients with a normal resting ABI will be misdiagnosed as having nonvascular limb pain when indeed the true etiology of their discomfort is PVD. A corollary to this is that many epidemiological studies use only resting ABIs as a diagnostic criteria for PVD, which leads to the underestimation of the true incidence of PVD. Another potential pitfall of ABIs

is vascular calcification. Severe calcification of the arterial wall eventually leads to an inability to compress the blood vessels, despite cuffs that are inflated to suprasystolic pressures; this is particularly common among patients with diabetes and among those undergoing chronic hemodialysis.

Page: 769

Question #51

Answer: B

Rationale: Routine aerobic exercise is recommended for all patients with PVD. The benefit of walking programs has been clearly established to increase time-to-claudication and maximal walking distance. The four primary categories of pharmacologic therapy are as follows: (1) antiplatelet therapy; (2) lipid-lowering therapy; (3) antihypertensive therapy; and (4) glycemic-lowering therapy. Specific therapies and therapeutic targets are listed elsewhere in this chapter. It should be kept in mind that these therapies are complementary and that they confer additive benefit. Pentoxifylline (Trental) is a drug that was approved by the U.S. Food and Drug Administration for claudication in 1984. However, there are no randomized data that demonstrate it to be any better than placebo. Therefore, there is no recommendation to use this agent for the treatment of claudication. Peripheral arterial revascularization is indicated for the relief of ischemic symptoms, including intermittent claudication and resting ischemic pain, and it is also recommended for limb preservation in the setting of critical limb ischemia.

Page: 778

Question #52

Answer: A

Rationale: Arising in the right atrium in the superior septal aspect at the junction of the lateral margin of the superior vena cava with the right atrium and the atrial appendage, the sinoatrial node extends laterally into the crista terminalis. The atrioventricular node lies at the apex of the triangle of Koch, and the distal portion of the atrioventricular node becomes the bundle of His.

Page: 781

Question #53

Answer: A

Rationale: Sinus bradycardia originates in the sinus node with a P wave that is indistinguishable from the normal sinus beat but that is at a rate slower than the established lower limit of 60 bpm. This is physiologically normal in patients during sleep, in athletic individuals, and as a consequence of many adrenergic-blocking drugs, such as β-blockers.

Page: 782

Question #54

Answer: B

Rationale: The electrocardiogram findings of atrial fibrillation are the absence of organized atrial activity with an irregular, usually rapid ventricular response. Atria are depolarized from widespread regions of both the left and right atriums, and this results in chaotic activation at rates exceeding several hundred beats per minute.

Page: 785

Question #55

Answer: C

Rationale: First-degree atrioventricular block is demonstrated as a PR interval of more than 200 msec. Type 1 second-degree atrioventricular block is characterized by a progressive prolongation of the PR interval followed by failure to conduct and depolarize the ventricle. Type 2 second-degree atrioventricular block is the abrupt failure of conduction through the AV node and the absence of a QRS complex. The PR intervals should be similar both before and after block. Third-degree atrioventricular block results from the failure of atrial impulses from the sinus node to conduct down to the ventricle.

Page: 788

Question #56

Answer: E

Rationale: Long QT syndrome, which is a disorder of myocardial repolarization, occurs as a result of abnormalities in membrane ion channels. Syncope and life-threatening polymorphous ventricular tachycardia and fibrillation may result. Autosomal-dominant inheritance patterns and variable phenotypic penetrance may be seen. Diagnosis in affected individuals is difficult, because the QT interval may occasionally be normal. Provocative maneuvers by a trained specialist may be necessary. Genetic testing for some (but not all) of the genetic abnormalities is available for confirmation.

Families with a history of sudden cardiac death or syncope should be evaluated carefully to determine the need for treatment, including β-blockers and implantable defibrillators.

Page: 788

Question #57

Answer: B

Rationale: In the AFFIRM trial, patients randomized to rhythm control had more hospitalizations and adverse drug effects, which were mostly related to antiarrhythmic drug therapy. Among patients undergoing the restoration of sinus rhythm, the use of direct current cardioversion is safe and effective. Anticoagulation with an international normalized ratio goal of 2 to 3 in nonvalvular atrial fibrillation is recommended for a minimum of 3 weeks before a cardioversion.

Page: 789

Question #58

Answer: D

Rationale: Patients with refractory clinical CHF have a 6- to 9-fold increase in sudden cardiac death as compared with the general population. The placement of a pacing device capable of pacing in the right ventricle and additionally at the lateral left ventricle has resulted in significant reductions in both morbidity and mortality. The addition of a defibrillator results in the further reduction of the mortality rate.

Pages: 795, 796

Question #59

Answer: D

Rationale: Studies have demonstrated a mortality benefit from implantable defibrillators as compared with drug therapy in primary prevention trials. Specific groups of patients have demonstrated the superiority of device therapy as compared with drugs: (1) patients with asymptomatic ventricular ectopy with inducible ventricular tachycardia; (2) patients with prior myocardial infarction and ejection fractions of less than 30%; and (3) patients with ejection fractions of less than 35% with New York Heart Association class II or III heart failure of more than 3 months.

Pages: 796, 797

40 Answers

Question #1

Answer: B

Rationale: Myoglobin released from damaged muscle can induce renal failure. The intratubular precipitation of myoglobin pigments causes tubular injury. Vigorous hydration, along with the addition of bicarbonate to the fluid, protects the kidneys. Urine will test positive for hemoglobin, and a definitive test for myoglobin is needed. Fasciotomy is required for compartment syndrome.

Page: 813

Question #2

Answer: D

Rationale: Poor tissue perfusion results in the failure to meet the metabolic requirements of the tissue, ischemia, and the accumulation of toxic byproducts. Hypoperfusion may be the result of many causes: fluid loss, pump failure, sepsis, anaphylaxis, spinal cord trauma, and medications.

Page: 818

Question #3

Answer: C

Rationale: Diagnostic peritoneal lavage is a useful—although invasive—test for free blood within the peritoneal cavity. It does not assess the retroperitoneal space, and it is not a replacement for the physical examination or clinical assessment of the patient. The trauma patient who is hemodynamically unstable requires active resuscitation, and diagnostic peritoneal lavage should only be performed when definitive treatment is within the capabilities of the institution. Therefore, diagnostic peritoneal lavage should only be performed when considering the need for exploratory laparotomy.

Pages: 812–813

Question #4

Answer: A

Rationale: Children are able to maintain their blood pressure despite significant blood loss (up to 25%–30%), at which point they may acutely decompensate. The high ratio of surface area to body volume makes hypothermia a major risk when treating pediatric trauma. The disproportionate size of the cranium, as well as the immature musculature and the lean body habitus, makes the risk of multisystem injury more significant. Oral intubation is the most reliable means of airway management.

Page: 814

Question #5

Answer: C

Rationale: Endotracheal tubes are preferred for airway stabilization. Cuffed endotracheal tubes are rarely needed for children who are less than 12 years old. The use of cuffed tubes increases the risk of subglottic edema and scarring.

Page: 814

Question #6

Answer: D

Rationale: The best care for the fetus is the proper care and resuscitation of the mother. Pregnancy does not preclude the need for a complete primary and secondary survey; however, special attention does need to be paid to the gravid patient. The administration of fluids and oxygen and the placement of the patient in the left lateral decubitus position are appropriate. Kleihauer-Betke testing is useful for assessing the degree of fetal-maternal hemorrhage in Rh-negative patients. Fetal heart rate should be assessed as a measure of uteroplacental function and fetal oxygenation.

Page: 815

Question #7

Answer: D

Rationale: Although many surgical techniques related to trauma are based on military experience, aggressive management and resuscitation in the emergency department were not fully developed until the 1970s. Unfortunately, the majority of traumas occur in patients who are less than 45 years old, with disability exceeding death by a factor of three. The death rate from trauma is approximately 150,000 annually.

Page: 802

Question #8

Answer: B

Rationale: Despite the desire to immediately address what appears to be the most obvious injury in the trauma patient, control of the airway is the single most important task for resuscitation. The primary ABCDE survey should be initiated, and this should be followed by the orderly identification and simultaneous treatment of the most lethal injuries.

Page: 808

Question #9

Answer: D

Rationale: Emergency assessment of the gravid female includes assessment of the fetus. The abdominal examination is useful to determine a sense of due date (if unknown), contractions, fetal movement, and localization and assessment of pain or tenderness. Fetal heart rate provides an assessment of fetal oxygenation. The sterile speculum examination allows the physician to visualize the cervix, note any fluid (i.e., clear, mucous, or bloody), and obtain specimens for pH and ferning. Although fetal ultrasound can be valuable for assessing position, placental location, amniotic fluid status, and fetal well-being, it is not generally part of the initial screening.

Page: 815

Question #10

Answer: B

Rationale: High-pressure injection injuries can result in infection, inflammatory reaction, and compromise of tissue perfusion. Digital block may worsen tissue perfusion by increasing tissue pressure. Early consultation and aggressive treatment are recommended. Imaging can prove useful for assessing the spread of injury.

Page: 816

Question #11

Answer: D

Rationale: Traumatic dislocation of a joint in close proximity to major vascular structures raises the question of occult vascular injury. In addition to detailed physical examination (including neurologic status and distal pulses), angiography is useful to assess the vascular structures.

Pages: 813

Question #12

Answer: D

Rationale: The Trendelenburg position is contraindicated because of possible increases in intracranial pressure. Decompression sickness affects the gases in the hollow and viscous organs as well as the gases dissolved in the blood. During ascent, gas bubbles may be liberated faster than the lungs can clear them. Failure to equalize pressure in the noncompressible spaces may result in pain and tissue damage.

Page: 831–832

Question #13

Answer: B

Rationale: Neurologic examination does not exclude a cervical spine injury. Protection of the spine and spinal cord is important for the management of trauma patients. Stabilization should be maintained until lateral neck films are obtained. If the patient exhibits mental status changes, assume a cervical injury until it is proven otherwise. If unable to obtain definitive radiographs, computed tomography scanning can be useful.

Page: 808

Question #14

Answer: D

Rationale: Patients with closed head injuries may have a lucid interval followed by neurologic decompensation. Prior to completing a secondary survey or progressing to advanced tests such as CTs, it may be necessary to return to the primary survey and to confirm that the patient has a secure airway, adequate ventilation and oxygenation, and adequate cerebral perfusion.

Pages: 808–809

Question #15

Answer: B

Rationale: Head injury may induce the Cushing reflex with resulting bradycardia and hypertension. The symptoms presented are more likely associated with hypovolemia due to acute hemorrhage, or hypotension from inflammatory mediated vasodilatation, capillary leakage seen in sepsis anaphylaxis. Sepsis is associated with DIC and anaphylaxis with mast cell degranulation.

Page: 821

Question #16

Answer: A

Rationale: Cardiogenic shock, most commonly seen with acute myocardial infarction, results in a reduction in the cardiac output, causing elevated central venous pressure and a reflex increased systemic vascular resistance and narrow pulse pressure.

Page: 860

Question #17

Answer: D

Rationale: The most common fibinolytic disorder is DIC. It can be caused by many processes including sepsis, trauma, cancer and infection. Treatment of DIC is focused on treatment of the underlying disease or process. This can be followed by replacement of coagulation factors (platelet, fresh frozen plasma, and perhaps cryoprecipitate transfusions) and even heparin therapy if there is significant thrombosis.

Page: 861

Question #18

Answer: A

Rationale: Urine output is a key indicator of fluid status. Placement of a Foley catheter is an inexpensive and easy method of visualizing urine production while eliminating any chance of mechanical obstruction to flow. Central lines and catheters are not routinely used in the initial management of shock.

Page: 819

Question #19

Answer: B

Rationale: Initial fluid replacement in the patient with an isotonic electrolyte solution. Crystalloid solutions include normal saline and lactated Ringer's solution. Albumin containing solutions are colloid solutions.

Free water is hypotonic. Blood is reserved for anemic patients who fail fluid resuscitation.

Page: 819

Question #20

Answer: A

Rationale: Synthetic monofilament (nylon) poses the least risk of surgical infection. In addition, nonabsorbable sutures are less reactive, and they may provide a better-appearing scar. Wounds closed with woven sutures are more susceptible to infection because of the possibility of bacteria being trapped in the weave.

Page: 822

Question #21

Answer: D

Rationale: The management of poisoning requires stabilization of the patient, starting with the airway. Poisoning patients can present with altered mental status, respiratory depression, metabolic derangement, and cardiac problems, all of which can affect proper ventilation. After the patient has been stabilized/resuscitated, definitive diagnosis and treatment can begin.

Page: 823

Question #22

Answer: C

Rationale: Although acetaminophen poisoning does have nonspecific gastrointestinal symptoms early during its course, followed by right-upper-quadrant pain, most damage is done during the third stage of poisoning, which occurs between 48 and 96 hours after ingestion. At this time, liver enzymes (serum aspartate aminotransferase/serum alanine aminotransferase) often rise to levels of more than 10,000; this may result in fulminant hepatic failure and death.

Page: 825

Question #23

Answers: C and D

Rationale: Acetaminophen is the most commonly reported pharmaceutical overdose. Treatment includes supportive care and gastrointestinal decontamination with charcoal. An acetaminophen level should be drawn a minimum of 4 hours after ingestion and applied to the Rumack-Matthew nomogram to determine if Mucomyst is indicated. The nomogram is based on a known time of ingestion. If the time is in question, serial levels may need to be drawn.

Page: 825

Question #24

Answer: D

Rationale: Toxic overdose with the tricyclic antidepressants requires cardiac monitoring as a result of the slowing of conduction, the widening of the QRS, the prolonged QT, and the potential for torsades de pointes and other arrhythmias. Serum levels are generally not helpful; the patient is followed clinically and monitored. Treatment is supportive, with gastrointestinal decontamination and alkalinization of the urine.

Page: 825

Question #25

Answer: A

Rationale: The body surface area method of evaluating the extent of a burn is only used for adults, and it is only calculated for individuals with second- or third-degree burns.

Page: 827

Question #26

Answer: A

Rationale: Although all of these burns require evaluation and may be very painful, the circumferential burn poses a risk of compartment syndrome, with secondary distal ischemia as well as a loss of function. Electrical burns of more significance can result in cardiac disturbances and rhabdomyolysis.

Page: 828

Question #27

Answer: B

Rationale: In the United States, normally behaving domestic dogs and cats, rodents, squirrels, hamsters, and rabbits do not usually transmit rabies. However, patients bitten by bats, coyotes, foxes, opossums, or skunks require rabies immunoglobulin and rabies vaccine. Dog, cat, and human bites generally require empiric antibiotics as well as the evaluation of tetanus status.

Page: 830

Question #28

Answer: D

Rationale: Augmentin provides excellent cover for *Staphylococcus* and *Streptococcus* species, *Pasteurella multocida*, and *Eikenella corrodens*; in addition, it is cost effective and readily available. Gentamicin and vancomycin are given intravenously, and they are not good choices for the ambulatory setting. Levaquin is a fluoroquinolone, and it is not suitable for children.

Page: 830

41 Answers

Question #1

Answer: C

Rationale: Detecting life-threatening or disabling medical conditions is the primary goal of the pre-participation physical examination.

Page: 835

Question #2

Answer: B

Rationale: Syncope during exercise and not after is a very concerning event and should be worked up. All diastolic murmurs and any murmur that increases with the Valsalva maneuver should also be evaluated. Chest pain on exertion can be a sign of heart disease and should be evaluated.

Page: 836

Question #3

Answer: B

Rationale: Despite several studies conducted in the United States using an electrocardiogram and/or echocardiography during the athletic screening of high school and college athletes, no definitive cases of a lethal cardiovascular abnormality were found.

Page: 836

Question #4

Answer: B

Rationale: Tachyarrhythmias in the athlete are abnormal, and they require further evaluation and treatment before the patient participates in strenuous exercise. Ventricular arrhythmias are particularly life threatening, and they usually occur in the presence of a structural heart problem.

Page: 837

Question #5

Answer: B

Rationale: Commotio cordis is most common among younger athletes (<13 years) because of more compliant chest walls. The most common cause of cardiac death among individuals who are more than 35 years old is coronary artery disease; among those less than 35 years old, it is structural heart disease. Sudden cardiac death is rare, occurring in 1 in 100,000 to 1 in 300,000 individuals.

Page: 837

Question #6

Answer: D

Rationale: The term *concussion* is defined as a traumatically induced disturbance of neurologic function, with variable symptoms. Cognitive function and cranial nerve examination are necessary for concussion evaluation. A loss of consciousness is not a marker of the severity of the concussion. Return to play is a medical decision, and the opinion of a coach or parent who wants the patient to stay in the game should not matter.

Page: 838

Question #7

Answer: B

Rationale: The term *stinger* is defined as a unilateral upper extremity pain and paresthesias resulting from a blow to the neck and shoulders. Stingers are very common in American football, and they rarely cause *axonotmesis*. Bilateral symptoms may indicate a cervical spine problem, and they warrant further workup.

Page: 839

Question #8

Answer: A

Rationale: The risk of spinal cord injury and quadriplegia is too high for a patient with a history of transient neuropraxia with functional or anatomic spinal stenosis to return to a contact or collision sport.

Page: 839

Question #9

Answer: B

Rationale: Because a cervical spine injury cannot be ruled out in an unconscious player and because removing the helmet puts the player's neck in extension, the helmet should not be removed. However, the face mask should be removed to gain access to establish airway control.

Page: 840

Question #10

Answer: B

Rationale: Heat stroke is not a common problem. Fluid replacement on a hot day should be about 500 mL taken less than 2 hours before the event and about 250 mL every 20 minutes during the event. Fluid replacement should be scheduled, and thirst is not a good indicator of hydration status. Evaporation is the primary mechanism for heat dissipation.

Page: 841

Question #11

Answer: A

Rationale: There is an ongoing argument about the exact pathophysiology of hyponatremia, but the condition develops in the setting of excessive hypotonic fluid replacement, during which time sodium is progressively lost in sweat. Patients usually do not have high core body temperatures, and they should be promptly sent to the hospital for monitoring normalization of the sodium. Patients do not have any sodium or hydration problems at rest. The typical patient is an inexperienced marathoner who will finish the race in more than 4 hours.

Page: 842

Question #12

Answer: C

Rationale: The innermost layer of clothing should wick the sweat away from the body, and the outermost layer should be windproof. Dehydration increases the risk of frostbite. Moisture is the most dangerous variable.

Page: 842

Question #13

Answer: A

Rationale: Finding shelter from the wind and moisture and removing wet clothes are standard treatments for hypothermia. In severe cases, warm intravenous fluids can be used in the hospital setting. Warming and refreezing are more damaging to tissue than just freezing.

Page: 842

Question #14

Answer: C

Rationale: Altitude illness is rare below 8000 feet, and the speed of ascent is a major factor among patients who get acute mountain sickness. Physical fitness is not protective. Previous acute mountain sickness is predictive of future problems.

Page: 842

Question #15

Answer: B

Rationale: Rapid descent is the immediate treatment for high-altitude pulmonary edema.

Page: 844

Question #16

Answer: A

Rationale: Pulp involvement in tooth avulsion requires an urgent dental referral to protect the tooth and to avoid infection. Enamel fractures can be managed with a dental referral within 48 hours. Luxation should be repositioned as long as there is no jaw fracture. Avulsed teeth should be transferred in saline-soaked gauze.

Page: 843

Question #17

Answer: B

Rationale: Anterior packing should only be performed with appropriate visualization to avoid further injury to the patient. Nasal pinching and a topical decongestant can be used for epistaxis.

Page: 843

Question #18

Answer: A

Rationale: Any athlete with trauma around the eye should be evaluated for visual acuity, globe rupture, extraocular movements, pupil reactivity, and hyphema.
Page: 844

Question #19

Answer: C

Rationale: Splenic rupture almost exclusively happens during the first 3 weeks of mononucleosis, whereas splenomegaly happens in half of the cases and usually resolves by week 4 to week 6. The majority of the time, mononucleosis is a 4-week illness. Ultrasound can be considered, but it is not required for return to playing a sport.
Page: 844

Question #20

Answer: B

Rationale: Herpes gladiatorum has a prevalence of up to 40% among college wrestlers, and it can be difficult to evaluate because of trauma over the area. Herpes outbreaks usually occur 2 to 5 days after exposure. Although some team physicians will treat the entire team, this has not been proven to stop all outbreaks.
Page: 845

Question #21

Answer: A

Rationale: EIB is difficult to diagnose, but spirometry before and after an exercise challenge should be performed. A 10% to 15% drop in forced expiratory volume is noted among patients with EIB. First-line treatment would be an inhaled β_2-agonist. No sports limitations are put on these patients.
Page: 846

Question #22

Answer: C

Rationale: Sports anemia does not represent a true pathology but rather an increase in plasma volume.

Athletes with this condition should be tested for iron deficiency with any amount of anemia, not just when the hemoglobin is below 10.
Page: 846

Question #23

Answer: B

Rationale: Sickle-cell trait does occur in 6% to 8% of black Americans, and it does involve an increased risk of sudden death.
Page: 847

Question #24

Answer: B

Rationale: Although hematuria is a common problem in endurance athletes, evaluation is still warranted to rule out infection or other problems.
Page: 848

Question #25

Answer: B

Rationale: Previous injury to the low back is the strongest predictor for a back injury in an athlete. Although most cases of back pain can resolve without treatment, treatments such as physical therapy have shown to produce quicker recovery times and less recurrence of back pain. Diagnostic imaging is rarely needed in the acute setting. Oral steroids are not used to treat the stress injury spondylolysis.
Page: 848

Question #26

Answer: A

Rationale: Eccentric loads place a muscle at higher risk of injury. Nonsteroidal anti-inflammatory drugs have not been proven to shorten the healing time of a muscle. Tendinosis, which is a histopathological change in the tendon, is thought to be the main contributor to tendon injuries. Immobilization causes muscle atrophy, and it does not promote healing.
Page: 850

Question #27

Answer: D

Rationale: Chondromalacia is the breakdown of the cartilage on the patella; it usually does not cause shin pain.

Page: 851

Question #28

Answer: C

Rationale: Although stress fracture pain typically does not occur at rest, it can occur at that time. About half of lower-extremity stress fractures are in the tibia. Certain stress fractures have a higher risk for not forming a union (e.g., femoral neck, navicular, anterior tibia); these stress fractures should be managed by a sports medicine specialist. Relative rest and activity modification are the mainstays of treatment.

Page: 851

Question #29

Answer: B

Rationale: Open physes in long bones and apophyses at tendon attachments of bone provide "weak links" at which acute and repetitive overuse injuries can occur. Treatment will vary, depending on the extent of the injury to the physes.

Page: 852

Question #30

Answer: B

Rationale: Athletic amenorrhea is caused by hypothalamic pituitary axis suppression, and it is a diagnosis of exclusion. Other causes of amenorrhea must be ruled out, including pregnancy, hyperthyroidism, hyperprolactinemia, primary deficiency of gonadotropin-releasing hormone, and hyperandrogenic anovulatory syndrome. Athletic amenorrhea is an energy deficit problem, and strenuous activity with adequate energy intake usually does not disrupt the menstrual cycle. Psychological stress does play a role.

Page: 853

Question #1

Answer: B

Rationale: The human bony skeleton does not provide motor power. Muscles and ligaments provide motor power, whereas the bony skeleton provides structural attachments for muscles and ligaments.

Page: 857

Question #2

Answer: D

Rationale: In children, cortical bone is more pliable, like green wood in a growing tree, which can lead to a greenstick fracture when angular force is applied. In this situation, there is failure on the convex side of the bend, but the concave side undergoes plastic deformation and does not completely fracture. Rotational forces applied to bone are associated with spiral fractures. Elderly patients with osteoporotic thinning of cortical bone are typically more likely to suffer complete fractures or compression fractures.

Page: 857

Question #3

Answer: A

Rationale: In this scenario, the possibility of an open or compound fracture cannot be ruled out. Open fractures are surgical emergencies, and they require immediate irrigation and debridement. Even a small puncture wound over a fracture may allow skin flora to get into the fracture site and initiate a cascade of events leading to infection. Because deep bone infections are particularly difficult to treat and may lead to nonunion or chronic disability, they must be addressed proactively and aggressively to reduce the risk of infection.

Page: 857

Question #4

Answer: A

Rationale: The epiphyseal plate is a cartilaginous plate that is present in the long bones. It is the area of a growing long bone where length is added to the metaphysis and the diaphysis. During growth, the epiphyseal cartilaginous plate is weaker than the surrounding bone, and it is often weaker than the ligaments and tendons that attach nearby. The epiphyseal plate, therefore, is the "weak link" of the musculoskeletal chain in skeletally immature individuals. Because of this, injuries that typically cause ligament sprains or musculotendinous injuries among adults may lead to growth plate fractures among children.

Page: 858

Question #5

Answer: B

Rationale: The shoulder serves as the connection between the upper extremity and the axial skeleton. Therefore, the true functional shoulder joint is not just the glenohumeral joint but also the scapular thoracic joint, the acromioclavicular joint, and sternoclavicular joint.

Page: 859

Question #6

Answer: B

Rationale: This is a classic description of a Salter–Harris type II injury. This is the most common form of growthplate fracture. The intact nature of the periosteum makes reduction relatively easy, and the prognosis is excellent for future growth.

Pages: 858–859

Question #7

Answer: B

Rationale: The patient in this case most likely has a fracture of his clavicle, as suggested by localized pain, swelling, and palpable crepitus. This mechanism of injury is characteristic for clavicular fractures. A fall during which a person lands on the edge of the shoulder can also result in AC joint separation; however, in this case, the child is not tender over the AC joint, and swelling is localized to the middle third of the clavicle.

Page: 859

Question #8

Answer: C

Rationale: This is a classical description of a grade 2 AC joint separation. A grade 1 injury involves only a partial injury to the acromioclavicular ligaments, and no displacement is visualized either on x-rays or stress views. A grade 2 injury involves the complete injury of the acromioclavicular ligaments, but coracoclavicular ligaments are intact. This allows for the subluxation or dislocation of the distal clavicle superiorly to a mild degree. The height of the subluxation in grade 2 injuries is generally no thicker than the thickness of the clavicle itself. A grade 3 injury involves the complete rupture of the acromioclavicular ligaments as well as the coracoclavicular ligaments. The distal end of the clavicle and the acromion are now separated by more than a full clavicular width (almost 1–2 cm). There is no grade 0 AC joint separation.

Page: 860

Question #9

Answer: B

Rationale: Injury of the long thoracic nerve and its resulting serratus anterior weakness is the most common cause of scapular winging. Provocative maneuvers including active protraction, retraction, and elevation in various planes may illicit scapular winging or scapular dyskinesia. The spinal accessory nerve innervates the trapezius muscle, along with the rhomboids. The deltoid nerve provides muscular innervation to the deltoid muscle. The median nerve supplies muscular innervation to the flexor compartment of the forearm as well as some intricate muscles of the hand.

Page: 860

Question #10

Answer: C

Rationale: The rotator cuff is a group of four muscles—the supraspinatus, the infraspinatus, the teres minor, and the subscapularis—that originate from the scapular surface, traverse just outside of the glenohumeral capsule, and insert onto the tuberosities of the humerus. The rotator cuff initiates motion in the shoulder, positions the humeral head in the glenoid, maintains depression of the humeral head in the glenoid socket, and serves as secondary and active restraints to instability. The supraspinatus muscle is most commonly described as an abductor of the shoulder. However, it can be appreciated that the primary function of the supraspinatus is not to abduct the shoulder but rather to compress the humeral head into the glenoid fossa and to prevent excessive superior translation of the humeral head during functional activities. The infraspinatus and the teres minor are both described as lateral rotators of the shoulder. The subscapularis is described as a medial rotator of the shoulder.

Page: 863

Question #11

Answer: D

Rationale: The patient in this scenario has multiple features that suggest that a complete tear of the rotator cuff is present. The change in the nature of the pain suggests that a new pathology is present. Shoulder pain that is frequently exacerbated by overhead movements is indicative of rotator cuff tendinopathy. The marked weakness during the examination of the supraspinatus (resisted abduction) and of the infraspinatus and the teres minor (resisted external rotation with elbow flexed to 90 degrees) also suggests that the rotator cuff tendons are the source of his pathology. Most convincing, however, is the positive drop arm sign when performing the "empty can" test. If the patient is unable to maintain the empty can position, suspicion should be raised for a complete rotator cuff tear. For a complete rotator cuff tear with clinical dysfunction, management is often surgical. In this case, the patient is an elite athlete who will require correction of this tear to continue to compete in baseball.

Page: 863

Question #12

Answer: D

Rationale: For athletes who make repetitive overhead movements, like the one described in the question, developmental posterior capsular tightness has been appreciated; this leads to increased stresses over the anterior aspect of the shoulder and associated anterior instability. Current controversies exist regarding the ideal treatment for a first-time shoulder dislocator. In a young athletic or military population, the risk of recurrence and future shoulder problems approaches 90%. Surgical treatment in this population, with repair of labral detachments, has lead to a high return to play and to performance, with a less than 10% chance of recurrence. Primary repair for first-time shoulder dislocation may not be necessary in other populations.

Page: 867

Question #13

Answer: A

Rationale: Lateral elbow tendinopathy, which is commonly called "tennis elbow" or "lateral epicondylitis," is the most common elbow ailment seen in primary care offices. The injury is caused by the repetitive overuse of the wrist extensor and the forearm supinator muscles that originate at the lateral epicondyle of the humerus (more specifically, the extensor carpi radialis brevis). Once thought to be the result of inflammation, lateral elbow tendinosis is now thought to result from more chronic changes in the musculotendinous matrix, with very little inflammation being present. Microtears, chronic granulation tissue, and scar-tissue formation are commonly encountered in surgical pathological specimens from "tennis elbow." Patients present as a result of pain in the lateral aspect of the elbow. They may complain of weakness of the elbow or restricted motion, but this is not as common. Pain is worsened by gripping and lifting activities, particularly with the hand in a palm-down position, such as when lifting a suitcase, briefcase, or purse.

Page: 870

Question #14

Answer: D

Rationale: Injuries to the ulnar collateral ligament are most commonly noted in throwing athletes. The injury occurs because of the valgus force that the throwing elbow experiences during the acceleration phase of throwing. Most injuries are the result of repetitive forces to the ulnar collateral ligament, although a single valgus episode may lead to injury as well. Patients will present most commonly as a result of medial elbow pain mostly noted during throwing or other overhead activities. Other possible presenting complaints include loss of throwing velocity, painful elbow motion, or numbness in the fourth and fifth fingers as a result of increased traction forces across the ulnar nerve. Positive physical examination findings include tenderness on palpation of the medial aspect of elbow and tenderness with valgus stress testing. Actual instability on valgus stress testing may be very difficult to appreciate unless the ligament is completely torn.

Page: 871

Question #15

Answer: B

Rationale: Management of ulnar collateral ligament injury begins with pain control and an assessment of whether the injury is a partial or complete ligament injury. As with other musculoskeletal problems, relative rest, ice, medications, and protective splinting or bracing can all be helpful for relieving discomfort; this includes avoiding the inciting activity. Maintaining or regaining motion and strength are also important components of the rehabilitation process. When the patient is pain-free on examination and rehabilitation exercises have been completed, a slow reintroduction to throwing activities can begin. This may take 4 to 8 weeks even in cases of low-grade sprains. Return to full throwing activities can take up to 6 months; however, a majority of patients may not be able to return to their prior level of throwing. In higher-grade injuries and complete tears, surgical intervention to reconstruct the ligament is often needed, with a 70% to 90% success rate of returning athletes to their previous level of sport.

Page: 871

Question #16

Answer: C

Rationale: The patient in this case has a type 1 nondisplaced radial head fracture. Treatment of radial head fractures usually involves a short period of splint and sling immobilization followed by early mobilization. Type 1 fractures are only immobilized for several days before mobilization begins, provided that elbow pain is controlled. Type 2 fractures that are mildly displaced and that cause no mechanical blockade can be treated in a similar fashion to type 1 injuries, although the initial length of splinting may be longer. If mechanical blockade is present or if the patient is involved in high-demand activities, open reduction with internal fixation should be considered. Computed tomography scanning to delineate the fracture more completely is recommended in these cases. For patients with a type 2 fracture with mechanical blockade who place low demand on the elbow, complete radial head excision is often considered. Type 3 fractures are severely comminuted, and they are not felt to be reconstructible; therefore, excision is the treatment of choice.

Pages: 872–873

Question #17

Answer: C

Rationale: Fractures of the olecranon are not as common as radial head fractures, but they do happen with some frequency. The mechanism of injury is usually a direct fall onto a flexed elbow, but it may also result from being struck directly on the olecranon by a hard

Fracture Type	Fragment Size	Displacement
Type 1	Marginal injury	Non-displaced
Type 2	Larger fragment	>2 mm displacement
Type 3	Comminuted (3+ pieces)	Variable

In Rakel RE, editor: *Textbook of family medicine,* ed 7, Philadelphia, WB Saunders, 2007.

object. The most common examination finding is pain on palpation of the olecranon. Crepitus and even a palpable step-off deformity may be noted. Radiographs should be obtained in all cases of pain at the olecranon after direct trauma. Anteroposterior and true lateral projections should adequately reveal the fracture. The fracture is considered to be nondisplaced if there is less than 2 mm of displacement that does not increase with elbow flexion to 90 degrees and if the patient is able to extend the elbow actively against gravity, showing that the triceps mechanism is intact. Nondisplaced fractures may be treated in a conservative manner with a long-arm cast with the elbow at 45 to 90 degrees of flexion for up to 3 weeks. Although the fracture will not be completely healed for 6 to 8 weeks, most are stable in 3 weeks. All displaced fractures should be treated by an orthopedic surgeon.

Page: 873

Question #18

Answer: B

Rationale: Carpal tunnel syndrome is the most common nerve entrapment syndrome encountered in primary care. The most common etiology is tenosynovitis of the hand flexors that leads to median nerve compression; this leads to pain in the wrist or numbness into the hand. Reduced grip strength is also common. Numbness may be reported as occurring throughout the hand, although the median nerve only supplies sensation to the radial three and a half digits. Physical examination is usually negative. Tinel's test is performed at the wrist by tapping over the wrist flexor retinaculum. If the nerve is injured either by compression or traction, it may give off a signal when struck. Tingling or pain in the distribution of the tested nerve is considered a positive test. Phalen's test is performed by having the patient flex his or her wrists to a 90-degree position (holding the dorsal aspects of the hands back to back). The patient maintains this position for 1 minute or until symptoms develop; the lack of symptoms after 1 minute constitutes a negative test. Diagnostic imaging is not necessary to make a diagnosis of carpal tunnel syndrome.

Pages: 874–875

Question #19

Answer: D

Rationale: Treatment of carpal tunnel syndrome begins with attempts to avoid or to at least modify activities that are known to cause pain for the patient. This may involve ergonomic changes in the workplace, including wrist support pads for computer use. Wrist splinting, particularly at night, may prove helpful. Oral analgesic and nonsteroidal anti-inflammatory drug use may also lead to relief, but studies show that they are no more effective than placebos. Corticosteroid injection is a helpful adjunct for many patients, and it has been shown to relieve symptoms better than placebo. A majority of patients will experience good relief of symptoms if these conservative measures are followed.

Pages: 874–875

Question #20

Answer: C

Rationale: de Quervain's tenosynovitis is a painful condition of the abductor pollicis longus and extensor pollicis brevis muscles along the radial aspect of the wrist that is caused by overuse or repetitive use activities. Swelling may be noted along the side of the wrist as well. The classic clinical finding is a positive Finkelstein's test. This is performed by having the patient flex and adduct his or her thumb to the palm and then close the remaining fingers over the thumb. The examiner then passively takes the patient's wrist into ulnar deviation. Pain along the tendons with this maneuver is considered a positive test.

Page: 875

Question #21

Answer: C

Rationale: Fractures of the distal radius are among the most commonly encountered fractures in primary care. The most common mechanism of injury is a fall on an outstretched hand. Patients present with pain in the wrist, which usually occurs immediately after a fall. The pain is increased with attempted motion, and the patient may guard the wrist with the opposite hand. Many physicians prefer to obtain radiographs before this portion of the examination if the history and observation raise adequate suspicion of a distal radius fracture. For the patient described here, there is clear

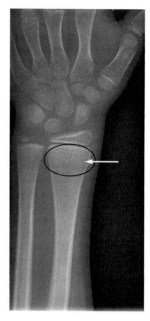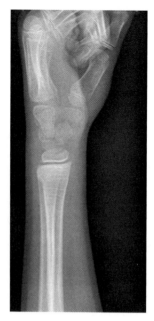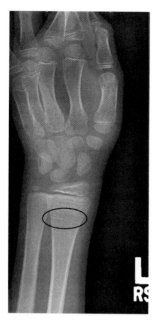

Figure 42-7 Copyright James L. Moeller, MD. In Rakel RE, editor: *Textbook of family medicine,* ed 7, Philadelphia, WB Saunders, 2007.

cortical interruption in the left-most image along with a distinct fracture line as delineated by the arrow and circle, as shown in Figure 42-7.

Page: 877

Question #22

Answer: B

Rationale: Scaphoid fracture is the most common fracture of a carpal bone and the second most commonly encountered fracture of the wrist region, after the distal radius. The blood supply to the scaphoid is retrograde, which means that the blood vessels enter the bone from the distal end and move proximally. Because of this, fractures of the proximal portion of the scaphoid generally take longer to heal than more distal injuries, and malunion or nonunion is not uncommon. The most common physical examination finding is tenderness with palpation over the scaphoid tubercle or the anatomic snuff box. Radiographs should be obtained in all cases of suspected scaphoid injury. Important views include anteroposterior, lateral, and oblique views as well as ulnar deviation or scaphoid views. Treatment of scaphoid fracture is initiated if suspicion is high, even if x-rays are initially negative.

Page: 878

Question #23

Answer: A

Rationale: This patient has a characteristic presentation of septic arthritis. Intraarticular joint infections are orthopedic emergencies, and they require urgent operative irrigation. The most common source of infection is *Staphylococcus aureus,* which is an aggressive bacteria, that, in a very short time, can soften and degrade the hyaline cartilage and leave the patient with permanent osteoarthritis.

Page: 884

Question #24

Answer: D

Rationale: If the skeletally immature patient has pain at the insertion of the patellar tendon on to the tibia, the most likely diagnosis is an apophysitis of the tibial tubercle or Osgood–Schlatter disease. Both problems are more common during active phases of growth, and they are generally treated conservatively with rest, flexibility exercises, and a gradual return to activity. Juvenile rheumatoid arthritis typically presents before the age of 4 years, with parents complaining that their children are irritable and lethargic and show a reluctance to play.

Page: 885

Question #25

Answer: B

Rationale: Patellar instability can be either acute or chronic in nature. Patients with an acute knee patellar dislocation will oftentimes present after a twisting or rotational motion during which they felt a significant pop on the anterior aspect of their knee. Their knee may swell up with a large hemiarthrosis, and they will have tenderness primarily over the medial retinaculum, either on the insertion of the patella or the medial patellofemoral ligament, where it originates from the medial epicondyle. In either case, the patient will have a positive apprehension sign, which occurs when the examiner makes an effort to displace the patella laterally and the patient has the sensation that the patella will go out of place again. The "chandelier sign" is an intense sensation of apprehension in which the patient grimaces and reaches for his or her knee or the ceiling (the chandelier) out of fear of redislocating the knee cap.

Page: 886

Question #26

Answer: A

Rationale: The term "terrible triad" often refers to the triad of injuries to the anterior cruciate ligament, the medial collateral ligament, and the medial meniscus. Injuries to these structures are often related, because their close anatomic and functional relationship leads them to be injured by similar mechanisms, such as twisting motions or valgus stresses. The posterior cruciate ligament is not associated with this triad, and it is typically injured as a result of a posteriorly directed force on the tibia.

Page: 887

Question #27

Answer: C

Rationale: The patient has a history of a high-impact motor vehicle accident during which her lower extremity struck the dashboard of her vehicle. This is a characteristic mechanism of posterior cruciate ligament injury. The posterior cruciate ligament is usually injured as a result of a posterior directed force on the tibia. If a posterior drawer test does not have significant posterior sag, conservative treatment is appropriate, with quadriceps rehabilitation as the primary goal. If the patient has significant posterior sag and instability with associated pain, surgical reconstruction of the posterior cruciate ligament is recommended.

Page: 891

Question #28

Answer: A

Rationale: Sprains are injuries to the ligamentous structures of the ankle. Eighty-five percent of ankle sprains involve the anterior talofibular ligament, the calcaneofibular ligament, or the posterior talofibular ligament. The most common mechanism of lateral ankle sprain is an inversion ankle injury. This usually occurs by stepping in a hole while walking or running, landing from a jump on another person's foot, or simply by "rolling the ankle" when trying to change direction. Inversion events with the ankle in a plantarflexed position (this is the most common) will often lead to anterior talofibular ligament injuries, whereas inversion events with the ankle in a dorsiflexed position will more typically lead to calcaneofibular ligament injuries

Page: 892

Question #29

Answer: A

Rationale: In the United States, patients presenting for ankle injury often undergo radiographic evaluation, but the use of routine radiographs to evaluate ankle injury is an area of debate. Well-designed studies from Ottawa, Canada, have shown that many patients with ankle injury can safely be managed without routine radiographs. Regarding the lateral ankle, indications for ankle radiograph include the following: (1) age of less than 18 years or more than 55 years, (2) inability to bear weight for four consecutive steps either immediately after the injury or while in the examination room, and (3) pain over the posterior portion of the distal 6 cm or at the tip of the fibula. If pain is noted in the proximal or midshaft fibula, tibia and fibula films should be obtained. Pain over the base of the fifth metatarsal is an indication for foot radiographs.

Page: 893

Question #30

Answer: B

Rationale: The ankle syndesmosis is the area of the distal tibia-fibula joint. Syndesmosis sprains account for 1% to 18% of ankle sprains, with a higher incidence among high-level athletes. Mechanisms of injury are forceful external rotation and hyperdorsiflexion injuries. A common adverse outcome of syndesmosis sprain is heterotopic ossification. Plain radiographs are adequate to make the diagnosis among patients with persistent pain. Heterotopic ossification, which is reported to occur in 25% to 90% of cases, may or may not be symptomatic. Ossification may cause pain from an inflammatory response during the early stages and then from pressure on adjacent bones. Fracture of the ossification is also a potential cause of pain (Figure 42-8). Conservative treatments may reduce the pain, but surgical excision may be required.

Page: 894

Question #31

Answer: C

Rationale: The test described is the Thompson test. This test is recommended for assessing the integrity of the Achilles tendon in suspected injuries. Lay the patient prone on the examination table with the knee flexed to 90 degrees and the ankle in a neutral position. Squeeze the mid gastrocnemius area, and observe for passive ankle plantarflexion. If the Achilles tendon is intact, the ankle will plantarflex (negative test). If the Achilles tendon is torn, the ankle will remain in a neutral position (positive test).

Page: 896

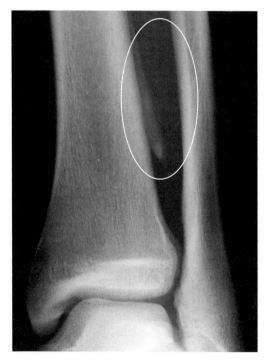

Figure 42-8 Copyright James L. Moeller, MD. In Rakel RE, editor: *Textbook of family medicine,* ed 7, Philadelphia, WB Saunders, 2007.

Question #32

Answer: B

Rationale: The injection of depot cortisone has been shown to improve all of the conditions listed. However, cortisone injection for Achilles tendonitis is not recommended as a result of the increased risk of Achilles tendon rupture and the subsequent morbidity of such an outcome. Cortisone injection has been shown to reduce pain from plantar fasciitis. There are risks to cortisone injection, including plantar fascia rupture and necrosis of the plantar fat pad (the natural heel cushion). These adverse potential outcomes should be reviewed with patients before injection. Both infrapatellar and trochanteric bursitis respond well to cortisone injection.

Page: 896

Question #33

Answer: C

Rationale: The patient described in this question likely has plantar fasciitis. The clues for this diagnosis are pain of a sharp, stabbing nature localized to the heel that is worse in the morning, worse upon rising from a seated position, and worse after the patient being on his or her feet for prolonged periods. The primary finding on physical examination reveals tenderness over the origin of the plantar fascia. A calcaneal fracture could present with similar pain complaints, but it would be unlikely to improve throughout the day.

Page: 896

Question #34

Answer: A

Rationale: The patient described in option A has the classical description of a scaphoid fracture. Scaphoid fracture is the most common fracture of a carpal bone, and it is the second most commonly encountered fracture of the wrist region, after the distal radius. The most common physical examination finding is tenderness with palpation over the scaphoid tubercle or over the anatomical snuff box. Radiographs are often negative shortly after injury; if this is the case, radiographs should be repeated after 2 weeks if suspicion remains high.

Page: 878

Question #35

Answer: C

Rationale: The figure shows the "lift off" test to isolate and test the subscapularis muscle. The supraspinatus muscle is isolated and tested by resisted flexion of the extended arm at an angle of 60 degrees from straight forward. The infraspinatus and the teres minor are tested as a group by resisted external rotation of the shoulder with the elbow flexed to 90 degrees.

Page: 865

Question #36

Answer: C

Rationale: Most clavicle fractures can be treated conservatively with a sling or a figure-of-eight dressing. For most patients, a simple sling for comfort is adequate for the first few weeks, and this should be followed by progressive range-of-motion activities. The nonunion of midshaft clavicle fractures is quite rare. A Salter–Harris type IV fracture is an intra-articular fracture. Open reduction with internal fixation is commonly needed to ensure anatomical alignment of the joint surface and apposition of the epiphyseal plate. Fractures of the base of the fifth metatarsal deserve special discussion. There is a watershed area of blood flow in the proximal portion of this metatarsal that puts it at particular risk for malunion and nonunion. Jones fractures occur in the proximal third of the metatarsal, and they do not involve the tarsometatarsal joint. Fractures of the distal fibula can be problematic. Largely displaced fractures and fractures that lead to a widening of the ankle mortise should be treated with open reduction and internal fixation.

Pages: 858, 860

Question #37

Answer: A

Rationale: Of the choices presented for this question, only a distal radial fracture should be treated with a short-arm cast for immobilization. The goal of immobilization in any fracture that requires such treatment should be to stabilize both sides of the joint nearest to that fracture. Thus, short-arm casting for a distal radial fracture would stabilize both sides of the wrist joint. Nondisplaced olecranon fractures should be treated with immobilization of the elbow joint (e.g., in a long-arm cast). Nondisplaced radial head fractures typically benefit from early mobilization; however, if they were to require immobilization, they too would be immobilized at the elbow with either a long-arm splint or cast. Finally, scaphoid fractures are a unique type of fracture that requires a variant of the short-arm cast known as a thumb spica cast. This type of cast, in addition to immobilizing the wrist joint, isolates and immobilizes the thumb to allow for better healing of the fracture.

Pages: 876, 877

Question #38

Answer: A

Rationale: Overall, the radius is the bone that is the most commonly fractured. The scaphoid is the most commonly fractured carpal bone, and it is the second most commonly fractured bone overall. The clavicle is the most frequently fractured bone in the pediatric population. Thankfully, femoral fractures are uncommon, because they carry a great deal of morbidity and mortality. For an otherwise healthy elderly patient who has suffered a femoral neck fracture, the 1-year mortality rate as a result of the bone injury and complications thereof approaches 50%.

Page: 876

Question #39

Answer: C

Rationale: Tenosynovitis of the digital flexor tendons is quite common, and it is more commonly known as "trigger finger." Although any finger can develop trigger finger, it is most commonly seen in the index, middle, and ring fingers. This can be a painful condition that makes gripping and fine motor control activities of the hand difficult to perform. Patients present with the complaint of a finger that "sticks" with motion, primarily flexion. The finger will stick in a partially flexed position, and, with continued attempts to flex the finger, the digit will suddenly complete the motion. Motion and activities may be associated with pain.

Page: 875

Question #40

Answer: B

Rationale: The procedure described is known as a hematoma block. It is common for acute traumatic fractures to develop a stable hematoma around the fracture site. Closed reduction of a fracture can be quite painful and traumatic to the patient. Despite the fact that bone itself does not contain pain sensory innervation, the periosteum surrounding the bone is highly innervated with pain-sensing fibers. Replacement of the old blood within the stable hematoma with 2% lidocaine or some other topical anesthetic uses the space already created in the soft tissue surrounding the fracture and achieves anesthetic block of the periosteum surrounding the fracture, thereby making closed reduction more comfortable for the patient and avoiding the complications of general anesthesia or systemic analgesics.

Page: 877

43 Answers

Question #1

Answer: B

Rationale: Eighty percent of patients with rheumatoid arthritis will have a positive RF.
Page: 918

Question #2

Answer: C

Rationale: Up to 5% of healthy individuals will have a positive RF. RF is also frequently positive in patients with chronic obstructive pulmonary disease, viral hepatitis, and sarcoidosis. However, the higher the RF titer, the more likely it is the result of rheumatoid arthritis.
Page: 918

Question #3

Answer: B

Rationale: Antinuclear antibody test results are positive in 95% of patients with lupus, and the test is often used to screen for systemic lupus erythematosus. However, the result is also positive in 5% of the normal population.
Page: 918

Question #4

Answer: B

Rationale: Urate crystals can be distinguished from calcium pyrophosphate dihydrate crystals under microscopy. Urate crystals are shaped like needles, and they are negatively birefringent. Calcium pyrophosphate dihydrate crystals are shaped like rhomboids, and they are weakly positively birefringent.
Page: 920

Question #5

Answer: B

Rationale: The iatrogenic infection rate is generally estimated at 1 in 10,000, making it much less common than the missed diagnosis of a septic joint.
Page: 920

Question #6

Answer: D

Rationale: It is estimated that arthritis affects 20% of the population. Roughly half of those affected have osteoarthritis.
Page: 921

Question #7

Answer: A

Rationale: A boutonniere deformity is characteristically seen with advanced rheumatoid arthritis. Heberden's and Bouchard's nodes are two types of deformities that are seen with osteoarthritis. Heberden's nodes affect the distal interphalangeal joints, and Bouchard's nodes affect the proximal interphalangeal joints.
Pages: 921, 922

Question #8

Answer: A

Rationale: Although anti-inflammatories are frequently used for the treatment of osteoarthritis, the condition is considered a noninflammatory type of arthritis that primarily affects the cartilage of the synovial joints.
Page: 921

Question #9

Answer: C

Rationale: Studies have shown that occupational kneelers have significantly greater frequencies of osteoarthritis affecting the knees than do control groups of clerical workers. Specifically, shipyard workers, miners, and carpet or floor layers have been shown to have greater frequencies of knee osteoarthritis. Although at one time felt to cause arthritis, long-distance running has not been associated with a greater frequency of arthritis.

Page: 922

Question #10

Answer: C

Rationale: The pain associated with osteoarthritis typically worsens as the day progresses and is relieved with rest. There is less than 30 minutes of localized morning stiffness, and there are no constitutional or systemic symptoms.

Page: 922

Question #11

Answer: A

Rationale: Marginal erosions are typically seen with rheumatoid arthritis. The radiographic abnormalities associated with osteoarthritis include osteophyte formation, asymmetric joint-space narrowing (defined as <3 mm on a weight-bearing knee), and subchondral bone sclerosis.

Page: 923

Question #12

Answer: B

Rationale: No currently available treatment has been shown to alter the natural history of osteoarthritis. Therefore, the goal of the management of the disease is primarily to relieve pain, stiffness, and swelling.

Page: 923

Question #13

Answer: A

Rationale: Exercise programs—including swimming, other aerobic conditioning, and walking—have been shown by numerous studies to be helpful. Weight control and, if necessary, weight reduction have also been shown to improve symptoms.

Pages: 923, 924

Question #14

Answer: B

Rationale: Acetaminophen is the initial drug of choice for symptom control associated with osteoarthritis. Traditional NSAIDs (beginning with ibuprofen) and non-acetylated salicylates are considered to be second-line options.

Page: 924

Question #15

Answer: A

Rationale: The recommended dose of acetaminophen for patients with osteoarthritis is 1000 mg four times daily (in the absence of liver disease). This is the recommended initial drug of choice for patients with osteoarthritis.

Page: 924

Question #16

Answer: D

Rationale: Risk factors for upper gastrointestinal bleeding include age of more than 65 years, history of peptic ulcer disease or upper gastrointestinal bleeding, concurrent use of oral corticosteroids and anticoagulants, and possibly smoking and alcohol consumption.

Page: 924

Question #17

Answer: B

Rationale: NSAIDs and a proton-pump inhibitor remain the treatment of choice for the prevention of NSAID-induced gastric ulcers.

Page: 924

Question #18

Answer: B

Rationale: Several studies have documented the efficacy of glucosamine for reducing symptoms associated with osteoarthritis. A meta-analysis of 11 studies found that SAMe was as effective as NSAIDs for reducing pain and functional limitations and that it has a somewhat better adverse-effect profile. A Cochrane review of herbal therapies found studies demonstrating that avocado/soybean unsaponifiables showed beneficial effects on function, pain, and the intake of NSAIDs. Lycopene has not been shown to improve symptoms associated with osteoarthritis.

Page: 925

Question #19

Answer: B

Rationale: Rheumatoid arthritis is a chronic, inflammatory, systemic disease in which cellular and autoimmune mechanisms result in the destruction of tissues (primarily the synovium).

Page: 925

Question #20

Answer: C

Rationale: The prevalence of rheumatoid arthritis is between 1% and 2% of adults, and it ranges from 0.3% of the population that is less than 35 years old to about 10% of the population that is more than 65 years old.

Page: 925

Question #21

Answer: A

Rationale: As compared with osteoarthritis, rheumatoid arthritis is associated with morning stiffness that lasts for more than 1 hour.

Page: 926

Question #22

Answer: B

Rationale: Cervical spine involvement in rheumatoid arthritis is common, and early symptoms are neck stiffness and decreased motion. However, symptoms can progress to result in neurologic complications from C1–2 instability resulting from tenosynovitis of the transverse ligament of C1. Radiographs of the cervical spine in flexion and extension may be needed to detect C1–2 involvement. If there is C1–2 involvement, caution is necessary during surgical procedures that require intubation.

Page: 926

Question #23

Answer: A

Rationale: As compared with osteoarthritis, rheumatoid arthritis usually spares the distal interphalangeal joints.

Page: 926

Question #24

Answer: A

Rationale: Felty's syndrome is associated with rheumatoid arthritis, splenomegaly, leukopenia, leg ulcers, lymphadenopathy, thrombocytopenia, and the human leukocyte antigen DR4 haplotype. It is more common among patients with severe, nodule-forming rheumatoid arthritis.

Page: 926

Question #25

Answer: D

Rationale: Periarticular osteoporosis is seen radiographically during the late stages of rheumatoid arthritis. Other radiographic abnormalities include marginal bone erosions and joint-space narrowing.

Page: 926

Question #26

Answer: B

Rationale: Almost 90% of the joints ultimately affected in a given patient with rheumatoid arthritis are involved during the first year of the disease. This allows the family physician to give the patient who has had rheumatoid arthritis for several years some assurance about which joints ultimately will be affected.

Page: 927

Question #27

Answer: B

Rationale: NSAIDs improve inflammation and pain, but they do not alter disease progression or improve prognosis.

Page: 928

Question #28

Answer: A

Rationale: Folic acid (1 mg/day) reduces methotrexate-induced mouth sores without decreasing the drug's efficacy. Methotrexate is considered by many rheumatologists to be the disease-modifying antirheumatic drug of choice, and it is the most frequently used of those types of drugs in the United States.

Page: 929

Question #29

Answer: A

Rationale: Methotrexate toxicities include hepatotoxicity, bone marrow suppression, the rare development of B-cell non-Hodgkin's lymphoma, subcutaneous nodules, opportunistic infections, and hypersensitivity pneumonitis.

Page: 929

Question #30

Answer: D

Rationale: It is estimated that up to one in three rheumatoid patients will either be hospitalized or die from a gastrointestinal bleed at some point. NSAID-associated gastrointestinal bleeding is a widespread problem. Patients on long-term nonselective NSAIDs should be monitored several times yearly for abnormalities in hematocrit levels, stool guaiac testing, renal function, and liver function.

Page: 931

Question #31

Answer: B

Rationale: The least-toxic NSAIDs were found to be coated or buffered aspirin, salsalate, and ibuprofen. The most toxic were indomethacin (Indocin), tolmetin sodium (Tolectin), meclofenamate sodium (Meclomen), and ketoprofen (Orudis, Oruvail). High-toxicity NSAIDs provide no more clinical benefit than do lower-toxicity NSAIDs.

Page: 931

Question #32

Answer: B

Rationale: Studies have shown that no one NSAID provides more clinical benefit than another. Selection is largely empirical, and it should be directed at minimizing toxicity.

Page: 931

Question #33

Answer: A

Rationale: Periodic measurements of erythrocyte sedimentation rate and C-reactive protein, plain radiographs, and functional status assessments in addition to serial joint examinations are important for patients with rheumatoid arthritis. RF titers are not helpful for following disease progression; when a patient is discovered to have a positive RF, repeating the test is of no value.

Pages: 932, 933

Question #34

Answer: B

Rationale: Hyperuricemia is a marker for gout, but each can exist without the other. Asymptomatic hyperuricemia is not a disease. The risk of gout, however, is proportional to the degree and duration of hyperuricemia. Hyperuricemia is present in 5% of adult men, and, of these, only 5% to 10% develop acute gout. It normally takes at least 20 years of hyperuricemia before a patient has his or her first episode of gouty arthritis. Lowering the uric acid level does not decrease the risk of gouty nephropathy. Because of the expense and the potential drug toxicity, the treatment of asymptomatic hyperuricemia is therefore generally not recommended.

Page: 933

Question #35

Answer: A

Rationale: Primary hyperuricemia results from two different inborn errors of metabolism: 90% of patients have reduced excretion of uric acid, whereas 10% of patients have increased production of uric acid.

Page: 933

Question #36

Answer: B

Rationale: Hyperuricemia is present in 5% of adult men, and, of these, only 5% to 10% develop acute gout. It normally takes at least 20 years of hyperuricemia before a patient has his or her first episode of gouty arthritis. Lowering the uric acid level does not decrease the risk of gouty nephropathy. Because of the expense and the potential drug toxicity, the treatment of asymptomatic hyperuricemia is therefore generally not recommended.

Page: 933

Question #37

Answer: B

Rationale: The two most important factors in the development of acute gouty arthritis are obesity and alcohol. Ethanol metabolism blocks the renal excretion of uric acid, and this leads to gouty attacks. Dietary excesses of purine-rich foods (e.g., sweetbreads, sardines, anchovies, kidney, liver) have traditionally been mentioned, but, in reality, they are rarely responsible for acute gouty attacks.

Page: 935

Question #38

Answer: C

Rationale: Colchicine, indomethacin (Indocin), and corticosteroids are all indicated for the treatment of acute gouty arthritis. However, allopurinol should never be initiated until an acute attack has subsided.

Page: 935

Question #39

Answer: B

Rationale: Although most of the spondyloarthropathies are linked to the human leukocyte antigen B27 gene, B27 by itself does not explain the development of these diseases; the pathogenesis of these conditions is still unknown. Most people with B27 do not develop these diseases, and these diseases also occur in the absence of B27.

Page: 936

Question #40

Answer: D

Rationale: Extra-articular manifestations of ankylosing spondylitis include acute uveitis (iritis), aortitis, and neurological complications resulting from C-spine fractures from even minor trauma.

Page: 936

Question #41

Answer: B

Rationale: The mainstay of the treatment of ankylosing spondylitis is NSAIDs. Corticosteroids have not been shown to be helpful. Physical therapy focusing on strengthening the back extensor muscles may improve functional status, and, at the very least, they may help maintain an erect posture if spinal ossification occurs. Etanercept (Enbrel), sulfasalazine (Azulfidine), and methotrexate (Rheumatrex) are considered second-line drug therapies; however, these drugs have demonstrated no clear effects on the progression of decreased spinal mobility. More studies are being performed to better assess these agents' effects on ankylosing spondylitis.

Page: 936

Question #42

Answer: C

Rationale: The classic triad of reactive arthritis (Reiter's syndrome) includes nongonococcal urethritis, conjunctivitis, and arthritis. Although classically described, these three symptoms are present in only one third of all patients with Reiter's syndrome.

Page: 937

Question #43

Answer: A

Rationale: The most common sites affected by acute septic arthritis are the knees (50%), followed by the hips (20%), shoulders (8%), ankles (7%), wrists (7%), elbows (6%), and other joints (5%).

Page: 938

Question #44

Answer: B

Rationale: Septic joints are typically quite painful, swollen, red, and warm. However, 20% of patients will be afebrile. Among elderly patients, fever is seen only 10% of the time.

Page: 938

Question #45

Answer: D

Rationale: Erythema migrans is associated with Lyme disease. The characteristic "target" rash of erythema migrans develops within 1 month (mean, 1 week) of a bite from an infected tick.

Page: 939

Question #46

Answer: A

Rationale: Treatment of early Lyme disease among adults includes doxycycline (100 mg twice daily) or amoxicillin (500 mg three times daily) for 20 to 30 days. Azithromycin is not indicated for the treatment of Lyme disease.

Page: 940

Question #47

Answer: B

Rationale: Transmission of Lyme disease is more likely with prolonged tick attachment. Infection occurs in only 1% of patients after tick attachment for less than 72 hours as compared with 20% after attachment of more than 72 hours. Therefore, frequent checks for ticks and their prompt removal can prevent Lyme disease.

Page: 939

Question #48

Answer: B

Rationale: Rheumatic fever appears to be linked only to pharyngitis; group A streptococcal impetigo does not seem to be associated with rheumatic fever.

Page: 940

Question #49

Answer: B

Rationale: Sjögren's syndrome is an autoimmune disorder that is most likely caused by T-cell–mediated exocrine gland destruction, which is characterized by dry eyes (keratoconjunctivitis sicca) and dry mouth (xerostomia). Constipation is not typically associated with Sjögren's syndrome.

Page: 944

Question #50

Answer: A

Rationale: The family physician should consider the diagnosis of giant cell arteritis for any patient who is more than 50 years old who is presenting with a new onset of headaches, elevated erythrocyte sedimentation rate, abrupt loss of vision, polymyalgia rheumatica, and prolonged fever.

Page: 945

Question #51

Answer: C

Rationale: Cardiopulmonary disease is the leading cause of death among patients with diffuse cutaneous systemic sclerosis.

Page: 947

Question #52

Answer: D

Rationale: Henoch–Schönlein purpura is a small-vessel vasculitis that is seen mostly among children. Immune complexes are deposited, which can cause petechiae, nephropathy or renal disease, and gastrointestinal bleeding. The purpura usually occurs in dependent areas, such as the buttocks and the lower extremities. Affected children often present with abdominal pain after an upper respiratory infection.

Page: 950

44 Answers

Question #1

Answer: D

Rationale: Diphenhydramine (Benadryl) and hydroxyzine (Atarax, Vistaril) are first-generation antihistamines that are relatively safe and very effective, although caution should be used among elderly patients. Second-generation antihistamines are similarly effective for reducing pruritus, but they may be less sedating for some patients. These include fexofenadine (Allegra), loratadine (Claritin), and cetirizine (Zyrtec).

Page: 955

Question #2

Answer: D

Rationale: When choosing a corticosteroid, keep in mind that these agents are better absorbed through damaged skin and the thin stratum of infants. In general, thin epidermis is more permeable to steroids than thick epidermis. In addition, occlusive dressings promote cutaneous hydration and increase absorption, and they may enhance steroid potency by as much as 100 times. To achieve maximal penetration and efficacy, topical corticosteroids should be applied to moist skin after bathing. Begin with the lowest-potency agent needed for the least amount of treatment time. Class I steroids are useful for severe dermatosis over nonfacial and nonintertriginous areas, especially the palms and soles.

Page: 956

Question #3

Answer: B

Rationale: Among infants, seborrheic dermatitis (cradle cap) is usually self-limited, and it resolves with the regular use of baby shampoos. Because psoriasis is rarely cured, the goal of therapy is to maintain control of the lesions. The etiology of pityriasis rosea is unknown; because no bacterial etiology has been associated with it, the effect of erythromycin is likely the result of its anti-inflammatory properties. Although infants are the most susceptible, miliaria may persist into adulthood for more than half of those affected.

Page: 956

Question #4

Answer: C

Rationale: Because no bacterial etiology has been associated with the disease, the effect of erythromycin is likely the result of its anti-inflammatory properties. Postinflammatory hyperpigmentation may occur with ultraviolet B radiation therapy, so some experts recommend against its use. Persistence of either the rash or pruritus beyond 12 weeks should prompt reconsideration of the original diagnosis, to consider biopsy to confirm the diagnosis, and to question the patient again about the use of medications that may cause a rash similar to that of pityriasis rosea. An important goal of treatment is to control pruritus, which may be severe. For these patients, treatment with zinc oxide, calamine lotion, topical steroids, oral antihistamines, and even oral steroids may be necessary.

Page: 958

Question #5

Answer: B

Rationale: Pemphigus vulgaris is an autoimmune bullous disease that, if not treated with appropriate immunosuppressive agents, may be fatal. Bullous pemphigus may last months to years; however, it is a self-limiting disease, and it is rarely fatal. Dyshidrotic eczema eruptions occur with variable severity, and it can be mild or debilitating; however, there is no associated mortality. Erythema multiforme minor is a localized eruption of the skin with only mild or no mucosal involvement.

Page: 959

Question #6

Answer: D

Rationale: Although often asymptomatic, most patients with dermatitis herpetiformis have an underlying gluten-sensitive enteropathy. The disease may occur at any age, although it most commonly appears in patients who are between 20 and 40 years old. Men are affected twice as often as women. Dermatitis herpetiformis rarely occurs in blacks and Asians; the lesions occur

in a symmetrical pattern on the extensor surfaces of the body, and mucous membranes are rarely affected.
Page: 960

Question #7

Answer: D

Rationale: Ninety percent of worker's compensation claims for skin conditions are the result of contact dermatitis.
Page: 962

Question #8

Answer: A

Rationale: The most frequent symptom of atopic dermatitis is pruritus, which can be severe and which can sometimes cause sleep disruption. It has been referred to as "the itch that rashes," and it is a common problem that affects up to 15% of all children. In the majority of cases, atopic dermatitis occurs before the age of 5 years, frequently during the first year of life. Antihistamines, topical corticosteroids, and topical doxepin are the mainstays of therapy.
Page: 962

Question #9

Answer: C

Rationale: Erythema infectiosum, or Fifth disease, is caused by human parvovirus B19. It has a prodrome of fever, anorexia, sore throat, and abdominal pain. After the fever resolves, the classic bright-red facial rash ("slapped cheek") appears. The exanthem progresses to a diffuse, reticular rash that may wax and wane for several weeks. Human parvovirus B19 infection is of particular concern among pregnant women, because it has been associated with fetal hydrops and subsequent fetal death.
Page: 964

Question #10

Answer: D

Rationale: Rubeola is distinguished by the presence of Koplik's spots on the oral mucosa.
Page: 964

Question #11

Answer: D

Rationale: The mainstay of therapy for urticaria is the avoidance of known triggering agents.
Page: 964

Question #12

Answer: C

Rationale: Erythema nodosum is more frequently seen among women, and it is most commonly caused by streptococcal infection and sarcoidosis. Many other causes have been reported, including tuberculosis, salmonella, and Campylobacter. Patients present with fever, malaise, and joint discomfort in addition to the characteristic painful nodules.
Page: 965

Question #13

Answer: D

Rationale: The hallmark of sarcoidosis is infiltration with noncaseating granulomas. Both papules and plaques can be a variety of colors, including red, violaceous, hyperpigmented, or translucent. When multiple lesions are present, they tend to occur symmetrically. Lesions appearing on the alar rim of the nose, which is also known as lupus pernio, may be associated with granulomatous infiltration of the upper airway. Lesions of cutaneous sarcoidosis may be difficult to treat, because they tend to recur. Topical corticosteroids are often ineffective, because they do not adequately penetrate the skin lesions.
Page: 966

Question #14

Answer: B

Rationale: Scabies is caused by the parasite *Sarcoptes scabiei,* which is an obligate human parasite. Patients with scabies usually present with a pruritic papular rash with linear excoriations or burrows. Scabies can survive apart from their human hosts for up to 4 days, making reinfestation a frequent occurrence. In adults, the head and neck are frequently spared.
Page: 966

Question #15

Answer: A

Rationale: Although the reasons for it are not well understood, foods associated with pruritus ani include tea, coffee, cola, chocolate, citrus fruits, and tomatoes. Pruritus in patients with lichen simplex chronicus is usually worse during periods of inactivity, such as at bedtime and during the night. The detection of a single live head lice louse is sufficient for the diagnosis of infestation. Lindane shampoo, which was once considered the treatment of choice, is now used infrequently because of concerns about neurotoxicity and parasite resistance.

Page: 967

Question #16

Answer: B

Rationale: Mupirocin ointment is the treatment of choice for impetigo, and it has been shown to be as effective as oral antibiotics for limited disease, including cases caused by methicillin-resistant *S. aureus* and group A β-hemolytic streptococcus.

Page: 968

Question #17

Answer: D

Rationale: If a pseudomonal infection is suspected and lesions persist for more than 5 days without treatment, ciprofloxacin (Cipro) should be considered.

Page: 970

Question #18

Answer: C

Rationale: The preferred treatment for erythrasma is a course of oral erythromycin plus daily cleansing with soap and water. Treatment of a furuncle often requires drainage of the lesion. Streptococci have been reported to be the cause of erysipelas in as many as 80% of cases, with approximately two thirds of those caused by group A streptococci and one fourth caused by group G streptococci. Methicillin-resistant *S. aureus,* which can be hospital or community acquired, has also been noted as a cause of impetigo.

Page: 971

Question #19

Answer: D

Rationale: HSV infection can be characterized by episodes of latency, with asymptomatic viral shedding. Both serotypes can be present at oral or genital sites. HSV infection increases the risk of human immunodeficiency virus transmission, and it is believed to play an important role in the heterosexual spread of human immunodeficiency virus. Recurrent episodes are less likely with the HSV-1 serotype than with the HSV-2 serotype.

Page: 971

Question #20

Answer: D

Rationale: Corneal involvement, which should be suspected when lesions appear on the tip of the nose, can cause temporarily or permanently decreased visual acuity or blindness. The incidence is much higher among individuals who are immunocompromised or elderly. Analgesics such as acetaminophen and even narcotics are sometimes required to control the discomfort caused by herpes zoster. The rash rarely crosses the midline of the body, and it is usually confined to a single dermatome.

Page: 972

Question #21

Answer: D

Rationale: Of the many subtypes of human papillomavirus, types 16 and 18 are especially associated with the development of carcinoma.

Page: 973

Question #22

Answer: C

Rationale: Oral antifungals, including griseofulvin, terbinafine (Lamisil), and itraconazole (Sporanox), are all effective for the treatment of tinea barbae when used for an adequate duration, which may be up to 4 weeks. Topical antifungals are ineffective for tinea barbae.

Page: 974

Question #23

Answer: C

Rationale: Lyme disease is a systemic infection caused by the spirochete *Borrelia burgdorferi*. The bacterium is inoculated into the skin by a tick bite, and the tick is almost always of the genus *Ixodes*. Oral antibiotics such as doxycycline, amoxicillin, cefuroxime (Ceftin), erythromycin, azithromycin (Zithromax), or amoxicillin-clavulanate (Augmentin) should be administered for 10 to 21 days. For patients with erythema migrans and a history that is suggestive of a tick bite, serologic testing is unnecessary, because the pretest probability of Lyme disease is high and the sensitivity of the serologic test is low during the early stages of infection.

Page: 977

Question #24

Answer: C

Rationale: Doxycycline is the agent of choice for both adults and children with Rocky Mountain spotted fever because of its effectiveness, its broad margin of safety, and its convenient dosing schedule. Vascular injury of the pancreas and the gastrointestinal tract—including the stomach, the small intestine, and the colon—may result in nausea, vomiting, diarrhea, and abdominal cramping. These common and nonspecific gastrointestinal symptoms that are present early in the course of the disease may complicate the diagnosis. Lesions typically begin on the wrists and ankles and then spread to cover the soles and palms. The rash continues to move centripetally, covering the extremities, the genitals, and the trunk and typically sparing the face. Indirect fluorescent antibody testing is the best and most widely used serologic test; it has a high specificity and sensitivity (94%). However, antibodies usually do not appear until 1 to 2 weeks after infection.

Page: 977

Question #25

Answer: D

Rationale: Isotretinoin (Accutane) is a known teratogen, and it should not be used by women of childbearing age unless the avoidance of pregnancy is ensured. By law, contraception counseling is mandatory, and two negative pregnancy test results are required before the initiation of therapy. Baseline laboratory examination should also include cholesterol and triglyceride assessments, a determination of the hepatic transaminase level, and a complete blood cell count. Pregnancy tests and laboratory examinations should be repeated monthly during treatment.

Page: 978

Question #26

Answer: C

Rationale: Nearly half of patients with acne rosacea develop ocular symptoms, including eyes that are itchy, burning, or dry; that have a gritty or foreign body sensation; and that involve erythema and swelling of the eyelid. The ocular changes can become chronic. Corneal neovascularization and keratitis can occur, and this leads to corneal scarring and perforation. Most patients respond well to long-term topical antibiotic treatment involving metronidazole, erythromycin, and clindamycin. Oral or topical retinoid therapy may also be effective. Common triggers include exposure to the sun, cold weather, sudden emotion (including laughter or embarrassment), hot beverages, spicy foods, and alcohol consumption.

Page: 978

Question #27

Answer: D

Rationale: Repigmentation therapy includes the use of corticosteroids, ultraviolet light, calcineurin inhibitors, and surgery. Genetic factors appear to play a role. The onset of vitiligo can be at any age, but it peaks during the 20s and 30s. Although vitiligo has the same prevalence among all races, it can be especially disfiguring among patients with highly pigmented skin.

Page: 978

Question #28

Answer: B

Rationale: Because xanthelasma are always benign, treatment is primarily cosmetic. In some instances, cholesterol reduction can induce the regression of the plaques. Surgery, carbon dioxide laser, or trichloroacetic acid may also be effective. Because hyperlipidemia is present in about half of patients with these lesions, a lipid profile should be obtained for all patients with xanthelasma. Lesions are also seen as a classic feature of primary biliary cirrhosis.

Page: 980

Question #29

Answer: A

Rationale: Seborrheic keratoses are hyperkeratotic lesions of the epidermis that often appear to be "stuck on" the surface of the skin and that are most commonly found on the trunk. Basal cell carcinoma is the most common human malignancy; it is usually slow growing, and it rarely metastasizes. Cutaneous squamous cell carcinoma is the second most common form of skin cancer. Actinic keratosis lesions have malignant potential, and they can transform into squamous cell carcinoma.

Page: 981

Question #30

Answer: D

Rationale: Incision and drainage at the edge of the nail plate markedly improves the associated discomfort of a paronychia, and it allows for rapid healing. Antibiotics are not necessary if the incision successfully achieves adequate drainage.

Page: 986

Question #31

Answer: B

Rationale: The shave biopsy technique is a good choice for lesions such as acrochordons, seborrheic keratoses, and some dermatofibromas. However, shave biopsy should never be used for pigmented lesions; punch biopsies are useful for the assessment of these lesions. Electrosurgery can be used for incisional techniques that produce full-thickness excision of nevi.

Page: 988

Question #32

Answer: D

Rationale: A vesicle is described as a circumscribed, elevated, fluid-containing lesion that is less than 0.5 cm in its greatest diameter, and it may be intraepidermal or subepidermal in origin. A macule is a circumscribed area of change in normal skin color with no skin elevation or depression; it may be any size. A papule is a solid, raised lesion that is up to 0.5 cm in its greatest diameter. A pustule is a circumscribed elevation of skin that contains purulent fluid of variable character (i.e., the fluid may be white, yellow, greenish, or hemorrhagic).

Page: 956

45   Answers

Question #1

Answer: D

Rationale: Along with the typical symptoms of hyperglycemia such as weight loss, polyuria, and polydipsia, one of the following criteria is required to confirm a suspected diagnosis of diabetes mellitus: more than two random serum glucose values of greater than 200 mg/dL, a fasting blood glucose level greater than or equal to 126 mg/dL that is confirmed on repeat testing, or a 2-hour glucose challenge level of greater than 200 mg/dL (i.e., a blood glucose value drawn 2 hours after a 75-mg oral glucose challenge). The hemoglobin A1c level reflects the average 3-month blood glucose level; it is useful for measuring the level of glycemic control, but it is unacceptable for diagnostic purposes.

Page: 989

Question #2

Answer: B

Rationale: A fasting serum glucose value between 100 and 125 mg/dL has been designated as demonstrating the condition that is now known as prediabetes. Patients with prediabetes have been shown to have an increased risk of progressing to non–insulin-dependent diabetes mellitus. It is yet to be determined what impact this condition will have on long-term complications, but early identification of this pre-disease state offers the physician valuable opportunities to provide education about nutrition, lifestyle modification, and other preventive strategies.

Page: 989

Question #3

Answer: B

Rationale: Metabolic syndrome is an extremely common condition that is believed to have a prevalence of more than 25% of the U.S. population. The Adult Treatment Panel guidelines define the components of metabolic syndrome as any three of the following: a fasting serum glucose level of more than 110 mg/dL, a blood pressure level greater than or equal to 130/85 mmHg, a fasting serum triglyceride level of greater than 150 mg/dL, a

high-density lipoprotein cholesterol level of less than 40 mg/dL in men or less than 50 mg/dL in women, and a waist circumference of more than 102 cm for men or 88 cm for women. The increased incidence of this condition is felt to be worsened by the obesity epidemic along with greater rates of hypertension and hyperlipidemia.

Page: 989

Question #4

Answer: A

Rationale: In some cases, it may be difficult to distinguish type 1 (juvenile) diabetes from type 2 (adult-onset) diabetes. The presence of hyperglycemia associated with the demonstration of anti-islet antibodies (namely, anti-glutamic acid decarboxylase) is specific to the diagnosis of type 1 diabetes mellitus. Depressed insulin levels are nonspecific, and they may be lowered by the presence of hyperglycemia, dehydration, or lipotoxicity. C-peptide levels may be normal in patients who have received antidiabetic therapy, which makes them less useful for diagnostic purposes.

Page: 991

Question #5

Answer: C

Rationale: The typical somatic signs and symptoms of diabetes mellitus often take years to develop during a prolonged latent phase. The most common method of diagnosing early type 2 diabetes is during a routine risk factor assessment for cardiovascular disease. Appropriate screening of fasting serum glucose levels and lipid profiles will detect many cases and help to guide further diagnostic workups.

Page: 992

Question #6

Answer: B

Rationale: The daily requirement of insulin for most patients with type 1 diabetes ranges from approximately 0.5 to 1 U/kg/day. A level of 0.5 U/kg/day is usually enough to prevent the development of ketosis, but higher levels are required for adequate levels of glucose control. This average dose may be initiated in newly diagnosed type 1 diabetics who are not in diabetic ketoacidosis.

Page: 994

Question #7

Answer: C

Rationale: The total calculated daily dose of insulin should be divided so that 50% is given as a long-acting preparation such as insulin glargine (Lantus) or ultra (Humulin U). This provides basal coverage to limit lipolysis. The remaining 50% of the daily insulin dose should be divided into multiple doses directed at ambient or anticipated glucose levels. These short-acting preparations, such as R (regular insulin), lispro (Humalog), and aspart (NovoLog), should be given before meals and based on anticipated carbohydrate content.

Page: 994

Question #8

Answer: B

Rationale: The use of home glucose monitoring is essential for the management and prevention of complications for all diabetics. The American Diabetes Association has released guidelines that state that the target fasting and premeal glucose level should be less than 120 mg/dL. This tight control will help to prevent many of the short- and long-term complications found in diabetic patients. In certain subpopulations that may be at risk for hypoglycemia, such as young children and the elderly, looser control with a fasting target of 150 mg/dL may be appropriate.

Page: 995

Question #9

Answer: A

Rationale: As published in the *American Diabetes Association Diabetes Care* supplements of January 2004 and January 2005, the Diabetes Control and Complications Trial Research Group[1] and the UK Prospective Diabetes

Study Group[2] state that type 1 and type 2 diabetic patients, when guided by self glucose monitoring, are able to accomplish excellent glucose control and near-normal hemoglobin A1c levels. Evidence shows that this tight glycemic control reduces the occurrence and progression of the microangiopathic complications of diabetes mellitus.

Page: 995

Question #10

Answer: C

Rationale: There are now significant level B evidence recommendations against the use of a specific diabetic diet. All recommendations should be based on a comprehensive plan of care that includes proper nutrition, healthy activity, home glucose monitoring, and appropriate medical management. A healthy meal plan with close control of carbohydrate intake along with decreasing fat will help patients achieve a healthy weight.

Pages: 995–996

Question #11

Answer: B

Rationale: The recommended daily caloric intake should be divided into specific contents of carbohydrate, fat, and protein. The current recommendation includes 60% carbohydrate, 30% fat, and 10% protein, with cholesterol limited to 300 mg/day.

Page: 996

Question #12

Answer: A

Rationale: Regular walking is an important exercise that may help improve circulation, promote weight loss, and assist with glycemic control. However, it should be noted that diabetic foot evaluation of the skin and circulation and neurologic examination are essential for

---

1. Diabetes Control and Complications Trial (DCCT) Research Group: The effect of intensive treatment of diabetes on the development and progression of long-term complications in insulin-dependent diabetes mellitus. *N Engl J Med* 329:977–986, 1993.

2. United Kingdom Prospective Diabetes Study (UKPDS) Group: Intensive blood-glucose control with sulphonylureas or insulin compared with conventional treatment and risk of complications in patients with type 2 diabetes (UKPDS 33). *Lancet* 352:837–853, 1998; and United Kingdom Prospective Diabetes Study (UKPDS) Group: Tight blood pressure control and risk of macrovascular and microvascular complications in type 2 diabetes: UKPDS 38, *BMJ* 317:703–713, 1998.

preventing diabetic foot injuries and ulcers. Adequate assessment to rule out peripheral neuropathy may be accomplished by evaluating the patient for a loss of microfilament touch sensation on the pronator surface of the foot. Prophylactic treatment with orthotics, foot lubrication, and adequate footwear are essential for the prevention of diabetic foot disease.

Page: 997

Question #13

Answer: B

Rationale: Data published by the American Diabetes Association in its diabetes care supplement dated January 2005, based on studies from the Diabetes Control and Complications Trial Research Group[1] and the UK Perspective Diabetes Study Group,[2] stated that the optimal therapeutic goal for the prevention of the microangiopathic complications of diabetes mellitus is achieving a hemoglobin A1c of less than 7% while avoiding the risk of hypoglycemia.

Page: 999

Question #14

Answer: A

Rationale: Although there are no specific guidelines recommending a drug of choice for the management of patients with non–insulin-dependent diabetes mellitus, the consensus of the authors and of most clinical authorities is that metformin should be the first-line drug, especially for overweight patients. Metformin acts by blocking glucose production by the liver, which leads to a reduction in insulin resistance. The drug is not associated with further weight gain, and it is usually well tolerated. It is contraindicated for patients with renal insufficiency, and lactic acidosis may occur if it is given inappropriately. The drug is available generically at a relatively low cost.

Page: 999

Question #15

Answer: B

Rationale: The class of glitazones, which are used by many physicians as first-line agents, are highly effective for the management of patients with non–insulin-dependent diabetes. These agents incite the production of cellular proteins that facilitate insulin's actions on the cytoplasm and the mitochondria; this leads to the significant improvement of insulin resistance. However, the medication may be associated with an unpredictable weight gain and the development of peripheral edema. In patients with renal insufficiency or diastolic dysfunction, glitazones are associated with an increased risk of pulmonary edema.

Page: 999

Question #16

Answer: D

Rationale: Sulfonylureas are the oldest class of oral medications used for the treatment of type 2 diabetes mellitus. Their mechanism of action leads to the stimulation of insulin secretion. In general, the class has a prolonged therapeutic duration, and it is the drug that is most often associated with hypoglycemic episodes. This hypoglycemic risk is increased if the hemoglobin A1c level is maintained at less than 7%, and it is also increased in patients with renal disease. The advantage of sulfonylureas as a first-line drug is that they may be combined with any of the other oral medications, and they are available as low-cost generic alternatives.

Page: 999

Question #17

Answer: E

Rationale: Supplemental insulin has now been proven to reduce the microangiopathic complications of non–insulin-dependent diabetics who have not achieved adequate control with the use of behavioral methods along with combinations of oral drugs. A long-acting insulin preparation given at bedtime is the most physiologic option, because it offsets the hyperglycemia of the dawn phenomenon. This results in "beta cell rest," which provides increased insulin to improve postprandial function and to restore control. In addition, glargine insulin is associated with less hypoglycemia than other preparations.

Pages: 999–1000

Question #18

Answer: C

Rationale: The use of insulin pump therapy is becoming readily available throughout the community. Use of the pump requires a highly motivated patient who is willing to do home glucose monitoring at least six to eight times per day. There are no data that pump therapy is superior to regular injections for patients who are well controlled. The major advantage is the decreased need for injections of insulin preparations and the improvement in glucose control for some patients. In addition to the extensive patient education that is required, complications include pump failure and recurrent localized infections at the site of needle entry.

Page: 1002

Question #19

Answer: B

Rationale: Diabetic ketoacidosis results when there is an absolute or relative lack of insulin that leads to hyperglycemia, dehydration, glycolysis, and ketoacidosis. It is often the presenting condition in new type 1 diabetic, and it may also present as a result of failure to administer insulin or septicemia in a known diabetic patient. Laboratory findings include elevation of blood glucose, hemoconcentration as a result of dehydration, and often a reduction in the PaO_2 tension. A reduction in serum bicarbonate along with a decrease in the pH and a respiratory compensation along with the presence of serum acetone is necessary for a diagnosis. Many patients will present with a potassium imbalance, with 30% of patients being hyperkalemic and up to 20% of patients being hypokalemic.

Page: 1003

Question #20

Answer: C

Rationale: Intravenous fluids are the cornerstone of the initial resuscitation if the patient is in diabetic ketoacidosis. Fluids are necessary to restore capillary perfusion. The first several liters of fluid should be normal saline, which is the best crystalloid volume expander. Generally healthy patients will tolerate 1 L/hour for the first several hours of resuscitation. As resuscitation progresses and the patient's hydration status improves, a change to 0.45% saline is indicated. As the glucose level reaches 200 mg/dL, the addition of glucose is required.

Page: 1004

Question #21

Answer: A

Rationale: Non-ketotic hyperosmolality syndrome usually occurs in type 2 diabetics who present with marked hyperglycemia associated with azotemia, severe dehydration, and a hyperosmolar state. With increasing concentrations of serum osmolality and subsequent cerebral fluid shifts, changes in mental status may occur, and they may sometimes lead to coma. Patients who are most susceptible to this syndrome are often elderly, they may have sustained a cerebrovascular accident or an acute myocardial infarction, or they may be septicemic. It is rare for type 2 diabetic patients to develop ketoacidosis.

Page: 1005

Question #22

Answer: D

Rationale: Most women with preconception diabetes mellitus have type 1 diabetes. Recent studies have shown that, with tight glycemic control, complications can be significantly reduced. This tight control is associated with decreased prematurity, reduced risk of fetal developmental anomalies, and a decreased risk of bronchopulmonary dysplasia. Women of advanced maternal age are at increased risk for the development of type 2 diabetes that is often unrecognized before conception. Developmental anomalies are less common among children of type 2 diabetic mothers, which may be related to the probable shorter duration of disease.

Page: 1006

Question #23

Answer: E

Rationale: Glargine insulin (Lantus), which is now widely used for the treatment of both type 1 and type 2 diabetes, is not approved for use during pregnancy. Humulin R and N insulins have been proven safe and effective, and they may be used in a multiple dosing schedule or through an insulin pump. Metformin is the drug of choice for the treatment of type 2 diabetics when they are pregnant. Regardless of therapy choice, tight glycemic control is essential for preventing maternal and neonatal complications.

Page: 1007

Question #24

Answer: D

Rationale: Diabetes that is diagnosed during pregnancy is commonly known as *gestational diabetes mellitus.* Fifty percent of the women who develop gestational diabetes will continue to evolve into type 2 diabetics. This condition may represent the first clinical manifestation of type 1 or type 2 diabetes in patients who were asymptomatic before pregnancy, or it may represent the activation of diabetic genes during pregnancy. Research has shown that the conversion rate of gestational diabetes to full-blown type 2 diabetes may be reduced with therapeutic lifestyle changes after pregnancy.

Page: 1007

Question #25

Answer: B

Rationale: With the increasing prevalence of diabetes mellitus, most professional societies recommend that all pregnant women (except low-risk patients) be screened for diabetes. Otherwise healthy white women who are less than 25 years old represent this low-risk category. Patients with a prior history of glucose intolerance, obesity, hypertension, or a positive family history of diabetes should all be screened.

Page: 1007

Question #26

Answer: C

Rationale: Careful preoperative evaluation of the diabetic patient is essential to minimize the risk of surgical procedures. Special attention to good glycemic control as well as the assessment of cardiovascular and renal pathologies should be performed. Immediately before the surgical procedure, all oral medications as well as short- and intermediate-acting insulins should be discontinued. Basal insulin coverage with long-acting insulin such as glargine (Lantus), along with the administration of glucose and potassium, is most effective.

Page: 1008

Question #27

Answer: C

Rationale: According to the landmark study of the Diabetes Control and Complications Trial, the rate of progression of the triopathy of diabetic microangiopathic complications, which includes neuropathy, nephropathy, and retinopathy, is reduced by 50% with tight glycemic control. In this study, hemoglobin A1c levels were reduced from 9% to 7%, and they continued to remain controlled throughout the 7-year trial. In addition, 8 years after the study, patients with a hemoglobin A1c level of 8% still showed lower rates of microangiopathic complications.

Page: 1009

Question #28

Answer: C

Rationale: Numerous studies have now confirmed the significant benefit of angiotensin-converting enzyme inhibitors and angiotensin receptor blockers for preventing the progression of or reversing the presence of microalbuminuria and diabetic nephropathy. Recent studies are showing that other agents may have similar effects. Clinical guidelines now suggest that a blood pressure below 130/85 mm Hg is also essential for preventing the progression of cardiovascular and renal disease. Diabetic patients should be checked for microalbuminuria at least annually. Any degree of microalbuminuria indicates a need for tighter glycemic control and the addition of an angiotensin-converting enzyme inhibitor or an angiotensin receptor blocker. Other important measures include weight control and the limitation of salt, potassium, and protein, along with adequate hydration. In general, angiotensin-converting enzyme inhibitors seem to be more effective for type 1 diabetics, whereas angiotensin receptor blockers are possibly better for type 2 patients.

Page: 1012

Question #29

Answer: A

Rationale: Although most clinicians have diabetic patients remove their shoes before they enter the examination room, this method is less likely to elucidate signs of early diabetic foot disease. The critical moment in the foot examination is immediately after the stocking is removed, when it should be observed for moisture resulting from heat generation within the patients' shoes. A moist foot will usually have good perfusion, and it is a more reliable early sign of diabetic foot disease. The typical findings of loss of hair along with a pale, cool extremity are later findings of diabetic microangiopathy. Patients at this early stage will most often have normal peripheral pulses. A neurological examination, including monofilament sensitivity testing, is also essential for detecting more advanced diabetic peripheral neuropathy.

Page: 1009

Question #30

Answer: B

Rationale: The feet are the most common area of the peripheral nervous system to be affected by diabetic complications. Paresthesias usually begin 5 to 10 years after diagnosis in patients who have a hemoglobin A1c level that remains above 8.5%. Typical symptoms begin in the evening as a result of decreased perfusion when supine or sleeping. These paresthesias are typically perceived as numbness, burning, or a "pins and needles" sensation in ether the toes or the bottom of the feet. Massaging the foot may improve microcirculation, which leads to the alleviation of symptoms. On physical examination, a dry, hairless foot with thickening of the skin and subcutaneous tissue is often found. With advanced disease, findings include decreased deep tendon reflexes, a loss of vibratory and position senses, and a loss of fine touch evidenced by microfilament testing.

Page: 1010

Question #31

Answer: E

Rationale: The prevention of diabetic neuropathy with tight glycemic control is the cornerstone of delaying the progression of foot disease. Careful diabetic foot care is essential to prevent limb-threatening diabetic foot infections. Patient education along with podiatry referral is important for all patients who are at risk for disease. As the condition progresses, nocturnal paresthesia can become debilitating, and medical intervention is often required for symptom control. Neurostabilizers such as gabapentin, amitriptyline, carbamazepine (Tegretol),

and duloxetine (Cymbalta) have been shown to be effective for the treatment of diabetic neuropathy. Acetaminophen and nonsteroidal anti-inflammatory drugs may be useful for mild disease or as adjunctive therapy. Narcotic analgesics should be a last resort, because they are of limited benefit and may lead to significant drug dependency in these patients.

Page: 1010

Question #32

Answer: D

Rationale: As the risk factors and signs of diabetes increase, so does the complication rate. Cardiovascular disease is the leading cause of death among diabetic patients. As the condition progresses, tight control of glucose, blood pressure, and lipids are essential to prevent further and more rapid degeneration. The threshold for using statins has greatly decreased. with recent data demonstrating that all patients should have their low-density lipoprotein levels lowered to less than 100 mg/dL, with a target of 70 mg/dL. Some more recent studies are indicating that statins may have protective actions irrespective of the low-density lipoprotein level and that they should be given to all diabetic patients. In addition to the use of statins, angiotensin-converting enzyme inhibitors, and angiotensin receptor blockers, aspirin in low doses should be prescribed to all diabetic patients, unless it is contraindicated.

Page: 1014

46 Answers

Question #1

Answer: C

Rationale: Approximately 80% of thyroid hormone produced by the thyroid gland is T4, whereas the rest is T3. T3 is believed to be the biologically active form, and most of it is formed from the deiodination of T4 in the peripheral circulation. A total T4 level measures the total amount of circulating T4, most of which is bound to a protein called thyroid-binding globulin (TBG). TBG levels can be affected by various drugs and conditions, which in turn can alter total T4 levels without affecting free T4. Estrogen-containing oral contraceptives increase TBG levels, and, hence, they increase the total T4 levels without altering the free T4 levels. Obtaining a free T4 level is preferred over a total T4 level for such patients. A thyroglobulin level helps differentiate factitious from endogenous hyperthyroidism. Thyroglobulin levels are low, and they accompany suppressed thyroid-hormone production in patients with factitious hyperthyroidism; alternatively, thyroglobulin levels are elevated in patients with endogenous hyperthyroidism.

Page: 1021

Question #2

Answer: B

Rationale: Subclinical hypothyroidism is defined as an elevated TSH level in the presence of a normal free T4 level. Patients who test positive for anti-tissue peroxidase are more likely to develop overt hypothyroidism. Patients with these antibodies also have a 2.5-fold increase in their risk of miscarriage. These antibodies can be present in both hyperthyroidism and hypothyroidism, and their presence suggests an autoimmune etiology. Their presence in a hyperthyroid patient suggests Graves' disease, and it suggests Hashimoto's disease in a hypothyroid patient.

Page: 1022

Question #3

Answer: D

Rationale: Radioiodine uptake is increased among patients with Graves' disease, but it is reduced in patients with hyperthyroidism that results from postpartum thyroiditis, subacute thyroiditis, silent (lymphocytic) thyroiditis, and factitious thyrotoxicosis.

Page: 1022

Question #4

Answers: (1), A; (2), A; (3), B; (4), B

Rationale: There are various modalities used to treat hyperthyroidism, including radioiodine (iodine-131), surgery (thyroidectomy), and antithyroid drugs. Of these, thyroid ablation using radioiodine is the most common form of therapy used in the United States; its efficacy is approximately 70% to 95% at 1 year after administration. Hypothyroidism is a side effect of therapy, and it develops approximately 3 months after starting therapy. Hence, most patients who are treated with radioiodine ultimately need to be on thyroid-hormone replacement therapy. Pregnancy should be ruled out before starting radioiodine therapy, because it is an absolute contraindication. Agranulocytosis is a rare but serious complication of antithyroid drugs (e.g., methimazole, propylthiouracil), and so patients on these medications should have their leukocyte count checked if they have a fever or complain of a sore throat.

Page: 1027

Question #5

Answers: (1), A; (2), A; (3), B

Rationale: Thyroid nodules are common in clinical practice, and they are seen more frequently among women (6%) than men (1%–2%). The functional status and the possibility of malignancy are two issues that need to be addressed in every patient with a thyroid nodule. Hence, obtaining a TSH level is the first step in the evaluation of such patients. Patients with a suppressed TSH level are highly unlikely to have a malignant nodule, and fine-needle aspiration is usually not necessary. Alternatively, when the TSH level is either normal or high, the next most cost-effective step is to obtain a fine-needle aspiration of the nodule. Although only 5% of thyroid nodules are malignant, the risk of malignancy is greater among patients who are less than 30 and more than 60 years old, among those with a history of head and neck radiation, and among those with a family history of thyroid cancer.

Page: 1029

Question #6

Answer: B

Rationale: Thyroid adenocarcinomas (papillary and follicular) are more common than medullary and anaplastic cancers, and they have a better prognosis. Adenocarcinomas arise from thyroid follicular tissue, and they produce thyroglobulin, which serves as a marker of current, residual, and recurrent disease. Anaplastic and medullary cancers do not produce thyroglobulin. The prognoses of patients with adenocarcinomas are very good (papillary has a better prognosis than follicular), although it is poor for the other two. Papillary adenocarcinomas are locally invasive, and they have the best prognosis. Follicular adenocarcinomas are more aggressive, and they are more likely to present with metastatic disease. Iodine-131 is used both as a diagnostic and therapeutic modality for thyroid adenocarcinomas.

Page: 1029

Question #7

Answer: D

Rationale: Thyroid hormone requirements are increased during pregnancy, and they return to prepregnancy levels after delivery. The average thyroid hormone requirement goes up by 50% during pregnancy. Thyroid status should be very closely monitored, typically by checking TSH levels every 1 to 2 weeks. TSH levels should be maintained within the normal reference range.

Page: 1030

Question #8

Answer: E

Rationale: Thyroid gland lymphomas are more common among patients with a long-standing history of Hashimoto's thyroiditis.

Page: 1028

Question #9

Answer: E

Rationale: The most common cause of hypercalcemia in the office setting is primary hyperparathyroidism, whereas, in a hospitalized patient, the main cause is malignancy. Other causes include milk–alkali syndrome, sarcoidosis, adrenal insufficiency, vitamin D intoxication, and medications (e.g., thiazide diuretics, lithium). (See the table below.)

Page: 1031

Question #10

Answer: D

Rationale: Of the listed antihypertensive agents, thiazide diuretics can cause hypercalcemia in an otherwise healthy individual by decreasing urinary calcium excretion. Other agents that are known to cause hypercalcemia include lithium and vitamin D intoxication. Loop diuretics promote urinary calcium excretion, and they are thus used for the treatment of hypercalcemia.

Page: 1031

Parameter	Malignancy	Hyperparathyroidism
Duration	Acute (recent onset)	Chronic (long history)
Serum calcium	Frequently >14 mg/dL	Usually <14 mg/dL
Serum chloride	Usually <103 mEq/dL	Usually >103 mEq/dL
Anemia	Frequent	Unusual
Serum PTH	Low	Mid-high normal or elevated
Urinary calcium	Normal or high	Normal or high
Sedimentation rate	Increased	Normal
Alkaline phosphatase	Increased	Normal or increased
Weight loss	Marked	Minimal
Serum phosphate	Low, normal, or high	Normal or low
Renal stones	Uncommon	Occasional
Response to steroids	Sometimes effective	Not responsive
Radiographic study	Soft tissue lesions, metastatic lesions	Subperiosteal bone resorption
HCO_3	Normal or high	Normal or low

PTH, Parathyroid hormone.
Modified from DeGroot LJ, Larsen PR, Hennemann E (eds): *The thyroid and its diseases,* ed 6. New York, Churchill Livingstone, 1996, p 346; data from Murray IPC: Personal communication. In Rakel RE [ed]. *Textbook of family medicine,* ed 7. Philadelphia: WB Saunders, 2007.

Question #11

Answer: C

Rationale: With the exception of raloxifene, all of the agents listed are effective for the reduction of vasomotor symptoms in postmenopausal women. Selective serotonin reuptake inhibitors and selective norepinephrine reuptake inhibitors (e.g., venlafaxine) are effective, generally well tolerated, and recommended as first-line agents for the treatment of vasomotor symptoms. They may also have a positive impact on menopausal mood changes. Venlafaxine is considered to be the most effective agent for the treatment of hot flashes in the reuptake inhibitor class, but it can elevate blood pressure. Common class side effects include sexual dysfunction and gastrointestinal disturbances (e.g., nausea, diarrhea). Clonidine and gabapentin are less effective, and they are hence used as second-line agents. Relaxation techniques and meditation are alternative forms of therapy that have been shown to be effective for the reduction of vasomotor symptoms. Black cohosh and other phytoestrogens have variable efficacy, and they are not regulated by the U.S. Food and Drug Administration. Raloxifene, which is a selective estrogen receptor modulator used for the treatment of osteoporosis, can cause hot flashes. Although estrogen–progesterone replacement therapy is most effective for the treatment of vasomotor symptoms, it is not recommended because the risks of therapy far outweigh the benefits. The U.S. Food and Drug Administration recently approved Angeliq, a combination of drospirenone and estrogen, for the treatment of moderate to severe vasomotor symptoms and vulvar/vaginal atrophy associated with menopause in women whose uteruses are intact.

Page: 1046

Question #12

Answer: C

Rationale: Raloxifene is a selective estrogen receptor modulator that has stimulatory as well as inhibitory effects on estrogen receptors. It causes a modest increase in bone mineral density, and it is used for the treatment of postmenopausal osteoporosis. However, it is less efficacious than bisphosphonates, and it also has the potential to decrease the risk of breast cancer. Like estrogen and tamoxifen, it increases the risk of venous thrombosis, but it does not increase the risk of endometrial cancer. Hot flashes and leg cramps are common side effects of therapy with this agent.

Page: 1046

Question #13

Answer: B

Rationale: Primary adrenal insufficiency is mainly autoimmune in etiology, and it should be suspected in a patient presenting with vague, nonspecific symptoms (e.g., the triad of decreased energy, anorexia, and weight loss) with a history of other autoimmune endocrinopathies (e.g., type 1 diabetes mellitus, Hashimoto's thyroiditis). Acute adrenal insufficiency can be fatal if it is not recognized, and it should be strongly suspected in a patient with refractory hypotension with or without a known adrenal pathology. Primary adrenal insufficiency is associated with a plasma adrenocorticotropic hormone level greater than 100 pg/dL, and a presumptive diagnosis can be made when the morning cortisol level is less than 3 µg/dL. Further diagnostic confirmation is made with adrenocorticotropic hormone stimulation tests. A morning plasma cortisol level greater than 19 µg/dL rules out adrenal insufficiency. The treatment of acute insufficiency consists of intravenous fluids to correct hypovolemia, intravenous dexamethasone, and treatment of the precipitating cause. Dexamethasone is usually preferred over hydrocortisone, because it does not interfere with tests that evaluate adrenal function, and its effects last for 24 hours.

Page: 1036

Question #14

Answer: B

Rationale: Plasma aldosterone concentration to plasma renin activity is considered to be the screening test of choice in suspected cases of hyperaldosteronism; a ratio of greater than 20 with a plasma aldosterone concentration of more than 15 ng/dL is considered to be positive. The diagnosis is confirmed by a 24-hour urinary aldosterone level of greater than 10 to 14 µg/dL after a period of potassium repletion and salt loading. A serum potassium level of less than 3.5 mEq/L in a patient with refractory hypertension suggests hyperaldosteronism; however, many such patients have normal serum potassium levels. Computed tomography scanning of the adrenals helps identify structural abnormalities of the glands, but it is not used as a screening test.

Page: 1040

Question #15

Answer: B

Rationale: Of the known causes of hypopituitarism, the most common cause is a pituitary adenoma. Other causes include extrapituitary tumors (e.g., craniopharyngiomas), infiltrative diseases (e.g., sarcoidosis, hemochromatosis, histiocytosis X), postpartum hemorrhage and shock (Sheehan's syndrome), mutation in the PROP-1 gene (the most common cause of congenital hypopituitarism), and surgery or radiation of or around the pituitary gland.

Page: 1043

Question #16

Answer: A

Rationale: Adults with growth-hormone deficiency have reduced life expectancy compared with age-matched controls. Decreased lean body mass, dyslipidemia, increased cardiovascular events, and decreased bone mineral density are some of the features that are seen among such patients.

Page: 1047

Question #17

Answer: A

Rationale: Ovarian failure is suggested by the presence of a high serum FSH level and by the absence of withdrawal bleeding after the administration of progesterone (i.e., the progesterone challenge test). (See Figure 46-1.)

Page: 1045

Question #18

Answer: B

Rationale: Serum IGF-1 levels are used to monitor the effectiveness of recombinant human growth hormone therapy. It is recommended that these levels be maintained in the middle of the normal range, because higher levels are associated with side effects. Side effects of therapy include glucose intolerance, edema, carpal tunnel syndrome, and paresthesias.

Page: 1047

Question #19

Answer: D

Rationale: A reversible cause for galactorrhea should be sought before further evaluation. Medications are the most common cause of hyperprolactinemia and galactorrhea. Common offending agents include metoclopramide, imipramine, selective serotonin reuptake inhibitors, H_2 antagonists, phenothiazines, haloperidol, and calcium channel blockers. If such an agent is identified, it should be discontinued (if possible) and the prolactin level rechecked. Imaging of the pituitary and the hypothalamus with magnetic resonance imaging is recommended for patients in whom the offending agent cannot be stopped or when a pathologic cause is suspected. If the prolactin level is increased, then further evaluation should include a serum TSH level, a thyrotropin-releasing hormone level, and a serum creatinine

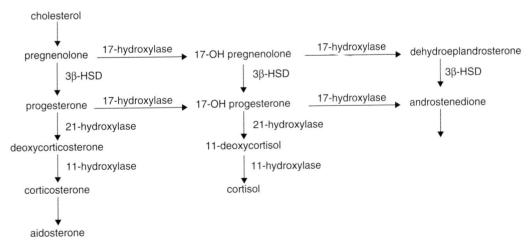

Figure 46-1 Modified from Carr BR: Disorders of the ovaries and female reproductive tract. In Wilson JD, Foster DW, editors: *Williams textbook of endocrinology,* ed 8, Philadelphia, 1992, WB Saunders. In Rakel RE, editor: *Textbook of family medicine,* ed 7, Philadelphia, WB Saunders, 2007.

level (renal insufficiency and failure results in decreased prolactin clearance).

Galactorrhea is a common manifestation of hyperprolactinemia in women, but it is less often seen in men. Amenorrhea or oligomenorrhea may also be present, and it can result from the prolactin-induced inhibition of gonadotropin-releasing hormone and, hence, the inhibition of luteinizing hormone and FSH. Other signs of gonadal failure including infertility, vaginal dryness, and decreased bone mineral density may be present.

Page: 1048

Question #20

Answer: B

Rationale: Acromegaly is caused by excessive growth-hormone secretion, typically from a growth-hormone–secreting pituitary adenoma. Growth hormone stimulates the release of IGF-1 from the liver. Growth hormone and IGF-1 (a potent growth and differentiation factor) stimulate the growth of various tissues and organs, resulting in skin thickening, coarsening of the facial features, macrognathia, and large hands and feet (i.e., acral bony overgrowth). Degenerative joint disease as a result of cartilage and bone overgrowth causes back and joint pain. A higher incidence of valvular heart disease, hypertension, cardiomyopathy, and arrhythmias is seen; cardiovascular disease is the cause of increased mortality among patients with acromegaly. Colonic polyps are also seen with an increased frequency among patients with this condition, and there is a possible increased risk of colon cancer. Pressure effects of the pituitary adenoma on surrounding normal pituitary tissue result in the hyposecretion of various other pituitary hormones, especially gonadotropins. Consequently, hypogonadism with resulting ovarian/testicular failure is often seen. Other metabolic effects include impaired glucose tolerance and abnormalities of calcium and phosphate metabolism. Serum IGF-1 levels are the single best screening test for acromegaly, because growth hormone levels fluctuate, and they are unreliable for the making of the diagnosis. The diagnosis is confirmed by an increased serum level of growth hormone after a glucose tolerance test (in normal individuals, the growth hormone level is 1 ng/mL or less at 1 to 2 hours after a 75-gm oral glucose load). A pituitary magnetic resonance image helps locate the source of the excess growth-hormone secretion. The preferred treatment is the surgical removal of the pituitary adenoma using a trans-sphenoidal approach, and it has a high rate of success. Octreotide (a somatostatin analog) is used

either as an adjuvant to surgery or when surgery is contraindicated. Radiotherapy is an option for patients in whom surgical and medical therapy fail.

Page: 1049

Question #21

Answer: B

Rationale: Patients with Cushing's disease have hypercortisolism with a myriad of clinical features. Hypercoagulability results from an increased production of clotting factors, and this results in an increased risk of thromboembolic events. Hypertension is common, and it is often multifactorial. Other features include proximal muscle weakness, impaired insulin resistance, decreased bone mineral density (resulting in osteopenia and osteoporosis), gonadal dysfunction (typically amenorrhea), depression, anxiety, and easy irritability. Postural hypotension is not a feature of Cushing's disease.

Page: 1050

Question #22

Answer: A

Rationale: A 24-hour urinary cortisol excretion is the first step in the evaluation of Cushing's syndrome. The overnight 1-mg low-dose dexamethasone suppression test is also used as a screening test, whereas the 2-day 2-mg dexamethasone suppression test is often used as a confirmatory test.

Page: 1050

Question #23

Answer: C

Rationale: Galactorrhea is defined as the inappropriate secretion of milk from the breast in the absence of parturition or when such secretion occurs more than 6 months after delivery in a non-breast-feeding woman. Common causes include certain medications, prolactinomas, chronic renal failure, excessive nipple stimulation, and thyroid disorders. In the vast majority of patients, the cause is unknown. Some medications that are commonly used and that can cause galactorrhea include psychotropic agents (e.g., risperidone, other dopamine receptor blockers) and oral contraceptives. Laboratory tests used for the evaluation of such patients include serum FSH, luteinizing hormone, TSH, and prolactin levels and a pregnancy test. Prolactin levels of greater than 200 ng/mL are usually seen in patients with a prolactinoma; further evaluation includes pituitary magnetic resonance imaging. Treatment consists of treating the underlying etiology or replacing the offending agent with a reasonable alternative.

Page: 1048

Question #24

Answer: C

Rationale: Of the causes listed, PCOS is the most common cause of hirsutism. It is diagnosed after excluding other conditions that cause androgen excess and irregular menstrual cycles and after the determination of at least two of the following: oligo-ovulation or anovulation, elevated levels of circulating androgens, clinical manifestations of androgen excess, and polycystic ovaries as defined by ultrasound.

Page: 1056

Question #25

Answer: B

Rationale: Patients with PCOS have a higher prevalence of impaired glucose tolerance and type 2 diabetes mellitus, and, hence, they should be screened with a 2-hour glucose tolerance test using a 75-gm glucose load. Steps to improve insulin sensitivity, such as weight loss, exercise, and drugs (i.e., metformin and thiazolidinediones), improve the chances of ovulation. Sulfonylureas do not improve insulin sensitivity. Other associated comorbidities include hypertension, obesity, vascular disease, and obstructive sleep apnea. Initial laboratory testing includes a fasting lipid profile, a serum total testosterone level, and a dehydroepiandrosterone-sulfate level. Patients also have an increased prevalence of endometrial hyperplasia and carcinoma, which can be reduced by cyclic progestins or oral contraceptives.

Pages: 1056–1057

Question #26

Answer: C

Rationale: Turner's syndrome is a chromosomal disorder that is characterized by the partial or total absence of the X chromosome. These individuals are phenotypi-cally females, and they have a short stature, wide-spaced nipples, a shield-like chest, and a webbed neck. Aortic root abnormalities are seen in up to 15% of individuals with this syndrome. These patients may also present for the evaluation of delayed puberty, primary or secondary amenorrhea, or recurrent pregnancy loss. Long-term hormone replacement therapy starting around the age of 14 years is usually required.

Page: 1058

Question #27

Answer: D

Rationale: Cryptorchidism is the most common endocrine disorder in the pediatric male. Its incidence is approximately 10% in term males, and it increases with prematurity (up to 30%). Imaging studies (computed tomography scanning and ultrasound) have poor accuracy for locating the testes, but a thorough examination may help. Differentiation from retractile testes is important. A palpable testis is pulled into the scrotum and kept there for a minute and then released; a retractile testis will stay in that position, whereas an undescended testis will return to its original position. Approximately 10% of undescended testes are intraabdominal; these carry the highest risk of testicular cancer. Treatment options include surgery and/or hormonal therapy with human chorionic gonadotropin or gonadotropin-releasing hormone. Hormonal therapy increases the likelihood of testicular descent. Treatment should be recommended as early as 6 months of age, and it should be completed by the age of 2 years. Early treatment helps to preserve fertility, and it increases the chance of detecting testicular malignancy.

Page: 1059

Question #28

Answer: A

Rationale: Varicocele is the most common cause of male infertility.

Page: 1060

Question #29

Answer: B

Rationale: Hyperglycemia with or without diabetic ketoacidosis, hyperproteinemia, and hypertriglyceridemia can cause hyponatremia with normal or high plasma osmolality. The syndrome of inappropriate antidiuretic hormone secretion also causes hyponatremia, but it is associated with a decrease in plasma osmolality, an inappropriately increased urine osmolality (>100 mOsm/kg), and urinary sodium level greater than 40 mEq/L. Diabetes insipidus is associated with hypernatremia.

Page: 1054

Question #30

Answer: B

Rationale: Desmopressin is the primary treatment for central diabetes insipidus. It is a potent antidiuretic that has minimal effects on blood pressure. Demeclocycline induces nephrogenic diabetes insipidus, and it is used for the treatment of the syndrome of inappropriate antidiuretic hormone secretion.

Page: 1054

Question #1

Answer: D

Rationale: Body fat percentage, although it is more precise than other measurements of adiposity, can be difficult to measure in the office setting. The BMI can be misleadingly high in a muscular person with a high level of lean body mass. The distribution of body fat has an impact on health risk; central obesity is associated with the greatest health risks.

Page: 1075

Question #2

Answer: A

Rationale: As the population as a whole becomes more overweight, the averages and percentiles will increase accordingly. The Centers for Disease Control and Prevention definition of overweight among children applies to the ages of 2 through 19 years. Between birth and the age of 2 years, overweight is assessed by the weight-for-length percentile; being at or above the 95th percentile is considered overweight or obese. Body weight tracks to some extent from child to adult, except during infancy. An obese adolescent has an 80% risk of becoming an obese adult.

Page: 1075

Question #3

Answer: C

Rationale: Blacks are at greater risk for obesity than whites. Black women are more likely than black men to be obese, whereas the differences between the sexes are not as obvious among whites. Immigrants to the United States begin to see an increase in the incidence of obesity starting about 10 years after their arrival. The prevalence of obesity is greater in rural than in urban areas.

Pages: 1077–1078

Question #4

Answer: B

Rationale: The genetic influence on obesity is polygenic, with more than 250 associated genes and chromosomal regions. Within a family, both genetic and environmental factors may play a role; however, a genetic predisposition is apparent in twins who are raised apart. Leptin is a protein that is produced in adipose tissue that provides negative feedback to appetite control centers; a deficiency of leptin or of leptin receptors may play a role in obesity. Overall, it is estimated that genetic factors are responsible for 30% to 40% of the variability in adult weight.

Page: 1078

Question #5

Answer: C

Rationale: Central obesity is believed to be the result of increased androgenic effects, and it is more common among men. When it is seen among women, it may be related to hyperandrogenic states, such as PCOS. Computed tomography scanning and magnetic resonance imaging of the abdomen have been used in research settings to assess visceral fat deposits, but they are not cost effective or practical in the clinical setting. Increased visceral fat is associated with metabolic syndrome, either as a cause or as a marker.

Page: 1075

Question #6

Answer: B

Rationale: Ghrelin is a peptide that is produced in the stomach and the duodenum that stimulates eating. Leptin is a protein that is produced in adipose tissue, and it provides negative feedback to appetite-control centers. Fluctuations in plasma glucose and vagal afferent activity also provide input to the brain. Central nervous system neurotransmitters are involved in appetite control, and they may be modulated with medication.

Page: 1079

Question #7

Answer: D

Rationale: The chief determinant of the BMR is the amount of lean body mass. Physical activity (both daily activities and exercise) is the most variable component of energy expenditure. Formal exercise levels have not changed significantly in the United States in several decades; it is thought most of the decrease in energy expenditure is the result of an overall more sedentary daily lifestyle.

Page: 1079

Question #8

Answer: C

Rationale: An increase in portion size has been attributed to "portion distortion" as larger-sized restaurant portions have become the norm for many Americans. Satiety is largely determined by the weight and volume of the food consumed. Per-capita sugar consumption increases correlated with increases in the prevalence of obesity in the United States. Eating frequent, smaller meals is associated with being less overweight, perhaps because larger meals are associated with greater insulin release.

Page: 1079

Question #9

Answer: D

Rationale: Antidepressants, antipsychotics, anticonvulsants, and hypoglycemic agents can all contribute to weight gain. Of the commonly used selective serotonin reuptake inhibitor antidepressants, paroxetine is the most likely to cause weight gain. The anticonvulsants valproic acid and gabapentin are more likely to cause weight gain, whereas lamotrigine is weight neutral, and topiramate may promote weight loss. Both older antipsychotics, such as the phenothiazines and haloperidol, as well as newer agents, such as clozapine and olanzapine, can increase weight. Metformin, which increases insulin sensitivity, may promote modest weight loss, and it may ameliorate the weight gain from other hypoglycemics.

Page: 1079

Question #10

Answer: A

Rationale: Endocrine or metabolic disorders account for less than 1% of cases of obesity. Hypothyroidism rarely presents with isolated weight gain; typically, cold intolerance, fatigue, obstipation, and hair loss are also seen. Children with endocrine causes of obesity are typically also short in stature. Conversely, childhood obesity from exogenous factors is associated with an increased rate of statural growth, an increased bone age, and early puberty. Cushing's syndrome presents with hypertension rather than hypotension.

Page: 1079

Question #11

Answer: C

Rationale: More than 50% of women with PCOS are obese. Insulin resistance may be seen, even in the absence of obesity. Whether PCOS is a cause or consequence of obesity is controversial. Typically, women with this disorder have irregular menses, hirsutism, insulin resistance, and elevated levels of testosterone and luteinizing hormone.

Page: 1080

Question #12

Answer: A

Rationale: Obesity is a well-established risk factor for hypertension; weight loss has been found to be the most effective lifestyle change to decrease blood pressure. Obesity is one of the factors that is associated with an age-related increase in hypertension, as demonstrated in the Nurses Health Study. The increased vascular tone may result from insulin resistance and subsequent increased insulin levels. Controlling weight may reduce the incidence of hypertension among whites by 48% and among blacks by 28%.

Page: 1080

Question #13

Answer: B

Rationale: Obesity is associated with elevated triglycerides and low high-density lipoprotein cholesterol levels; weight loss will improve these levels. Total and low-density lipoprotein cholesterol levels are only mildly affected by weight gain, but they may also improve with the same lifestyle changes that bring about weight loss. The favorable effect of aerobic exercise on lipids is greatest when it is associated with weight loss. Some—but not all—studies have found obesity to be an independent risk factor for coronary artery disease; it may be that it is simply associated with other, more well-established coronary artery disease risk factors. Obesity may also be an independent risk factor for congestive heart failure and cardiomyopathy.

Page: 1080

Question #14

Answer: B

Rationale: Up to 80% of cases of type 2 diabetes can be attributed to overweight and obesity. Overweight women are at a 40-fold increased risk for the condition, whereas overweight men are at a 60-fold increased risk. There is a time delay of about 10 years between the onset of being overweight and the development of diabetes; over time, insulin resistance surpasses the body's ability to increase insulin production, and blood glucose rises.

Page: 1080

Question #15

Answer: C

Rationale: NCEP-III requires three of five criteria to define metabolic syndrome, of which no single criteria is absolutely required. The World Health Organization and the American Association of Clinical Endocrinologists define metabolic syndrome differently, adding increased urinary albumin excretion as a criteria and requiring the presence of impaired glucose tolerance or type 2 diabetes. Approximately 40% of individuals who are more than 50 years old meet the NCEP-III criteria. Metabolic syndrome increases the risk of type 2 diabetes, coronary artery disease, and cerebrovascular disease.

Page: 1080

Question #16

Answer: C

Rationale: Smoking is the largest avoidable cause of cancer, and obesity is the second largest. An increased risk of death from several cancers is seen among obese patients, including esophageal, colon, kidney, gallbladder, and pancreatic cancer as well as non-Hodgkin's lymphoma and multiple myeloma; there is also a trend toward an increased risk of prostate, gastric, ovarian, and endometrial cancer. Breast cancer has been most closely associated with central obesity.

Page: 1081

Question #17

Answer: D

Rationale: Being overweight is a major risk factor for OSA. The increased risk is most likely the result of increased neck circumference and pharyngeal fat deposits. The primary health concerns are right ventricular dysfunction, systemic hypertension, pulmonary hypertension, and erectile dysfunction; and daytime somnolence may also put patients at an increased risk of various accidents. The risk of progressing to more severe OSA with a 10% weight gain is sixfold.

Page: 1081

Question #18

Answer: A

Rationale: Fatty liver disease is the most common cause of elevations in liver enzymes, and it affects 20% of the U.S. population. Nonalcoholic steatohepatitis may lead to fibrosis and cirrhosis, and it has been linked to insulin resistance. Because of changes in cholesterol flux, an obese person with gallstones may become symptomatic during rapid weight loss.

Page: 1081

Question #19

Answer: D

Rationale: The association between obesity and degenerative joint disease among adults is most often seen in weight-bearing joints such as the hips and knees. Obese children are at increased risk for scoliosis, pes planus, genu valga, and slipped femoral capital epiphysis. Obesity is associated with depression among adult women but not among adult men; it can also cause poor self-esteem in children and teens.

Page: 1081

Question #20

Answer: B

Rationale: An early adiposity rebound seen on BMI-for-age charts increases the risk of adult obesity. Risk factors for obesity include parental obesity, maternal smoking during pregnancy, sedentary lifestyle, and poor diet. Replacing sugary drinks with low-fat milk may help with weight loss as well as with overall nutrition. The goal of treatment should be a reduction in the BMI to less than the 95th percentile for age and to prevent or reverse comorbidities. A lipid panel and a fasting glucose level are indicated for children with a BMI that is over the 85th percentile for age if there is a family history of lipid disorders or early onset cardiovascular disease.

Page: 1082

Question #21

Answer: C

Rationale: Because overly restrictive dieting can interfere with growth rate, bone mineralization, and menstruation, a modest calorie restriction with increased physical activity should be employed. The goal, except in severe cases, should be to maintain a stable weight while height increases, thereby decreasing the BMI. Sedentary activities should be limited to 2 hours per day. Sibutramine is approved for use in patients who are more than 16 years old, but it is frequently associated with blood pressure elevations and tachycardia, which often result in discontinuation.

Page: 1082

Question #22

Answer: B

Rationale: The U.S. Preventive Services Task Force recommends screening for obesity in adults; this can be done with three simple steps: measuring BMI, measuring waist circumference, and identifying comorbidities. Calorie restriction without exercise results in less weight loss than do the two modalities combined, and it may result in a greater loss of lean body mass. Weight loss medications such as sibutramine or orlistat can be considered for patients with a BMI of 27 kg/m^2 or greater if comorbidities are present.

Page: 1082

Question #23

Answer: C

Rationale: The initial goal of weight-loss therapy should be 10% of baseline weight. However, some patients may respond better to working toward a healthier lifestyle rather than toward a specific goal weight. A weekly weight loss of 1 to 2 lb is achievable with a daily calorie deficit of 500 to 1000 calories, because 1 lb of fat contains 3500 calories. Patients should be aware that they need to maintain indefinitely the lifestyle changes that lead to weight loss.

Page: 1084

Question #24

Answer: A

Rationale: In a study that compared four different popular diets, all were equally effective with regard to resultant weight loss at 1 year. Low-carbohydrate diets may be difficult to adhere to long term, and they may adversely affect nutritional status. Very-low-calorie diets may produce more rapid initial weight loss, but they produce similar results as other diets over time. A low-calorie diet is most often employed. When the patient chooses less energy-dense foods, the volume of food eaten may stay about the same.

Page: 1084

Question #25

Answer: B

Rationale: Behavioral-based approaches have been found to be helpful with weight loss. Addressing emotional issues, such as stress and depression in particular, may be beneficial. To promote weight loss, 60 minutes a day of physical activity is recommended; to maintain weight loss, up to 90 minutes a day may be necessary. The use of a pedometer may help to change the lifestyle of a previously sedentary patient.

Page: 1084

Question #26

Answer: D

Rationale: Sibutramine is a nonselective inhibitor of serotonin, norepinephrine, and dopamine. Although it may raise blood pressure and heart rate, it is not absolutely contraindicated for people with coronary artery disease or well-controlled hypertension. As compared with placebo, patients receiving active drug lost 4.45 kg more in 1 year.

Page: 1085

Question #27

Answer: D

Rationale: Orlistat acts by inhibiting gastric and pancreatic lipase, thereby reducing the digestion and absorption of fats. Because of this, there is a risk of the decreased absorption of fat-soluble vitamins; patients taking orlistat should also take a daily multivitamin. Patients who follow a very-low-fat diet will receive little if any benefit from the medication. Gastrointestinal side effects occur in about 20% of patients; half of these patients will see a resolution of the side effects within 1 week.

Page: 1085

Question #28

Answer: B

Rationale: Green tea contains both caffeine (unless decaffeinated) and catechin; both may aid in weight loss. Increased soluble fiber may also have modest weight-reduction benefits. Caffeine may be present in many herbal preparations under the names of *guarana* or *gotu kola*. Ephedra, because of its serious side effects, is no longer on the market.

Page: 1085

Question #29

Answer: C

Rationale: To qualify for bariatric surgery, a patient should have a BMI of more than 40 kg/m^2 and weight-related complications. All procedures that are used currently can be performed laparoscopically. Gastric bypass is more effective than gastroplasty for weight loss; it is associated with fewer revisions, but it does involve more side effects. Vitamin and mineral supplementation is needed for the long term for patients who are undergoing malabsorptive procedures.

Page: 1086

Question #30

Answer: A

Rationale: BMI can also be calculated as weight (lb) $\times$ 703/height $(in)^2$. Tables are available if they are preferred over calculation. Obesity is defined as a BMI of 30 kg/m^2 or more. Extreme (morbid) obesity is defined as a BMI of 40 kg/m^2 or more.

Page: 1077

48 Answers

Question #1

Answer: A

Rationale: Improving the diet through public health education by promoting physical activity and balancing energy needs with intake is a focus on preventing chronic diseases in an aging population. Access to a computer is needed to take full advantage of this effort to improve health. Acquaint yourself with the information, and be proactive in the development of strategies to help your patient population benefit.

Page: 1089

Question #2

Answer: E

Rationale: A more in-depth assessment would be warranted if the patient has chronic illnesses or signs and symptoms related to poor nutrition. Such an assessment would include the consideration of anything purchased over the counter, such as multivitamins, herbals, nutritional supplements (common sports supplements), appetite suppressants, or stimulants and laxatives. Additionally, information about the consumption of alcohol and illicit drugs, about the financial and social status, and about any gastrointestinal symptoms would provide information to determine the patient's ability to obtain, ingest, digest, metabolize, and absorb nutrients.

Page: 1089

Question #3

Answers: A, B, and C

Rationale: Laboratory tests would confirm your suspicions of ongoing nutritional problems and direct treatment options. A complete blood cell count reveals changes in red blood cell production from insufficient levels of iron, vitamin B$_{12}$, folic acid, and other vitamins, and it is considered important for the assessment of nutritional status.

Page: 1098

Question #4

Answer: G

Rationale: Adolescents require more kilocalories per kilogram than any other age group, aside from infants. However, although they are gaining independence and should be accepting a role in how much is eaten, this does not necessarily translate to immediately understanding nutrient-dense calories or eating enough calories to match their energy needs. If nutritional assessments reveal certain needs, the coach should be advised, and adjunct training and education should be provided for the team.

Page: 1101

Question #5

Answers: A and B

Rationale: If your patient required a hospital stay for diverticular disease, then a complete blood cell count was most likely performed in the hospital. A transthyretin level, which is also known as a prealbumin level, would correlate with protein energy status in some patients with malnutrition.

Page: 1098

Question #6

Answers: B, C, and E

Rationale: Overall nutritional needs increase at conception and during pregnancy and lactation. Adequate calories will increase the opportunity for adequate nutrients; folic acid will help prevent neural tube defects (it also lowers homocysteine levels, thereby reducing cardiovascular disease), and iron will minimize chances of prematurity, low birthweight, and perinatal mortality.

Page: 1089

Question #7

Answers: A, B, and C

Rationale: A parent's role also includes providing a healthy range and variety of foods in a pleasant eating environment. Children then have the role to consume the food in the amounts that they need and want.

Page: 1099

Question #8

Answer: D

Rationale: An obese individual can be overfed but undernourished. Statistics from the National Health and Nutrition Examination Survey[1] demonstrate the prevalence of obesity in American adults as being 63.1 million. A BMI of 30 or greater is a measure of height to weight, and it delineates where obesity begins. An increased risk of hypertension, dyslipidemia, coronary artery disease, stroke, type 2 diabetes, gallbladder disease, osteoarthritis, sleep apnea, respiratory problems, and some cancers is seen among overweight and obese patients.

Page: 1097

Question #9

Answer: B

Rationale: C-reactive protein (CRP) is an acute-phase serum protein that indicates acute systemic inflammation. If the CRP level is low, there is more validity to the plasma protein levels of transthyretin or prealbumin, retinol-binding protein, albumin, and transferrin. According to the American Heart Association and the Centers for Disease Control and Prevention, an elevated CRP level determined by using a high-sensitivity CRP test may be a way to assess cardiovascular risk; however, this method is not widely accepted or used in routine office settings. A level of 3.0 mg/L represents a patient who is at high risk.

Page: 1098

Question #10

Answer: A

Rationale: Three steps currently recognized for the prevention of osteoporosis as a chronic disease are as follows: (1) eating a balanced diet that is rich in calcium and vitamin D; (2) performing weight-bearing exercise; and (3) living a healthy lifestyle, with no smoking or excessive alcohol intake. The focus of the study of adult nutrition is to optimize nutrition during this phase of the life cycle to improve the older adult's quality of life.

Page: 1101

1. National Center for Health Statistics: National Health and Nutrition Examination Survey (NHANES, 1999-2000), 2005. Available at http://www.cdc.gov/nchs/about/major/nhanes/nhanes99_00.htm. Accessed June 2, 2006.

Question #11

Answer: B

Rationale: Water is overlooked as a major nutrient. It can be found, of course, in water itself, and it is also found in beverages, fruits, vegetables, and nearly all foods. It functions as a medium for most of the body's reactions; it helps move materials to and waste from cells; it aids in the control of body temperature, and it lubricates the joints of the body. Infants, children, the elderly, and those with illnesses are susceptible to dehydration.

Page: 1091

Question #12

Answer: D

Rationale: Elderly patients have different nutritional needs. A nutritional assessment tool specific to the elderly, the Mini Nutritional Assessment, could provide the information needed to identify critical health problems.

Page: 1102

Question #13

Answer: A

Rationale: Lowering sodium intake is indicated as sufficient treatment for prehypertension and early stage I hypertension (with no comorbidities, such as diabetes or cardiovascular disease). Lifestyle modifications are also recommended, regardless of control with medications of any treatment level. These recommendations include 45 to 60 minutes of daily aerobic exercise (or at least 3 days per week), lowering salt and fat consumption, increasing fruit and vegetable intake, weight loss of 3% to 9%, and limiting alcohol intake to less than three drinks per day.

Page: 1102

Question #14

Answer: D

Rationale: There has been no percentage of daily value established for trans fats. Research has shown that trans fats increase low-density lipoprotein cholesterol levels, along with cholesterol and saturated fat. The U.S. Food and Drug Administration is requiring all food manufacturers, processors, and distributors to include the amount of trans fat on the Nutrition Facts panel of the food label as of January 1, 2006.

Page: 1106

Question #15

Answer: E

Rationale: The metabolic syndrome involves metabolic risk factors as defined by the NCEP ATP III. These improve with dietary management with an additional focus on modest weight loss and increased physical activity.

Pages: 1102–1104

Question #16

Answer: G

Rationale: The recommendation for fiber consumption is 20 to 35 g per day for adults; for children 2 years old and older, it is 5 g plus 1g for each year of their age per day, including both soluble and insoluble fiber. Increasing fiber in the diet also helps manage diverticular disease, constipation, irritable bowel syndrome, and some cancers.

Page: 1090

Question #17

Answer: C

Rationale: Although folate supplementation lowers the level of serum homocysteine (an elevated serum homocysteine is estimated to increase the risk of coronary heart disease), there is insufficient evidence indicating its use for coronary artery disease. Testing for plasma homocysteine levels can improve the assessment of risk for coronary heart disease.

Page: 1102

Question #18

Answer: B

Rationale: The glycemic index is an indication of the increase in blood sugars within 2 to 3 hours after the consumption of a food or beverage that contains carbohydrates. Studies have shown that the glycemic response is related to the total amount of carbohydrate consumed and that it does not depend on the type of carbohydrate. Controlling blood sugar in patients with type 2 diabetes relies on the quantity of food, the distribution of carbohydrates, and the inclusion of fiber, protein, and fat during the course of a day.

Pages: 1105–1106

Question #19

Answers: A, B, and C

Rationale: Achieving weight loss by consuming a lower amount of saturated fat (30% of calories totally from all fats) and less cholesterol also benefits blood sugar control and decreases the risk of coronary artery disease.

Page: 1105

Question #20

Answer: B

Rationale: A weight loss of 5% of body weight over 2 weeks designates the patient as mildly malnourished, and a 10% weight loss signifies severe malnutrition. A nutrition screen is to be done within 24 hours of admission to the hospital. The subjective global assessment has been validated as an instrument to assess nutritional status with trained clinicians.

Page: 1106

Question #21

Answers: A, B, and D

Rationale: An estimate of the calorie needs of a hospitalized patient can be calculated using the resting energy expenditure. The level of stress should also be considered to determine the number of calories that a patient requires.

Page: 1106

Question #22

Answers: B and E

Rationale: Nutrition support can be administered enterally or parenterally. Enteral nutrition is used if the gut is working, and it provides complex nutrients (e.g., fiber, intact proteins), with a beneficial effect on the mucosa of the gastrointestinal tract. It can be delivered nasogastrically and postpylorically with a duodenal or jejunal tube placement. Parenteral nutrition support can be delivered as peripheral parenteral nutrition for the short term (7–10 days) or as total parenteral nutrition through a central vein for the long term and for cases in which higher concentrations of glucose and protein needs are to be considered.

Page: 1108

Question #23

Answer: D

Rationale: The focus should be on the behavior change that is necessary to accomplish the outcome: in this case, limiting salt (sodium) intake to lower blood pressure. The behaviors are a way for the patient to accomplish the outcome.

Page: 1108

Question #24

Answer: E

Rationale: A health behavior change plan uses a step approach, starting with small goals in short time increments and escalating to long-term goals while the patient gains confidence in her ability to be successful with a new diet plan.

Page: 1109

Question #25

Answers: A, B, and C

Rationale: A systemic process that can be used—although it has not thoroughly tested for dietary interventions—is modeled after the tobacco-cessation interventions used in clinical care. It is called "the five As" construct: assess, advise, agree, assist, and arrange.

Page: 1109

Question #26

Answer: A

Rationale: A family history is the least expensive and most readily available tool to use in an office setting to appreciate the disease risk in an individual if a family member—especially a first-degree relative—has a history of a disease.

Page: 1111

Question #27

Answer: D

Rationale: The recommended weight gain for a biologically immature woman (i.e., one who becomes pregnant within 5 years of starting to menstruate) or one

with a BMI of less than 20 at conception is 31 lb, or 1.1 lb/week. The weight gain for a woman with a BMI of more than 20 but less than 27 is 20 to 26 lb, and the weight gain for a patient with a BMI of 27 or more or who is 35 years old or older is up to 20 lb, or 0.7 lb/week.

Page: 1099

Question #28

Answer: D

Rationale: In 2004, a review of the entire set of nutrients was completed. The term *dietary reference intake* refers to three types of reference values: the recommended daily intake, the tolerable upper intake level, and the estimated average energy requirement. The focus is still on the prevention of nutritional-deficiency diseases and the reduction of the risk of chronic diseases. The Nutrition Facts label uses the dietary reference intake values as daily values to represent the minimum needs of the general population.

Page: 1111

Question #29

Answer: B

Rationale: Fat supplies 9 Kcal/kg. It functions as a concentrated source of energy; it carries the fat-soluble vitamins (A, D, E, and K); it supplies essential fatty acids, and it is part of the integrity of the cell membrane and the transport process of the cells. A diet of excess fat results in weight gain and obesity in addition to increased blood cholesterol and triglyceride levels. When counseling patients about dietary strategies for weight reduction and lowering blood lipid levels, recommending a lower-fat diet and portion control is still sound advice.

Page: 1091

Question #30

Answer: B

Rationale: Your patient would benefit from a referral to a certified diabetes educator for assistance with educating her about the behavioral changes needed to manage her diabetes with diet and exercise. There is not enough time during an office visit to attempt this type of counseling. Consideration should also be given to managing the blood sugar levels with medication.

Page: 1104

Question #1

Answer: B

Rationale: There are no strict evidence-based guidelines for the management of acute abdominal pain in the office and emergency department settings. A consensus statement from the American College of Emergency Physicians on the initial evaluation and management of patients presenting with a chief compliant of nontraumatic acute abdominal pain accounts for the most widely accepted recommendations. This clinical policy recommends against using the location of pain or the presence of fever to restrict the differential diagnosis. All patients with abdominal pain should undergo stool occult blood testing, and female patients of reproductive age warrant a pelvic examination and a pregnancy test. Patients who are being evaluated for abdominal pain in the emergency department should be provided with appropriate narcotic analgesia. When the cause of the presenting abdominal pain is unclear, physicians should perform serial abdominal examinations over several hours in an effort to reach a diagnosis.

Page: 1118

Question #2

Answer: D

Rationale: Computerized tomography scanning has been shown to aid in the diagnosis of patients presenting with abdominal pain, especially when fever is also present; the American College of Radiology's Expert Panel on Gastrointestinal Imaging considers it the most useful imaging modality. Use of computed tomography has also been shown to reduce hospital admissions. Ultrasound, although useful for certain conditions (e.g., cholecystitis, diverticulitis, appendicitis), is not useful for the evaluation of many areas of the abdomen. Plain films of the abdomen can only provide useful information about bowel-gas patterns or the presence of intra-abdominal free air.

Page: 1118

Question #3

Answer: C

Rationale: For the infant or child with acute gastroenteritis, the early administration of oral rehydration solutions has been proven to decrease mortality. The World Health Organization recommends a hypotonic oral rehydration solution for global use. Fruit juices and sports drinks are hyperosmotic and should be avoided, because they can perpetuate diarrhea. When clinical dehydration is minimal, treatment should involve providing adequate fluids (orally, when possible) and maintaining an age-appropriate diet. Breastfed infants should continue nursing, whereas formula-fed infants should continue their standard formula upon rehydration. Children taking solid-food diets should continue during episodes of diarrhea, although foods high in simple sugars should be avoided, because the osmotic load may worsen diarrhea. Early refeeding decreases changes in intestinal permeability caused by infection, reduces illness duration, and improves nutritional outcomes.

Page: 1121

Question #4

Answer: C

Rationale: Family physicians must weigh the potential risks and benefits of treatment for cases of diarrhea. When managing traveler's diarrhea, prompt treatment with a fluoroquinolone or, in children, trimethoprim-sulfamethoxazole has been shown to reduce the duration of illness from 3 to 5 days to less than 1 to 2 days. In general, antibiotics should only be prescribed in documented bacterial stool infections, and they should not be used prophylactically to reduce the likelihood of secondary transmission. Antimotility agents should not be used to treat suspected or documented Shiga-toxin–producing *E. coli* infections. Antidiarrheal medications are not recommended for use in infants and children, because these agents may prolong the course of the diarrheal illness. For cases of *C. difficile*–associated diarrhea, oral metronidazole and vancomycin have been shown to be equally effective, although oral vancomycin is expensive, and it may select for colonization with vancomycin-resistant enterococci.

Page: 1121

Question #5

Answer: D

Rationale: Achalasia, which is the failure of the esophagus to relax, is characterized by the loss of esophageal peristalsis and incomplete relaxation of the lower esophageal sphincter. The etiology of this condition is not clear, and it occurs most commonly during the third to fifth decades of life. Dysphagia, regurgitation, weight loss, chest pain, and heartburn are common in most patients who present with achalasia. Odynophagia is not known to be commonly associated with achalasia.

Page: 1128

Question #6

Answer: A

Rationale: Infection with *H. pylori* is a major risk factor for the development of peptic ulcer disease. Populations with a standard of living lower than what is commonly found in the United States demonstrate a higher prevalence and association with peptic ulcer disease. Evidence dictates that patients younger than 45 years old with dyspepsia and no alarm symptoms should be tested for *H. pylori* and treated if they are positive. Alternatively, any patient more than 45 years old with dyspepsia, despite the presence of alarm symptoms (e.g., weight loss, anorexia, early satiety), should undergo prompt endoscopy. The empiric management of functional dyspepsia is recommended for *H. pylori*–negative patients who are less than 45 years old and who do not have alarm symptoms. Nonendoscopic *H. pylori* testing methods include a quantitative assay for serum immunoglobulin G antibodies, the radiolabeled urea breath test, and the stool antigen test. Comparatively, urea breath tests are more accurate than serologic tests.

Pages: 1131–1133

Question #7

Answer: C

Rationale: The use and overuse of NSAIDs and aspirin are the most common causes of peptic ulcer disease in *H. pylori*–negative patients. Up to 60% of unexplained cases of peptic ulcer disease are attributed to unrecognized NSAID use. During the first 3 months of NSAID use, studies have demonstrated a five- to seven-fold increase in the risk of gastric ulceration. Primary care providers need to complete a thorough evaluation of patients with peptic ulcer disease to determine the etiology of the disease.

Page: 1133

Question #8

Answer: B

Rationale: There are several evidence-based recommended pharmacological treatment regimens for the eradication of *H. pylori* infection. First-line therapy consists of a 14-day course of a proton-pump inhibitor, clarithromycin, and amoxicillin. Eradication rates for this regimen range from 80% to 90%. For penicillin-allergic patients, metronidazole instead of amoxicillin in this regimen yields eradication rates from 75% to 90%. The antibiotic choice in triple therapy has an impact on eradication rates, because antibiotic resistance must be taken into account. The current resistance rates for *H. pylori* in the United States are 33% for metronidazole, 11% for clarithromycin, and 0% for amoxicillin. There are no demonstrable differences among the available proton-pump inhibitors when they are used in triple-therapy regimens.

Page: 1133

Question #9

Answer: C

Rationale: The symptoms of GERD, including heartburn and regurgitation, occur as a result of the abnormal reflux of gastric contents into the esophagus. Because GERD is mainly a clinical diagnosis, a thorough history is essential. Treatment goals include symptom relief, quality-of-life improvement, avoidance of disease progression, and the prevention of complications, including erosive esophagitis, esophageal strictures, Barrett's esophagus, and adenocarcinoma of the esophagus. A cost-effective individualized approach to pharmacological therapy with H_2-receptor blockers or proton-pump inhibitors is appropriate. Diagnostic testing is recommended for patients with GERD who have an inadequate response to proton-pump inhibitor therapy, who need continuous chronic therapy to control frequent symptoms, who have had chronic symptoms lasting for more than 5 years, who have atypical or extraesophageal manifestations suggestive of complicated disease, or who have alarm symptoms suggestive of cancer. Extraesophageal manifestations of GERD include asthma, chronic cough, globus sensation, noncardiac chest pain, and recurrent laryngitis. The presence of alarm symptoms such as bloody stool, hematemesis, dysphagia, early satiety, weight loss, or iron-deficiency anemia requires prompt endoscopic evaluation.

Page: 1137

Question #10

Answer: D

Rationale: Upper gastrointestinal bleeding carries a significant mortality rate of 6% to 10%. Hospitalized patients who develop an upper gastrointestinal bleed are more likely to have coexistent medical problems and to have a higher mortality risk than an outpatient that develops a bleed. Risk stratification is essential to allow for the emphasis of preventive measures with patients. Risk factors for the development of upper gastrointestinal bleeding include aspirin and NSAID use, anticoagulant or antiplatelet therapy, *H. pylori* infection, erosive esophagitis, a prior history of upper gastrointestinal bleeding, the perioperative period, intensive care unit admission, and Zollinger-Ellison syndrome. A detailed history is important for stratifying patients with respect to bleeding severity risk.

Page: 1138

Question #11

Answer: A

Rationale: Stress ulceration is a form of hemorrhagic gastritis that may occur in patients who have suffered a moderate to severe physiologically stressful event. These stressful events include surgery (especially an intracranial procedure), trauma, organ failure, sepsis, thermal injury, or prolonged mechanical ventilation. There is no evidence to support the use of stress ulcer prophylaxis for adult general medical and surgical patients with fewer than two risk factors for a significant bleeding event when they are not in the intensive care unit setting. Current guidelines recommend a cost-effective approach to pharmacological stress-ulcer prophylaxis that is institution specific.

Page: 1139

Question #12

Answer: B

Rationale: The clinical symptoms of gastroparesis often include nausea, vomiting, and postprandial abdominal fullness. The condition is commonly related to poorly controlled diabetes mellitus, autonomic neuropathies, and postsurgical states. A careful history and physical examination are important. The best testing method for suspected gastroparesis is gastric emptying scintigraphy of a radiolabeled solid meal performed 2 hours after ingestion. Primary treatment includes dietary recommendations along with the use of antiemetics and prokinetic agents. Dietary guidelines include eating more frequent and small meals, consuming more liquids than solids, and eating foods that are low in fat and fiber content.

Pages: 1139–1140

Question #13

Answer: C

Rationale: When evaluating a patient with suspected biliary colic, the physician must determine acuity and choose from among expectant management, a workup with laboratory testing and diagnostic imaging, or an immediate surgical evaluation. Although they are not adequately predictive, certain laboratory findings are more common in cases of acute cholecystitis. Expected laboratory results include moderate leukocytosis, normal amylase, lipase, alkaline phosphatase, transaminases, and bilirubin. With associated pancreatitis, serum amylase and lipase may be elevated, whereas, with a common bile duct stone causing obstruction, alkaline phosphatase, liver transaminases, and bilirubin may be increased.

Page: 1141

Question #14

Answer: C

Rationale: Currently, abdominal ultrasound, which has a sensitivity and specificity of more than 90%, is the best screening imaging modality for the evaluation of gallstones. Findings on ultrasonography include gallbladder wall thickening along with the presence of sludge. The presence of gallstones alone is not adequate for making a diagnosis of cholecystitis. Computed tomography scanning of the abdomen may miss a significant amount of cholesterol stones, and it should only be used when ultrasound is nondiagnostic. Biliary scintigraphy or cholescintigraphy is reserved for patients in whom the diagnosis cannot be made by routine testing. Endoscopic retrograde cholangiopancreatography is useful for identifying and treating common bile duct stones. However, the procedure is invasive, and it may be complicated by iatrogenic pancreatitis.

Page: 1143

Question #15

Answer: D

Rationale: Most physicians recommend observation for most patients with asymptomatic cholelithiasis. Various nonsurgical treatments are available, including extracorporeal shockwave lithotripsy and gallstone dissolution using bile-acid therapy and contact solvents such as methyl-tert-butyl ether. Acute cholecystitis should be considered for surgical intervention with persistent or worsening pain and fever, increasing leukocytosis, or a worsening of the physical examination. Pain relief with narcotic analgesics is indicated with the exception of morphine, which may precipitate a spasm of the sphincter of Oddi. Laparoscopic cholecystectomy is now considered the procedure of choice, with a rare complication being common bile duct injury. With this procedure, the abdominal scar is minimized, the hospital stay is short, and the degree of pain is significantly less than with an open procedure.

Page: 1144

Question #16

Answer: C

Rationale: Jaundice is the clinical description of yellow-bronze skin and sclera, which is the result of an elevation of serum bilirubin levels. The vast majority of patients presenting with evidence of jaundice have some form of hepatitis. Most patients are symptomatic with anorexia, nausea, or fatigue. Rarely, asymptomatic patients may present with a diagnosis of either cholestatic jaundice or pancreatic carcinoma. Patients presenting with jaundice should have a comprehensive history and physical examination along with liver function testing and abdominal ultrasonography.

Page: 1144

Question #17

Answer: A

Rationale: Hepatitis is an acute inflammation of the parenchyma of the liver. Viruses are the most common etiology of infectious hepatitis in the United States. Less-common causes include bacterial and fungal infections, autoimmune and metabolic disorders, toxic exposures, and hepatotoxic medications, including acetaminophen. Serologic testing is crucial in the accurate diagnosis of the viral hepatitides. Hepatitis B surface antigen is the earliest indicator of acute hepatitis B infection. It may remain positive for up to 6 months, but persistence of this antigen may indicate a chronic carrier state. Antibody to hepatitis B surface antigen is an indicator of clinical recovery and subsequent immunity; it appears 1 to 2 months after the antigen disappears, and it is usually present for life. Hepatitis B e antigen indicates that the patient is highly contagious with an acute infection. The hepatitis B e antibody indicates the resolution of infection and a low likelihood of infectivity in the chronic carrier state.

Page: 1144

Question #18

Answer: E

Rationale: Serum transaminases as well as bilirubin and alkaline phosphatase may be markedly elevated in all forms of acute hepatitis. The level of elevation of these studies does not correlate well with the degree of hepatic dysfunction or the prognosis of illness. Alarm symptoms of severe parenchymal destruction include mental status changes, asterixis, ascites, and prolongation of prothrombin time. These patients should be hospitalized, with emphasis on improving nutritional status and hepatology consultation.

Page: 1145

Question #19

Answer: C

Rationale: Serum transaminases are elevated in cases of hepatic injury. Minor elevations of less than 300 IU/mL are often indicative of chronic viral hepatitis, metabolic disorders, and alcoholic hepatitis. In more than 70% of patients with alcoholic hepatitis, the AST-to-ALT ratio is greater than 2, which coincides with an elevation of gamma-glutamyl transpeptidase. Acute viral hepatitis correlates with elevations that are often in the range of 1500 to 3000 IU/mL. Higher elevations of transaminases are most commonly seen with hepatic injury resulting from exposure to hepatotoxins, medications, or significant ischemia.

Page: 1144

Question #20

Answer: B

Rationale: Viral hepatitis A is endemic worldwide, with 100% of preschool children being seropositive in areas of poor sanitation and 10% of U.S. children being seropositive. The virus is spread via the fecal–oral route, and it is often associated with outbreaks in restaurants from undercooked meat and vegetables. The disease is generally self-limited, with less than 5% of patients developing significant complications. Vaccination against hepatitis A is recommended for high-risk groups or as prophylaxis before travel to endemic areas. The incubation period is generally 2 to 6 weeks, and most patients fully recover.

Page: 1145

Question #21

Answer: D

Rationale: Hepatitis C affects more than 4 million people in the United States. The diagnosis is made by testing for antibodies against hepatitis C, because there is no laboratory test for the hepatitis C antigen. Transmission occurs through the contamination of blood and body fluids, and it is most common among intravenous drug abusers and health care workers after occupational exposures. The presence of concomitant human immunodeficiency infection increases the risk of transmission of hepatitis C. Therapy with a combination of pegylated interferon and ribavirin can achieve the sustained viral eradication of hepatitis C in almost 50% of treated patients.

Page: 1146

Question #22

Answer: B

Rationale: Cirrhosis is the term that is used to refer to a progressive, diffuse, fibrosing, and nodular condition that disrupts the normal architecture and function of the liver. It is currently the twelfth leading cause of death in the United States. Most cases of cirrhosis in the United States are the result of excessive alcohol consumption, hepatitis B and C, and obesity in the form of nonalcoholic fatty liver disease. Theoretically, these are all preventable etiologies. Ultimately, the chronic destruction of the liver architecture leads to a dysfunction in protein synthesis and an increased resistance to blood flow leading to portal hypertension and multiple complications, including ascites, bleeding varices, spontaneous bacterial peritonitis, encephalopathy, and hepatorenal syndrome.

Page: 1146

Question #23

Answer: D

Rationale: Most cases of acute pancreatitis can be described as a mild parenchymal interstitial edema with a rapid recovery. The most common causes of acute pancreatitis are, by far, gallstones and alcohol. Other, less-common causes include hypertriglyceridemia, trauma, medications, endoscopic retrograde cholangiopancreatography, viral infections, neoplasms, perforated peptic ulcer disease, and idiopathic causes. The most common presenting symptom is a gnawing epigastric pain that may radiate to the back and that is constant, lasting from hours to days.

The pain is usually worsened by food or alcohol, and it can be precipitated by binge drinking. Nausea, vomiting, and a low-grade fever commonly accompany the pain.

Page: 1148

Question #24

Answer: D

Rationale: Despite the high sensitivities and specificities of the serum markers of acute pancreatitis, they are not useful for predicting the severity or course of disease. Amylase and lipase, although they are released at approximately the same time after pancreatic insult, are cleared from the bloodstream at different rates. Amylase is almost totally cleared within 48 to 72 hours, whereas lipase can be detected as many as 14 days after the acute event. Amylase may be elevated in other non-pancreatic conditions. C-reactive protein and urinary trypsinogen seem to have the ability to serve as prognosticators of disease severity. The C-reactive protein assay is inexpensive, readily available, and relatively sensitive. A cutoff of 150 mg/L seems to be useful for differentiating between mild and severe acute pancreatitis.

Page: 1149

Question #25

Answer: E

Rationale: Inflammatory bowel disease, which is the collective term used to describe ulcerative colitis and Crohn's disease, carries significant symptom burden. The induction of remission and achieving a symptom-free state are the main goals of pharmacological treatment. The mainstay of remission-induction therapy has been systemic steroids, which have been shown to produce remission rates as high as 70%. For mild flares of ulcerative colitis, 5-aminosalicylic acid derivatives are commonly used, including mesalamine and sulfasalazine, although systemic steroids have been more successful for patients with Crohn's disease. For Crohn's disease, immunosuppressants—namely azathioprine—have been proven to be effective. Metronidazole and ciprofloxacin have also been used, but the use of antibiotics remains controversial. Methotrexate is also effective for the induction of remission in patients with Crohn's disease, but it requires laboratory monitoring and the avoidance of pregnancy. An antitumor necrosis factor-α antibody, infliximab, is effective for steroid-resistant patients with Crohn's disease, but it has significant side-effect risks to be considered.

Page: 1155

Question #26

Answer: B

Rationale: Irritable bowel syndrome is a common condition, and it represents approximately 12% of visits to primary care physicians and 28% of referrals to gastroenterologists. The prevalence ranges from 14% to 24% in women and from 5% to 19% in men. The disease is characterized by the presence of multiple gastrointestinal symptoms that may be exacerbated by psychological stressors. The physical examination is usually unremarkable. A workup consisting of multiple diagnostic screening tests—including complete blood cell count, erythrocyte sedimentation rate, serum chemistries, thyroid function studies, stool cultures, fecal occult blood testing, and colonoscopy—should be performed to rule out the presence of other disease.

Page: 1156

Question #27

Answer: D

Rationale: Lower gastrointestinal bleeding is a significant source of morbidity and mortality. Rapid decompensation and hemodynamic instability often occur in patients, as evidenced by orthostatic hypotension, pallor, palpitations, tachypnea, tachycardia, and chest pain. Immediate resuscitation with intravenous fluids and blood transfusions is necessary. Initial laboratory testing includes a complete blood cell count, a chemistry panel, and a coagulation profile, along with blood typing and cross matching. A careful history and a physical examination are essential for accurate and early diagnosis. The American Society for Gastrointestinal Endoscopy Standards of Practice Committee recommends colonoscopy as the procedure of choice for the evaluation and treatment of lower gastrointestinal bleeding.

Page: 1158

Question #28

Answer: C

Rationale: Diverticulitis is the most common complication of diverticulosis, and it occurs as a result of microperforation of the diverticulum, which may become infected and form intra-abdominal abscesses. The American Society of Colon and Rectal Surgeons Standards Task Force states that, with a typical history and physical presentation, a diagnosis can be made with clinical criteria alone. Abdominal and pelvic computed tomography scanning with oral and intravenous contrast is rapidly becoming the procedure of choice when the diagnosis is in question or when an intra-abdominal mass is suspected. Endoscopy in the acute setting should be avoided to prevent the risk of colonic perforation.

Page: 1162

Question #29

Answer: B

Rationale: Colorectal cancer is the third most common cancer and the second leading cause of cancer death in the United States. Risk factors include increasing age, family history, obesity, sedentary lifestyle, a diet high in red meat and low in vegetables, and excessive alcohol and/or tobacco use. The risk among the black population is 50% higher than it is among whites. Currently accepted methods for screening include the digital rectal examination, fecal occult blood testing, double-contrast enema, flexible sigmoidoscopy, and colonoscopy. The procedure of choice remains controversial. However, randomized studies show that all testing aids in the detection of disease. Level-A evidence shows that screening with annual fecal occult blood testing beginning at age 50 with three stool samples significantly reduces mortality from colorectal cancer. Colonoscopy provides the most complete visualization of the colon, and it is the gold-standard test for screening and continued patient monitoring. Newer tests, such as virtual colonoscopy and capsule endoscopy, are not yet approved for this use.

Page: 1165

Question #30

Answer: A

Rationale: Hemorrhoids are varicosities that arise from the perianal veins. External hemorrhoids originate distal to the dentate line, and internal hemorrhoids are located proximally. Risk factors include increasing age, chronic diarrhea, pregnancy, pelvic tumors, prolonged sitting, straining, and constipation. The most common presentation is asymptomatic bleeding, which is most often described as red spotting on toilet tissue or blood dripping into the bowl, normally at the end of defecation and separate from the stool. Pain with external hemorrhoids occurs in the event of thrombosis. Diagnosis is made by digital rectal examination, with the most accurate method being the use of an anoscope.

Page: 1167

Question #1

Answer: A

Rationale: An increase in the number of women smokers is partially to blame for this. Until the mid-1980s, breast cancer was the leading cause of cancer death among women. The poor survival of patients with lung cancer (10%–13% 5-year survival for non–small-cell lung cancer) is also a major factor.

Page: 1174

Question #2

Answer: D

Rationale: Primary prevention is aimed at preventing the disease from ever developing (e.g., preventing skin cancer by wearing sunscreen). Secondary prevention involves detecting and treating early disease or precursors to prevent more extensive disease (e.g., finding early breast cancer on mammography). Tertiary prevention involves the management of curable disease or improving quality of life after treatment (e.g., using tamoxifen for women with estrogen-receptor–positive breast tumors to prevent recurrent disease).

Page: 1175

Question #3

Answer: C

Rationale: Tomatoes (and tomato skins) are the best source of lycopene.

Page: 1177

Question #4

Answer: B

Rationale: Adenomatous polyps have the greatest malignant potential. Hyperplastic polyps, diverticula, and melanosis coli (as a result of laxative abuse) are not thought to have malignant potential.

Page: 1178

Question #5

Answer: A

Rationale: Neoadjuvant chemotherapy can be used before surgery for a number of locally extensive tumors (e.g., breast cancer, rectal cancers) in an effort to make the disease more easily resectable.

Page: 1182

Question #6

Answer: E

Rationale: Flutamide is an antiandrogen that is used for the treatment of prostate cancer. Tamoxifen is an estrogen antagonist/agonist; it has estrogen-antagonist effects in the breast and estrogen-agonist effects on the bone and the endometrium (hence the increased risk of uterine cancer). These are examples of hormonal therapies.

Page: 1182

Question #7

Answer: A

Rationale: Extensive small-cell lung cancer has a very poor prognosis. Aggressive chemotherapy has somewhat improved the outlook for limited-stage disease, with many patients living for 2 years.

Page: 1183

Question #8

Answer: C

Rationale: More patients are choosing lumpectomy over modified radical or simple mastectomy now that it is known that this does not have an impact on survival in properly selected patients. The condition of the breast (prior radiation) and the size of the tumor must be such as to make this therapeutically and cosmetically feasible.

Page: 1184

Question #9

Answer: F

Rationale: All of the items listed are risk factors in prostate cancer, and many of them are also linked to each other (e.g., high-fat diet, obesity, and physical inactivity).
Page: 1184

Question #10

Answer: A

Rationale: The Gleason score is a histologic differentiation scoring system that has a strong association with prognosis. Grade 1 indicates well-differentiated disease, whereas disease considered to be grade 5 is poorly differentiated. The score is determined by adding the values for the two most prevalent patterns. Disease with a score of 2 to 4 is considered well differentiated; that with a score of 5 to 7 is considered moderately differentiated, and that with a score of 8 to 10 is considered poorly differentiated.
Page: 1185

Question #11

Answer: C

Rationale: Women who have had a hysterectomy for benign disease and women who are more than 65 years old without risk factors who have had three consecutive negative Pap smears are no longer felt to require Pap smears. It is important to remind women that this does not mean that they no longer need breast and pelvic examinations (especially with intact ovaries), mammograms, and other health-maintenance care.
Page: 1185

Question #12

Answer: C

Rationale: Early cervical cancer is highly curable, and the disease is also largely preventable. However, the 70% 5-year survival rate reminds us that patients can still die of this disease when it is not diagnosed at an early stage.
Page: 1186

Question #13

Answer: C

Rationale: The age of 50 years is the generally accepted age to begin screening patients who have an average risk for colon cancer. Patients at higher risk (e.g., those with positive family history, familial adenomatous polyposis, or hereditary non-polyposis colorectal cancer) require more aggressive recommendations.
Page: 1186

Question #14

Answer: A

Rationale: Patients who have an adenomatous polyp found on sigmoidoscopy have an increased risk of additional adenomas in the more proximal colon, beyond the reach of the sigmoidoscope. Because adenomatous polyps have malignant potential, colonoscopy is recommended.
Page: 1186

Question #15

Answer: F

Rationale: All of these factors are indications of extensive colon cancer.
Pages: 1186–1187

Question #16

Answer: G

Rationale: Early ovarian cancer causes few symptoms, which is one reason why this disease has such a poor prognosis. However, as the tumor enlarges, it can cause more symptoms than previously thought. For instance, it can mimic irritable bowel syndrome or gall bladder disease. It is important to consider ovarian cancer as a possibility for women with nonspecific gastrointestinal symptoms.
Page: 1187

Question #17

Answer: A

Rationale: CA 125 is not considered a good screening test for ovarian cancer, but it may be useful for the diagnostic workup and evaluation of selected patients. CA 19–9 is most commonly associated with pancreatic cancer, whereas CEA is associated with colorectal cancer and PSA with prostate cancer.

Page: 1187

Question #18

Answer: B

Rationale: Testicular cancer is the most common cancer in men between the ages of 15 and 44 years. This disease can be found during a self- or a physician examination, and follow-up sonographic evaluation should be performed. It is usually highly curable.

Page: 1187

Question #19

Answer: D

Rationale: CA 19–9 is associated with pancreatic cancer.

Page: 1187

Question #20

Answer: E

Rationale: Seminomas tend to have a better prognosis than non-seminomas. Non-seminomas that originate in extragenital locations (e.g., the mediastinum) have a worse prognosis.

Page: 1187

Question #21

Answer: D

Rationale: It is important to wait 6 months after surgery to obtain the first follow-up mammogram. This allows the distortion produced by surgery and/or radiation to subside, and it makes the study easier to interpret. Follow-up bone scans (in the absence of symptoms) are not felt to be helpful.

Page: 1187

Question #22

Answer: D

Rationale: During pregnancy, breast tissue becomes more dense, thereby making diagnosis by mammography

more difficult; sonography is helpful for overcoming this. The suggested intervals after treatment before trying to conceive are to help ensure that the patient has a good prognosis as well as to minimize effects of the treatment on the fetus.

Page: 1187

Question #23

Answer: D

Rationale: Every patient should have both a living will and a durable power of attorney for health care to ensure that his or her treatment wishes are honored and that the person of his or her choice is empowered to make decisions if the patient is unable to do so.

Page: 1188

Question #24

Answer: E

Rationale: The listed factors take into account the known hormonal, genetic, and environmental correlates of breast cancer. Coffee consumption has not been proven to be a factor.

Page: 1184

Question #25

Answer: E

Rationale: These factors reflect the fact that cervical cancer is a sexually transmitted disease and also that tobacco consumption plays a role.

Page: 1185

Question #26

Answer: E

Rationale: Obesity is also considered a risk factor for endometrial cancer. Many of these factors are also correlated with increased estrogen levels.

Page: 1175

Question #27

Answer: D

Rationale: The role of PSA interpretation is very complex. However, the test can be very useful if it is properly evaluated. The physician must take the time to explain the pros and cons and the factors involved in interpretation of this test to his or her patient.

Page: 1185

Question #28

Answer: D

Rationale: Thermography has been tried as a screening test for breast cancer in the past. It is based on the premise of increased temperature over the areas that are involved with the cancer. However, it has generally been abandoned as being too insensitive and not specific enough.

Page: 1184

Question #29

Answer: A

Rationale: The only curative treatment for lung cancer is surgery. Patients who have localized disease and who are in good enough medical condition for surgery should be given the benefit of this treatment. Patients with small-cell lung cancer are not often surgical candidates, because the disease is usually too widespread at the time of diagnosis.

Page: 1183

Question #30

Answer: D

Rationale: It is important to keep the possibility of leukemia in mind for children with bone and joint pain or any unexplained limp.

Page: 1174

Question #1

Answer: B

Rationale: Stem cells are pluripotent hematopoietic cells that can be transplanted to give rise to both myeloid and lymphoid cells. T cells and natural killer cells differentiate during lymphopoiesis, whereas monocytes and macrophages arise from myelopoiesis.

Page: 1191

Question #2

Answer: C

Rationale: The prevalence of iron deficiency in 1999 to 2000 is not reported for Asian Americans. It is 10% for whites and 19% for blacks, and it is highest for Mexican Americans, at 22%.

Page: 1193

Question #3

Answer: D

Rationale: Red cell mass represents the oxygen-carrying capacity of the body. As red cells traverse the circulation, the oxygen available within them is detected by specialized peritubular capillary lining cells in the kidney. This sensing mechanism is mediated by hypoxia-inducible factor 1 alpha.

Page: 1192

Question #4

Answer: A

Rationale: Anemia is the most frequent hematologic disorder seen in a family medicine practice, and it is of sufficient prevalence that knowledge of red cell function, the classification of red cell disorders, the evaluation of laboratory date, and the treatment of common anemias are important parts of the knowledge base of the competent family physician.

Page: 1193

Question #5

Answer: C

Rationale: The hypoproliferative anemias include aplastic anemia, anemia of inflammation, chronic renal insufficiency, hypothyroidism, and mild iron deficiency. Myelodysplasia is considered to be a maturation disorder; adequate erythropoietin stimulation is present with erythroid hyperplasia, but premature cell death is occurring within the marrow, and red cell production is ineffective.

Page: 1195

Question #6

Answer: D

Rationale: Inflammation causes hypoproliferation, and it is the most common form of anemia seen in hospitalized patients. Sometimes called anemia of chronic disease, it is more appropriately called *anemia of chronic inflammation.*

Pages: 1194–1195

Question #7

Answer: C

Rationale: Serum ferritin is the best laboratory test for making a distinction between iron deficiency and anemia resulting from inflammation. Ferritin is typically normal or increased with inflammation, and it is low with true iron deficiency. The serum iron level, the total iron-binding capacity, and the red blood cell protoporphyrin levels are the same in both conditions.

Page: 1196

Question #8

Answer: B

Rationale: Theoretically, the addition of intrinsic factor should correct the absorption defect that is associated with pernicious anemia. However, if the absorption defect is the result of disease of the terminal ileum, both stages of the Schilling test will be positive.

A host of surrogate markers for pernicious anemia include the measurement of intrinsic-factor antibodies or antiparietal cell antibodies. Unfortunately, these are positive in an increasing percentage of patients as they grow older, and, consequently, they cannot be considered definitive for the diagnosis.

Page: 1196

Question #9

Answer: B

Rationale: The treatment of iron deficiency is not always straightforward. There are numerous oral iron preparations to choose from, but ferrous sulfate and ferrous gluconate are among the most commonly used and the least expensive. The best regimen is to give three iron tablets a day; this provides about 150 mg of elemental iron. If the patient is compliant and absorption is normal, this will result in reticulocytosis within a week and an increase in the hemoglobin level of at least a gram within 2 weeks.

Page: 1197

Question #10

Answer: D

Rationale: Most patients who have the clinical phenotype of homozygous thalassemia are, in fact, compound heterozygotes. Homozygous alpha thalassemia is not seen in adults, because it results in hydrops fetalis in the newborn. However, beta-thalassemia trait and alpha-thalassemia trait are quite common, but they are usually associated with only mild anemia.

It is important to be aware of the fact that, with increasing numbers of immigrants from Southeast Asia, an increasing number of individuals who will have a form of thalassemia called hemoglobin Constant Spring might be seen in a primary care practice. Certifying the diagnosis is important so that iron or other therapies will not be inappropriately prescribed.

Page: 1197

Question #11

Answer: C

Rationale: An inherited condition that predisposes patients to intravascular hemolysis is the Mediterranean form of glucose-6-phosphate dehydrogenase (G6PD) deficiency. G6PD deficiency is the most common inborn error of red cell metabolism in the world, affecting nearly half a billion members of the world's population.

Because it is an X-linked genetic disorder, it is most severe in men. The Mediterranean abnormality of G6PD deficiency is associated with moderate chronic hemolysis, but this may become overwhelming and even fatal when the red cells are exposed to oxidative stress. Any oxidative stress in these individuals may have severe clinical consequences, and it may require transfusion or exchange transfusion as part of the therapy.

Page: 1197

Question #12

Answer: A

Rationale: Congenital forms of extravascular hemolysis include inherited hemoglobinopathies (e.g., the thalassemias, sickle cell disease), inherited membrane defects (e.g., hereditary spherocytosis, hereditary elliptocytosis), and enzyme defects. Defects of the metabolic machinery of the red cell usually cause hemolysis by creating unstable hemoglobin or by failing to generate adequate amounts of adenosine triphosphate to maintain red cell membrane plasticity. An example of the latter is pyruvate kinase deficiency. This is an autosomal recessive disorder, and it is the most common enzyme deficiency of the glycolytic pathway. Most patients with pyruvate kinase deficiency have a mild anemia, and they generally do not require transfusions.

Page: 1198

Question #13

Answer: A

Rationale: Sickle cell anemia is an inherited autosomal condition in which glutamic acid in the sixth position on the beta globin chain is replaced by a valine (Glu6Val). This results in hemoglobin SS in the homozygous state. Sickle cell trait, or hemoglobin AS, is found in 8% to 10% of blacks in the United States, and sickle cell anemia occurs in about 1 in 400. The gene for hemoglobin SS is very prevalent in sub-Saharan Africa. Persons of Mediterranean descent from India or Saudi Arabia have varying but somewhat lower percentages of the carrier state for hemoglobin SS. Sickle cell anemia is distributed worldwide, but it predominates in the Mediterranean, Saudi Arabian, and Indian populations. This distribution appears to be associated with independent mutations in these geographic regions. People with hemoglobin AS and SS are somewhat protected against malaria, because their erythrocytes are resistant to invasion by malarial parasites.

Page: 1199

Question #14

Answer: B

Rationale: A patient with sickle cell disease usually has chronic hemolysis producing a moderate anemia, intermittent jaundice, and a marrow with a thinned, bony cortex. Vaso-occlusive episodes and the appearance of Howell-Jolly bodies occur by the time the patient becomes an adult. The Howell-Jolly bodies reflect the fact that the patient has undergone an autoinfarction of the spleen.

Page: 1198

Question #15

Answer: B

Rationale: For a sickle cell preparation, blood is mixed with 2% sodium metabisulfite, which produces sickling; this would be inappropriate to administer to a patient. Lowering the blood pH would produce enhanced sickling of the red blood cells. Patients with sickle cell anemia are particularly susceptible to salmonella infections because of the associated decreased complement activation, and patients who are asplenic are also subject to an increased likelihood of infection from encapsulated organisms, such as the pneumococcus. Patients with sickle cell anemia should be given Pneumovax vaccine to prevent streptococcal pneumonia and sepsis. *Haemophilus influenzae* causes a high percentage of pneumonia among patients with sickle cell anemia.

Page: 1199

Question #16

Answer: D

Rationale: Neurologically, patients with sickle cell anemia are subject to stroke. Particularly disturbing is the fact that children with severe sickle cell anemia will have evidence by the age of 10 years of multiple small strokes that can be seen by magnetic resonance imaging or computed tomography scanning of the head; this has been associated with learning impairments in affected children. Aggressive transfusion protocols have been tested to try to reduce the incidence of this complication, and they have shown success. Thrombosis is peculiarly more common among children, whereas hemorrhage is more common among adults. The reason behind this observation is thought to be the occlusion of small vessels in hypoxic situations. Additionally, there is an increased attraction of sickled cells to the endothelium; this causes proliferation of the endothelial intimal surface, which can contribute to vascular occlusion. There is a high rate of recurrent stroke within 3 years of the initial event. Parvovirus infection can also cause pure red cell aplasia in these patients, and it can lead to a devastating exacerbation of the anemia.

Page: 1199

Question #17

Answer: C

Rationale: Autoimmune hemolytic anemias are very uncommon, but they can be dramatic upon presentation. About half of the patients have no associated disease. The diagnostic test for autoimmune hemolytic anemia is the Coombs' antiglobulin test. This is performed in both the direct and indirect manner, and it determines the presence of antibody coating the patient's red cells or free antibody in the plasma that is capable of binding to red cells. The autoantibodies may fix complement, or they may target the red cell for phagocytosis by the reticuloendothelial system.

Page: 1199

Question #18

Answer: A

Rationale: During the evaluation of patients with polycythemia or suspected polycythemia, it is important to first establish that the red cell mass is increased. This is achieved through a direct measurement of the red cell mass using isotope dilution techniques, which can be performed at most large hospitals. It is important to determine whether the polycythemia is primary or secondary in nature through the determination of the circulating erythropoietin level in the patient. If elevated, then the causes of the increased erythropoietin production need to be considered. These include heart or chronic pulmonary disease or other causes that are less frequent, such as renal cysts, hepatic or cerebellar tumors, uterine leiomyoma in women, or impaired hemoglobin function, such as that caused by heavy smoking (which results in elevated levels of carboxyhemoglobin, a form of hemoglobin that is essentially inert as an oxygen transporter).

Page: 1199

Question #19

Answer: B

Rationale: Two different kinds of cells with differing functions make up the white blood cell count. Phagocytic cells consisting of neutrophils, eosinophils, monocytes, and macrophages are primarily responsible for the ingestion and killing of microorganisms. Lymphocytes are responsible for cellular-mediated immunity and humoral immunity expressed through the production of antibodies.

Page: 1200

Question #20

Answer: C

Rationale: Peripheral blood neutrophils have specific granules and three to four lobes to their nuclei. When increased numbers of lobes are found, this suggests a nuclear maturation defect, such as vitamin B_{12} deficiency.

Page: 1202

Question #21

Answer: D

Rationale: In patients with Hodgkin's disease, Reed-Sternberg cells produce interleukin-5, which increases eosinophil presence and leads to the nodular sclerosing type of the disease.

Page: 1201

Question #22

Answer: A

Rationale: According to evidence-based medicine recommendations,[1] the highest specificity for the presence of infection occurs when more than 20% of the total white count is made up of band neutrophils. The highest sensitivity for infection is the presence of Dohle bodies, toxic granulations, and cytoplasmic vacuoles when the peripheral smear is examined. The highest predictor of the presence of acute inflammation is a total white cell count of greater than 10,500.
Strength of recommendation: A

Page: 1202

Question #23

Answer: C

Rationale: See following table.
Page: 1200

Absolute Neutrophil Count	Result
500–1000	Some risk of infection; fever can occasionally be managed on an outpatient basis
<500	Significant risk of infection; fever should always be managed on an inpatient basis with parenteral antibiotics; clinical signs of infection

Reproduced with permission from Baehner RL: Overview of neutropenia. In Rose BD, editor: Waltham: Up to Date, 2006. For more information, visit www.uptodate.com.

Question #24

Answer: C

Rationale: Evidence-based recommendations have been made by the American Society of Hematology for the management of idiopathic thrombocytopenic purpura, and they include the following[1]:

1. Patients with platelet counts above 50,000/µL do not routinely require treatment.
2. Treatment is indicated for patients with platelet counts in the 20,000/µL to 30,000/µL range and for patients with platelet counts below 50,000/µL with significant mucosal bleeding or risk factors for bleeding.
3. Patients with platelet counts below 20,000/µL need not be hospitalized if they are asymptomatic or if they have only mild purpura.
   Strength of recommendation: A

Page: 1205

Question #25

Answer: B

Rationale: Inherited disorders of platelet function are uncommon. Perhaps the most common is Glanzmann's thrombasthenia. This is a congenital disorder with identified mutations in the GPIIb/IIIa complex. Adenosine-diphosphate–induced platelet aggregation and platelet contribution to clot retraction are both abnormal. Abnormalities involving impaired granular release and the relative absence of granules characterize Bernard-Soulier syndrome and the Wiskott-Aldrich syndrome. These are very rare, and they are also associated with

1. Neutrophilia, 2005. Available at http://www.uptodate.com. Accessed June 2, 2006.

1. Dale DC, Federman DD (eds): ACP Medicine. New York, WebMD, 2004. 23.

thrombocytopenia. Von Willebrand's disease is an example of impaired platelet adhesion and aggregation as a result of the deficiency of von Willebrand factor, which significantly affects platelet function.

Page: 1206

Question #26

Answer: B

Rationale: Lymphocytosis varies somewhat with age. In individuals who are more than 12 years old, the upper limit of normal is 4000 cells/μL. Neonates and young children may have normal absolute lymphocyte counts of up to 8000 cells/μL. The absolute lymphocyte count can be calculated by multiplying the white blood cell count by the percentage of lymphocytes in the differential. When an absolute lymphocytosis is encountered, the peripheral smear should be examined for the presence of atypical lymphocytes, granular lymphocytes, blasts, smudge cells, and other abnormalities of morphology and diversity.

Page: 1207

Question #27

Answer: D

Rationale: Reactive lymphocytosis can sometimes be mistaken for a primary or malignant lymphocytosis when examining the peripheral blood smear, particularly in cases of infectious mononucleosis, when there may be a marked increase in lymphocytes that are larger, atypical, and/or transformed. Other causes of secondary lymphocytosis may generate small lymphocytes such as those seen in pertussis. Viral infections are the most prevalent cause of secondary lymphocytosis including Epstein-Barr virus, cytomegalovirus, herpes simplex virus, varicella, rubella, human immunodeficiency virus, adenovirus, and hepatitis. Occasionally, toxoplasmosis and pertussis in children can cause a lymphocytosis that is extremely high (up to levels of 50,000/μL–70,000/μL).

Page: 1207

Question #28

Answer: D

Rationale: Virchow's node is an enlarged left supraclavicular node that is usually infiltrated with a metastatic tumor from below the diaphragm, especially one of gastrointestinal origin. A matted node that is enlarged could be the result of a local phenomenon such as an infection, a bite, or a trauma to the arm, but it may also represent a melanoma, a lymphoma, or metastatic breast cancer in a young woman. Bilateral hilar adenopathy and the enlargement of nodes in the femoral triangle are more likely to be seen with systemic disease, with generalized infection, or, on occasion, with lymphoma.

Page: 1208

Question #29

Answer: A

Rationale: Acute myelogenous leukemia (AML) arises from the malignant transformation of myeloid progenitor or stem cells in the bone marrow, which are the precursors of granulocytes, erythrocytes, and megakaryocytes. Acute lymphoblastic leukemia (ALL) arises from precursor cells of the B and T cell lines.

AML and ALL have a similar overall incidence, but ALL is found predominantly among children, and AML is seen predominantly among adults. The peak age for the diagnosis of ALL is between 3 and 5 years, and the median age for the diagnosis of AML is 60 years. Both acute leukemias are more common in white than black populations, and Jews are more likely to be affected than non-Jews.

Page: 1209

Question #30

Answer: B

Rationale: Radiation is a potential inciting agent for acute leukemia, particularly among people who have received large doses of radiation in the past for the treatment of ankylosing spondylitis or Hodgkin's lymphoma. The radiation exposure used for diagnostic x-ray imaging does not appear to increase the risk of leukemia.

Page: 1210

Question #31

Answer: A

Rationale: Because the patient's condition was discovered by chance and because she is asymptomatic and without lymphadenopathy or splenic enlargement, she is in the initial or indolent phase (stage 0), and no treatment is indicated. As the disease advances, monoclonal antibody therapy may be tried; it is increasingly being used to try to bring about longer survival times.

Page: 1211

52 Answers

Question #1

Answer: B

Rationale: Although the urinalysis can detect occult disease, evidence of the benefit of routine urinalysis is limited. Most positive results do not identify occult disease, and false-positive results can cause patient suffering and result in potentially dangerous medical evaluations. Thus, screening is not recommended for asymptomatic adults. Microalbuminuria screening is recommended routinely for patients with diabetes. There is a good chance of false-positive or false-negative results with dipstick testing.

Page: 1217

Question #2

Answer: B

Rationale: Although the urine culture is the gold standard for diagnosing UTIs, the value of the midstream, clean-catch collection method is uncertain. Urine should not be obtained from a catheter bag, because bacterial contamination is typical. Urine cultures for women with typical UTI symptoms and colony counts of Enterobacteriaceae (e.g., *E. coli*) as low as 10^2 signify infection. Likewise, colony counts as low as 10^3 may signify infection in men with typical symptoms.

Page: 1222

Question #3

Answer: C

Rationale: Ultrasound is the method of choice for imaging renal cysts and the renal parenchyma. Likewise, it is the test of choice for evaluating scrotal and testicular disorders, and it is nearly 100% sensitive for testicular tumors. Computed tomography scanning is a better choice for imaging solid renal masses, and it is the test of choice for renal calculi.

Page: 1222

Question #4

Answer: D

Rationale: Hematuria is often an incidental finding on urinalysis, and most patients with this finding do not have significant pathology. The American Urological Association Best Practice Policy defines hematuria as 3 or more red blood cells per high-powered field for adults. Greater than 5 red blood cells per high-powered field on at least two weekly samples is generally considered abnormal in children. Warfarin should not cause hematuria if the international normalized ratio is within the goal treatment range. Initial laboratory testing usually includes a urinalysis, a urine culture (if indicated), and a serum creatinine level. Patients with an initial evaluation that does not suggest primary renal disease should be evaluated with upper urinary tract imaging, urine cytology, and cystoscopy.

Pages: 1224–1226

Question #5

Answer: C

Rationale: Risk factors for urologic malignancy include an age of more than 40 years, tobacco use, analgesic abuse, pelvic irradiation, occupational exposures, prior urologic disease, irritative voiding symptoms, a history of UTIs, and cyclophosphamide use.

Page: 1225

Question #6

Answer: D

Rationale: Nocturia is more common among the elderly, and studies of this population indicate that it increases the risk of falling. Nocturia is common among both men and women. Although the treatment of benign prostatic hypertrophy may help nocturia, it is common among men without benign prostatic hypertrophy. Therefore, clinicians should consider the contribution of nocturnal polyuria. Treating sleep apnea may help alleviate the increased urine production associated with an increased production of atrial natruretic peptide.

Page: 1227

Question #7

Answer: C

Rationale: Proteinuria is a marker of kidney disease, and it contributes to renal impairment. Although orthostatic proteinuria may occur in adults, it is uncommon after the age of 30 years. Most proteinuria is transient in children. Persistent proteinuria is confirmed by at least two of three weekly urine samples.

Pages: 1227–1228

Question #8

Answer: A

Rationale: Hydronephrosis is more commonly diagnosed prenatally now that fetal ultrasonography is widely used. Infants with fetal hydronephrosis require an ultrasound during the first week of life. After the diagnosis has been confirmed, the evaluation begins with a urinalysis, a urine culture, a basic metabolic panel (if bilateral), and a voiding cystourethrogram. If the voiding cystourethrogram is normal, a furosemide renogram is needed to evaluate for obstruction. In the absence of severe obstruction or high-grade vesicoureteral reflux with evidence of renal injury, a conservative approach including regular evaluations and serial renal ultrasounds is appropriate.

Page: 1229

Question #9

Answer: D

Rationale: Hypospadias is seen infrequently, but it must be recognized early (preferably at the initial newborn examination). Circumcision should be withheld in all cases of hypospadias, and a urology consultation should be obtained. Hypospadias can occur with or without chordee (curvature).

Page: 1230

Question #10

Answer: D

Rationale: Labial adhesions are not uncommon among young girls, and they may contribute to the development of UTIs. Retrospective data and case series do support the treatment of labial adhesions with estrogen cream to the adhered areas with gentle traction until the adhesions have separated. *Phimosis* is the inability to retract the foreskin over the glans, and *paraphimosis* is the inability to return the retracted foreskin over the glans; both are conditions of uncircumcised males. Acute paraphimosis requires urgent medical attention, because vascular engorgement can lead to necrosis of the glans.

Page: 1230

Question #11

Answer: D

Rationale: Testicular torsion is most commonly seen during adolescence, and it is a true medical emergency. Testicular viability declines to 0% if detorsion occurs 24 hours after the onset of symptoms. The diagnosis can be made by physical examination, at which time the testis may be noted to lie more horizontally (i.e., the bell-clapper deformity), and there may be a loss of cremasteric reflex. Color Doppler ultrasound with a sensitivity of 89% to 100% and a specificity of 77% to 100% may be of assistance. Testicular torsion can occur with systemic illnesses, such as Henoch-Schönlein purpura, and it can mimic other conditions, such as appendicitis or nephrolithiasis.

Page: 1231

Question #12

Answer: B

Rationale: Most patients with Peyronie's disease do not require any treatment and thus can be reassured. The management of hydroceles in young children is supportive, and most hydroceles resolve by the age of 2 years. Torsion of the appendix testes is less severe than testicular torsion, and it can be managed supportively with analgesia and scrotal elevation. Undescended testis occur in 2.7% to 5.9% of full-term male infants. Patients with truly undescended testes generally require urologic evaluation. Even after orchiopexy, testicular self-examination should be taught to patients, because they have a slightly increased risk of testicular cancer in either testicle.

Page: 1230

Question #13

Answer: A

Rationale: Renal disease is a very significant public health problem in the United States; it affects nearly 20 million people.

Page: 1231

Question #14

Answer: C

Rationale: The risk for chronic kidney disease is increased by diseases such as diabetes, hypertension, autoimmune disorders, genetic syndromes, urinary infection, urinary obstruction, and renal calculi. Pharmacologic toxicity and social factors such as age, ethnicity, and lower socioeconomic status can also elevate risk.
Page: 1231

Question #15

Answer: B

Rationale: Patients with type 2 diabetes and nephropathy clearly benefit from therapy with either class of medications. However, the evidence supporting ARBs for the prevention of end-stage renal failure among patients with advanced nephropathy is stronger. The overall evidence base is more extensive for ACE inhibitors, which are also less expensive, and they have been proven to be beneficial for more comorbidities. Thus, ACE inhibitors are generally the best initial choice for most patients.
Page: 1233

Question #16

Answer: A

Rationale: Interventions that have been found to be beneficial for the management of nocturnal enuresis include dry-bed training with positive reinforcement, decreasing fluids at night, medication (e.g., desmopressin, tricyclics), and conditioning therapy with bed-wetting alarms. A systematic review has reported that desmopressin plus an alarm is better than an alarm alone or than an alarm plus placebo.
Page: 1233

Question #17

Answer: C

Rationale: Sexual dysfunction does not decline with age. Nevertheless, normal erectile function depends on multiple body systems, including the cardiovascular, endocrine, and nervous systems; and disorders of these systems increase with advancing age. As many as 30 million men have erectile dysfunction. Although prevalence increases with age, 7% of men ages between the ages of 18 and 30 years are reported to have erectile dysfunction. Risk factors include diabetes, cardiovascular disease, and depression.
Page: 1234

Question #18

Answer: C

Rationale: Interstitial cystitis is a chronic, noninfectious bladder disorder. The symptoms of this condition are similar to those of a UTI, with the addition of chronic pelvic pain and/or dyspareunia. It is a disorder that is almost exclusively found among middle-aged women. Pentosan polysulfate sodium is approved by the U.S. Food and Drug Administration for the treatment for this condition. Prospective data on dietary interventions for interstitial cystitis are lacking.
Page: 1236

Question #19

Answer: B

Rationale: Although anticholinergic agents have been demonstrated to be effective for the treatment of overactive bladder, important differences in the effectiveness of the agents within this class of medications have not been demonstrated.
Page: 1236

Question #20

Answer: D

Rationale: White men have the highest risk of kidney stones. The study of choice for diagnosing renal calculi is the helical, noncontrast computed tomography scan. It is more sensitive than intravenous urography; it provides a quicker diagnosis, and it is of about equal cost. Stones that are less than 5 mm will likely pass without intervention.
Page: 1237

Question #21

Answer: A

Rationale: In men under the age of 35 years, epididymitis usually coexists with asymptomatic urethritis. Gram-negative enterics may also be noted in association with insertive anal intercourse or among men who are more than 35 years old who have had invasive procedures, such as cystoscopy.

Page: 1238

Question #22

Answer: A

Rationale: Prostatitis is more likely than UTI to be found among otherwise healthy men with UTI symptoms. As is also found with UTI, gram-negative enterics (e.g., *E. coli*) are the most likely etiologic organisms. Most experts advise against prostate massage because of its associated discomfort and theoretic potential to disseminate infection. Urine culture is typically positive for the causative organism.

Page: 1238

Question #23

Answer: E

Rationale: Chancroid is caused by infection with *Haemophilus ducreyi*, and it is associated with painful genital ulcers and adenopathy. The genital ulcers of syphilis, on the other hand, are typically painless. Coinfection with gonorrhea and chlamydia is common. Adults with syphilis are treated with a single dose of 2.4 million units of penicillin intramuscularly, and children are treated with a single dose of 50,00 units/kg intramuscularly up to a maximal dose of 2.4 million units.

Page: 1239

Question #24

Answer: C

Rationale: Women presenting with at least one symptom of UTI have a 50% chance of having a UTI. Combining the symptoms of dysuria and frequency (without vaginal symptoms) increases that likelihood to 90%. Although there is growing resistance to trimethoprim-sulfamethoxazole, many women treated with this agent achieve clinical cure despite evidence of a resistant organism on culture. Randomized trials support the use of cranberry juice as a preventive treatment for recurrent UTI; its effect is likely the result of the inhibition of bacterial adherence to uroepithelial cells.

Pages: 1240–1241

Question #25

Answer: E

Rationale: The major risk factors for prostate cancer are age, being black, and family history. Uncertainty and controversy surround prostate-specific antigen testing, and a large, randomized screening trial (The Prostate, Lung, Colorectal, and Ovary Trial) is underway to address this important issue. The U.S. Preventive Services Task Force found the evidence insufficient to make a recommendation for or against screening. In view of the debate surrounding prostate-specific antigen screening, it is recommended that patients be fully informed about the risks, benefits, and limitations of the test before making a decision to have it performed. Renal cancers are twice as common among men as they are among women. Heavy tobacco use is a risk factor for men, and severe obesity is a risk for both sexes.

Pages: 1244–1245

Question #1

Answer: C

Rationale: Subconjunctival hemorrhage is usually the result of a sudden rise in intrathoracic pressure caused by coughing, sneezing, or straining associated with constipation or heavy lifting. The usually white sclera, which is visualized through the nearly transparent conjunctiva, is hidden by a subconjunctival collection of blood that has extravasated from conjunctival vessels as a result of decreased venous return caused by transient increase in intrathoracic pressure. A subconjunctival hemorrhage will usually resolve in 2 to 3 weeks. Iritis, acute angle closure glaucoma, and ophthalmia neonatorum pose a serious threat to vision, and they require immediate referral to an ophthalmologist.

Page: 1252

Question #2

Answer: E

Rationale: Every patient who calls the office with the complaint of a red eye should be asked about all of the listed symptoms as well as about any history of recent ocular trauma, ocular surgery, or contact lens use. The presence of any of these may indicate a serious ocular disorder and should result in prompt evaluation.

Page: 1253

Question #3

Answer: D

Rationale: Ophthalmia neonatorum, acute dacryocystitis, and congenital glaucoma can cause serious vision loss, and they can even be life threatening (ophthalmia neonatorum and acute dacryocystitis). These conditions usually present with one or more of the following findings: very swollen lids, red eyes, copious and purulent discharge, and a cloudy cornea. If an infant presents to your office with these findings, immediately refer him or her to an ophthalmologist. By comparison, with chronic dacryocystitis or nasal lacrimal duct obstruction, the infant has a chronic history of tearing and crusty lids without eye redness and, if present, only a very mild amount of lid swelling. Most of these cases will resolve by 9 to 12 months of

age. However, if the condition is still present at 6 months, referral to an ophthalmologist should be considered.

Pages: 1253–1254

Question #4

Answer: D

Rationale: Topical steroids are very useful to the ophthalmologist who is treating patients with severe ocular allergy and iritis. However, topical steroids can cause cataracts, glaucoma, and the progression of viral, bacterial, or fungal ocular infections. Accordingly, topical steroids should be prescribed only by ophthalmologists.

Page: 1258

Question #5

Answer: D

Rationale: For cases of chemical injury, minutes do matter: the faster that the ocular surface can be cleaned of the offending chemical, the better. After the on-site 15-minute irrigation, the patient should either come in to the office or go to the nearest emergency department for immediate evaluation.

Page: 1260

Question #6

Answer: A

Rationale: Hyphema can cause many long-term ocular problems, including corneal blood staining, optic nerve atrophy, and anterior and posterior synechiae. The risk of these is increased if the patient has sickle cell disease, but a hyphema does not increase the risk of a systemic sickle crisis.

Page: 1262

Question #7

Answer: D

Rationale: Frequently, mild post-traumatic abrasions and black eyes will resolve without ocular complications.

However, lacerations of the lids and of the ocular surface require careful evaluation and treatment to minimize the long-term problems, and these should be referred to an ophthalmologist.

Page: 1261

Question #8

Answer: A

Rationale: Any of the listed condition can cause serious long-term vision loss or even death (in the event of a missed retinoblastoma). Accordingly, the American Academy of Ophthalmology and the American Association of Pediatric Ophthalmology and Strabismus recommend that children be screened in the newborn nursery, at 6 months old, at 3 years old, and at 5 years old.

Page: 1263

Question #9

Answer: D

Rationale: Retinoblastoma is the most common intraocular malignancy found in children. If it is not diagnosed, it will cause a loss of vision and possibly death. Leukocoria and strabismus are common presentations. Immediate referral to an ophthalmologist is needed for a child with leukocoria.

Page: 1264

Question #10

Answer: B

Rationale: The terms *myopia* and *nearsightedness* mean the same thing: the patient sees better at close range. Likewise, *hyperopia* and *farsightedness* also mean the same thing: the patient sees better at a distance. Both can be detected with screening, and they may need to be corrected with a refraction if they are determined by an ophthalmologist to be significant.

Page: 1265

Question #11

Answer: A

Rationale: Children or adults who have eyes that are not aligned have strabismus. If the eyes turn in, it is called *esotropia;* if they turn out, it is called *exotropia.*

A family history is common with both of these conditions. If they are left uncorrected, amblyopia or lazy eye may develop. Esotropia is more common than exotropia.

Page: 1266

Question #12

Answer: B

Rationale: Amblyopia is a condition in which an eye does not see well despite a normal examination. Causes include strabismus, refractive error, and cataract. It can be reversed but only effectively so before the age of 7 to 9 years. *Strabismus* is a condition in which the eyes are not aligned. Strabismus is usually primary, but it can also be caused by amblyopia.

Page: 1266

Question #13

Answer: A

Rationale: Depending on the type and severity of myopia (nearsightedness) or hyperopia (farsightedness), LASIK or PRK could be preformed. Both LASIK and PRK are considered types of refractive surgery.

Page: 1273

Question #14

Answer: E

Rationale: Physicians who treat patients who are taking ocular medications need to be aware of their potential side effects.

Page: 1273

Question #15

Answer: B

Rationale: Because the major causes of vision loss occur more commonly as one ages (i.e., cataracts, glaucoma, macular degeneration, and diabetic retinopathy), adults who are more than 65 years old should have a complete eye examination every 1 to 2 years, and adults who are more than 40 years old should have such an examination at least every 3 years.

Page: 1273

Question #16

Answer: A

Rationale: During the aging process, the lens in the eye becomes more still, and it does not as readily change shape to focus on near objects. This is a normal age-related event for most adults in their 40s and 50s and certainly among even older adults; reading glasses will be required to see near objects clearly.

Page: 1275

Question #17

Answer: A

Rationale: Currently, the most common technique to remove cataracts during cataract surgery is with a small needle applying controlled pulses of ultrasonic power to break up or emulsify the lens—hence the term *phacoemulsification*. In nearly every case, a replacement intraocular lens is placed in the eye to optimize visual acuity.

Page: 1275

Question #18

Answer: D

Rationale: Glaucoma is the most common cause of permanent vision loss among black patients. Blacks are four times more likely to have glaucoma and eight times more likely to go blind. Cataracts are more common among this population, but they are a reversible cause. Retinal detachment is not more common than glaucoma. Diabetic retinopathy is also a common cause of permanent vision loss, and it increases the risk of glaucoma.

Page: 1275

Question #19

Answer: E

Rationale: Depending on the severity of the glaucoma, all or only a few of the listed treatments may be required. Usually, topical medications or lasers are used for glaucoma that has been detected early or that is mild; oral medication or incisional surgery may be required for more advanced or severe cases.

Page: 1276

Question #20

Answer: A

Rationale: Macular degeneration causes the loss of central or reading vision but not a loss of side vision. Diabetic retinopathy is a common cause of the loss of all vision in adults. Retinal detachment causes a loss of side vision first. Temporal arteritis is frequently associated with scalp and jaw pain and sudden vision loss, but, overall, this is a rare finding.

Page: 1278

Question #21

Answer: C

Rationale: The dry or nonexudative type accounts for 90% of macular degeneration, but it is the wet or exudative type that accounts for 90% of the severe vision loss.

Page: 1278

Question #22

Answer: A

Rationale: All of the current treatment options for macular degeneration—vitamins, laser, and ocular injections—only attempt to slow the progression of the disease.

Page: 1278

Question #23

Answer: A

Rationale: Overall, diabetic patients have a 25-times higher risk of going blind as compared with patients without diabetes. The risk decreases with better glucose control.

Page: 1279

Question #24

Answer: A

Rationale: A vitreous detachment is more common, but a retinal detachment can cause a loss of vision. With the symptoms of flashers, floaters, and a veil over the vision, the patient should see an ophthalmologist within 24 hours.

Page: 1280

Question #25

Answer: A

Rationale: Amaurosis fugax is the ocular version of a transient ischemic attack. The patient should be evaluated for carotid and cardiac valvular disease. Optic-neuritis–associated vision loss is transient, but vision takes days to weeks to return, and it is usually associated with retro-ocular pain. Temporal arteritis presents in a way that is very similar to optic neuritis, except the pain is in the jaw and the scalp, and the vision loss is permanent. Retinal detachment vision loss is painless, but vision does not return.

Page: 1281

Question #26

Answer: E

Rationale: The Age-Related Eye Disease Study showed a statistically significant decrease in progression when adults with intermediate or advanced age-related macular degeneration took the above-listed combination of supplements. There was no significant benefit for those with no or only mild age-related macular degeneration. Cupric oxide (2 mg) was also included to offset the potential side effect of anemia that may result from the zinc supplementation.

Page: 1279

Question #27

Answer: B

Rationale: The Optic Neuritis Treatment Trial revealed the importance of 3 days of intravenous steroids first followed by oral steroids for hastening visual recovery and delaying the onset of multiple sclerosis symptoms. It also revealed that oral steroids should not be used before intravenous steroids or alone, because this resulted in a more frequent relapse of symptoms. The Controlled High-Risk Avonex Multiple Sclerosis Trial showed that patients with a high risk of developing multiple sclerosis—including patients with high-risk symptoms or findings on a magnetic resonance image—experienced a significant reduction in the rate in developing multiple sclerosis when they were taking Avonex.

Page: 1281

Question #28

Answer: A

Rationale: This clinical picture described here is very suggestive of temporal arteritis: the correct symptoms, signs, and laboratory abnormalities are listed, and the patient is in the correct age range. Temporal arteritis will involve the second eye within 10 days in 65% of patients, and the vision loss is usually permanent. Accordingly, start treatment with steroids before planning biopsy. The clinical picture is less likely than that which is commonly associated with optic neuritis.

Page: 1280

Question #29

Answer: B

Rationale: Dermatochalasis is an age-related loss of skin elasticity, and the affected skin of the upper eyelid begins to droop over the edge of the lid and lashes; it can even block the superior visual field. This drooping, baggy skin can be removed with surgery. *Ptosis* is a drooping eyelid that is caused by a weakening of the eyelid muscles, and it can also cause a significant loss of the superior visual field. This is more common among the elderly, but it can occur at any age, and it can frequently accompany dermatochalasis. It requires a different type of eyelid surgery for repair. If the superior visual field is significantly affected by either dermatochalasis or ptosis, the surgical repair is considered functional rather than cosmetic.

Page: 1274

Question #30

Answer: E

Rationale: Parents and the general public have many misconceptions about strabismus surgery, so all of the listed topics should be discussed.

Page: 1269

Question #1

Answer: C

Rationale: Reading and writing are impaired in patients with both Wernicke's and Broca's aphasias, and this results from damage to the dominant cerebral hemisphere. Among patients with Wernicke's aphasia, there is poor comprehension but fluent (and often meaningless) speech. By contrast, among patients with Broca's aphasia, there is good comprehension, but the speech is meaningless.

Page: 1278

Question #2

Answer: D

Rationale: The deep tendon reflexes are graded from 0, which means they are absent, to 4, which means they are increased and pathologic reflexes with one or more beats of clonus. A rating of 2 represents a normal reflex; 1 means that the reflex is present with reinforcement, and 3 means that the reflex is normal but more brisk than average.

Page: 1285

Question #3

Answer: B

Rationale: Features of the patient's history that should warn of an ominous cause for headache include a sudden onset of "first headache"; a claim that this is the worst headache that the patient has ever experienced; a late onset of new headaches (after the age of 50 years); a headache associated with fever, rash, or stiff neck; a progressively worsening headache; and a headache associated with neurological signs and symptoms other than aura.

Page: 1285

Question #4

Answer: A

Rationale: To establish a diagnosis of migraine without aura, there must have been at least five attacks fulfilling the following criteria:

1. Headache attacks lasting 4 to 72 hours.
2. Headache with at least two of the following characteristics: unilateral location, pulsating quality, moderate or severe intensity (inhibits or prohibits daily activities or causing avoidance of routine), and/or aggravated by physical activity such as walking or climbing.
3. During the headache, the patient experiences nausea and vomiting and/or photophobia and phonophobia.

Page: 1286

Question #5

Answer: C

Rationale: For mild migraine attacks, combination medicines such as aspirin, acetaminophen, and caffeine are a grade A treatment recommendations. Triptans should be reserved for more severe headaches; they are not indicated for basilar migraines or paraplegic migraines. Dihydroergotamine mesylate and aqueous lidocaine can also be used for more severe headaches.

Page: 1286

Question #6

Answer: A

Rationale: The criteria for the diagnosis of cluster headaches include at least five attacks involving the following elements:

1. Severe unilateral orbital or supraorbital pain lasting from 15 to 180 minutes.
2. Headache associated with at least one of the following ipsilateral signs in addition to the headache: conjunctival infection, lacrimation, nasal congestion, miosis/ptosis, eye edema, forehead and facial sweating, or a sense of restlessness/agitation.
3. Frequency from every other day to eight per day.

Page: 1287

Question #7

Answer: D

Rationale: Rebound headaches are characterized by a diffuse, bilateral, almost daily headache aggravated by mild physical or mental exertion. These headaches are frequently present on awakening, and they can be associated with restlessness, nausea, forgetfulness, and depression.

Page: 1288

Question #8

Answer: A

Rationale: The major risk after a TIA or a minor stroke is the subsequent occurrence of a myocardial infarction. Patients with a previous TIA or stroke have a 4.5% to 6.6% annual risk of subsequent stroke. The risk for stroke after a retinal TIA (amaurosis fugax) is much less than that after a hemispheric TIA.

Page: 1289

Question #9

Answer: B

Rationale: It is important to determine the exact timing of the onset of symptoms to make determinations about the use of tissue plasminogen activator. If a patient awakens from sleep with a neurological deficit, the stroke must be assumed to have had its onset at the time that sleep commenced, and decisions involving the use of tissue plasminogen activator should be based on this assumption.

Page: 1290

Question #10

Answer: C

Rationale: Areas of cerebral ischemia lose their normal autoregulatory capacity, and tissue perfusion is directly linked to mean arterial pressure. When cerebral ischemia occurs, blood pressure elevations are often transient, and spontaneous declines are common. Therefore, overzealous treatment of blood pressure can convert an area of ischemia that retains the potential for recovery into an area of frank infarction with no potential for recovery. Thus, during the first few days after an ischemic stroke, elevated blood pressure should not be treated unless the systolic blood pressure is consistently greater than 220 mm Hg or the diastolic blood pressure is consistently greater than 120 mm Hg. Patients who have received tissue plasminogen activator should have their blood pressures maintained below 185/110 mm Hg, and patients with myocardial infarction, heart failure, aortic dissection, or renal failure should have more aggressive blood pressure control.

Page: 1292

Question #11

Answer: A

Rationale: Delirium is a transient, global disorder of cognition and consciousness. The changes in consciousness typically develop over a relatively short period of time, and they fluctuate during the course of the day. This is in contrast with dementia, in which cognitive impairment develops gradually. A history of dementia does not preclude the diagnosis of delirium, but dementia is a known risk factor for the development of delirium.

Page: 1293

Question #12

Answer: C

Rationale: Haloperidol's advantages for the treatment of delirium include the fact that it is less anticholinergic, less sedating, and less likely to cause hypotension or arrhythmias than thioridazine. Lorazepam (Ativan) is the chief anxiolytic agent used for the treatment of delirium.

Page: 1293

Question #13

Answer: C

Rationale: End-of-life care issues are an important aspect of the treatment of patients with dementia. Family members should be informed that studies show that feeding tubes do not prolong life, that they are associated with discomfort and medical complications, and that they are generally not recommended for patients who are in the final stages of a dementing illness. The role of hospice care should also be discussed early during the course of illness.

Page: 1295

Question #14

Answer: D

Rationale: Defining altered states of consciousness helps with the process of determining appropriate care. *Coma* describes a state of sustained unresponsiveness to external stimuli. *Stupor* describes the state of a patient who is arousable with vigorous and repeated stimuli but whose response is slow or inadequate. *Obtundation* describes a lesser state of decreased arousal with some responsiveness to voice or touch. *Lethargy* is a state of diminished arousal that can be maintained spontaneously or by light repeated stimulation. *Confusion* and *delirium* refer to states of alertness with impaired cognition.

Page: 1296

Question #15

Answer: B

Rationale: In the comatose patient, certain signs, including the odor of the breath, can help elucidate the cause of the condition as well as the appropriate treatment. Most cases of alcohol intoxication will be readily apparent. Diabetic ketoacidosis has a fruity odor; uremia has a urine-like smell, hepatic failure has a musty fetter; arsenic has a garlic aroma, and cyanide poisoning has the scent of almond.

Page: 1297

Question #16

Answer: C

Rationale: In the comatose patient, the ABCs of acute resuscitation are initiated. The "coma cocktail"—thiamine, glucose, and naloxone—can be administered. Glucose is useful for treating possible hypoglycemia, and thiamine is coadministered with glucose to prevent Wernicke's encephalopathy. Naloxone will temporarily reverse opiate narcosis, but, in addicted patients, withdrawal symptoms including vomiting may occur. This can be minimized by starting at low doses and increasing up to 10 mg if opiate poisoning is suspected.

Page: 1299

Question #17

Answer: A

Rationale: Narcolepsy is a REM-dissociative disorder that is characterized by excessive daytime hypersomno-

lence; it is associated with cataplexy, sleep paralysis, and hypnagogic hallucinations. Patients with narcolepsy have episodes of REM that occur at the wrong time. *Cataplexy* is the sudden, brief loss of muscle tone that occurs with a strong emotion, such as intense laughter. *Sleep paralysis* is the inability to move skeletal muscles voluntarily during the sleep–wake transition. *Hypnagogic hallucinations* are vivid visual or auditory events that are associated with normal dreaming.

Page: 1300

Question #18

Answer: B

Rationale: Sleep studies are helpful for characterizing the nature of sleep disorders. During a sleep study, the patient is monitored for episodes of apnea. An apnea is obstructive if there is no airflow with respiratory effort. Central apnea is characterized by the absence of airflow and respiratory effort. Hypopnea is a 50% reduction in airflow, and the respiratory distress index is a measure of severity of episodes of apnea. The respiratory distress index refers to the number of events that last longer than 10 seconds that occur during an hour. Sleepiness seems to correlate more with fragmented sleep than with the respiratory distress index.

Page: 1301

Question #19

Answer: A

Rationale: Febrile seizures are seizures without a definite cause that are associated with fever. Approximately one third of children who experience a first febrile seizure will experience at least one more, but less than 5% of children who experience a febrile seizure develop epilepsy. Risk factors for first febrile seizure include a family history of febrile seizures, developmental delays, very high fever, and child-care attendance. The younger the child is when the first febrile seizure occurs, the more likely the child is to have another febrile seizure. A family history of febrile seizures also increases the likelihood of recurrence. Most recurrences of febrile seizure are within 1 year.

Page: 1303

Question #20

Answer: D

Rationale: Deciding whether to initiate an antiepileptic drug after a first nonfebrile seizure is controversial. The rate of recurrence after a single, unprovoked, nonfebrile seizure ranges widely, but there are certain findings and characteristics that increase the likelihood of recurrence, including electroencephalogram abnormalities, previous neurological injury, partial seizures, and a family history of seizures.

Page: 1304

Question #21

Answer: D

Rationale: Most adult patients with meningitis present with the classic triad of fever, headache, and neck stiffness. Other symptoms include nausea and vomiting, seizures, cranial nerve palsies, and other focal neurological deficits. Meningismus maybe detected with Kernig's sign (resistance to knee extension after flexion of the patient's hip and knees by the examiner) or Brudzinski's sign (involuntary flexion of the knees in a supine patient in response to rapid neck flexion by the examiner). Other symptoms include nuchal rigidity, lethargy, photophobia, confusion, sweats, and rigors. Papilledema occurs in less than 1% of patients during the early phases of the disease.

Page: 1305

Question #22

Answer: C

Rationale: *H. influenzae, N. meningitidis,* and *S. pneumoniae* account for 80% of cases of meningitis in the United States. Group B streptococcus is the most common cause among infants during the first months of life.

Page: 1306

Question #23

Answer: B

Rationale: The theoretical goal of using corticosteroids for patients with bacterial meningitis is to minimize meningeal inflammation, thereby decreasing the severity and incidence of brain injury. However, its use does remain a controversial issue. Dexamethasone should be given to infants and children with *H. influenzae* type B meningitis if it can be initiated 10 to 20 minutes before (or at least continently with) the first doses of antibiotics at a dose of 0.15 mg/kg every 6 hours for 2 to 4 days. Adjunctive dexamethasone should not be given to infants and children who have already received antimicrobial therapy, because administration in this situation is unlikely to improve patient outcome. Dexamethasone should also be administered 10 to 20 minutes before (or at least concomitant with) the first dose of antibiotics in all adult patients with suspected or proven pneumococcal meningitis. Dexamethasone should not be given to adult patients who have already received antibiotics. These are all grade A recommendations.

Pages: 1306–1307

Question #24

Answer: D

Rationale: Although diabetes and alcoholism are the most common causes of peripheral neuropathy among adults in developed countries, leprosy is still the primary treatable cause of peripheral neuropathy worldwide. Human immunodeficiency virus is one of the fastest growing causes.

Page: 1314

Question #25

Answer: B

Rationale: Guillain-Barré syndrome is a rapidly progressive paralytic syndrome that affects persons of all ages. The traditional description of a rapid progression of ascending, symmetric weakness starting in the lower extremities and moving to the upper extremities is useful, but variations are common. In the majority of cases, recovery is complete or nearly complete; however, in about 10% of cases, permanent disability develops, and, in 3% to 5% of cases, patients die. Treatment usually consists of either plasmapheresis or intravenous human immunoglobulin. There is no role for steroids in the acute treatment of Guillain-Barré syndrome.

Page: 1320

Question #26

Answer: A

Rationale: Bell's palsy affects cranial nerve 7 (facial nerve), and it is probably the most common isolated cranial neuropathy. The forehead is involved, and any indication that the forehead is spared should prompt a search for a central cause. Bilateral Bell's palsy is rare, and it should also prompt the consideration of other illnesses. Some evidence suggests that corticosteroids, if they are started early, may hasten recovery and reduce the incidence of sequela.

Page: 1322

Question #27

Answer: C

Rationale: Duchenne's muscular dystrophy is an X-linked recessive disorder, and it is rarely seen in girls. Symptoms typically present between ages of 3 and 7 years. Pelvic girdle and thigh weakness forces these children to rise from the floor by placing their hands on their knees and walking up their thighs (Grower's sign). Firm pseudohypertrophy of the calves results from the replacement of muscle with fibrous and fatty tissue. Cardiac muscle is also affected, with involvement ranging from asymptomatic electrocardiogram changes to arrhythmias and congestive heart failure.

Page: 1322

Question #28

Answer: A

Rationale: Myotonic dystrophy is the most common adult muscular dystrophy. It is characterized during its early stages by distal as opposed to proximal weakness and atrophy. Another key feature is the presence of myotonia, which is the slow relaxation of a normal muscle contraction; this is evident in the inability to immediately release a handshake. Systemic features can include frontal balding and testicular atrophy.

Pages: 1323–1324

Question #29

Answer: B

Rationale: The hallmark clinical features of Parkinson's disease include tremor, rigidity, and bradykinesia. Poor postural reflexes are also commonly observed. Tremor is the presenting symptom of up to 70% of patients, and it is an asymmetric resting tremor that is often described as "pill rolling" because of the manner in which the wrist and fingers flex. *Bradykinesia* refers to the slowness of movements, and rigidity is often associated with "cog wheeling," which is a ratchety quality to the passive movement of a limb.

Page: 1326

Question #30

Answer: D

Rationale: No studies clearly demonstrate a best initial treatment for Parkinson's disease. In addition, medications also do not appear to slow the progression of the disease. Levodopa-carbidopa is the most frequently used agent, but, after a few years of treatment, some patients develop dyskinesias, an unpredictable on-off response, or a "wearing-off" response before the next dose. Monoamine oxidase type B inhibitors are relatively contraindicated for patients with peptic ulcer disease or cardiovascular disease. Thalamotomy, posteroventral pallidotomy, and deep brain stimulation with implanted electrodes are possible surgical treatments for patients with Parkinson's disease.

Page: 1327

Question #31

Answer: C

Rationale: The clinical symptoms of multiple sclerosis vary, depending on which part of the nervous system is affected, but three symptoms are highly suggestive of the condition: optic neuritis, nystagmus resulting from internuclear ophthalmoplegia, and Lhermitte's sign, which is an electrical sensation that extends down the back and the legs with the flexion of the neck.

Page: 1328

Question #32

Answer: A

Rationale: The diagnosis of amyotrophic lateral sclerosis is based on the characteristic clinical signs of progressive weakness, atrophy, fasciculations, and hyperreflexia. Amyotrophic lateral sclerosis almost never presents with fasciculations alone. There are no specific laboratory tests for amyotrophic lateral sclerosis, and it is almost universally a fatal disease.

Page: 1330

55 Answers

Question #1

Answer: C

Rationale: Patients are typically quite receptive to questions about their sexual health. Physicians, on the other hand, may be uncomfortable or hesitant to address this topic. According to survey data, although 49% of women and 43% of men reported experiencing at least one sexual problem, fewer than 20% had sought medical assistance. Another study demonstrated that physicians only documented issues relating to patients' sexual problems 3% to 4% of the time. It is important to remember that each individual will have differing goals and expectations about his or her sexuality, and it is the task of the physician to individualize care accordingly.

Page: 1335

Question #2

Answer: E

Rationale: Many factors influence sexual problems, including medical illness, medications, relationship difficulties, and past sexual abuse. In addition, alcohol and drug abuse, toxic exposures, prior surgeries, sexual orientation, and gender identity also influence sexual dysfunction. Birth order in the family is not a contributing factor.

Page: 1338

Question #3

Answer: C

Rationale: Sexual aversion disorder is characterized by the severe avoidance of all or nearly all sexual contact. Patients who are voluntarily celibate do not fall into this diagnostic category, because their situation does not cause distress or difficulty.

Pages: 1339–1340

Question #4

Answer: A

Rationale: ED has multiple causes and contributing factors. Causes may involve the vascular, neurologic, endocrine, and psychological systems. Comorbid medical conditions such as diabetes, cancer, stroke, and hypertension are strongly associated with ED. The prevalence is quite high, with 40% of men between the ages of 60 and 69 years and 60% of men 70 years old or older experiencing ED. Physical examination and laboratory evaluation to assess vascular risk should be obtained, including serum glucose level, creatinine level, blood urea nitrogen level, and lipid profile. Additional laboratories may be needed, depending on the patient's risk factors.

Pages: 1340–1341

Question #5

Answer: C

Rationale: Taking a thorough history is the most important diagnostic tool when assessing a patient who presents with premature ejaculation. Multiple factors contribute to this phenomenon, including the patient's past sexual history, an understanding of sexual functioning, and relationship issues. Family physicians are ideally suited to take this comprehensive history and to direct further treatment options.

Page: 1343

Question #6

Answer: E

Rationale: Helping the couple shift the focus of sexual satisfaction from achieving partner orgasm with intercourse to one of mutual pleasuring is a most helpful intervention when addressing the issue of premature ejaculation. The squeeze technique, the stop-and-start technique, and masturbation training are behavior modification tools that can assist the patient with improving ejaculatory control. SSRIs are highly effective for delaying ejaculation, and sildenafil is also being studied for this condition.

Page: 1343

Question #7

Answer: B

Rationale: Although some patients who report dyspareunia do indeed have a history of sexual abuse, there are many other causes. Among men, Peyronie's disease, neuropathy, and infection can be the causative factors. Among women, vaginal septae, atrophic vaginitis, and infectious vaginitis can be causative factors. *Dyspareunia* is a term that can be applied to both men and women. For both genders, relationship issues are often a contributing aspect as well.

Page: 1343

Question #8

Answer: C

Rationale: Less than 50% of women can reach orgasm with vaginal intercourse alone; this does not represent a form of female orgasmic disorder. Additional clitoral stimulation during intercourse or other forms of pleasuring may be necessary for a woman to be able to climax.

Page: 1344

Question #9

Answer: A

Rationale: Female orgasmic disorder is divided into two categories: primary and secondary inhibited orgasm. In primary inhibited orgasm, the woman has never been able to achieve orgasm. Many factors are potential contributors to this, including lack of sexual knowledge, neurologic or gynecologic pathology, and inhibitions surrounding sexuality from strict religious or cultural traditions. Marriage is no guarantee that orgasmic disorder will resolve. Secondary inhibited orgasm is characterized by the inability to achieve orgasm despite prior ability to climax. After the cause of female orgasmic disorder is identified and the underlying issue(s) are addressed, many women can go on to successfully have orgasms.

Page: 1344

Question #10

Answer: D

Rationale: Vaginismus is an involuntary spasm of the pelvic musculature of the outer third of the vagina. The cause is often idiopathic, although it can sometimes be the result of vaginal septae or other anatomic abnormalities. Many cases develop after pelvic trauma, infection, or sexual abuse. Treatment is complicated, and it may require the intervention of a sex therapist

or a specially trained physical therapist for pelvic floor biofeedback.

Page: 1345

Question #11

Answer: B

Rationale: Youth Risk Behavior Surveillance survey data from the Centers for Disease Control and Prevention show that 47% of high-school-aged teenagers have experienced sexual intercourse. Although they may be embarrassed by the topic, the majority of adolescents would like their health care provider to ask them directly about sexual knowledge and experience. Data from the National Longitudinal Study of Adolescent Health revealed that 88% of teens who had made consistent virginity pledges (i.e., promising to remain abstinent until marriage) and 99% of teens who had not done so had experienced sexual intercourse before marriage. Even among teens who do not report rape or sexual assault, there is always a possibility that this has occurred, and family doctors should be alert to this risk. According to 2003 data, only 63% of teens reported condom use with last intercourse, and so this educational message should be reinforced with adolescent patients.

Page: 1347

Question #12

Answer: E

Rationale: Unfortunately, nonheterosexual youth are at higher risk for experiencing earlier age of substance abuse, dropping out of high school, becoming homeless, and being subjected to harassment and violence as compared with their heterosexual peers. Censure, alienation, and abandonment by the family of origin are devastating and not uncommon consequences for gay and lesbian teens.

Page: 1348

Question #13

Answer: A

Rationale: To many older adults, maintaining sexual intimacy is important. It is often assumed that, as people age, they will inevitably lose all interest in sex. Certain factors can influence participation in sexual relationships, such as sequelae from medical illnesses, side effects of medications, and some physiologic changes. Lack of an available partner is a common issue as a result of the greater longevity of women in the United States.

Page: 1349

Question #14

Answer: C

Rationale: From midlife to old age, testosterone levels decrease, reaching 50% of young adult levels. Because of the potential risks of hepatotoxicity and lipid abnormalities, only patients with a documented low serum testosterone level should be considered as candidates for testosterone replacement therapy. Periodic laboratory tests, including hemoglobin, liver function, lipid, and prostate-specific antigen testing, should be performed for a patient who is receiving testosterone replacement therapy, and these patients should be monitored for potential adverse side effects. Oral testosterone products often do not provide adequate replacement without hepatotoxicity. Therefore, transdermal replacement is the preferred method, which misses the first-pass effect on the liver.

Page: 1350

Question #15

Answer: A

Rationale: Homosexual and bisexual sexual orientations have existed from ancient times, so they are certainly not a modern phenomenon. The American Psychiatric Association declassified homosexuality as a mental disorder in 1974. The cause is most likely a combination of genetic and social factors, and it does not represent developmental impairment. Same-sex sexual behavior has been documented in many species of mammals and nonhuman primates, so it is not exclusive to humans.

Page: 1351

Question #16

Answer: B

Rationale: When taking a sexual or social history, the words a physician chooses can either facilitate or limit communication. By asking the patient what kind of birth control he or she uses, the physician makes the assumption that the patient is in an exclusively heterosexual relationship. This can be a message to homosexual or bisexual patients that the doctor is not open or comfortable discussing issues regarding same-sex relationships. The remainder of the questions listed are gender neutral, and they will encourage open communication.

Page: 1351

Question #17

Answer: D

Rationale: In the past, sexual reorientation therapy was advocated to attempt to change a person's sexual orientation from homosexual to heterosexual. Not only did this not work, it was associated with significant negative mental health consequences, including increased feelings of guilt and shame. Therefore, psychotherapy to change sexual orientation is no longer recommended. In addition to other minority populations, GLB persons are a target group for hate crimes and violence. Most persons in same-sex couples are not eligible for spousal health insurance benefits, and this often leaves a partner who is not working or who is not employed full time without insurance coverage. In 2005, the American Psychiatric Association endorsed legal recognition for same-sex unions and marriages, citing the mental health benefits of stable marital and family relationships.

Page: 1351

Question #18

Answer: A

Rationale: Although there have been case reports of female–female transmission of human immunodeficiency virus, it is less efficient than female–male transmission. That being said, all sexually active patients should be counseled about risk-reduction practices. Lesbians have the same breast and cervical cancer screening needs as heterosexual women. Unfortunately, lesbians may have a lower incidence of screening, because these tests are often performed at contraception, prenatal, or postpartum visits. Gay men are actually more likely to exercise regularly and less likely to be obese than heterosexual men. When a male patient presents with urethritis, it is appropriate to ask specifically about participation in oral–genital sex or receptive anal intercourse, because some treatment regimens for urethral gonorrhea and chlamydia are not effective against pharyngeal and anal infections. GLB patients do report experiences of provider prejudice, and this may hinder them from seeking necessary health care.

Page: 1351

Question #19

Answer: D

Rationale: Sex is not the same as gender. Sex is assigned by the appearance of genital anatomy, whereas gender is someone's psychological self-perception of maleness or femaleness. Although gender and sex are generally concordant, in a small percentage of persons, gender and sex are discordant. There is a continuum of gender variance. Cross-dressers are persons who sometimes dress as the other sex to be perceived as such or for sexual pleasure, whereas transsexuals are those who actually desire to live full-time as the opposite sex (i.e., as the sex that is concordant with their gender), often using hormone therapy and having sex-reassignment surgery. Although Western culture has accepted the gender binary of male or female only, many non-Western cultures recognize the existence of more than two genders.

Page: 1352

Question #20

Answer: D

Rationale: The Harry Benjamin International Gender Dysphoria Association is an organization of health professionals that care for transsexuals and that publish the standards of care for these patients. The standards of care are guidelines for professionals to determine appropriate candidates for hormone therapy and sex-reassignment surgery. The other organizations listed are very helpful for providing useful information for caring for transgendered persons, but they do not issue the standards of care.

Page: 1352

Question #21

Answer: A

Rationale: Sexual education is sometimes the only intervention a patient needs to help overcome sexual problems. This is especially true at times of physiologic change, such as puberty, menopause, pregnancy, the elder years, preoperatively and postoperatively, and in the context of a progressive medical illness.

Page: 1337

Question #22

Answer: E

Rationale: Past history of urinary tract infections does not influence male orgasmic function. Alcohol use may lower inhibitions and increase sexual interest, and it later may cause difficulty with sustained arousal or orgasm. SSRIs are well-known medications that inhibit orgasm. Diabetes and any other systemic illness that affects the nervous system or the vascular system can contribute to male orgasmic disorder. Relationship issues are also a common contributing factor.

Page: 1343

Question #23

Answer: E

Rationale: For the treatment of vulvar vestibulitis, the use of topical creams, topical or oral antibiotics, laser treatments, and vestibulectomy is controversial. The cause of vulvar vestibulitis is currently unknown. The first three answer options given are the diagnostic criteria for vulvar vestibulitis. It is important to distinguish this condition from vaginismus, because the approaches to management are quite different.

Page: 1345

Question #24

Answer: C

Rationale: The Kinsey Scale is a seven-value scale that ranges from 0 to 6 that classifies sexual orientation on a continuum. Although exclusive homosexuality and exclusive heterosexuality are at either end of the scale, there are varying degrees of behavior in between. These range from incidental homosexual or heterosexual experience to more-than-incidental experience or equivalent homosexuality and heterosexuality.

Page: 1348

Question #25

Answer: B

Rationale: Peak testicular elevation—not descent—is associated with male orgasm. Testicular descent does not occur until the resolution phase of the male sexual response. The other statements given are all part of the normal physiology of the male orgasm.

Page: 1336

Question #26

Answer: D

Rationale: The coadministration of nitrates or α-adrenergic blockers with PDE5 inhibitors can lead to profound hypotension; therefore, this combination should be avoided. The length of effect of the medications varies with the brand, with sildenafil and vardenafil lasting 3 to 5 hours and tadalafil lasting 24 to 36 hours. These medications are metabolized by the liver; therefore, potent cytochrome P450 3A4 inhibitors can really increase serum levels. Dose-reduction recommendations vary by agent, but they may be recommended on the basis of age or of hepatic or renal function.

Page: 1341

Question #27

Answer: A

Rationale: Siberian ginseng is used in traditional Chinese medicine as an aphrodisiac, but it has not been evaluated scientifically for use for the treatment of ED.

All of the other therapies listed are available treatments for ED.

Page: 1341

Question #28

Answer: A

Rationale: Transsexual people do require lifelong hormone therapy, although later in life a lower dose may decrease the risk of complications from hormones. The general rule is that any intact organ should have appropriate screening. Therefore, a female-to-male patient with an intact cervix and a male-to-female patient with an intact prostate both need appropriate cancer screening. Among female-to-male patients who have undergone chest reconstruction, all of the glandular tissue may not be removed; therefore, at a minimum, self breast examinations should be continued. If a legal name change is pending, the patient should be asked how he or she wants to be addressed; cross-reference filing of the chart under both names may be required.

Page: 1352

56 Answers

Question #1

Answer: B

Rationale: Genetics is the study of single genes and what they do. An example is the substitution of valine at the sixth position of the hemoglobin β chain, which causes sickling of the red blood cell wall; two copies of this defect result in disease. Genomics looks at the functions and interactions of all genes in the genome. This includes multiple factors that affect gene expression as well as the social and ethical implications of the genetic information available.

Page: 1357

Question #2

Answer: B

Rationale: The Human Genome Project began in 1990, and the genome has mapped the 30,000 genes that humans have. Previously, it was thought that humans had 100,000 genes, but it was found that one gene can produce multiple proteins.

Page: 1358

Question #3

Answer: B

Rationale: The new genomic information has many benefits. Understanding diseases and developing prevention and treatment are advantages. Although it may demonstrate that one is at risk for a disease, it does not give information about when a disease will develop or its subsequent severity.

Page: 1358

Question #4

Answer: A

Rationale: Family physicians more often see diseases like diabetes, which are multifactorial and which do not lend themselves to specific genetic testing and prognosis. Geneticists tend to see single-gene disorders that are rarely seen in the family physician's office.

Page: 1358

Question #5

Answer: D

Rationale: Of the conditions listed, heterozygote Factor V Leiden is the most common, with an estimated prevalence of 1 in 20 to 1 in 100. Klinefelter's syndrome in males has an estimated prevalence of 1 in 500, whereas cystic fibrosis affects 1 in 2500 to 1 in 3300. Huntington's disease is the least prevalent at 1 in 14,000 to 1 in 33,000.

Page: 1358

Question #6

Answer: B

Rationale: Family physicians tend to use a shared decision-making model with patients. Multiple visits may be used, and advice is formulated within the context of an ongoing relationship. Geneticists adhere to nondirective counseling whereby they provide information and do not offer guidance; this practice is rooted in reaction to the eugenics movement of the 20th century.

Page: 1358

Question #7

Answer: C

Rationale: Because a physician's time and resources are limited, a national collaboration of primary care and genetics professionals developed mnemonics to help clinicians think genetically. *FamilyGENES* highlights red flags to alert the physician, and it includes multiple affected family members, groups of anomalies, disease presentation, and surprise laboratory values. The mnemonic *SCREEN* identifies a set of family history questions, and it includes patients' concerns, reproductive information, early disease, death, disability, and ethnicity.

Page: 1358

Question #8

Answer: A

Rationale: The study of genomics has demonstrated that many chronic conditions involve multiple genes as well as other factors. These may include viruses, environmental toxins, nutrition, hormones, and DNA damage repair. Diabetes, coronary artery disease, depression, hyperlipidemia, and asthma are all multifactorial.

Page: 1359

Question #9

Answer: A

Rationale: Venous thromboembolism involves multiple genes and is multifactorial. The genes involved include Factor V Leiden, protein C, protein S, prothrombin G20210A, and anticoagulant deficiency. Breast cancer involves BRCA1 and BRCA2, whereas cystic fibrosis involves CFTR and early onset Alzheimer's disease involves APP, PSEN1, and PSEN2.

Page: 1360

Question #10

Answer: D

Rationale: Only early onset Alzheimer's disease is autosomal dominant. The high-risk population is individuals with multiple family members with Alzheimer's disease who were diagnosed when they were younger than 65 years old. Patients will present with dementia, and there are no recommendations for early screening.

Page: 1360

Question #11

Answer: C

Rationale: Ashkenazi Jews and whites of northern European ancestry are at increased risk for cystic fibrosis, with the carrier rate of 1 in 25 among whites. Tay-Sachs disease has long been known to affect Ashkenazi Jews, and it has a carrier rate in high-risk groups of 1 in 30. The Amish, Cajun, and French-Canadian populations are also at higher risk. The incidence of Alzheimer's disease has not been found to be increased in any particular ethnic group.

Page: 1360

Question #12

Answer: A

Rationale: Only in diabetes is there some information about the gene involved and the gene frequency. For type 1 diabetes, there are human-leukocyte-antigen–associated genes, and 8% of patients with high-risk genotypes develop disease. For patients with non–insulin-dependent diabetes, linkage studies have demonstrated that there are three loci that confer susceptibility to disease.

Page: 1362

Question #13

Answer: A

Rationale: Cystic fibrosis, which is an autosomal-recessive disease, has a carrier rate among whites of 1 in 25. Prenatal testing and newborn screening are currently available. As a result of newborn screening, it is known that many patients have only mild disease.

Page: 1360

Question #14

Answer: B

Rationale: Adult hemochromatosis is an autosomal-recessive disease that involves the HFE gene. It affects 3 to 5 of every 1000 people, with the high-risk population being whites of northern European ancestry. Patients will have high serum ferritin levels and high iron saturation. They can present with cardiomyopathy, arthropathy, cirrhosis, diabetes, and skin pigmentation. Patients with sickle cell disease present with anemia, abdominal pain, stroke, infections, and aplastic crises. Patients with β-thalassemia present with anemia and hepatomegaly. Patients with Down syndrome have characteristic facies as well as cardiac disease.

Page: 1360

Question #15

Answer: B

Rationale: Although there are familial predispositions to many multifactorial diseases, there are many cases in which no specific genes have been identified; therefore, no genetic testing is available, and so a risk-assessment approach is used. An example is the Framingham risk score, which identifies patients who are at high risk for coronary artery disease. Even after adjusting for known risk factors, family history remains an independent predictor of coronary artery disease.

Page: 1359

Question #16

Answer: C

Rationale: The high-risk populations for breast cancer include women of Ashkenazi Jewish descent and women with a family or personal history of breast or ovarian cancer. A family history in a first-degree relative doubles the personal risk. These women may benefit from early detection, and families may benefit from BRCA testing. Although family history increases risk, an autosomal-dominant pattern of inheritance is found in only 5% to 10% of women with breast cancer.

Page: 1359

Question #17

Answer: C

Rationale: Although genetic testing for mutations in the BRCA1 and BRCA2 genes may be helpful for some individuals who are at risk for breast cancer, the decision to test is complex, and it requires counseling before the test is performed. Counseling may be done be a geneticist or a family physician with genetics training. It is possible that, in the future, this counseling will be part of primary care practice.

Page: 1359

Question #18

Answer: A

Rationale: A woman with a BRCA mutation can approach an 80% lifetime risk of breast cancer and a 50% risk of ovarian cancer. Even with these increased odds, there is little evidence that aggressive strategies at early detection have significant benefit. Chemoprevention, surgery, and early detection modalities are available to these high-risk women. Further research is needed to determine which strategies are the best.

Page: 1359

Question #19

Answer: D

Rationale: Current recommendations for colorectal cancer screening include early screening at the age of 40 years or 10 years before the age of onset of a family member. If there are multiple family members with colorectal cancer—especially in more than one generation or with an onset before the age of 50 years—then a pattern of autosomal dominant inheritance is suggested. Most of these families will have hereditary nonpolyposis colon cancer mutations, which confer an 80% lifetime risk of cancer. Individuals with familial adenomatous polyposis have a 100% lifetime risk.

Page: 1363

Question #20

Answer: B

Rationale: Although a clear advantage to early screening is the prevention of colorectal cancer, the early removal of adenomatous polyps has made determining family history risk more difficult. With genetic testing availability, the detection of a specific mutation can be very helpful for guiding patients with regard to screening. If a specific mutation is found in the family and the patient does not have that mutation, he or she does not have to continue with early screening. If a mutation is not found in the family, then all members should continue earlier screening and more frequent evaluation than the general population.

Page: 1363

Question #21

Answer: D

Rationale: For both early onset and normal late-onset Alzheimer's disease, the medical presentation and the clinical criteria develop as dementia. The high-risk population includes those with multiple family members, especially those with onset before the age of 65 years for the early onset type. Research has identified the genes involved as APP, PSEN1, and PSEN2 for the early onset type and a mild correlation with APOE for normal late-onset Alzheimer's disease. The pattern of genetic transmission is autosomal dominant.

Page: 1363

Question #22

Answer: B

Rationale: There is little evidence that the treatment of Alzheimer's disease is very effective or that genetic testing has a high predictive value. Therefore, there is no recommendation for screening for the disease. About 25% of normal late-onset Alzheimer's disease is familial.

Page: 1363

Question #23

Answer: C

Rationale: Iron overload may lead to hemochromatosis, but it is not synonymous with the condition. Hemochromatosis is the excessive accumulation of iron in target organs that leads to organ damage and clinical disease. Iron overload is diagnosed by the laboratory evaluation of serum iron studies. To prevent progression to hemochromatosis, an individual with iron overload should have phlebotomy at regular intervals. Iron overload is autosomal recessive, and it is present in populations with and without HFE mutations.

Page: 1363

Question #24

Answer: C

Rationale: The Centers for Disease Control and Prevention recommends against routine screening for hemochromatosis for a variety of reasons. One reason is that iron overload does not necessarily lead to hemochromatosis. Hemochromatosis is associated with mutations in the HFE gene, although having the mutation does not guarantee the onset of disease. Testing positive could lead to the false labeling of a patient who will not develop a disease.

Page: 1363

Question #25

Answer: A

Rationale: Serum iron testing (specifically serum ferritin and iron saturation) is a relatively low-cost and low-risk way to screen family members who are at risk for hemochromatosis. The prevalence of iron overload increases with age, so periodic serum iron testing is warranted to detect disease early. Testing for HFE mutation is not recommended, because even the presence of two HFE mutations does not confer disease; this is probably the result of low genetic penetrance.

Page: 1363

Question #26

Answer: D

Rationale: For a broad array of psychiatric disorders such as substance abuse, depression, schizophrenia, and autism, a positive family history increases the personal risk of disease. If multiple family members are affected, the risk is increased beyond that predicted from twin studies. Studies with identical twins have found that both twins are not always affected and that, in some cases, the unaffected twin's child has the same risk as the affected twin's child; this has led to the thought that there may be incomplete genetic penetrance.

Page: 1364

Question #27

Answer: B

Rationale: One standard for the diagnosis of cystic fibrosis is the presence of CTFR mutations. To get cystic fibrosis, a person must receive two copies of a mutated CTFR gene. There are more than 1000 mutations of this gene, and, yet, some individuals with cystic fibrosis have no recognized mutation. Therefore, it is important to test the family member first, because the current prenatal testing panels do not cover all ethnic groups; they only address the mutations that are commonly found among northern Europeans.

Page: 1364

Question #28

Answer: D

Rationale: Newborn screening has identified patients with cystic fibrosis with only mild disease, and it has since been shown that different mutations cause different disease severity. This leads to some dilemmas with regard to newborn screening, because it is not known whether diagnosing disease before the onset of symptoms will improve outcomes. In addition, the consequences of informing parents that a child has a disease—which may be mild or severe—before any clinical signs appear are unknown.

Page: 1364

Question #29

Answer: C

Rationale: When it was discovered in 1956 that sickle cell disease resulted from a mutation in one codon, sickle cell disease became the first genetic disorder with a known molecular basis. It is believed that sickle cell disease is common because carriers (heterozygotes) have a natural resistance to malaria. All women of African descent should have access to testing before or during pregnancy. Other hemoglobinopathies include α- and β-thalassemia. In Southeast Asia and Africa, the highest prevalence of α-thalassemia is found, with about 30% of the population affected. α-Thalassemia results from the underproduction of α-globin chains. There are four possible genotypes, because each person carries four genes for α-globin (two from each parent's chromosomes).

Page: 1364

Question #30

Answer: A

Rationale: There are several causes of microcytosis on a blood count; however, iron-deficiency anemia and hemoglobinopathies account for the majority of cases. α-Thalassemia and β-thalassemia can cause microcytosis. Asymptomatic individuals with mutations in two α-globin genes have the α-thalassemia trait. β-Thalassemia is an autosomal-recessive disease; only patients with the β minor are asymptomatic. Patients with β thalassemia major usually present during the first 2 years of life with severe anemia and hepatosplenomegaly.

Page: 1365

Question #31

Answer: B

Rationale: There are five gene variants that increase the risk of venous thromboembolism: Factor V Leiden, prothrombin G200210A, protein C deficiency, protein S deficiency, and deficiency of antithrombin. Factor V Leiden is the most common, and 5% of people of European descent are heterozygotes with this condition. Factor VIII deficiency results in bleeding.

Page: 1365

Question #32

Answer: C

Rationale: Genetic testing has important ramifications for patients and their families. Results can lead to depression, negative lifestyle behavior changes, and altered relationships with family members, including survivor's guilt for someone who tests negative. It is often important to test the affected family member first to ensure proper testing for specific mutations. Otherwise, a negative test may not be meaningful.

Page: 1365

Question #33

Answer: B

Rationale: Counseling before testing is very important when a family physician orders a genetic test. The test may reveal a mutation that can cause disease; however, this finding will not definitively predict that the disease will occur, its time of onset, or its severity. Most diseases have multiple factors that involve risk, including genetic and environmental factors, and very few diseases have 100% penetrance. For common diseases, the absence of a mutation does not change the baseline population risk of the disease.

Page: 1365

Question #34

Answer: D

Rationale: Hemoglobin electrophoresis can detect hemoglobinopathies, whereas testing for cystic fibrosis can identify some mutations in certain ethnic groups. Both of these tests can identify asymptomatic carriers. The quadruple serum test compares assays of the levels of four biochemical markers to standards at the gestational age to identify patients who are at risk for Down syndrome and neural tube defects. Chorionic villous sampling is an invasive test that is performed late during the first trimester. It is more accurate; however, there are higher incidences of associated spontaneous abortions and minor anomalies, so it is not routinely performed.

Page: 1366

Question #35

Answer: D

Rationale: Pharmacogenetics considers the genetically determined variations in response to medicines. The cytochrome P450 system is at the forefront of current applications of pharmacogenetics. Of the 14 types of cytochrome P450 identified, only CYP1, CYP2, and CYP3 seem to be instrumental in drug metabolism. Both terfenadine and ketoconazole interact with macrolide antibiotics. These drugs inhibit the cytochrome P450 3A4 pathway and prolong the QT interval, leading to the fatal torsades des pointes.

Page: 1367

Question #1

Answer: D

Rationale: Anxiety and depressive disorders are the two most common mental health problems encountered in everyday medical practice. In the Epidemiologic Catchment Area Study,[1] anxiety disorders occurred in 15.4% of the community, second only to substance abuse, which occurred in 16.7% of the population. According to a more recent National Comorbidity Study,[2] the lifetime prevalence of anxiety disorders was 24.9%, second only to substance abuse, which occurred in 26.6% of the population.[3]

Page: 1371

Question #2

Answer: B

Rationale: Anxiety is a subjective feeling of heightened tension and diffuse uneasiness that is conceptualized as internally derived and unrelated to an external threat. It is not merely fear, because it lacks a specific object.

Page: 1371

Question #3

Answer: B

Rationale: Anxiety disorders occur among those patients with strong support systems and much psychological strength as well as those who lack social support and who have many maladaptive personality traits.

Page: 1371

Question #4

Answer: D

Rationale: Panic attacks are of sudden onset, and they become "full blown" immediately. The attack is associated with all of the other symptoms listed, and it can be associated with a fear of going crazy or losing control during an attack.

Page: 1372

Question #5

Answer: C

Rationale: To meet the DSM-IV criteria for a panic disorder, the attack must be followed by at least a 1-month persistent concern about having additional attacks, by worry about the implications of the attack, or by a significant change in behavior related to the attack. Panic disorder may be diagnosed after one attack occurs. However, other causes of the related symptoms need to be ruled out.

Page: 1372

Question #6

Answer: E

Rationale: The onset of panic disorder is generally between the ages of 17 and 30 years, with a mean of 22.5 years. The highest 6-month prevalence was in the 25- to 44-year-old age group,[4] whereas, in the National Comorbidity Study, the highest prevalence was in the 15- to 24-year-old age group.[2]

Page: 1372

Question #7

Answer: B

Rationale: Panic attacks often happen after one or a series of life events overwhelms the patient's coping mechanisms. Anticipatory anxiety often begins to occur after subsequent attacks; this is related to the anxiety between attacks that another attack will occur. This behavior leads to the second and third stages of panic—anticipatory anxiety and agoraphobia.

Page: 1372

1. Regier DA, Myers JK, Kramer M, et al: The NIMH Epidemiologic Catchment Area program. Historical context, major objectives, and study population characteristics. *Arch Gen Psychiatry* 41:934-941, 1984.
2. Magee WJ, Eaton WW, Wittchen HU, et al. Agoraphobia, simple phobia, and social phobia in the National Comorbidity Study. *Arch Gen Psychiatry* 53:159-168, 1996.
3. Kessler RC, McGonagle KA, Zhao S, et al. Lifetime and 12-month prevalence 1982. of DSM-III-R psychiatric disorders in the United States. Results from the Roy-Byrne PP: Integrated treatment of panic disorder. *Am J Med* 92(1A):5, 1994.
4. Myers JK, Weissman MM, Tischler GL, et al. Six-month prevalence of psychiatric disorders in three communities, 1980–1982. *Arch Gen Psychiatry* 41:959-967, 1984.

Question #8

Answer: E

Rationale: Patients with panic disorder often develop stage III panic-agoraphobia with which they are unable to leave the house except in the presence of a protector or a significant other. They often cling regressively to their caretaker and require his or her presence at all times. They may actually become more attached to family members and need their support to leave the house.

Page: 1372

Question #9

Answer: A

Rationale: Patients with chest pain with negative cardiac workup suffered panic disorder nearly 50% of the time; this was documented in three separate studies.[5-7] Two studies have documented that one quarter to one third of primary care patients with palpitations meet the criteria for panic disorder. Labile hypertension develops in some patients with panic disorder during an attack; this may lead to a negative workup for other causes, such as pheochromocytoma.

Page: 1373

Question #10

Answer: A

Rationale: Nearly all patients with agoraphobia have panic attacks.

Page: 1374

Question #11

Answer: C

Rationale: Most if not all specific phobias and nearly all social phobias develop after some situation in which the patient had an unpleasant or dangerous experience, such as a dog bite or a social situation in which he or she was intensely scrutinized and/or criticized. Those with social phobias avoid situations in which unfamiliar people or situations are present, because they fear that they may act in a manner that might be humiliating or embarrassing.

Page: 1374

Question #12

Answer: B

Rationale: Persons with average-severity social phobia have 10% lower levels of earned wages and graduation from college and a 10% lower probability of holding a technical professional or managerial job than those without social phobia.

Page: 1374

Question #13

Answer: B

Rationale: All of the listed symptoms except delusional thinking can occur in patients with GAD, along with other symptoms, such as becoming easily fatigued, restlessness, or feeling "keyed up" or on edge.

Page: 1374

Question #14

Answer: B

Rationale: A very small subset of patients has primary GAD. GAD is nearly always the result of another major DSM-IV disorder such as panic disorder, major depression, alcohol abuse, or an axis II personality disorder. These disorders and organic disorders must be screened for and ruled out before a patient is treated for primary GAD.

Page: 1375

Question #15

Answer: E

Rationale: Patients with PTSD tend to have an exaggerated awareness state signified by all of the listed symptoms, along with an increased startle response.

Page: 1375

5. Bass C, Wade C. Chest pain with normal coronary arteries: A comparative study of psychiatric and social morbidity. *Psychol Med* 14:51-61, 1984.
6. Beitman BD, Basha I, Flaker G, et al. A typical or nonanginal chest pain. Panic disorder or coronary artery disease? *Arch Intern Med* 147:1548-1552, 1987.
7. Katon W, Hall ML, Russo J, et al. Chest Pain: Relationship of psyciatric illness to coronary arteriographic results. *Am J Med* 84:1-9, 1988.

Question #16

Answer: C

Rationale: Patients with PTSD often cannot recall the important aspects of the prior trauma. They may avoid thoughts, feelings, or conversations associated with the trauma, and they may have a sense of a foreshortened future. Diagnosis requires three of the listed characteristics.

Page: 1375

Question #17

Answer: D

Rationale: Approximately 60% of patients with major depression also have an anxiety disorder, and 20% of patients with major depression have panic disorder. Patients with panic disorder have a 50% to 90% chance of having major depression during their lifetimes.

Page: 1376

Question #18

Answer: D

Rationale: Patients with anxiety often have sweaty, moist palms. Other increased motor activity is also present, such as rapid, shallow respirations; multiple, frequent movements; and muscle or facial tics. Dilated pupils may be an autonomic sign of anxiety.

Page: 1377

Question #19

Answer: E

Rationale: Patients with heart disease may have angina, tachycardia, and dyspnea similar to an anxiety attack. Other organic causes include all of the listed diseases in addition to hypoglycemia and other forms of central nervous system disease.

Page: 1376

Question #20

Answer: B

Rationale: The likelihood that a patient will present the problem of anxiety to his or her primary care practitioner is great, because anxious patients usually perceive the problem to be primarily medical rather than psychological. The family physician often sees emotional problems in their early stages, before fixed patterns of illness have been set; this is why it is important to diagnose anxiety early and to treat it before it develops into a long-term problem.

Page: 1378

Question #21

Answer: E

Rationale: The physician should do an adequate workup to confidently assure the patient of an absence of organic disease. If reassurance is given too early during the workup, the patient will discount the physician's diagnosis of anxiety as the cause of his or her condition. Physicians should always take into account their own feelings about this type of patient. Patience and a nonjudgmental attitude are required on the physician's part, along with the capacity to identify and encourage the particular interests and goals that are important to the individual patient. After the diagnosis of anxiety has been made and explained to the patient, it is counterproductive to continue ordering laboratory and diagnostic tests. This creates doubt in the patient's mind about the diagnosis of anxiety.

Page: 1378

Question #22

Answer: B

Rationale: It is important that the physician not tell the patient that nothing is wrong with him or her or that the condition is all in his or her head. The physician should seek explanatory statements about what the patient thinks is going on. The physician should explain how the autonomic nervous system is often responsible for the physical manifestations of anxiety, such as the spasm of smooth muscle in irritable bowel syndrome.

Page: 1378

Question #23

Answer: D

Rationale: Cognitive-behavioral therapy has been shown to be very beneficial in panic disorder. Medication should be used to totally block panic attacks as soon as possible. After the panic attacks have been totally stopped, the patient should be encouraged to resume the activities that may have initiated the panic attack. For cases in which the patient encounters activities that precipitated the attack, relaxation techniques may be helpful for preventing future attacks.

Page: 1379

Question #24

Answer: E

Rationale: All of the listed medications are useful for panic disorder, along with the serotonin norepinephrine uptake inhibitors. The first line of treatment in primary care should be SSRIs. In addition, up to 50% of patients with panic disorder have major depression, and the SSRIs are effective for the treatment of both panic disorder and depression. However, in controlled trials, cognitive-behavioral therapy has been equally as effective for the treatment of mild to moderate panic disorder.

Page: 1379

Question #25

Answer: D

Rationale: With SSRIs, treatment should start at a very low dose. Doubling of the initial dose should occur every 5 days as tolerated. The goal of treating panic attacks is to totally alleviate the attacks with the medication. Explain to patients that they will have jitteriness, nausea, and headache but that these symptoms will usually resolve within 1 to 2 weeks of starting treatment. Anorgasmia occurs in 20% to 35% of patients who are taking SSRIs. If this occurs, the dosage may have to be decreased or the medication changed.

Page: 1380

Question #26

Answer: B

Rationale: Patients do better with counseling if they know how counseling works and if they have had a

previous successful counseling experience. Awareness that their problem is psychological in nature and the presence of "signal anxiety" personality traits such as perseverance, dependability, non-impulsiveness, and trusting are all signs that counseling will work for these patients.

Page: 1381

Question #27

Answer: E

Rationale: Benzodiazepines have a lower potential for dependence and abuse among patients with anxiety disorder, except in those with a history of anxiety and substance abuse disorders. Their lethality rate, even in cases of overdose, is much lower than many other drugs that are used for anxiety. There are lower rates of side effects and allergic reactions among people taking benzodiazepines. These drugs do not tend to activate liver microsomal enzymes, and, therefore, they do not change the metabolism of other drugs as often. However, many patients with anxiety have difficulty stopping these medications. They often have rebound anxiety and withdrawal. Therefore, when attempting to stop these medications, it may be beneficial to withdraw the drug slowly; to offer frequent, short, regular office visits until symptoms subside; or to convert therapy from benzodiazepines with a short half-life to those with a longer half-life.

Page: 1382

Question #28

Answer: A

Rationale: In vivo exposure to a phobic stimulus, either by gradual exposure or by "flooding," has been found to be more effective for total efficacy and rapidity of cure than desensitization by imagery.

Page: 1382

Question #29

Answer: E

Rationale: Mellman and Davis[8] demonstrated all of the listed characteristics in patients with PTSD.

---

8. Mellman TA, Davis GC. Combat-related flashbacks in posttraumatic stress disorder: Phenomenology and similarity to panic attacks. *J Clin Psychiatry* 46:379-382, 1985.

Medications dampening the sympathetic nervous system have been found to be effective for patients with PTSD. These include monoamine oxidase inhibitors, clonidine, and high-dose propranolol. SSRIs have been shc•vn to be effective for civilian populations but not for veterans.

Page: 1383

Question #30

Answer: C

Rationale: SSRIs have been found to be effective for civilian populations with PTSD. However, they were not efficacious for veteran populations. Prazosin has been shown to be effective for nightmares. Clonidine diminishes the release of norepinephrine.

Page: 1383

58 Answers

Question #1

Answer: B

Rationale: There are more than 100 million prescriptions written each year for antidepressants, and only a minority are written by psychiatric specialists. Clinical depression falls well within the scope of primary care practice, which is a major, critical component of the nation's mental and behavioral health delivery system. Psychiatry's contribution to managing this condition in ambulatory settings occurs more often for resistant, hard-to-treat forms of depressive disorders. The economic and emotional costs of untreated or undertreated depressive disorders are hard to overestimate.

Page: 1387

Question #2

Answer: A

Rationale: Although there is some variation internationally, the prevalence of depression in the United States among the general population is 2% to 4%. The prevalence increases to 6% to 10% among ambulatory medical patients, and it increases even more among hospitalized medical patients to as high as 14%. Regardless of setting, however, at least half of patients suffering from depression remain untreated. Family physicians are obligated to be on the lookout for signs and symptoms, given the sheer numbers of medical patients they encounter who suffer from depression.

Page: 1387

Question #3

Answer: E

Rationale: The interconnections between emotionality, humor, outlook, and the outcome of many medical illnesses are complex, and the mechanisms are not well understood. What is clear, however, is that depression worsens the morbidity and mortality of several major diagnoses, including cardiovascular disease, diabetes, several types of cancer, soft-tissue disease, reactive headache, and asthma. It has not been shown to contribute to the severity of osteoporosis or inflammatory joint disease.

Pages: 1387–1388

Question #4

Answer: A

Rationale: The lifetime prevalence for depression is about 17%, with 8 million cases diagnosed annually; however, this makes up only about half of the number that is theorized to exist. In fact, depression rates are increasing as the age of onset is decreasing. Formal psychiatric training in residencies often takes place in inpatient psychiatric units or in the presence of psychiatric-liaison services, with little real-world crossover for the ambulatory care family medicine office. Patients often do not recognize or admit their own emotional state, and they prefer a strictly physical cause for their presenting problem. Depression is often equated with feeling sorry for oneself or not being tough enough to face life. Trained to diagnose physical ailments, family physicians as well as other primary care providers may not routinely consider psychological causes or contributions, especially during the early phases of evaluating a problem.

Page: 1387

Question #5

Answer: C

Rationale: Risk factors for depression include age; population studies demonstrate a trend for younger patients to develop depression and a risk trend that also increases with age. Peak incidence is seen between young and early middle adulthood (20–40 years of age), with proportionally more geriatric patients suffering from depression than any other cohort. Women are twice as likely as men to develop depression, and 1 in 10 pregnant women develops postpartum depression. Although family history is a more robust predictor for bipolar disorder, the relative risk is still two to five times greater if a first-degree relative has ever had a major depressive episode, with a doubling of risk if both parents were ever affected. Nutritional status is often a symptom of depression, with depressed patients often either under- or overeating. Nutritional intake is itself not considered causal.

Page: 1387

Question #6

Answer: B

Rationale: Although depression is often missed in women, they are the easiest cohort in which depression is identified. Depression is more prevalent among women, and women are more likely to be forthcoming about complaints that involve their affective states. In addition, such reporting is more socially acceptable. Depressed men often feel stigmatized and like they are not being manly enough, and they are much more likely to self-medicate symptoms with alcohol or drugs. Children and adolescents are as likely to present with irritability, anger, and oppositional attitude as sadness and depressed mood.

Page: 1387

Question #7

Answer: D

Rationale: After patients have had a major depressive episode, they are at increased risk to develop a recurrence. This is even more true of women who have experience postpartum depression, because biological and hormonal factors play a more significant role. About 1 in 10 pregnant women will suffer from depression within 3 to 4 weeks after giving birth, with symptoms ranging from mild to severe, as they do in major depressive disorder. Although antidepressant pharmacotherapy must be carefully considered, most antidepressants are considered to be safe during pregnancy.

Page: 1387

Question #8

Answer: A

Rationale: Although environment clearly contributes to both the development of major depressive disorder and how rapidly it can be successfully treated, the strongest evidence for depressive causes lies in genetics. Twin studies show that monozygotic twins have a 65% concordance, which is about four times greater than the dizygotic concordance. Adoption studies show that children raised in homes in which one family member suffers from depression are not significantly more likely to develop depression than the general population. Conversely, adopted children who have a known depressed first-degree relative remain at two to five times greater risk, even if no one else in the home has ever suffered from depression. Children who are biologically related and who are raised in homes with one depressed parent are also at two to five times greater risk. For a child who is biologically related to and raised by two depressed parents, there is a five- to ten-times greater relative risk.

Page: 1388

Question #9

Answer: E

Rationale: Although the most potent predictor of suicide risk is the presence of a prior attempt, many factors also influence this potential: serious, long-term chronic illness; high levels of physical pain; divorce; premature death of a parent; family dislocation; early trauma; and chemical abuse. Ironically, patients with severe major depression rarely attempt suicide, because they typically lack enough initiative and energy to carry it out. Patients who were severely depressed but who have improved to a point where they are moderately or mildly depressed are actually at much greater risk.

Page: 1388

Question #10

Answer: B

Rationale: Although suicidal ideation, especially among the medically chronically ill, is common, actual attempts are relatively rare. Nevertheless, suicide was the eleventh leading cause of death in the United States in 2001, and it is the third leading cause of death in the 15- to 24-year-old age group, after accidents and homicides. Although women attempt suicide more often than men, more men complete the attempts, because the lethality of their attempts is greater. Of those who attempt suicide for the first time and survive, 1 in 100 will kill himself or herself within the subsequent year, although the increased risk continues throughout their lifespan. Of those who completed suicide, between 1 in 2 and 1 in 4 had attempted it previously.

Page: 1388

Question #11

Answer: A

Rationale: Physician-assisted suicide is hotly disputed in many states, but it is only legal in Oregon when strict criteria are followed. Family physicians are ethically bound to explore and ascertain the reasons that patients request help with ending their lives.

Page: 1389

Question #12

Answer: C

Rationale: Observed—as opposed to subjectively experienced—psychomotor agitation or retardation is one of the nine primary symptoms in major depression; five of these symptoms must be present for the diagnosis. Specifically excluded from consideration are symptoms related to a physical illness like hypothyroidism, one's self-reproach or inappropriate guilt about having a medical illness, and the loss of a loved one. During the occurrence of a manic or hypomanic episode, the presumptive diagnosis of bipolar disorder I or II is made, even if there has never been a depressive episode.

Page: 1389

Question #13

Answer: E

Rationale: Depression screening can provide critical information about severity of symptoms and how they change in response to treatment or lack of treatment, but it does not diagnose depressive illness. Practice-based screening measures are administered during the general annual or biannual examination; case-finding measures are administered only when there is a suspicion of depressive illness. Depressed patients are more likely to present with physical symptoms such as insomnia, hypersomnia, loss of appetite, pain, and fatigue than to present with emotional difficulties. Each instrument is assessed for the psychometric properties of validity and reliability, and this necessitates instrument-specific statistical cutoffs. Although self-reporting instruments are quickly scored, they are not appropriate for use with everyone. Interviewer-administered instruments are required for those who are mentally challenged.

Page: 1389

Question #14

Answer: A

Rationale: There are several screening inventories that can be used with children and adolescents, including the Children's Depression Inventory, the Child Depression Scale, the Adolescent Depression Scale, and the Patient Health Questionnaire for Adolescents. Even armed with these instruments, diagnosing depression in youth can be formidable. Adults and children often report quite different signs, all of which can have multiple causes. Children and adolescents describe internalizing symptoms that are not necessarily specific to depression, such as "I don't like anyone in my class" or "I don't want to go out with my friends anymore; they've all become jerks." Parents, teachers, and coaches describe externalizing symptoms that can also have a variety of causes, such as "He's gotten lazy and isn't studying anymore" or "She's become so moody, I can't even talk to her without her losing her temper with me."

Page: 1390

Question #15

Answer: C

Rationale: The USPSTF concluded that brief interventions designed to fit into everyday family practice have been found to produce clinically meaningful changes, particularly when addressing risk behaviors. Although longer counseling sessions can be effective and are often used as part of the treatment of depression and other disorders, the USPSTF does not make any conclusion about these sessions. It does recommend the routine screening of depression in adults, and it acknowledges that family physicians and primary care providers play a significant role in the treatment of depression in the United States.

Page: 1390

Question #16

Answer: D

Rationale: BATHE is a rapid screening tool that allows for insight into psychosocial issues and that may also be used as a therapeutic intervention. It takes about 5 to 7 minutes to complete, and it is best used when there is little time for counseling but psychosocial issues are of concern. The acronym *BATHE* stands for the following:

*B*ackground: what is happening that is of concern to the patient;

*A*ffect: how the patient feels about what is happening;

*T*rouble: what troubles the patient about what is happening and how he or she feels;

*H*andling: how the patient is handling the situation; and

*E*mpathy: the physician provides a concluding empathetic remark about the situation to the patient.

Page: 1392

Question #17

Answer: A

Rationale: The SPEAK technique is used to motivate depressed patients, and it is more effective when it is used in conjunction with the BATHE technique. The BATHE technique can be thought of as the assessment part of the visit, because it helps define issues and sentiments, whereas the SPEAK technique is part of the plan, because it helps design a plan to activate the patient. The acronym *SPEAK* stands for the following:

Schedule: the patient prepares a written daily schedule of activities;

Pleasant: at least one of the daily activities should be pleasant to the patient;

Exercise: the patient commits to increasing the level of physical activity;

Assertion: the patient is encouraged to be more assertive and to take control of his or her own life; and

Kind: the patient should think kind thoughts about him- or herself.

Page: 1392

Question #18

Answer: D

Rationale: The DIG technique is used to help patients create solutions to their problems. It is not a screening or diagnostic tool but rather a therapeutic behavioral tool. *DIG* is an acronym for *D*ream, *I*nitiate, and *G*et going. The first step is to have patients dream of the miracle that would solve their problems. The next step is for patients to initiate a process that will make that miracle happen and to make changes in themselves that the miracle would cause. This is the first small step in making a change. The third step is getting going and implementing activities to have the process of change occur. The DIG technique takes about 15 minutes to complete during the typical office visit.

Pages: 1392–1393

Question #19

Answer: C

Rationale: Medications generally provide a rapid response to depression in the outpatient setting. However, this response does not reduce the risk of relapse after the medication is withdrawn. Depression generally responds more slowly to behavioral therapy, but longer-term studies have shown that behavioral therapy tends to be as effective as medication. Cognitive-behavioral therapy has been shown to reduce the subsequent risk for relapse of depression. Often a combination of medications and behavioral therapy is used, especially for patients with chronic depression, because combined treatment produces a higher improvement rate than drug therapy or behavioral therapy alone.

Page: 1394

Question #20

Answer: E

Rationale: Most patients with depression are treated by their primary care providers, and most never see a mental health care provider. In fact, the majority of antidepressant medications are prescribed by primary care providers. However, there are times when a consultation with a mental health care provider is warranted. These times include the referral of patients with comorbid psychiatric disease or personality disorder, when at least two trials of medications have failed, when the patient requests such a referral, and when the physician lacks expertise for or interest in treating the depression.

Page: 1387

Question #21

Answer: D

Rationale: Cognitive behavioral therapy is a well-documented and effective approach to the treatment of depression. It employs a short-term, goal-oriented approach. The thought is that dysfunctional thinking can be modified, and, therefore, the emotions produced by the dysfunctional thinking will be changed. If there is a stressor or an experience that caused a negative feeling, the approach to this stressor can be changed. Interpersonal psychotherapy is a separate approach to behavioral changes involving sessions that last about 20 minutes. It is effective for all phases of treatment.

Page: 1393

Question #22

Answer: C

Rationale: Antidepressant therapy is commonly prescribed by the primary care provider. Responses to therapy, although they are variable, usually are seen within 3 to 4 weeks; this is true for all classes of medications. Continued and improved responses can be seen with further continuation of the medication and dosage adjustments. Patients should be given a trial of therapy for 4 to 6 weeks before determining that there is treatment failure.

Page: 1393

Question #23

Answer: B

Rationale: SSRIs have a relatively safe side-effect profile, but there are some side effects or situations that may be of concern. Sexual dysfunction is one of the side effects of SSRIs. It can be treated with weekend holidays (for those medications with short half-lives), with the addition of bupropion, or with the reduction of the dose of the SSRI. Other common side effects of SSRIs include gastrointestinal disturbances, akathisia, and hyperhydrosis. Arrhythmias are of significant concern with TCAs, as are anticholinergic side effects such as urinary retention and dry mouth. Neuropathy is sometimes treated with TCAs. Interaction with foods that contain tyramine is of concern when prescribing monoamine oxidase inhibitors.

Page: 1395

Question #24

Answer: E

Rationale: About 80% to 90% of patients will ultimately have some response to medications for the treatment of depression. Approximately 60% to 70% will respond to the initial treatment choice, regardless of what drug it may be, and up to 90% will respond to a second medication trial. The choice of medication must be individualized; and side effects, pharmacokinetics, previous responses to a medication, and comorbid conditions must be considered. Often, starting with a low dose and increasing the medications gradually is prudent.

Page: 1394

Question #25

Answer: A

Rationale: TCAs tend to have significant and potentially lethal side effects. However, not all TCAs are created equally. TCAs are either secondary or tertiary amines, and the secondary amines are associated with less severe side effects. Examples of secondary amines are nortriptyline and desipramine. Examples of tertiary amines are imipramine and amitriptyline. Bupropion and fluoxetine are not TCAs. Significant side effects

associated with TCAs include arrhythmias, sedation, and anticholinergic side effects such as dry mouth and eyes and urinary retention.

Page: 1395

Question #26

Answer: B

Rationale: SSRI discontinuation syndrome is a common phenomenon that is caused by the rapid withdrawal of an SSRI. Patients present with flu-like syndromes 3 to 4 days after the abrupt cessation of the SSRI. Patients also experience nausea, dizziness, paresthesia, headache, and anxiety. It is more commonly seen after the withdrawal of SSRIs with short half-lives (e.g., fluoxetine), and it can be treated by reinstituting the medication. This syndrome can be prevented with a tapering of the SSRI over a couple of weeks when discontinuing the medication.

Page: 1395

Question #27

Answer: D

Rationale: Hypericum extract, which is also known as St. John's wort, is an herb that is frequently used for the treatment of depression. Some studies have demonstrated beneficial effects of St. John's wort, whereas others have not. Currently, it is felt that evidence regarding hypericum extract for the treatment of depression is inconsistent and confusing. Phytoestrogens have been used for the treatment of menopausal symptoms, and saw palmetto has been used for the treatment of prostate disease. Echinacea has been suggested to be beneficial for the common cold, and garlic has been tried for the treatment of hypertension. All of these extracts have not been sufficiently studied to make recommendations or to reach any conclusions about their effectiveness.

Page: 1395

Question #28

Answer: E

Rationale: Exercise has been shown to lower levels of depression. In fact, some studies have shown it to be as effective as individual or group psychotherapy or cognitive therapy. The benefits of exercise are also noted with other mental health disorders, including anxiety, panic disorder, and reducing disruptive behavior in disabled individuals. Exercise is also part of the treatment of other disorders, such as chronic fatigue syndrome and fibromyalgia. The exact mechanism by which exercise improves symptoms of depression is not clearly understood.

Page: 1395

Question #29

Answer: B

Rationale: ECT is an effective treatment for depression, especially if medications do not provide a sufficient and satisfactory response. For this type of treatment, seizures are induced three times per week over a 6- to 12-week period in a controlled setting with anesthesia. Subsequently, patients receive outpatient ECT and antidepressant medications. ECT is actually quite humane, despite its stigma in society. It has a response rate of nearly 87%. Patients will usually try two medications before medication is considered as having failed. Therefore, those patients with contraindications to SSRIs may be given a trial of TCA antidepressants.

Page: 1396

59   Answers

Question #1

Answer: D

Rationale: The number of individuals who experience a traumatic event during their lifetime is becoming increasingly more common. A trauma may be a violent event, such as rape or a motor vehicle accident, or it may be a natural disaster like an earthquake, a hurricane, or a tsunami. Approximately 66% of patients will experience traumatic events during their lifetimes. All forms of trauma carry a 1-year prevalence rate of 20%. Post-traumatic stress disorder is a common sequela of these events; it occurs in approximately 8% of Americans, and it is twice as common among women.

Page: 1400

Question #2

Answer: C

Rationale: The comprehensive evaluation and assessment of a crisis, trauma, or disaster involve an understanding of multiple elements, including the following: the normal equilibrium state, the stressor or precipitant, the personal interpretation or meaning of events, the crisis state, preexisting psychiatric conditions, selective past history, social support system, and the effects on community resources. Crisis intervention theory offers a systematic comprehensive approach to a patient who has experienced a traumatic event.

Page: 1400

Question #3

Answer: D

Rationale: Hobson and Kamen[1] have revised the original social readjustment scale described by Homes and Rahe.[2] The scale includes more than 50 external life stressors that cause significant stress for most individuals. The top items are separated into five domains: (1) death and dying, (2) health care issues, (3) stress related to crime and the criminal justice system, (4) financial

and economic issues, and (5) family stresses. The list represents the most common precipitants that cause a crisis.

Page: 1401

Question #4

Answer: C

Rationale: The crisis state can be defined as a brief psychological upheaval, precipitated by a stressor, that produces an intense state of inner turmoil or disorganization that overwhelms a person's ability to cope and adapt. Patients experience this state in different ways, and they may present to their family physicians with various and oftentimes confusing complaints. Symptom clusters may be physical complaints, thought disturbances, and uncomfortable feelings, or they may be behavior related.

Page: 1401

Question #5

Answer: A

Rationale: The *Diagnostic and Statistical Manual of Mental Disorders IV* classifies the initial 1-month period of a crisis during which there is impaired functioning as an *acute stress disorder*. It further specifies that the acute symptoms must last more than 2 days and less than 4 weeks. The event must cause a significant impairment in social or occupational functioning. The four possible outcomes are successful coping, a return to previous baseline functioning, partial resolution, and unresolved crisis. Unresolved crises predispose the patient to relapses of acute stress disorder.

Page: 1402

Question #6

Answer: E

Rationale: Most patients who suffer a major crisis event as a result of trauma or disaster will usually recover within 4 to 6 weeks. Prognostication depends on pretraumatic, traumatic, and post-traumatic risk factors. Pretraumatic risk factors include psychiatric history, genetics, coping styles, gender, and culture. Traumatic risk factors depend

1. Hobson CJ, Kamen J, Szostek J, et al: Stressful life events: A revision and update of the social readjustment rating scale. *Int J Stress Manag* 1:123, 1998.
2. Holmes TH, Rahe RH: Social readjustment scale. *J Psychosom Res* 2:213,1967.

on the type, severity, and duration of trauma. Post-traumatic risk factors include coping styles, individual and community resources and responses, capacity for problem solving, and adaptation.

Page: 1402

Question #7

Answer: B

Rationale: A patient's past medical history is extremely important when performing an evaluation status after a suicide attempt. Physicians must understand the dynamics of the crisis that led to the attempt, and they must search the patient's past for significant clues that may help elucidate suicidal ideology. Helpful clues include marital problems, severe medical or psychiatric history (e.g., drug and alcohol abuse), and personal or family suicide attempts.

Page: 1403

Question #8

Answer: D

Rationale: Individual support through a network of social systems such as family and community is essential to daily functional status. A stable social support system is the most important mechanism for preventing the common sequelae associated with crises and disasters of all types. A patient is most likely to become dysfunctional as the result of a crisis that threatens his or her immediate social environment. Examples include divorce, employment loss, or an eviction notice.

Page: 1403

Question #9

Answer: E

Rationale: The family physician should take a basic and standard approach to evaluating a patient in a crisis situation. The who, what, where, and why are parts of a rapid assessment that can help formulate the cause of the crisis and identify specific interventions and problem-solving approaches. This initial approach must be geared toward helping the patient deal with the acute psychosocial effects of the crisis itself. A comprehensive assessment includes evaluating the crisis precipitants and looking at the personal meaning of the event, the crisis state itself, and the individual's available social support network.

Page: 1405

Question #10

Answer: B

Rationale: An eco map is a pictorial representation of the patient's entire support network. The map includes a genogram, which consists of current family and family of origin for three generations. In addition, the map includes the immediate support network and consists of the patient's living environment, including neighbors, churches, schools, and employers. The family physician must explore this eco map to determine who is available for, interested in, and capable of assisting the patient in crisis.

Page: 1405

Question #11

Answer: D

Rationale: The patient who presents in crisis will usually have numerous symptoms and multiple problems that need to be addressed. In addition to the patient's immediate concerns, the most important primary issue to focus on urgently is safety. Food, clothing, shelter, and the assessment of risk for suicide and violence must be given priority. The physician must set a priority list to formulate specific treatment and management plans.

Pages: 1407, 1409

Question #12

Answer: E

Rationale: A problem-focused or symptom-oriented treatment plan is essential for the immediate management of the patient in crisis. Using the timeline and the eco map for evaluation, the physician may then begin crisis intervention treatment. The three main approaches to crisis intervention include the following: (1) fostering coping skills and adaptive problem solving; (2) using a crisis-resolution strategy; and (3) using appropriate medication for symptom control or psychiatric disorders.

Page: 1406

Question #13

Answer: B

Rationale: Each individual has his or her own way of dealing with stressful situations. Various coping skills and styles are the unique ways that individuals respond to stress. Those individuals who can use multiple styles of coping are the ones who are the most successful when dealing with a crisis. Diverse adaptive coping styles, such as intuitive, trial and error, wait and see, emotional, and manipulative, are positive ways of dealing with stress. Pathological coping styles, such as antisocial, impulsive, random, and chaotic, should be avoided, especially during the crisis period.

Page: 1408

Question #14

Answer: C

Rationale: When dealing with crisis intervention, the physician must teach various coping styles and skills to the patient in need. A crisis-resolution strategy based on crisis principles is composed of the following 16 steps:

1. Recognize early warning signs.
2. Set expectations.
3. Normalize symptoms.
4. Talk the problem over.
5. Discuss painful feelings and emotions.
6. Identify the specific symptoms and problems of those most affected by the crisis.
7. Identify precipitants.
8. Create an eco map.
9. Prioritize.
10. Develop a treatment plan.
11. Obtain information.
12. Teach coping styles.
13. Make a specific plan.
14. Implement the plan.
15. Assess the results.
16. Try again or consult.

Page: 1408

Question #15

Answer: D

Rationale: For patients who suffer from crisis events, the best psychological treatment is often no treatment at all. If the patient's social and occupational functioning has remained intact, no treatment is the best option for the first 6 weeks of the crisis period. Recent trends of mandatory debriefing after mass traumas have not been shown to be helpful for the prevention of post-traumatic stress disorder, and they should be avoided. Literature has shown that compulsory treatment may make patients worse by requiring a reliving of the experiences

before the patients are ready to deal with them. However, patients who are showing signs of a psychiatric disorder such as post-traumatic stress disorder should be offered therapy when it is voluntarily requested.

Page: 1408

Question #16

Answer: A

Rationale: Psychotherapeutic techniques should be used as first-line crisis intervention for most patients. There have been no evidence-based recommendations for the use of medications to prevent post-traumatic stress disorder among these patients. The use of medications for symptom control may be helpful and appropriate when dealing with severe anxiety, insomnia, or psychotic symptoms.

Page: 1408

Question #17

Answer: B

Rationale: The presence of insomnia and other sleep disturbances is common during crisis or during the immediate post-traumatic state. Lack of sleep may markedly affect an individual's ability to cope with these stressful situations. First-line pharmaceutical intervention for the treatment of sleep disturbances should be with the use of a nonbenzodiazepine hypnotic agent such as zolpidem, zaleplon, or eszopiclone. Benzodiazepines should be avoided, because they may inhibit effective coping mechanisms.

Page: 1409

Question #18

Answer: A

Rationale: Sertraline was the first medication approved by the U.S. Food and Drug Administration for the treatment of posttraumatic stress disorder. Recently, other SSRIs such as paroxetine and fluoxetine have also been proven to be effective. No medications are approved for the treatment of acute stress disorders. Some patients may require adjunctive therapy with mood-stabilizing agents or sedative hypnotics. Others may also present with global psychotic symptoms requiring the use of low doses of atypical antipsychotic agents.

Page: 1409

Question #1

Answer: B

Rationale: For patients with personality disorder with psychotic symptoms, the typical or atypical antipsychotics would be the right choice. Risperidone, which is an atypical drug, would be a good choice. Divalproex is a mood stabilizer, and sertraline is an antidepressant; they would best be used for a patient with mood symptoms. Lithium would best be used for a patient with a personality disorder with irritability and impulsivity.

Page: 1421

Question #2

Answer: A

Rationale: Amitriptyline, which is a tricyclic antidepressant, could be used for patients with personality disorders with mood symptoms. It would not be useful for patients with psychotic symptoms or for those with irritability or impulsivity. Selective serotonin reuptake inhibitor antidepressants may be helpful for patients with irritability or impulsivity.

Page: 1421

Question #3

Answer: E

Rationale: Many features of the borderline patient are similar to those of the narcissistic patient. One difference is that the narcissistic patient does not have mini-psychotic breaks. However, both of these types of patients are prone to splitting, projection, acting out, and projective identification.

Page: 1418

Question #4

Answer: C

Rationale: All of the listed items are features of patients with personality disorders, except for acting out, which is more often a feature of borderline, narcissistic, or antisocial patients. It is best not to confront the delusions of the paranoid personality disordered patient, but it is acceptable to correct their distortion of reality.

Page: 1417

Question #5

Answer: A

Rationale: Patients with personality disorders are very difficult to treat, and they require a lot of time from both the physician and the office staff. They contribute significantly to practice dissatisfaction for some physicians. The result may be poor medical care for these patients.

Page: 1411

Question #6

Answer: A

Rationale: Many features that are attributed to personality style are also features of personality disorder; it is sometimes a matter of degree. However, personality disorders are much harder to modify, if they can be changed at all. Personality style can be modified to fit the environment, and it is likely to be somewhat like the personality of one of the patient's parents. Both personality style and personality disorder can be stable over time.

Page: 1411

Question #7

Answer: D

Rationale: The three clusters of personality disorders are (1) odd and eccentric, (2) dramatic, emotional, and erratic, and (3) anxious and fearful. These clusters are useful for differentiating among personality disorders. Although some patients with personality disorders are suspicious, this characteristic is not one of the three designated clusters that are used for definition and diagnosis. These patients are complex, and so some of them may meet the criteria for two cluster groups or even for more than one personality disorder.

Page: 1412

Question #8

Answer: C

Rationale: Patients with personality disorders may generate feelings that cause a physician to act in an atypical fashion; this is called *patient-generated countertransference*. These could be reactions such as intense feelings of love, hate, or even sexual arousal; fantasies or dreams; ordering tests that are not needed; or giving discounts. These reactions should alert the physician to the possible diagnosis of personality disorder. None of the other responses is appropriate to describe patient-generated countertransference.

Page: 1412

Question #9

Answer: B

Rationale: Beck introduced cognitive-behavioral therapy in 1990. The theory is that people have core beliefs, a worldview, and personality-specific fears that can be identified and influenced by conscious awareness. Irrational thinking can occur when stressors act on the background of those core beliefs. This may create irrational fears or mood changes and subsequent behaviors that may be negative. The other responses do not fall under the definition of cognitive-behavioral therapy or any other documented therapy.

Page: 1415

Question #10

Answer: C

Rationale: Borderline patients may use devaluation as a defense mechanism. They do feel abandoned, and it is best to tell them that you understand their feelings. It this case, it would be useful to focus on the fact that your vacation does not affect your future desire to care for this patient, and it may help to clarify that construing your vacation as a personal abandonment is a distorted belief. It does not help to become angry with this patient, and asking her to visit with your partner while you are away would be unfair to both parties.

Page: 1419

Question #11

Answer: C

Rationale: Most personality disorders are not recognized until after an unpleasant interpersonal interaction with either a close contact or a physician when typical psychiatric symptoms are noticed. At other times, patients with these conditions may seem peculiar, but they may not exhibit symptoms of psychiatric illness.

Page: 1411

Question #12

Answer: C

Rationale: Patients with type A disorders will tend to underuse medical services, whereas those with type B disorder may misuse, overuse, or underuse medical recommendations. Only those with type C disorders are likely to adhere to medical advice out of fear that something bad could happen if they do not. Type D is not a cluster label.

Pages: 1411–1412

Question #13

Answer: A

Rationale: Patients with neurotic personality organization have the most stable view of themselves, and they use a higher level of defense mechanisms. Those with borderline personality organization often use splitting as a defense mechanism. Patients with psychotic personality organization have the most primitive defense system, because they often have a loss of reality. Psychosomatic personality organization is not a recognized type of personality organization.

Page: 1415

Question #14

Answer: B

Rationale: The confrontation of patients' contradictory beliefs and behaviors is suggested as the first step in psychotherapy in an effort to empathize with and acknowledge patients' fears. This is followed by the clarification of misunderstandings and then interpretations of beliefs and behaviors.

Pages: 1419–1420

Question #15

Answer: E

Rationale: It is wise to empathize with the patient's core beliefs. A good technique is to modify the patient's surroundings by bringing friends or family into the care plan. It is not unusual to have to set limits. Persons with personality disorders do not make changes quickly or easy. It is more effective to discuss and accept the patient's limitations with regard to coping skills and to modify them slowly over time. You may want to allow illogical feelings or thoughts unless they are part of a delusional system; then it would be unwise and counterproductive.

Page: 1420

Question #16

Answer: A

Rationale: Patients with borderline personality disorders fear separation, and they may often react with panic or anger. They often make intense demands of health care professionals. Dealing with these fears and demands can drain a physician. Realistic limit setting is important for both the patient and the physician.

Page: 1413

Question #17

Answer: B

Rationale: Pharmacotherapy has been shown to be an effective adjunct to psychotherapy to decrease impulsivity and psychotic symptoms in patients with borderline personality disorder.

Page: 1418

Question #18

Answer: D

Rationale: Patients with self-defeating personality disorder can be helped by the physician empathizing with them and discussing realistic symptoms and improvements.

Page: 1414

Question #19

Answer: A

Rationale: Physician reactions are very useful for recognizing and diagnosing patients with personality disorders. These patients may cause physicians to react in atypical ways; that abnormal response should alert the physician to think about the possibility of a personality disorder in the patient.

Page: 1412

Question #20

Answer: A

Rationale: Amitriptyline is the only nonantipsychotic on the list. It is an antidepressant, and it would not be useful to treat psychosis.

Page: 1421

61 Answers

Question #1

Answer: A

Rationale: A symptom is defined as a subject complaint or reports from the patient. Symptoms cannot be observed; they are not determined by the physician's point of view, and they may include mental complaints such as depression in addition to physical complaints.
Page: 1427

Question #2

Answer: C

Rationale: Impairment is more often associated with somatization than with any other psychiatric disorder.
Page: 1429

Question #3

Answer: C

Rationale: Patients with multisomatoform disorder are rated as being nine times more difficult to deal with; depressed and anxious patients are felt to be three times more difficult to treat as compared with nonsomatic controls.
Pages: 1428–1429

Question #4

Answer: C

Rationale: Somatization tends to run in families, particularly among females, males with substance abuse, and individuals who have experienced childhood sexual and physical abuse.
Page: 1429

Question #5

Answer: B

Rationale: Patients who are suspected of somatization disorder usually meet the criteria for mental disorder, and it is recommended to have them try an antidepressant as treatment at some point in time.
Page: 1431

Question #6

Answer: B

Rationale: Encouragement to schedule frequent, brief visits is the most effective strategy, and it may discourage the patient from developing new symptoms.
Page: 1431

Question #7

Answer: A

Rationale: The recommendation for the evaluation of a patient with multiple complaints is to conduct a focused physical examination and to pursue workups only if physical findings are present.
Page: 1430

Question #8

Answer: D

Rationale: Empathizing with the patient with somatoform disorder by reassuring him or her that the symptom is common can be disabling; telling him or her that it may not have an explanation can be beneficial.
Page: 1430

Question #9

Answer: E

Rationale: The listed therapies have been shown to be modestly effective in several trials, but there is no specific mention of any worth of family therapy.
Pages: 1431–1432

Question #10

Answer: D

Rationale: The listed medications have some evidence of effectiveness, except for benzodiazepines.

Page: 1431

Question #11

Answer: B

Rationale: Somatization is the most likely diagnosis with no physical findings or causal mechanisms but prolonged symptoms of pain.

Page: 1430

Question #12

Answer: A

Rationale: Most patients with somatoform disorder complain of some type of pain. The other complaints listed are also likely, but pain is the most common.

Page: 1428

Question #13

Answer: B

Rationale: Patients with somatization disorder will have multiple complaints with no physical findings, and their symptoms are not likely to resolve. It is best to focus on one symptom, to focus on functionality rather than symptom resolution, and to avoid blood work and imaging without physical findings. It may be appropriate to base the appointment primarily on time.

Page: 1430

Question #14

Answer: C

Rationale: Patients with somatization disorder often have chronic pain complaints but normal physical examination, imaging, and laboratory studies. Performing a workup would likely disclose a brain malignancy, diabetes, or a vision problem; however, the chronicity of the problem makes somatization disorder, which often begins during childhood, a more likely diagnosis.

Pages: 1427–1428

Question #15

Answer: B

Rationale: School phobia could be a diagnosis if the pain was only occurring during the school year. All of the listed diagnoses are possible for a 9-year-old, with no findings pointing to an organic cause of the pain. Somatization is more likely because of the fact that pain is the complaint and that it is has not changed.

Page: 1428

Question #16

Answer: D

Rationale: Somatization is associated with very high levels of health care use, even apart from the use associated with comorbid conditions.

Page: 1429

Question #17

Answer: A

Rationale: Parallel diagnostic inquiry is the strategy that begins by explaining that all symptoms, all illness, and all diseases are produced, sustained, and amplified by both physical and psychosocial factors that interplay with one another.

Page: 1430

Question #18

Answer: A

Rationale: The PRIME-MD or the self-administered PHQ-15 questionnaires are emerging as the most commonly used instruments to diagnose somatization disorder. These tools are being used both in research and in the clinical setting.

Page: 1430

Question #19

Answer: C

Rationale: The emotion-focused interviewing technique is the most effective for use with somatization patients.

Page: 1430

Question #20

Answer: A

Rationale: Emotion-focused interviewing involves exploring emotionally charged situations and observing the response. This allows for the classification of the patient into a somatization category for specific short-term psychotherapy.

Page: 1430

Question #21

Answer: C

Rationale: Emotion-focused interviewing allows for the classification of the patient into a somatization category for specific short-term psychotherapy. This does not assist with medication choice; it is not used for research specifically, and it does not resolve the symptoms.

Page: 1430

Question #22

Answer: E

Rationale: Somatization disorder is categorized into four main patterns of somatization: (1) striated muscle tension, (2) smooth muscle tension, (3) cognitive perceptual disruption, and (4) conversion. Emotion-focused interviewing may allow for the determination of the classification.

Page: 1428

Question #23

Answer: A

Rationale: Although the patient does have somatization disorder, chest pain—especially in a 65-year-old male—should never be dismissed on the basis of a normal physical examination. An electrocardiogram would be paramount for establishing the diagnosis of a myocardial infarction.

Page: 1428

Question #24

Answer: C

Rationale: Scheduled, frequent, brief visits have been shown to improve health and reduce costs among patients with somatization disorder.

Page: 1429

Question #25

Answer: D

Rationale: Somatization disorder often manifests as multiple, difficult-to-explain complaints of pain. Low back pain is common without injury, as are some shoulder pains. Multiple musculoskeletal complaints would be expected after a motor vehicle accident.

Page: 1429

Question #26

Answer: A

Rationale: An experienced physician's clinical judgment about whether an explanation will be found for the patient's complaints is accurate 90% of the time.

Page: 1430

Question #27

Answer: A

Rationale: Polypharmacy, multiple drug reactions or allergies, multiple drug failures, and prior use of psychotropic drugs and controlled substances may suggest somatization.

Page: 1429

Question #28

Answer: C

Rationale: This patient likely has somatization disorder and would potentially benefit from a trial of antidepressant therapy, frequent scheduled visits, and cognitive-behavioral therapy. Shockwave therapy may be used for chronic tendinosis pain, which usually has physical findings that are consistent.

Page: 1431

Question #1

Answer: A

Rationale: Many people mistake normal age-associated memory decline with the development of dementia. Age-associated memory decline usually entails slower accessing of memories. Thus, forgetting where you placed the keys is not associated with dementia, because most people will eventually remember where the keys are. However, dementia involves memory loss that has a directly impact on activities of daily living and instrumental activities of daily living. Aphasia (language difficulty), apraxia (inability to perform a motor function), and agnosia (failure to recognize common objects) are common features of dementia.

Page: 1435

Question #2

Answer: D

Rationale: Secondary causes of dementia are rare. However, there is general consensus regarding a basic workup. Among the tests to be checked are the complete blood cell count, the thyroid-stimulating hormone level, the vitamin B_{12} level, and the syphilis serology. Serum electrophoresis is used to detect such entities as multiple myeloma.

Page: 1436

Question #3

Answer: B

Rationale: Visual hallucinations, fluctuating course, and confusion are all common symptoms of both dementia and delirium; onset and the presence of other disease states in these settings will help differentiate the two. However, in patients with dementia, attention is often preserved, whereas in patients with delirium it is compromised. This can be easily tested by having the patient recite the days of the week in reverse order or by performing the letter test (the patient is given a random series of letters and instructed to give a signal when he or she hears a specific letter, such as "A").

Page: 1435

Question #4

Answer: B

Rationale: This is a very common scenario. Although AD is a strong consideration, the cognitive screening is out of proportion with the clinical picture. There is no indication of cancer. Lewy body dementia usually presents with hallucinations either preceding or in concordance with dementia. The most likely diagnosis is depression and dysphoric depression specifically. Although this patient's functioning has certainly declined, he should not be scoring a 0/30 on a Mini Mental State Examination. This patient is not putting forth any effort during the testing, whereas a patient with AD will make excuses to cover up any noticeable deficits.

Page: 1435

Question #5

Answer: B

Rationale: The genetics of AD are just beginning to be worked out. Although it is known that having the e4 allele of the APOE gene confers a definite risk of developing AD, it is not a direct relationship. Because one set of genes is inherited from each parent, there are numerous homozygotes for e4. However, the majority of these patients do not develop AD. Therefore, routine screening for the APOE genotype is not recommended.

Page: 1437

Question #6

Answer: D

Rationale: In addition to all of the listed factors, age and family history of a first-degree relative with AD are also risk factors.

Page: 1437

Question #7

Answer: C

Rationale: Lewy body dementia accounts for 20% of all dementia cases, and it shares many common features with other dementias. Early hallucinations are one of the hallmark signs that help differentiate this disease. The deficit of choline acetyltransferase is even greater in cases of Lewy body dementia, and so the response to acetylcholine-esterase inhibitors may be even more robust than that seen among patients with AD. Fluctuating cognition is another hallmark feature of LBD. Stairstep progression is associated with vascular dementia.

Page: 1439

Question #8

Answer: D

Rationale: Relying solely on the computed tomography image of the head to make the diagnosis of AD is problematic at best. Although it is true that all of the mentioned findings are associated with AD, they are also equally associated with normal age-associated changes. The purpose of the head imaging is to find possible causes for the cognitive impairment, such as tumor or bleed. The findings need to be correlated with the clinical picture of the patient. Patients with Pick's disease will have anterior temporal lobe atrophy on imaging. Central pontine myelinolysis is associated with neuronal death to hyponatremia that has been corrected too quickly; it is fatal.

Page: 1437

Question #9

Answer: B

Rationale: Acetylcholine is the most prominent neurotransmitter deficiency in dementia. This is evident in the lower center, such as in the hippocampus and the nucleus basalis of Meynert. The deficiency seen here translates to increased atrophy in the cerebral cortex and a resultant cognitive deficit. Acetylcholine neither negatively affects norepinephrine nor is it neurotoxic.

Page: 1438

Question #10

Answer: A

Rationale: One study did show a modest effect from ginkgo biloba for the prevention of AD. However, subsequent studies have been equivocal. Therefore, the National Institute of Aging is funding a study to answer the question. Interestingly, other hopeful preventative treatments such as nonsteroidal anti-inflammatory drugs, hormones, and vitamin D have not been shown to have

an effect. Saw palmetto is used for benign prostate hyperplasia, and black cohosh is used for menopausal symptoms. Ginseng is used by some to improve concentration.

Page: 1438

Question #11

Answer: C

Rationale: Determining the terminal phase of AD is problematic at best. Some argue that the start of the phase is nonremedial weight loss. All the rest of the symptoms are also on the Local Coverage Determinations (LCD) list, except calling out. This can occur at any time during the course of dementia, but it is more common during the moderate phase, and it increases in frequency as the patient enters the severe phase.

Page: 1438

Question #12

Answer: C

Rationale: Lewy body dementia and Parkinson's disease share a similar histopathological feature: Lewy bodies. These are cytoplasmic inclusion bodies that are found throughout the paralimbic, the temporal, and the parietal cortex and preferentially in the substantia nigra in patients with Parkinson's disease. This helps explain the shared movement impairments, including the pill-rolling tremor, bradykinesia, and masked facies. However, the progression and extent of the neuronal damage are responsible for the dementia in patients with Parkinson's disease, in whom this has a later onset. Alternatively, dementia and hallucinations are early manifestations of Lewy body dementia as a result of the more widespread distribution of the Lewy bodies. Many patients with Lewy body dementia are misdiagnosed with Parkinson's disease if the presenting history is not known.

Page: 1438

Question #13

Answer: D

Rationale: Although gait disturbance, urinary incontinence, and dementia are known as the classic triad of normal-pressure hydrocephalus, because of the multiple comorbidities associated with aging, they are very commonly found in the other dementias as well. The key to this diagnosis is the combination of the computed tomography findings with the improvement in symptoms with a spinal tap. This is one of the alternative diagnoses that you are ruling out with head imaging during your initial workup. The study will comment on the ventricular enlargement that is out of proportion with cerebral atrophy. Remember that cerebral atrophy is a normal finding in an aging brain; however, the noted ventriculomegaly will be proportional to the atrophy seen on the scan. If it is not proportional, you should consider a diagnostic spinal tap. In a patient with normal-pressure hydrocephalus, you will see improvement in the gait disturbance and some cognitive improvement. However, this will be short lived, because the spinal fluid will reaccumulate. Correction of this dementia is with a surgical shunt. Patient selection is key.

Page: 1441

Question #14

Answer: A

Rationale: There are four described forms of Creutzfeldt-Jakob disease: (1) infectious/iatrogenic, (2) sporadic, (3) genetic, and (4) new variant. Sporadic is the most common form that is encountered. It is associated with a long preclinical phase but with rapid progression and death after it becomes clinically evident. The infectious/iatrogenic form is associated with prions, and it is the result of exposure to infected dura mater or of a corneal transplant; it has also been seen after injection with human growth hormone or pituitary gonadotropin. Genetic Creutzfeldt-Jakob disease has an earlier onset and a slower course. It has an autosomal-dominant mode of expression, and is uniformly fatal. New-variant Creutzfeldt–Jakob disease is associated with bovine spongiform encephalopathy, which is also called mad cow disease.

Page: 1441

Question #15

Answer: C

Rationale: Screening for dementia remains an area of controversy. Neither the U.S. Preventive Services Task Force nor the Canadian Task Force recommends screening asymptomatic patients, regardless of age. The key to this recommendation is the asymptomatic status. Even in a patient with a recent cerebral vascular accident or other head trauma, if neither the patient nor the family is concerned, then screening is not recommended. This does not apply to a patient without complaint but who is having obvious cognitive difficulties during the visit encounter. It is recommended to screen any patient with either overt personal concern or family concern about memory loss.

Page: 1436

Question #16

Answer: D

Rationale: This is a very common office scenario. AD often has a paranoid phase. This is the result of the patients misplacing items or giving them away and then forgetting about doing so. Thus, they often think that people are stealing from them. Furthermore, the focus of the blame is often a family member. They will often claim to hear the person in the house but will not see him or her; this is known as misinterpreting environmental cues. Frank visual hallucinations are also very common. Psychotic depression often involves delusions of persecution or guilt. Personality disorder involves behavior patterns more than hallucinations, except of course for schizophrenia. Manic episodes will usually involve ideas of grandiosity and increased activity, neither of which is hinted at in this clinical situation.

Page: 1441

Question #17

Answer: B

Rationale: Mild cognitive impairment will present in the manner described in this scenario. The primary feature of this disorder is the perception of memory problems, verified by cognitive screening, that does not have an impact on daily functioning. This differentiates it from AD and vascular dementia, because the cognitive deficit directly affects the daily functioning of patients with these disorders. Creutzfeldt-Jakob disease has a subacute preclinical phase, but it then presents with rapid decline.

Page: 1435

Question #18

Answer: B

Rationale: Staging dementia can be problematic. Several grading systems have been used in the past to place patients. Recently, mild, moderate, and severe impairment have been used. The degree of impairment is based on the predominant systems at the time. Mild impairment involves memory deficits and some mild personality and behavior changes. Later mild impairment is characterized by aphasia and apraxia, progressive memory loss, and disorientation. Severe impairment involves the inability to recognize family members, bowel and bladder incontinence, and unintelligible speech. The terminal phase involves certain LCD criteria set forth by Medicare.

Page: 1437

Question #19

Answer: C

Rationale: This case illustrates the difficulty of diagnosing vascular dementia. The first area to look at is the presenting history. AD will present with a gradual decline, whereas Lewy body dementia presents with hallucinations and a fluctuating course. Frontotemporal dementia will present with personality changes that either precede or occur in concordance with the dementia. Parkinson's disease has a late onset of dementia after the movement difficulties have been established. As this case shows, there does not have to be either a history of cerebral vascular accident nor radiologic evidence of strokes. Periventricular changes can be associated with normal aging. However, ischemic changes in the basal ganglion, the thalamus, the white matter, or the cortical regions are strongly associated with vascular dementia.

Page: 1440

Question #20

Answer: E

Rationale: Both the Mini Mental State Examination and the clock draw have been validated for screening for dementia. Adding a three-item recall to the clock draw is called a "mini-cog," and it is not sensitive to educational level or cultural differences, as the Mini Mental State Examination is. The Katz Index deals with the functionality of the patient.

Page: 1436

Question #21

Answer: C

Rationale: AD is the most prevalent dementia in the United States. It currently accounts for 70% of all dementias, and it affects roughly 4 million people. This is projected to increase to 13 million by the year 2050. Vascular dementia and Lewy body dementia account for roughly equal numbers of cases, and they are the second most common forms of dementia in the United States. Pick's disease is a frontotemporal dementia, and it is relatively uncommon.

Page: 1436

Question #22

Answer: D

Rationale: In this patient, his out-of-context behaviors are the distressing symptom. Although memory loss is present, behavioral changes are not usually prominent among patients with AD. Vascular dementia is a possibility, but, again, behavioral changes are not usually this drastic. Hallucinations are the presenting symptom for patients with Lewy body dementia. Frontotemporal dementia presents mainly with drastic behavior changes and social disinhibition.

Page: 1440

Question #23

Answer: C

Rationale: Dementia associated with human immunodeficiency virus was a very common aliment among this patient population. However, since the advent of treatment with highly active antiretroviral therapy, this dementia takes a very slowly progressing or static clinical course.

Page: 1441

Question #24

Answer: A

Rationale: Vascular dementia translates to neuronal injury and death. Although cerebral vascular accidents are one of the most common causes, an often-overlooked cause is repetitive hypoxic injury as a result of systemic hypotensive episodes. Head injury is a risk factor for the development of AD. Lewy bodies are found in both Lewy body dementia and Parkinson's disease. Tau protein phosphorylation is one of the pathologic consequences of AD.

Page: 1440

Question #25

Answer: D

Rationale: Treating the psychotic symptoms associated with dementia is problematic. There are no major tranquilizers approved by the U.S. Food and Drug Administration for this indication. Additionally, there is now a black-box warning on atypical antipsychotics warning of increased mortality when they are used to treat the frail elderly. Benzodiazepines are associated with respiratory depression and occasional death. The safest remedies so far are redirection and treating unmet physical needs, such as pain or constipation.

Page: 1441

Question #1

Answer: E

Rationale: Alcohol abusers use all of these services as well as emergency room services more than the general population. Comorbid conditions such as hepatitis C and pancreatitis are increased, and there is also an increased incidence of motor vehicle accidents, family violence, homicides, and injuries in this population.

Page: 1445

Question #2

Answer: B

Rationale: There is no single causative factor ascribed to alcoholism, although genetic markers play a significant role. However, the final expression of the disorder is ultimately determined by the environment, genetics, personality, and social circumstances.

Page: 1445

Question #3

Answer: E

Rationale: Alcoholism is defined as a repetitive but inconsistent and sometimes unpredictable loss of control of drinking. Drinking daily is not a necessary criterion. The DSM-III listed nine criteria for addiction: (1) tolerance; (2) withdrawal avoidance; (3) withdrawal; (4) inability to limit use; (5) preoccupation; (6) continued use despite problems; (7) socially dysfunctional use; (8) salience; and (9) inability to stop. The DSM-IV went further to divide alcohol-related disorders into alcohol abuse, alcohol dependence, and alcohol withdrawal.

Page: 1446

Question #4

Answer: A

Rationale: Evidence for screening for alcoholism is weighed as B by the UK's Scottish National Guideline from the Scottish Intercollegiate Network of 2003. The

diagnosis of alcoholism often rests on the history. Answering positive to any of the CAGE questions suggests that further information is necessary. History of driving under the influence, motor vehicle accident, repeated trauma, new-onset pancreatitis, upper gastrointestinal bleeding, or family or marital violence are also clues to take seriously. Further alcohol evaluation should be pursued.

Page: 1447

Question #5

Answer: F

Rationale: Elevation of pulse, blood pressure, and respiration may be clues to the severity of alcohol withdrawal. Skin changes in alcoholics include rhinophyma, palmar erythema, a red and swollen face, and porphyria cutanea tarda.

Page: 1448

Question #6

Answer: F

Rationale: The cause of alcoholism is related to chromosomes 1, 2, and 7. A parent with alcoholism increases the risk of alcoholism fourfold, even if the child is adopted. Both GABA and opiate receptors are implicated as alcohol reward pathways.

Page: 1445

Question #7

Answer: F

Rationale: Heavy alcohol use is more frequent among men than women. Alcohol abuse ranks nearly as high as hypertension and much higher than diabetes mellitus. The prevalence of binge drinking is 14.2%.[1]

Page: 1445

---

1. Winick C: Epidemiology. IN Lowinson JH, Ruiz P, Milliman RB, et al (eds): *Substance Abuse: A Comprehensive Textbook*, 3rd ed. Baltimore, Williams & Wilkins, 1996, p 13-50.

Question #8

Answer: E

Rationale: The Institute of Medicine recognizes all of the listed options as potential effects of alcohol use during pregnancy and during the periconception period.[2]

Page: 1453

Question #9

Answer: D

Rationale: The effects of alcohol on a fetus depend on the amount of alcohol consumed at one time, the timing of alcohol consumption during gestation, and the duration of alcohol use during pregnancy.[1] The controversy is regarding whether or not there is a safe threshold of consumption.

Page: 1453

Question #10

Answer: E

Rationale: Family history, personal history, and the CAGE assessment are important screening tools for adolescents. Urine drug screening is controversial, and the American Academy of Pediatrics recommends screening only if it is volunteered by the teen, if the teen has acute medical problems that may put him or her in grave danger, or if court-ordered monitoring is in place.

Page: 1453

Question #11

Answer: F

Rationale: Screening clues for alcoholism include a history of driving under the influence, domestic violence, unexplained trauma, family stress, or loss of employment and new-onset hypertension, gastritis, pancreatitis, or tremor.

Page: 1447

Question #12

Answer: F

Rationale: Diagnostic clues from the laboratory include a complete blood cell count with an elevated mean cell volume, an elevated gamma-glutamyl transpeptidase level, an aspartate aminotransferase level that is greater than the alanine aminotransferase level, unexplained leukopenia or thrombocytopenia, and a positive response to the carbohydrate-deficient transferring level.[3]

Page: 1447

Question #13

Answer: B

Rationale: At an alcohol level of 80–100 mg/dL, delayed reaction time and slurred speech may occur; thus, 80 mg/dL is the generally accepted level that is considered to be unsafe for driving.

Page: 1448

Question #14

Answer: A

Rationale: According to the U.S. and Scottish Intercollegiate Network Guidelines, benzodiazepines are the treatment of choice for alcohol withdrawal, with an evidence level of A.

Page: 1449

Question #15

Answer: E

Rationale: Delirium tremens is usually preceded by minor withdrawal symptoms, and it begins 3 to 4 days after the last drink. Severe and potentially life-threatening autonomic hyperactivity leads to tachycardia, hypertension, and diaphoreses, frequently with a low-grade fever. The patient's sleep activity is typically disturbed with excessive motor activity rather than somnolence.

Page: 1449

Question #16

Answer: E

Rationale: Two brief and simple questionnaires are the TWEAK and CAGE assessments. Longer screening

2. Muchowski K, Paladine H: An ounce of prevention: The evidence supporting periconception health care. *J Fam Pract* 53:126-133, 2004.

3. Borg S, Beck O, Helander A, et al: Carbohydrate-deficient transferrin and 5-hydroxytryptophan: Two new markers of high alcohol consumption. In Litten RZ, Allen JP (eds): *Measuring Alcohol Consumption. Psychosocial and Biochemical Methods.* Totowa, NH, Humana Press, 1992, p 148.

questionnaires include the AUDIT and MAST assessments; both of these are considered higher in predictive value, but they are more difficult to administer.

Page: 1447

Question #17

Answer: C

Rationale: Gastric emptying is rarely helpful because of the rapid absorption of alcohol, but it may be considered if the ingestion has occurred within 60 minutes.

Page: 1448

Question #18

Answer: B

Rationale: All of the listed items except vitamin B_{12} can be used to treat alcohol-induced coma, although fructose is rarely used. Obviously, protecting the airway and performing basic cardiopulmonary resuscitation are the priorities for a patient in an alcohol-induced coma. Fructose can enhance elimination, but it is rarely used. Thiamine and glucose should always be administered, because chronic alcoholism is associated with hypoglycemia and thiamine-deficient states.

Page: 1448

Question #19

Answer: A

Rationale: Outpatient treatment is safe for mild-to-moderate alcohol withdrawal in patients with no serious psychiatric or medical co-morbidities.

Page: 1449

Question #20

Answer: D

Rationale: Seizures tend to occur as one isolated seizure or a brief cluster of seizures, and they are frequently preceded by tremors. They tend to recur in the same general pattern in the same patient. Seizure activity is most common 24 to 48 hours after alcohol cessation, but it can occur as early as 24 hours or as late as 1 week after cessation. Withdrawal seizures are typically generalized, grand mal, and self-limited. Dilantin is not an effective treatment.

Page: 1449

Question #21

Answer: D

Rationale: The CIWA-Ar is a validated 10-item assessment tool used to quantify the severity of alcohol withdrawal syndrome. Patients with moderate withdrawal symptoms should receive treatment to reduce the risk of seizures and delirium tremens during outpatient detoxification. Benzodiazepines are the treatment of choice, with an evidence level of A for alcohol withdrawal according to both U.S. and Scottish Intercollegiate Network Guidelines.

Page: 1449

Question #22

Answer: F

Rationale: Delirium tremens occurs in less than 5% of alcoholics during withdrawal. It is usually preceded by minor withdrawal symptoms, but it may appear frankly. It usually begins 3 to 4 days after the last drink, and it is characterized by a marked change in sensorium. Risk factors for delirium tremens include a rise in the blood alcohol level, an alcohol withdrawal seizure early in the withdrawal syndrome, and a previous history of delirium.[4]

Page: 1449

Question #23

Answer: D

Rationale: Both chlordiazepoxide and diazepam are effective agents for the treatment of withdrawal. Additionally, β-blockers such as atenolol may decrease tremulousness and sympathomimetic symptoms if there are no contraindications to their use.

Page: 1449

Question #24

Answer: A

Rationale: According to the Scottish National Guideline published in 2003,[5] brief interventions in primary care can be very successful, with an evidence level of A.

Page: 1450

4. Victor M: Diagnosis and treatment of alcohol withdrawal states. *Pract Gastroenterol* 7:6-15, 1983.

5. Scottish Intercollegiate Guidelines Network (SIGN): The management of harmful drinking and alcohol dependence in primary care, 2003. SIGN Publication No. 74. Accessed July 23, 2006. Available at http://www.sign.ac.uk.

Question #25

Answer: E

Rationale: The six stages of change are as follows: (1) precontemplation; (2) contemplation; (3) preparation; (4) action; (5) maintenance; and (6) relapse.
Page: 1450

Question #26

Answer: B

Rationale: Confrontation by providing an overwhelming amount of evidence and feedback to the alcoholic patient needs to be carefully orchestrated by professionals who are trained in the treatment of chemical dependency. The family physician may be an appropriate member of the intervention group, but, unless he or she is actively involved in the treatment of alcoholism, a professional should be consulted for assistance.
Page: 1450

Question #27

Answer: B

Rationale: Best-evidence recommendations state that patients with alcohol problems in addition to anxiety and depression should be treated for the alcohol problem first; this has a level of evidence of B.[5]
Page: 1451

Question #28

Answer: D

Rationale: Only naltrexone and acamprosate have a level B recommendation. Antabuse receives a level C recommendation.
Page: 1452

Question #29

Answer: D

Rationale: Naltrexone is an opioid antagonist that is given as a daily 50-mg tablet. It is not an aversive agent, but it provides a surmountable opioid blockage, and many alcoholic patients report a less-than-expected pleasurable experience with alcohol consumption. Naltrexone undergoes first-pass hepatic metabolism, and it is hepatotoxic in excessive doses.
Page: 1452

Question #30

Answer: D

Rationale: Women have lower rates of alcohol abuse and dependency than men. They generally have more psychiatric symptoms, and they are more likely to be concomitantly abusing prescription medications. They also have move hidden drinking than men. Screening tests such as the CAGE assessment are less sensitive for women. The TWEAK assessment has performed better for women than the CAGE assessment. Women have better treatment outcomes if they are referred to all-female recovery programs.
Page: 1452

Question #1

Answer: A

Rationale: The habituating constituent of tobacco is nicotine, and it causes a typical withdrawal syndrome after smoking cessation. It is more addictive than cocaine and heroin. A person who smokes one pack per day gets approximately 100,000 reinforcing hits per year, which is far more than the number of hits obtained by a typical cocaine or heroin user.

Page: 1457

Question #2

Answer: D

Rationale: The leading avoidable cause of death in American society is cigarette smoking. Eighteen percent of the total deaths in the United States are the result of smoking. More people die from cigarettes than alcohol, car accidents, suicide, acquired immunodeficiency syndrome, homicide, and illegal drugs combined. On average, smokers die 10 years earlier than nonsmokers.

Page: 1457

Question #3

Answer: C

Rationale: About 40% of all deaths from cancer and 21% of deaths from cardiovascular disease are attributable to smoking. Approximately 400,000 people die each year from the effects of tobacco: 33% are from cardiovascular disease; 28% are from lung cancer; 22% are from respiratory disease, and at least 7% are from cancers other than lung cancer. Almost 1 in 10 of these deaths is caused by secondhand smoke.

Page: 1457

Question #4

Answer: B

Rationale: Every year, smoking kills 10,000 more women than breast cancer. Currently, more young women smoke than young men. Each day, 3000 children and adolescents start using tobacco products regularly.

Page: 1457

Question #5

Answer: A

Rationale: Approximately 35% of smokers try to quit each year, but less than 5% are successful. People who have a college education are twice as likely to be successful as those with less education. There is increased success with the number of attempts.

Page: 1457

Question #6

Answer: B

Rationale: Male smokers are 22 times more likely to develop lung cancer as compared with nonsmokers; females are 12 times more likely. People who smoke more than a pack of cigarettes per day have a risk that is at least 20 times that of a nonsmoker.

Page: 1458

Question #7

Answer: D

Rationale: Early detection does not seem to improve the survival rate for lung cancer. The risk of death from lung cancer decreases if the person stops smoking. Decreasing the amount that one smokes daily from 20 cigarettes to less than 10 cigarettes decreases the risk of lung cancer by 25%. At the time of diagnosis, 75% of patients with lung cancer already have metastases.

Page: 1458

Question #8

Answer: B

Rationale: The amount of tar in cigarettes has decreased in recent years, but the risk of lung cancer has not changed. According to surveys, most people feel that smoking

low-tar cigarettes is less dangerous than smoking regular cigarettes; they also erroneously believe that regular cigarettes are much more likely to cause illness.
Page: 1458

Question #9

Answer: A

Rationale: The risk for the development of cancer of the larynx is as much as 75% higher among people who use both tobacco and alcohol as compared with those who are only exposed to either substance alone.
Page: 1459

Question #10

Answer: B

Rationale: Smoking increases the risk of bladder cancer by three to four times. The kidney and the bladder make up the final pathway of the concentrated toxic byproducts of tobacco smoking, and they also provide the longest direct exposure to the radioactive substances and carcinogens.
Page: 1459

Question #11

Answer: B

Rationale: Smoking causes more than 50% increased mortality from leukemia. Smoking more than one pack per day results in a twofold increased risk as compared with nonsmokers. A person's risk for leukemia is increased by 30% by smoking. Approximately 14% of all cases of leukemia in the United States may be the result of cigarette smoking.
Page: 1459

Question #12

Answer: A

Rationale: The main cause of chronic obstructive pulmonary disease is cigarette smoking. The more one smokes, the more changes are observed in the bronchi and the lung parenchyma. The number of cigarettes smoked is inversely proportional to lung function. Smokers who quit even after 60 years have better pulmonary function than those who continue to smoke. A person who quit smoking at the age of 40 who is now 65 years old has similar lung function to that of someone who never smoked.
Page: 1459

Question #13

Answer: A

Rationale: More than half of all deaths from coronary artery disease are sudden deaths that result from cardiac arrhythmia. Nicotine increases serum catecholamine levels and thus is arrhythmogenic. The decline from sudden death is time dependent after smoking cessation, and, within a few years of quitting smoking, the risk of myocardial infarction decreases to a level similar to that of a nonsmoker.
Pages: 1459–1460

Question #14

Answer: D

Rationale: There is no safe level of smoking. The more one smokes, the greater the risk. The risk of myocardial infarction increases progressively to as high as a 20-fold among people who smoke 35 or more cigarettes a day. A woman has a 2.5-times greater risk of coronary artery disease from smoking only 1 to 4 cigarettes per day. Smoking and using oral contraceptives work together to cause a CAD risk that is 10 times greater than that of women who do neither.
Page: 1460

Question #15

Answer: B

Rationale: The third most common cause of death in the United States is stroke, and hypertension is the greatest risk factor. Overall, the incidence of stroke is 50% higher among smokers than nonsmokers: 40% in males and 60% in females. The risk increases in proportion to the amount of smoking that is done; it is twice as great in someone who smokes 40 cigarettes per day as compared with someone who smokes 10 cigarettes per day.
Page: 1460

Question #16

Answer: A

Rationale: Smokers inhale more frequently and more deeply to maintain their nicotine blood levels when smoking low-nicotine cigarettes. Because of this compensation, the tar intake also increases, and, thus, it changes a low-tar cigarette to a high-tar cigarette. A smoker who takes 14 puffs per cigarette as opposed to the standard 8.7 puffs per cigarette inhales 58% more tar.

Page: 1462

Question #17

Answer: B

Rationale: Warnings are required for cigarettes and smokeless tobacco but not for cigars, despite the increased risks associated with them. One large cigar has the nicotine of four or five cigarettes and more carcinogens in the sidestream smoke. Cigar smokers have a higher risk of coronary artery disease and of cancer of the oropharynx, nose, larynx, esophagus, and lung than nonsmokers. In addition, there appears to be a synergistic relationship between alcohol use and cigar smoking.

Page: 1462

Question #18

Answer: D

Rationale: There are two types of smokeless tobacco: snuff and chewing tobacco. Approximately 18% to 64% of users of these products have leukoplakia. The same carcinogens that are in cigarette tobacco are in smokeless tobacco, although some are found at even higher level. A powerful carcinogen, nitrosamine, is present in smokeless tobacco at levels up to 14,000 times higher than those allowed by the federal government to be present in beer and bacon.

Page: 1462

Question #19

Answer: C

Rationale: Because of the lower combustion temperature and the lack of filtration through the cigarette, sidestream smoke contains greater amounts of toxic substances than mainstream smoke. Sidestream smoke contains more than 4000 different chemicals, of which at least 60 are known carcinogens. The Environmental Protection Agency has determined that sidestream tobacco smoke is a class A human carcinogen that is in the same class as asbestos, mustard gas, arsenic, and benzene. It is estimated that, each year, 3000 people

die from lung cancer and 40,000 people die from heart disease as a result of secondhand smoke.

Page: 1463

Question #20

Answer: D

Rationale: Passive smoking has one third to one half the risk of direct smoking. There is a direct dose–response relationship to the amount of passive smoke. A study found that the annual mortality from lung cancer was 8.7 per 100,000 women whose husbands only smoked occasionally and 18.1 per 100,000 for those women whose husbands smoked 20 or more cigarettes per day.

Page: 1463

Question #21

Answer: B

Rationale: As many as 46,000 deaths of nonsmokers annually in the United States could be the result of passive tobacco smoke in the home and workplace. Secondhand smoke exposure causes people to have higher white blood cell counts and elevated levels of C-reactive protein, oxidized low-density lipoprotein cholesterol, homocysteine, and fibrinogen. The risk of fatal and nonfatal coronary heart disease is increased by about 30% with exposure to secondhand smoke.

Pages: 1462–1463

Question #22

Answer: B

Rationale: Seventy-five percent of adults who smoke had at least one parent who smoked. For each additional adult family member who smokes, the chance of a child taking up smoking doubles. There is at least one adult smoker in more than 50% of homes with children who are less than 5 years old.

Page: 1464

Question #23

Answer: C

Rationale: Small children inhale larger amounts of the harmful substances of secondhand smoke because they breathe more rapidly. Several studies have shown that children's increased risks of cough, bronchitis, and pneumonia are proportional to the number of cigarettes that their parents smoke, especially their mothers.

Page: 1464

Question #24

Answer: A

Rationale: The more that a pregnant woman smokes, the lower her newborn's weight is likely to be. A pregnant mother to be who quits by the fourth month of gestation has the same risk of having a baby with a low birth weight as a nonsmoker. On average, there is a 10-gm decrease in weight for each cigarette smoked per day during pregnancy. High passive smoke exposure among pregnant women who do not smoke doubles their risk of having low-birth-weight infants as compared with women with low exposure to secondhand smoke.

Page: 1464

Question #25

Answer: A

Rationale: Women who smoke during pregnancy have an increased risk of the premature rupture of membranes, bleeding during pregnancy, placenta previa, and placental abruption. The incidence of premature births and perinatal deaths is also increased among pregnant smokers.

Page: 1464

Question #26

Answer: B

Rationale: Women who smoke are three to four times more likely to take more than 1 year to get pregnant; the more a woman smokes, the more difficulty she will have. In addition, the spermatozoa of male smokers have more morphologic abnormalities and less motility as compared with the spermatozoa of nonsmokers.

Page: 1464

Question #27

Answer: B

Rationale: The tobacco industry spent $6.7 billion on marketing cigarettes in 1998, and this increased to $15.2 billion in 2003. They agreed to not advertise in

magazines that have more than 15% young readers or more than 2 million readers who are less than 18 years old. However, they have violated the spirit of the agreement by targeting magazines with circulations that are just under 2 million or for which the percentage of young readers is just under 15%.

Page: 1465

Question #28

Answer: A

Rationale: The intensity of counseling and its effectiveness have a clear relationship. The persistence of the physician and the eagerness of the patient to try different treatment regimens lead to successful cessation. Most smokers require multiple attempts to be successful, and the chance of success increases with each attempt. A 22% success rate is associated with intense counseling, and a 13% quit rate is associated with minimal counseling. The physician should take advantage of a teachable moment, such as when the patient is seen for a respiratory or cardiovascular concern.

Page: 1467

Question #29

Answer: D

Rationale: According to the latest edition of *Treating Tobacco Use and Dependence,* sustained-release bupropion, nicotine inhalers, and nicotine nasal spray have been added to the list of recommended first-line medications. However, they are only available by prescription. The only two recommended drugs in the original guidelines in 1996 were nicotine gum and transdermal nicotine. Clonidine and nortriptyline are on the list as second-line agents. Benzodiazepines and α-adrenergic–blocking agents have not been shown to be effective for smoking cessation.

Page: 1467

Question #30

Answer: B

Rationale: It is a common myth that smoking relieves stress. This can easily be shown to be false by pointing out that the stress that is being relieved is what resulted from the dependence on the cigarette, which is the essence of addiction. One can point out that deep breathing has a relaxing effect.

Page: 1469

Question #31

Answer: A

Rationale: Children and teenagers represent the market that is the most carefully nurtured by tobacco-industry advertisers. Unfortunately, more than 3000 teenagers start smoking in the United States each day. Marlboro cigarettes are the choice of almost three fourths of this population.

Page: 1457

65 Answers

Question #1

Answer: B

Rationale: In 2003, an estimated 19.5 million American adults—or 8.2% of Americans who are more than 12 years old—reported using illicit drugs during the preceding month.

Page: 1473

Question #2

Answer: C

Rationale: Approximately 14.6 million Americans reported using marijuana in the past 12 months. This was followed by 6.3 million users of psychotherapeutics, of which 4.7 million reported abusing prescription pain medications.

Page: 1473

Question #3

Answer: D

Rationale: *Abuse* is the use of a drug in a manner that deviates from approved social or medical patterns. *Intoxication* is a reversible syndrome caused by a specific substance that effects mental, behavioral, social, and occupational functioning. *Tolerance* is the need for increased amounts of a substance to achieve the desired effect or a diminished effect with continued use of the same amount.

Page: 1473

Question #4

Answer: A

Rationale: Heroin is an opioid that is derived from poppies and that can be injected subcutaneously, intramuscularly, or intravenously. It can also be snorted, smoked, or ingested. Because of its short half-life, several doses are required per day to avoid withdrawal. New users tend to be urban and noninjecting users.

Page: 1474

Question #5

Answer: D

Rationale: Short-acting medications containing hydrocodone and oxycodone are the most commonly abused prescription medications. Long-acting medications such as OxyContin are sometimes touted as having a lower potential for abuse. However, by crushing and snorting or injecting these medications, the time-release properties of the medication can be bypassed, and the potential for abuse and addiction increases significantly. OxyContin abuse has surpassed heroin abuse in some areas. The appropriate use of opioids for cancer and other chronic pain is not likely to result in addiction.

Page: 1474

Question #6

Answer: B

Rationale: Methamphetamine can be easily synthesized using pseudoephedrine and household chemicals. As a result, many states are passing laws regulating the dispensing of pseudoephedrine-containing medications by pharmacies. Methamphetamine use is growing most rapidly in urban areas among young, white users. Some urban areas, like Newark, NJ, reported an increase in methamphetamine-related emergency room visits of more than 500% in 2003. Methamphetamine can be smoked, snorted, injected, or ingested orally or anally. Although the initial intoxication from the drug typically lasts 8 to 13 hours, the effects of use can persist for several weeks and can include irritable or aggressive behavior and psychosis.

Page: 1475

Question #7

Answer: C

Rationale: The withdrawal or abrupt termination of benzodiazepines produces an unpleasant and potentially life-threatening withdrawal syndrome. Physicians often initially prescribe benzodiazepines for legitimate purposes. Because of the addictive potential of benzodiazepines and their use to counteract the side effects of other drugs of abuse, it is important to screen patients for a history of abuse before prescribing them.

Page: 1476

Question #8

Answer: A

Rationale: Methamphetamine often is associated with dental decay. Tachycardia, hypertension, anxiety, and acute psychosis can be associated with either acute intoxication or withdrawal. Skin abscesses and track marks can be associated with intravenous drug use or "skin popping."

Page: 1476

Question #9

Answer: B

Rationale: Approximately 11.2% of teenagers between the ages of 12 and 17 years report current drug use. Between 1991 and 2003, the abuse of steroids among teens increased 126% among boys and 350% among girls. The abuse of prescription medications, particularly opioids, is common among teens, with nearly 1 in 10 reporting the abuse of a prescription medication. Teens who smoke are about eight times more likely to use drugs than nonsmokers.

Page: 1479

Question #10

Answer: D

Rationale: Physicians often overestimate the risks of patients becoming addicted to prescription pain medications. Patients who have a history of drug abuse are at increased risk, and providers should document any substance abuse history for patients who are receiving chronic pain medications. Medication contracts are commonly used, and they may be helpful for educating patients and for obtaining informed consent.

Page: 1479

Question #11

Answer: B

Rationale: There are seven DSM-IV criteria for substance abuse, and at least three of these must be present for the definition to be met. Two of these criteria are tol-

erance and withdrawal. If either tolerance or withdrawal is present, then physiologic dependence is present. However, a patient can have substance abuse without experiencing tolerance or withdrawal.

Page: 1480

Question #12

Answer: A

Rationale: Primary care physicians may prescribe methadone for chronic pain, but only licensed centers can prescribe it for maintenance therapy. Methadone is a long-acting opioid that prevents withdrawal symptoms and that partially blocks the euphoric effects of heroin. Methadone maintenance therapy is one example of a harm-reduction strategy for treatment of drug abuse.

Page: 1482

Question #13

Answer: D

Rationale: Unlike methadone, buprenorphine is a class III medication that can be prescribed by primary care physicians who have received special certification. Buprenorphine is useful for both withdrawal and maintenance therapy, and it has been shown to be effective in well-designed trials.

Page: 1482

Question #14

Answer: B

Rationale: Clonidine is an α-receptor blocker that is used to treat hypertension and anxiety from opioid withdrawal. Tapering doses of long-acting narcotics like methadone can be used as part of detoxification programs or for maintenance therapy. Other medications, like nonsteroidal anti-inflammatory drugs, antiemetics, and sleep medications, are often used as adjuncts to therapy. Antidepressants may be used to treat coexisting mental illness, but they are not a mainstay of detoxification.

Page: 1482

Question #15

Answer: E

Rationale: Methadone therapy has been shown to reduce criminal activity, the use of illicit opioids, and human immunodeficiency virus risk activities, and it also controls cravings for opioids. Because of Drug Enforcement Administration regulations, methadone prescriptions for maintenance therapy are generally restricted to specially certified clinics and not permitted to be written by primary care physicians.

Page: 1482

Question #16

Answer: C

Rationale: Benadryl has not been known to cause false-positive benzodiazepine results. The other medications listed are all potential causes of false-positive urine drug screen results. Additional causes are shown in Table 5. Confirmatory testing can be ordered to verify positive results.

Page: 1478

Question #17

Answer: B

Rationale: Amphetamines are rapidly metabolized, and they are typically only detectable for 2 to 3 days after use. Marijuana is detectable for 1 to 7 days after typical use, but, because of a reservoir in fatty tissues, it can be present for up to 30 days with heavy use. Cocaine is detectable for 2 to 3 days, and phencyclidine may be present for 7 to 14 days.

Page: 1478

Question #18

Answer: F

Rationale: The last question in the CRAFFT questionnaire is, "Have you ever gotten into TROUBLE while using alcohol or drugs?" The need to take more of a drug to get the same effect is part of the DSM-IV criteria for substance abuse, not the CRAFFT questionnaire.

Page: 1478

Question #19

Answer: B

Rationale: The *R* in FRAMES stands for *responsibility.*

Page: 1483

Question #20

Answer: E

Rationale: The last DSM-IV criterion for substance abuse states the following: "...the substance use is continued despite the knowledge of having a persistent or recurrent physical or psychological problem that is likely to have been caused or exacerbated by the substance." The other answer options listed are taken directly from the DSM-IV criteria.

Page: 1480

Question #1

Answer: C

Rationale: The *confidence interval* is the probability range that describes the likelihood that a given hypothesis is true. The *positive predictive value* is the percent likelihood of a test reporting positive results in the presence of disease. The *reference interval* is frequently defined by the results that are obtained between chosen percentiles (e.g., the range of results between the 2.5th and the 97.5th percentiles). The most frequent reference value is the reference interval. The *laboratory directive* is an administrative instruction or communication with policy and procedure implications. The *odds ratio* is a statistical comparison of the occurrence probabilities of two groups.

Page: 1485

Question #2

Answer: B

Rationale: From the same person at different times, one can obtain different results as a result of a number of factors. *Biologic variability* is the variation of a test result of the same person at different times.

Page: 1485

Question #3

Answer: B

Rationale: *Biologic variability* is the variation of a test result of the same person at different times. Physiologic processes can produce biologic variability. Constitutional factors can produce biologic factors, and, likewise, they can cause biologic variability. By contrast, *analytic variation* is the variation in repeated tests of the same specimen. Analytic variation relates to analytic technique and specimen processing. Analytic variation is not related to the personal factors that affect biologic variability.

Page: 1485

Question #4

Answer: B

Rationale: With current technology, biologic variation plays a larger role than analytic variation in most laboratory tests. The consistency of analytic technique and specimen processing contributes to reductions in analytic variability. Biologic variations of physiologic, constitutional, and extrinsic sources contribute more greatly to the variability of results.

Page: 1485

Question #5

Answer: C

Rationale: The reference interval is most frequently defined by results that are between chosen percentiles. The most frequently cited range: from the 2.5th to the 97.5th percentiles.

Page: 1485

Question #6

Answer: A

Rationale: CLIA 1998 defined three requirements for reference values. The normal or reference ranges must be made available to the ordering clinician, and they must be included in the laboratory manual. The laboratory must establish specifications for the performance characteristics of each test. The performance characteristics must include the reference range, and the reference range must be established before and communicated with the patient's reported test results. Different visual cues can enhance the reader's perception of results as compared with reference ranges, including color differences to emphasize abnormal values and alert values, but these enhancements are not stipulated by CLIA 1998.

Page: 1485

Question #7

Answer: D

Rationale: Lipase and amylase levels both increase at 3 to 6 hours after the onset of acute pancreatitis. Although they both peak at 24 hours, each returns to normal at different rates. Amylase levels return to normal in 4 to

7 days, whereas lipase levels return to normal in 8 to 14 days.

Page: 1490

Question #8

Answer: D

Rationale: Hypertriglyceridemia can induce pancreatitis. Interestingly, pancreatitis caused by hypertriglyceridemia might not cause an increase in amylase. Therefore, a normal amylase level does not exclude a diagnosis of pancreatitis, especially if the episode is induced by hypertriglyceridemia. One would usually expect the amylase level to be more reliably elevated in patients with acute pancreatitis caused by alcohol, medications, or obstruction.

Page: 1490

Question #9

Answer: B

Rationale: Immunoglobulin M rheumatoid factor is the mainstay of laboratory testing to support the clinical diagnosis of rheumatoid arthritis. The anticyclic citrullinated peptide enzyme-linked immunosorbent assay shows promise for the diagnosis of rheumatoid arthritis. The anti-DNA test is highly specific for systemic lupus erythematosus. Likewise, the anti-Smith test is highly specific for systemic lupus erythematosus. Gilbert's syndrome is a form of unconjugated hyperbilirubinemia that does not generally indicate significant liver disease. Erythema multiforme is a disease of skin reaction and basal layer necrosis for which a specific laboratory test is not available, other than skin biopsy.

Page: 1490

Question #10

Answer: C

Rationale: In patients with drug-induced lupus, elevated antinuclear antibody titers decrease after the offending drug is discontinued. Hydralazine (Apresoline) can induce a lupus-like syndrome. Other drugs that can cause lupus-like syndrome are procainamide (Pronestyl), carbamazepine (Tegretol), phenytoin (Dilantin), and isoniazid. Hydrochlorothiazide should be avoided in patients with sulfa allergy. The antihistamine diphenhydramine treats hives, which often arise from allergic reaction. The muscle relaxant cyclobenzaprine can cause drowsiness, hypotension, and myalgias.

Page: 1491

Question #11

Answer: A

Rationale: Hepatic function, when normal, can usually maintain bilirubin levels below 5 mg/dL. The liver hepatocytes conjugate bilirubin, which is excreted in the conjugated water-soluble form in the bile. Bilirubinuria is a fairly sensitive marker for biliary obstruction, and it may occasionally be found before jaundice is evident. Thus, urinalysis may contribute to diagnosis before the patient appears clinically jaundiced.

Page: 1491

Question #12

Answer: E

Rationale: BUN is a byproduct of protein metabolism. The normal BUN reference value is approximately 7 to 18 mg/dL. BUN is produced by the liver, and it is "carried" through the circulation. The brain can be adversely affected by moderately to severely elevated BUN, a condition called *azotemia*. Hepatic encephalopathies include altered brain functions in the setting of elevated BUN. Congestive heart failure can raise BUN levels, and worsening renal function can contribute to a rise in BUN. However, at low flow rates, the renal tubules will increase the reabsorption of urea, thereby elevating BUN proportionally more than creatinine.

Page: 1491

Question #13

Answer: D

Rationale: Adrenal glands secrete mineralocorticoids, which affect the body's salt and water balance, and glucocorticoids, which affect glucose metabolism and related mechanisms. Prerenal and postrenal explanations are expected from BUN-to-creatinine ratios of greater than 20:1. Intrinsic renal pathology is implicated by a BUN-to-creatine ratio of 10:1.

Page: 1491

Question #14

Answer: A

Rationale: Low albumin is the most common cause of a low total calcium level. Formulae exist to mathematically correct the total calcium by accounting for the extent of hypoalbuminemia. Malignancy is associated with elevated calcium levels. In fact, calcium levels of more than 14 mg/dL are usually associated with malignancy. Hyperparathyroidism is among the differential diagnoses for hypercalcemia. A family history of reduced calcium excretion and subsequently elevated total calcium levels is found in patients with familial hypocalciuric hypercalcemia.

Page: 1491

Question #15

Answer: D

Rationale: Albumin-bound calcium is potentially available, but it is not physiologically active while bound. Total blood calcium includes at least 50% calcium in its bound, inactive form. Chelated fraction of calcium would be another form of bound, inactive calcium. Only the free or ionized portion of calcium is physiologically active.

Page: 1491

Question #16

Answer: D

Rationale: Carcinoembryonic antigen (CEA) is an oncofetal glycoprotein antigen, and it is nonspecific. CEA is one of the original tumor markers, and it is elevated in a variety of tumor types, including (but not limited to) colorectal tumors. A rising CEA level predicts liver metastases after colon resection. The CA-125 tumor marker is closely associated with ovarian cancer.

Page: 1491

Question #17

Answer: C

Rationale: The partial prothrombin time (activated partial prothrombin time) and the prothrombin time are poor screening tests for postoperative bleeding in patients without historical risk factors. Partial prothrombin time prolongation is found among patients with lupus anticoagulant and vitamin K deficiency, and it is significantly shortened by hemolysis. Platelet dysfunction and thrombocytopenia do not affect the partial prothrombin time.

Page: 1493

Question #18

Answer: A

Rationale: The Schilling test remained the gold standard for confirming the diagnosis of pernicious anemia for decades. Pernicious anemia is the specific form of vitamin B_{12} deficiency with macrocytic anemia that results from the failure of gastric mucosa to produce intrinsic factor. The absence of intrinsic factor leads to a lack of vitamin B_{12} absorption. The test for antibodies to intrinsic factor is the test that has largely replaced the Schilling test. Atrophic gastritis may occur from other explanations beyond antibody-mediated ones. Although vitamin B_{12} deficiency can lead to elevated levels of homocysteine, the deficiency is not the sole differential for elevated homocysteine. *H. pylori* antibodies are associated with the urease-producing bacterium that is implicated in 90% of duodenal ulcers.

Page: 1495

Question #19

Answer: B

Rationale: The carbon dioxide content of blood is mainly composed of bicarbonate. Blood also contains smaller amounts of carbonic acid and dissolved carbon dioxide. Lactate reflects the presence of lactic acid, which contributes to metabolic acidosis.

Page: 1495

Question #20

Answer: C

Rationale: Lactic acidosis causes an increased anion gap, and ketoacidosis contributes to an increased anion gap. Multiple myeloma can occasionally cause a low anion gap, and ethylene glycol poisoning contributes to a widened anion gap.

Page: 1495

Question #21

Answer: E

Rationale: The term *thrombocytopenia* refers to a low platelet count; it would not be part of the five-part white blood cell differential. *Hemolysis* refers to the destruction of red blood cells. Mean corpuscular volume and red cell distribution width are parameters that pertain to red blood cells. The cell types that make up the white blood cell differential are neutrophils, lymphocytes, monocytes, eosinophils, and basophils.

Page: 1498

Question #22

Answer: C

Rationale: Mild anemia is the most common abnormality found by a complete blood cell count (CBC). By contrast, polycythemia can also be observed in a CBC; it is an elevated hematocrit. Band forms are characteristics of neutrophils, and leukocytosis is an elevated white blood cell count. Thrombocytopenia is a low platelet count. All of these conditions can be shown by a CBC and observed in a peripheral smear.

Page: 1495

Question #23

Answer: D

Rationale: Bands are immature neutrophils. Segmented band forms are characteristic of mature neutrophils. Lymphocytes, basophils, monocytes, and eosinophils are subtypes of white blood cells.

Page: 1495

Question #24

Answer: B

Rationale: Valproic acid, heparin, and sulfa drugs can reduce platelets by destroying them. Vitamin B_{12} deficiency causes the decreased production of platelets. Disseminated intravascular coagulation also reduces the platelet counts by destroying platelets.

Page: 1496

Question #25

Answer: C

Rationale: Sickle cell disease decreases the erythrocyte sedimentation rate. Likewise, polycythemia, microcytosis, spherocytosis, extreme leukocytosis, excessive anticoagulant, low room temperature, and a clotted blood sample can decrease the ESR. Among conditions that can increase the ESR are anemia, hypoalbuminemia, macrocytosis, and advanced age. Aspirin and recent meals have no effect on the ESR.

Page: 1499

Question #26

Answer: B

Rationale: Male gender (rather than female gender) and niacin are associated with elevated homocysteine levels. Hypothyroidism is also associated with higher homocysteine levels, whereas hyperthyroidism is not. Although trimethoprim is associated with elevated homocysteine levels, sulfamethoxazole is not.

Page: 1502

Question #27

Answer: B

Rationale: C-reactive protein (CRP) is an acute-phase reactant that is associated with inflammation. CRP is one of the first proteins to increase at the start of an inflammatory process. CRP levels are not reduced by aspirin. Bacterial infections can raise CRP levels to more than 100 mg/L. CRP does not exhibit significant circadian variation, and it is not affected by age, race, food intake, or diet.

Page: 1499

Question #28

Answer: D

Rationale: Diabetes mellitus is characterized by hyperglycemia. The American Diabetes Association has redefined the normal fasting plasma glucose as less than 100 mg/dL. Prediabetes is present when the fasting plasma glucose level is between 100 and 125 mg/dL. Diabetes mellitus involves a fasting plasma glucose level of 126 mg/dL or greater.

Page: 1501

Question #29

Answer: C

Rationale: Glycosylated hemoglobin A1c is not currently recommended for the diagnosis of diabetes mellitus. Variability exists in the standardization of hemoglobin A1c measurement, and this test is not as sensitive as the fasting glucose or the glucose tolerance test for mild hyperglycemia. Insulin tests are used for the detection of insulin-secreting tumors and specifically for identifying insulin resistance. Fasting plasma glucose is the test that is recommended for the diagnosis of diabetes mellitus. The glucose tolerance test can detect mild hyperglycemia. Because it can induce hypoglycemia in hypoglycemic patients, the glucose tolerance test should not be routinely ordered for the evaluation of hypoglycemia. Lipase testing exhibits sensitivity and specificity for pancreatic disease to a greater extent than amylase testing. Lipase is not specifically a test for diabetes mellitus.

Page: 1501

Question #30

Answer: D

Rationale: *H. pylori* is a spiral urease-producing bacteria that is associated with nearly 90% of duodenal ulcers.

Page: 1501

Question #31

Answer: D

Rationale: The Hepatitis B surface antigen is the earliest serologic marker of hepatitis B infection. The Hepatitis B virus e antigen is only found in the presence of the hepatitis B surface antigen, and it is a marker for infectiousness. The antibody to the hepatitis B core antigen can be detected in blood during the "window period." The antibody to hepatitis B surface antigen is used to evaluate the effect of previous immunization. The antibody to hepatitis C is used to diagnose hepatitis C infection. Its presence does not differentiate between acute and chronic infection, and it does not indicate immunity to the hepatitis C virus.

Page: 1501

Question #32

Answer: D

Rationale: Hepatitis A deaths are rare. An increased mortality rate from hepatitis B can be expected in the presence of the hepatitis delta virus. Antibodies to the hepatitis B core antigen and to immunoglobulins M and G are used to distinguish between recent infection and previous infection, respectively. The hepatitis delta virus is present in about 4% of patients with hepatitis B infection, and it carries with it an increased mortality rate. The hepatitis B virus e antigen is a marker for infectiousness.

Page: 1501

Question #33

Answer: D

Rationale: The new rapid oral test for HIV is not yet recommended for neonates of HIV-infected mothers.

Quantitative RNA polymerase chain reaction testing is useful for evaluating indeterminate Western blot results and acute HIV infections before a patient's seroconversion. HIV-2 is rare and not statistically prevalent among HIV-infected mothers. HIV-1 DNA polymerase chain reaction testing is recommended for detecting HIV infection in the neonates of HIV-infected mothers. Because maternal antibodies are present for months in these neonates, the HIV-1 DNA polymerase chain reaction can identify neonates themselves who are infected with the HIV-1 virus from the presence of HIV-1 DNA in the neonatal blood.

Page: 1502

Question #34

Answer: D

Rationale: Lipid levels contribute to the evaluation of cardiovascular risks. Physiologic variation can result in lipid measurements from 13% above to 13% below an individual's usual results. Physiologic variations contribute more to the variation of results than do analytic variations in lipid measurements.

Page: 1504

Question #35

Answer: C

Rationale: The spirochete *Borrelia burgdorferi* is the responsible cause of Lyme disease. The spirochete is transmitted by an ixodid tick biting an animal (including a human). Early stages of Lyme disease may be seronegative, and seroconversion may take up to 8 weeks. About 5% of the normal population has false-positive antibodies for Lyme disease.

Page: 1505

Question #36

Answer: B

Rationale: Potassium is the most abundant cation in the body. The concentration of potassium is much higher in the intracellular space than in the extracellular fluids. Magnesium is the second most common intracellular cation. There is a poor correlation between serum magnesium levels and total body magnesium. Total calcium and ionized calcium correspond well in healthy, nourished individuals. In critically ill patients and malnourished patients, ionized calcium better reflects the amount of physiologically available calcium. Sodium is the major component of extracellular osmolarity.

Page: 1505

Question #37

Answer: B

Rationale: Alkalosis causes hypokalemia by shifting potassium intracellularly. Hypomagnesemia causes hypokalemia via the renal loss of potassium. Adrenal insufficiency causes hyperkalemia via the reduced excretion of potassium. Diuresis causes hypokalemia by promoting the renal excretion of potassium. Periodic paralysis causes hypokalemia via the nonrenal movement of potassium from the extracellular to the intracellular space.

Page: 1506

Question #38

Answer: C

Rationale: The third-generation ultrasensitive thyroid-stimulating hormone is the best test to confirm or exclude thyroid disease in an ambulatory patient. Thyroid-stimulating hormone is produced by the pituitary gland. Circulating triiodothyronine and thyroxine inhibit thyroid-stimulating hormone. The triiodothyronine resin uptake test is being replaced by the current accurate testing for free thyroxine and free triiodothyronine.

Page: 1511

Question #39

Answer: B

Rationale: It is important to recognize the limitations of drug detection assays. For example, most immunoassays for opiates are designed to detect heroin by measuring codeine, which is a byproduct of the metabolism of both heroin and morphine. It is important to remember that synthetic opioids such as oxycodone and methadone do not cross-react with most codeine immunoassays. With most of these assays, a negative result will be reported because of the lack of the immunoassay's detection of the synthetic opioid.

Page: 1512

Question #40

Answer: C

Rationale: The ESR is one of the oldest clinical laboratory tests. Its results increase with inflammation, infection, neoplasms, and collagen vascular diseases. The C-reactive protein is an acute-phase reactant. The likelihood of the radiologic progression of rheumatologic disease occurs among patients who are positive for anticyclic citrullinated peptide. The immunoglobulin M rheumatoid factor is not specific for rheumatoid arthritis. The rapid plasma reagent test is used to detect syphilis.

Page: 1508